ISSUES
IN HEALTH ECONOMICS

Contributors

Brian Abel-Smith

Jan Paul Acton

Kenneth J. Arrow

Richard Auster

Thomas W. Bice

Kenneth E. Boulding

W. John Carr

William O. Cleverley

Rosanna M. Coffey

Karen Davis

Alain Enthoven

Pamela J. Farley

Martin S. Feldstein

Paul J. Feldstein

Victor R. Fuchs

Paul B. Ginsburg

Jeffrey E. Harris

Herbert E. Klarman

Judith R. Lave

Lester B. Lave

Maw Lin Lee

Myron J. Lefcowitz

Samuel Leinhardt

Irving Leveson

Nelda McCall

Larry M. Manheim

Joseph P. Newhouse

Mark V. Pauly

Ira E. Raskin

Michael Redisch

Milton I. Roemer

David S. Salkever

Deborah Sarachek

Anne Scitovsky

William Shonick

John S. Spratt, Jr.

Kenneth E. Warner

William D. White

Henry W. Zaretsky

ISSUES
IN HEALTH ECONOMICS

Edited by

Roice D. Luke, Ph.D.
and
Jeffrey C. Bauer, Ph.D.

University of Colorado Health Sciences Center

AN ASPEN PUBLICATION®
Aspen Systems Corporation
Rockville, Maryland
London
1982

Library of Congress Cataloging in Publication Data

Issues in health economics.

Includes bibliographies and index.
1. Medical economics—Addresses, essays, lectures.
2. Medical economics—United States—
Addresses, essays, lectures.
I. Luke, Roice D.   II. Bauer, Jeffrey C.
RA410.I87   362.1   81-20674
ISBN: 0-89443-381-4   AACR2

Library of Congress Catalog Card Number: 81-20674
ISBN: 0-89443-381-4

Printed in the United States of America

1 2 3 4 5

Table of Contents

Preface

As teachers of graduate and undergraduate courses in health economics, we have regularly engaged in the ultimate academic frustration—trying to assemble a collection of supplemental readings that is simultaneously *comprehensive* with respect to the subject and *accessible* to the students. The task always involves making constant trade-offs among academic rigor, thoroughness of treatment, costs to students, and similar factors. However, our consciences were bothered most by the constant temptations to photocopy articles from our own collections and to sell them at cost directly to students. Copyright laws and campus bookstores were becoming less and less tolerant of this practice.

We informally asked our colleagues at other universities how they resolved this dilemma. The universality of the problem became obvious; teaching health economists did not have a convenient *and* legal way to share with students their preferred articles from the published periodical literature. The need for a comprehensive book of readings was readily apparent.

Consequently, we followed our informal inquiries with a formal survey to determine the readings that were assigned to students of health economics. The response to this survey was impressive. Approximately 40 teachers, including many of the established experts in the field, responded with copies of their syllabi, reading lists, and additional references to significant articles. We catalogued all references and counted the frequency of occurrence for each one. This procedure enabled us to rank and select the nontext readings assigned most frequently in health economics classes at colleges and universities throughout the United States.

We supplemented this quantitative analysis with editorial review to ensure balance and breadth. A small number of commonly assigned articles were deleted due to their similarity with other articles that fit better into the overall collection, and a few less common references were included to provide some coverage of topics that were listed in the syllabi more often than in the reading lists. (In other words, the editorial task required identification of situations where an important topic was supplemented with enough different articles that no one article emerged with substantial frequency.)

We also gave careful consideration to selection of articles dealing with both "health" and "medicine." The emphasis in the literature obviously favors the medical side of health care; this point was revealed very clearly in our analysis of reading lists. Nevertheless, we felt some attention should be given to the "health alternative," so we included in the book several readings on this subject.

The only other editorial prerogative was exercised in the case of highly quantitative studies. When the implications of empirical analyses were also addressed in the less mathematical literature, the nonquantitative articles were generally selected, so that the readings would be intellectually accessible to the widest possible range of readers.

The articles are organized in broad groups that roughly correspond to basic subject areas of economics. However, our review of course syllabi revealed enormous diversity in topical approaches to teaching health economics; teachers should assign the articles in an order that suits their own purposes. On the other hand, nonstudents should find some conceptual cohesiveness within each of the six sections of this book.

The formal survey and ensuing editorial selection have resulted in this book of readings, providing a collection of articles recommended by the nation's teaching health economists. As such, the book has obvious usefulness to students at all levels in a wide range of courses that deal, directly or indirectly, with health economics. This collection of "classics" and other faculty-endorsed articles should also provide an excellent resource to health care providers, administrators, legislators, policy analysts, consumers, journalists, and anyone else interested in the economics of health care. Above all, it will hopefully ease the burden of teachers like us who want to assign supplemental readings without risking the wrath of the publishers and bookstores that provide academicians with the protection they want and deserve when they are the authors.

Since we did not include our own publications in this book, we do not issue the usual disclaimer that all errors are ultimately ours. Each of the authors of the included articles would surely provide such a disclaimer if given the opportunity. However, we do accept responsibility for the final results of our selection process. Having identified several hundred articles, we know that many readers will note the absence of one or two of their favorites. We hope that the richness of the overall collection will compensate for the inevitable omissions.

The task could not have been completed without the excellent research assistance of Mary Keyser and the strong secretarial support of Tica McCollum. We thank them both.

Roice D. Luke
Jeffrey C. Bauer
December 1981

ECONOMIC AND POLITICAL CONTEXT

1. Is Medical Care Different?

MARK V. PAULY

Reprinted from *Competition in the Health Care Sector: Past, Present, and Future*. Copyright © 1978, Aspen Systems Corporation, 11-35.

As the title suggests, this paper will address the question of whether medical care is different from other goods and services, in the sense that a different kind of analysis or different kinds of supply and demand models are appropriate for medical care. At present, in the literature the answer to this question is a definite "yes." Both Selma Mushkin and Kenneth Arrow have argued that medical care is indeed different from other goods and services. Broadly speaking, the differences they list can be grouped under three headings: (1) greater *uncertainty* on the part of demanders; (2) *risk* associated with the random occurrence of illness; and (3) *absence of profit-seeking behavior* by providers of care. Arrow goes on to assert that these intrinsic differences explain the peculiar organization of the real-world medical care industry, with its set of governmental and quasi-governmental restrictions.[1]

In what follows I will assert that reality and theory are actually much less forthright than this literature suggests. I will not even say that the appropriate answer to the question is "yes or no"; it is rather, "yes, no, and maybe." In particular, I want to argue (1) that yes, there are currently some kinds of medical care and some kinds of situations in which the economist can use the same or similar methods of analysis as he uses for other industries reasonably well; but (2) no, there are other kinds of medical care for which the usual tools are not appropriate; while (3) there may be still other kinds of medical care for which competition (or more precisely an analogue to competition), and the usual analysis of competition, might not work perfectly, but might work reasonably well.

Competition currently may not work here because of restrictions on the actions of some of the participants. I also need to sound a pessimistic note, however; because we have not yet developed the appropriate method to handle group (3), and because that group may be large, we are at present

* I am grateful to Uwe Reinhardt, Gerald Goldstein, Barry Friedman, and members of the student-faculty seminar at Northwestern for suggesting a number of ideas and saving me from a number of errors. Remaining errors are my own.

nearly powerless to make any useful normative a priori statements, or many useful positive ones, about much of the medical-care sector. I will suggest that Arrow's assertion that the special characteristics of the industry arise from attempts to achieve optimality is at least open to serious question. I will also consider the effect of insurance coverage and supplier motivation on the distinctiveness of this industry. The main emphasis, however, will be on uncertainty, both because it seems most distinctive, and because the peculiarities on the supply side may not arise from anything intrinsic to the activity of supplying medical care, but, rather, from the way the supply side has adapted to uncertainty-generated restrictions on demand.

In what follows, I will first make some important distinctions among types of medical care. Then I will indicate why the economist's use of the competitive model as a tool of analysis is useful for some kinds of care, but why neither it nor the orthodox analyses of what to do when competition is absent is appropriate for other kinds of care.

TYPES OF MEDICAL CARE

It is, I believe, a grave mistake to try to characterize all of the services we lump under the general name of "medical care" in a similar way. There are several groupings of those services which should be distinguished: One may, for example, group by the extent of consumer experience.

Group (1)—Services which are purchased relatively frequently by most households.

Group (2)—Services a typical producer produces relatively frequently but which a typical consumer can consume relatively infrequently, perhaps once in a lifetime.

Group (3)—Services which a typical producer produces and a typical consumer consumes relatively infrequently.

In group (1) I would include such services as pediatric care, normal deliveries (especially after the first child), most of routine dental cavity repair and prevention, prescription drugs for common or chronic conditions, most non-prescription drugs, and routine care for persons with chronic conditions. In group (2) I would include such procedures as appendectomies, hysterectomies, hospitalization for acute gastrointestinal distress, pneumonia and many other common reasons for hospitalization. In group (3) I would include experimental and unusual procedures, including most of those undertaken in severe medical emergencies. There are no clear dividing lines among these groups, but rather various shades of gradation; the general notion of the distinctions should be clear.

There is another kind of threefold classification that will also be relevant for the following discussion. Some kinds of medical care are what might be called "diagnostic"; the critical elements are (1) the "care" consists primarily of information but (2) this information is usually peculiar to particular individuals. What one purchases is not a statement of what kinds of symptoms or test results are generally related to what kinds of conditions, but rather an assessment of what *his* symptoms and test results suggest. Another kind of care is what may be called "prescriptive-informative." This consists of general statements on the outcome of various courses of treatment on individuals with a particular diagnosis. Information is also being purchased here, but it is of somewhat more general nature than in the first case. How general it is depends on whether the diagnosis is common or rare. The third classification of care is that which is "active-therapeutic." This involves some time-consuming action by the provider: administration of an injection, a surgical procedure, or a normal delivery. Most medical-care contacts will have elements of some or all of these three types, but, again, the conceptual distinction among them will be useful.

ECONOMIC ANALYSIS AND INDUSTRY DIFFERENCES

With these distinctions in mind, let us turn to considering the types of analysis that might be applied. An economic analysis of an industry usually involves both positive and normative discussion, although the ultimate purpose for worrying about competition is normative. In positive analysis the critical characteristic of the "typical" industry is that suppliers maximize profit, or something analogous to profit. The normative question is usually couched in terms of efficiency or Pareto optimality. The strategy is usually to inquire whether competition is feasible, and, if it is, whether a competitive equilibrium would be efficient. If efficiency could be achieved, suggested Government intervention takes the form of insuring that the competitive preconditions are (approximately) present. If competitive equilibrium is infeasible, or if production with a large number of sellers would not be efficient, suggested intervention is usually the public utility model, with Government enforced barriers to entry and price regulation.

The primary reason for departure from the competitive model is the possible existence of unexploited economies of scale or of natural monopoly. In medical care, economies of scale are generally not important. In some rural markets natural monopoly may still occur, and hospitals probably display increasing returns to scale over some small sizes. In the urban and suburban areas in which the great bulk of the population lives, economies of scale either in ambulatory or hospital care are probably not very important, except for uncommon specialized procedures. Likewise, in such areas the number of sellers of medical services is large, again, except for the rare specialized service. On these grounds, then, the competitive market, with all of its nice optimality properties, should be expected to emerge once any governmental or cartel restrictions are removed.[2]

The missing condition in the medical care industry is surely not the absence of large numbers of sellers and buyers in most markets or for most types of care. Rather, if there is a missing condition, it is the absence of *consumer information.* The problem is even more complex. What consumers buy, in their diagnostic or prescriptive-informative transactions, is primarily information itself to be used in guiding future transactions. So we have a multiproduct industry in which the quality, quantity, and characteristics or content of one of the products—information—affects the demand of other products.

Consumer ignorance would have two consequences for efficiency. First, it may prevent the emergence of competitive equilibrium, because a seller may continue to sell some output even if his price is higher or his quality lower than that of some other sellers; firm demand curves are not perfectly elastic. Second, without any information necessary to determine quality, consumers may be purchasing a quality level lower than the utility-maximizing one.

So there are two alleged differences on the demand side between medical care and a typical industry: (1) Consumers are not informed and (2) what is demanded is not a typical commodity, but is information itself. We do have an attempt to analyze the medical-care industry which does make specific and clear reference to these characteristics: Arrow's classic article. I will argue that, where it is applicable, Arrow's discussion is unhelpful and possibly misleading in answering the question of appropriate analysis. I will assert that the appropriate analysis is surely more difficult, and certainly less conclusive, than what Arrow presents. While this is a negative conclusion, it is surely desirable, at this conference, to face up to the difficulties we are likely to encounter.

CONSUMER INFORMATION ABOUT TYPES OF MEDICAL CARE

It is generally alleged that consumers of medical care are very poorly informed. Karen Davis, for example, presents a typical argument:

> The nature of health care is such that the consumer knows very little about the medical services he or she is buying—possibly less than about any other service purchased. Some choices about medical care are made solely by patients. But a very large part of the decision making is done by physicians — diagnosis, treatment, drugs and tests, hospitalization, frequency of return visits are all substantially under the physician's control. . . . While the consumer can participate in policing the market, that participation is much more limited than in almost any other area of private economic activity. (Karen Davis, pp. 22, 23.)

The surprising thing about this statement, considering its strength, is that no evidence is provided, nor is there any suggestion as to how large a part is "a very large part." The statement that consumers are not well-informed about medical care may seem so obvious as not to require empirical documentation. But I will argue that things are not so easy.

Some information about the price and quality of medical care is costly, but it does not necessarily follow that consumers are poorly informed about all types of care. For some types, information may be relatively cheap (and so relatively extensively obtained). For some types, individuals may generate a substantial amount of information as a by-product of other activities. We do acquire a considerable amount of information simply by random contacts as consumers or as observers. For instance, a person who uses a particular physician's services necessarily acquires some information from the experience he has with the outcomes of those services. He may well want to incur costs to obtain additional information, even to the extent of purchasing more services than he otherwise would to generate more information, but it is possible that he may "automatically" be well informed.

Most of medical care, like most services, is an experience rather than a search good, to use Philip Nelson's terminology. Still, there may be some information on price or quality obtainable by search at relatively low cost. A consumption unit can tap not only its experience, but also the experience of friends. If each household's experience provides a relatively good estimate of quality, a given household can have both an idea of the quality of provider it is currently using, and, by contacting friends at a nominal cost, a good idea of the quality and price of some other providers as well.[3] If people select the highest quality provider for a given price in the subset of providers on which they have information, each household is likely eventually to become informed about high quality providers, so that information will become fairly complete. Of course, not all persons have friends, and so not all persons will face a low price for information. But, as has been suggested by Steven Salop, and by Sanford Grossman and Joseph Stiglitz, if enough people are well-informed, the remainder can appropriately judge quality by price and so there is no need for them to become well-informed.

It is not possible in this study to provide a definite measure of the types of medical care on which consumers are reasonably well informed. No large-scale empirical work has been done on this question; "reasonably well-informed" (like workable competition) is not even easy to define. However, I believe that it is possible to offer some numerical conjectures about that portion of total national health expenditure that might, as a starting point, be suggested as impossible to disprove as being the "reasonably well-informed" portion. Roughly, these types would be ones for which individual consumption units are likely to have fairly extensive experience, or whose outcomes are easy to judge either during or soon after the performance of the service.

In another sense, these estimates may understate the extent of reasonably well-informed purchases. Referrals from a primary care physician are the primary determinant of type of provider for many of those procedures with which an individual consumer does not have extensive experience.

If the consumer does have a reasonable amount of information on the quality of referrals provided by the primary care physician, he may still be effectively informed. This point will be discussed more extensively later.

Approximately what fraction of total medical-care spending goes for the types of care described above? Of all non-hospital physician visits, approximately 10 percent were made to pediatricians in 1971. About 10 percent of all other visits were for general checkup, immunization and vaccination, or pre- or post-natal care. Half of all physician visits were made for chronic conditions. While there is surely some overlap between these categories, it seems reasonable to conclude that at least half of ambulatory care physician visits are made by persons who might be reasonably well informed. On average, physicians spend approximately one-quarter to one-third of their time at the hospital; physicians' services were about 23 percent of all health-care spending,[4] so "informed" ambulatory care physician purchases are about 8 percent of total spending (.5x.75.x.23). For hospital care, about 10 percent of all discharges are for normal delivery, and this is about 5 percent of total spending. Total expenditure on all drugs was 10 percent of total personal health-care expenditures in 1973, and a reasonable approximation of the well-informed part would be about 5 percent. Routine dental care would add perhaps another 4 percent. A final, and somewhat more questionable category, is that of nursing home care which is about 7 percent. In total, then, perhaps one-fourth or more of total personal health-care expenditures might be regarded as "reasonably informed." [5]

I do not contend that consumer information is perfect; for most final consumption goods that is rarely so. What I suggest is that information is sufficiently extensive to permit an outcome at least as close to the competitive equilibrium as might occur with other "usual" services. This is not to imply that the information could not be improved; removal of institutional barriers to information might still produce an improvement in welfare, though that improvement need not be very large.

What might one mean by a "reasonably" or "appropriately" well-informed purchaser? The consumer seeks informaton on both price and quality. There appears to be no important intrinsic difference between medical care and other industries in generating or transmitting price information. Of course, existing laws prohibiting advertising may limit actual consumer knowledge of prices, and there may be some questions of product homogeneity which need to be answered for valid comparisons. The critical uncertainty is that about *quality*—both the quality of therapeutic performance, and the quality (accuracy) of diagnostic or prescriptive information. Without such information available to consumers, sellers can perhaps continue to sell even if they raise prices above the "going" level because they can convince consumers that they provide higher quality or because the customers of the seller who raises prices would prefer paying a higher price for a more certain level of quality rather than using a lower priced service whose quality is more uncertain.

It may be so obvious that consumers are ignorant about medical care quality as not to require proof. It is important to note, however, that there are two reasons why it is not the *total* amount of perceived consumer ignorance that is relevant to a discussion of the desirability and feasibility of competition. First, not everyone agrees on how quality is to be defined or measured. In particular, the qualities that particular consumers value may not be the qualities that experts measure. So consumers may not seek information about qualities which are irrelevant to them, appear to the experts to be uninformed, and yet be appropriately informed.

The second, and more important, reason is that everyone, including the experts, is imperfectly informed on much of medical care quality. Quality could be defined as the relationship between various characteristics of the medical-care process and differences in health outcomes. Consumers do not know, for example, whether board-certified surgeons are likely to produce better outcomes than non-board-certified ones, whether tonsillectomy on average improves children's health, or whether a particular laboratory test is useful. Consumers cannot evaluate quality. *But neither can anyone else.* No one knows whether board certification, tonsillectomies, or some lab tests will improve health outcomes or not. I would argue that much of the uncertainty that the consumer has about medical care quality, even (or especially) in the narrow sense of the relationships between characteristics and expected health outcome, is of this type.

In this sense, medical care is different from many other goods: The relationship of use of the good to the outcome is much more certain for, say, sugar or baking powder, than it is for medical care. It is this *irreducible* uncertainty that we often think of, *but this kind of uncertainty may be mostly irrelevant to any notion of competition.* (It is necessarily relevant only in the sense that some form of insurance may be desirable to deal with it.) The kind of uncertainty that is relevant is that which represents information about quality which the seller has but the buyer does not. Arrow has, of course, remarked on this asymmetry of information, noting that it is information about outcome (what will happen), not process (how things work) which is relevant. One should add, however, that there may not be more *reducible* intrinsic uncertainty in this type of medical care than elsewhere. For the types of care discussed in this section, there may still be considerable ignorance (say, about whether well-baby checkups really make a difference). But this is primarily irreducible uncertainty.

Paradoxically, for irreducible uncertainty to be irrelevant, it is necessary not only that consumers know that they are ignorant, but also that they know that those from whom they purchase are ignorant as well. For example, consumer uncertainty about the indications for tonsillitis or the value of board certification will not interfere with the proper functioning of the market if and only if consumers know that physician experts are themselves ignorant on these questions. The physician must not be able to persuade the consumer that medical knowledge is greater than it actually is. The ironic conclusion is that one of the most useful types (and probably one of the least expensive types) of information that could be provided to patients is information on what is *not* known by medical science and physicians.

CONSUMER IGNORANCE AND SECOND BEST

Another type of care is that which occurs rarely for any individual, so that his own experience, or even that of his necessarily limited contacts and friends, conveys relatively little information. Without incurring costs which are large enough to matter, he cannot become very well informed. At least at present, markets in this type of care may depart considerably from the competitive one. How much of currently observed consumer ignorance is intrinsic to the service and how much is due to the present set of institutional arrangements is unknown. We do not even know how great the extent of ignorance is. It does seem clear, however, that (a) with sufficient expenditure of real resources, any purchaser could become well informed but (b) information is sufficiently costly that it would not pay to become approximately well informed. The fundamental problem is that we have no notion, or even a suspicion, of what the equilibria in markets with imperfectly informed consumers would be like, and what is more important, whether there are institutional restrictions that could be put on the market to improve matters. (We do not even know if equilibrium necessarily exists.) As it stands, we can show that almost anything could be optimal, but we cannot show that anything actually is. Some examples: Restricting consumer choice is ordinarily not desirable. As will be shown, however, if information itself is costly, barring types of outputs or types of providers that few people would choose anyway may be cheaper and more desirable than providing information. A second example: It is ordinarily desirable that potential purchasers know prices. But if it is cheap to become informed about price, but expensive to become informed about quality, it is possible that more consumers may mistakenly purchase lower priced but even inappropriately lower quality care when price information is available than would occur if provision of information on price or quality were limited, as by advertising restrictions. Some information may be worse than no information.[6] All these things could occur, and a priori reasoning cannot distinguish the real from the possible. This is equivalent to saying that we are dealing with a second best problem, with imperfect markets, imperfect consumers, and an imperfect regulator. What is the appropriate method of analysis?

Arrow has considered this problem most directly in his paper. He begins by stating the two fundamental theorems of welfare economics: (1) Competitive equilibrium is Pareto optimal, and (2) every Pareto optimum is a competitive equilibrium for some distribution of income. He then argues that medical care is different: Because of lack of consumer information and the absence of markets, principally in insurance, the present peculiar institutional arrangements have arisen to improve matters. "The special structural characteristics of the medical-care market are largely attempts to overcome the lack of optimality. . . ."

While this is surely possible, the problem is that such arrangements do not *necessarily* improve matters; we have no assurance that these characteristics really are attempts by politicians and medical trade associations to do what the welfare economist would suggest. Where the market would achieve competitive equilibrium, we know that public intervention *could not* improve matters. When it seems reasonable to suppose that the market would not satisfy the usual competitive conditions, we only know that public intervention *might* improve matters. But it is a big step from "might" to "will."

Whether lack of consumer information provides an explanation for existing institutional arrangements, with competitive restrictions as an unfortunate by-product, or whether it simply furnishes an excuse for what would otherwise be unacceptable use of Government to preserve monopoly, is impossible to say. Arrow is misleading in arguing that "the first step in the analysis of the medical-care market is a comparison between the actual market and the competitive model." The competitive model is irrelevant to an analysis of the medical-care market; the relevant comparison is between the actual market and what equilibria could be achieved under alternative institutional arrangements.[7] In such a world, welfare economics cannot furnish reasons; it can only furnish excuses. While it is surely true that the optimal equilibrium might be achieved by chance, or by a government mystically endowed with the appropriate knowledge and incentives, the relevant model is one in which information has a real cost, and all organizations face the same information production technology.

What is obviously necessary, and has not been developed, by Arrow or anyone else, is a theory which shows why and how welfare-increasing restrictions would be expected to emerge from the interaction of self-interested providers and consumers. That is, we need a theory to explain why and how a desirable "social contract" would be expected to be chosen. One can, of course, invoke the vague notion that whenever Pareto optimal moves exist, institutions will emerge to facilitate these moves, but any satisfactory explanation would surely require more. One would like to know, for example, whether the circumstances surrounding the Abraham Flexner report (or the medieval medical guilds) might reasonably be interpreted as the welfare economist's social contract. One would also want a theory to predict what specific *kinds* of restrictions would be expected to emerge from such bargaining: What are the desirable "constitutional" rules?

The second-best model is more relevant; it is also enormously more difficult. I will argue that without developing it, we are really fighting with shadows, and may cheapen what work we do perform. One of the attractive features of the competitive model is that strong welfare predictions can be derived without information on what demand and production functions look like. We shall not get off nearly so cheaply here; whether or not a rearrangement can improve matters depends on the actual magnitudes of costs and benefits. One important element in the development of such a theory is the notion that the configuration of equilibrium depends upon the empirical technology for the production of information.

Searching for Price and Quality

In this section I first provide some discussion of a possible positive model of equilibrium. Then I consider the normative analysis of ways to produce welfare improvements on this equilibrium.

It is clear that in part this model will be similar to existing search models, and in part it will be a kind of monopolistic competition model, except that neither free entry nor economies of scale are necessarily assumed. Unfortunately the monopolistic competition theory for even the simple model in which only price is uncertain is far from complete, and the multiplicity of monopolistic competition models, equilibria, and welfare evaluations of outcomes is an embarrassment of riches. While the theory of a consumer searching from a distribution of prices is fairly well settled, how that distribution comes into existence has not been fully explained (Michael Rothschild).

One way of sorting out the problem is to consider alternative reasons for departures from optimality and alternative corrective policies. There are two sorts of corrective policies I will discuss: (1) policies to correct prices or entry, given information; and (2) policies to correct information or compensate for incorrect information, given prices and entry.

In this section I wish to assume that information is given to be less than full, and ask how the market might be expected to perform. If consumers are not fully aware of the quality of all providers, providers may be able to raise prices above the competitive level. To the extent that this power differs in different submarkets, providers may move in response to income differentials. The sort of result one can get is presented in a particularly striking way by M. Satterthwaite. He develops a model in which the information a consumer has on any individual physician's price or quality depends upon the experience that the consumer and his friends have had with that physician. In a town with, say, two doctors, there will be relatively extensive experience, and each consumer will have a reasonably good idea of the quality level provided by each doctor. Now let the number of physicians increase. On the average, the number of experiences (his own and friends') per physician will decrease, and so the consumer will be less well-informed about any physician. This can cause individual physician demand curves to become less elastic, and price to increase when the number of physicians increases. No recourse to a non-maximizing or target income model is necessary.

From the welfare viewpoint, this model suggests possible gains from regulating prices or from limiting mobility, because free entry may lead to higher prices. A. M. Spence makes the argument that price limitation is likely to be infeasible in general in monopolistic competition, but even the notion of maximizing welfare subject to a profit constraint may suggest that some restriction on entry may be desirable.

But again "maybe" is not "will be"; the power of a priori reasoning is limited to posing questions, not answering them. This type of result seems to be what one gets out of most of the "new" monopolistic competition literature; the extent of monopoly is something that needs to be known before one can judge empirically whether the monopolistic competition equilibrium is or is not subject to improvement.

Knowing About Knowledge: Implications for Licensing

The previous section asked the question of possible welfare improvements, given some level of less-than-perfect information. In this section I want to concentrate on information itself. I want, first, to suggest a somewhat different way of evaluating the performance of an industry in which much of the output is information. Consider the three classifications or stages of care: diagnosis, prescription, and therapy. (Ordinarily they will follow in this order.) From the consumer's viewpoint, the three are obviously related, in the sense that his demand for therapy depends upon the quantity and the content of the other types of care purchased for an episode of illness. But suppose that each seller at a prior stage thinks that he cannot affect demand *from him* by the content of the advice he provides. Finally, and this is critical, assume that the consumer can perfectly evaluate the *quality* of each kind of care. By quality here I mean the usefulness of outcome from each stage. For example, for diagnosis, quality would mean the accuracy of diagnosis. For prescription it would mean the accuracy of advice about the outcomes to expect from various courses of therapy, given some diagnosis. For therapy, quality refers to the outcomes expected from performance of given therapeutic procedures on patients with given diagnoses.[8] Outcomes here means all the outcomes or characteristics that the consumer values, and is not limited to morbidity or mortality.

If the consumer was fully informed about these qualities, then the outcome would, I conjecture, be Pareto optimal. This differs from the usual notion of consumer information in that knowledge of "quality" applies not to the advice, but to the advisor, not the performance, but to the performer. The consumer is still ignorant about specifics, but he can judge which provider sells the high quality advice; he knows the provider's reputation.

There are some implications here for the notion of agency. If the consumer is well informed about primary-care physicians' general performance as agents, the referring physician will be a perfect agent. It is not necessary that the consumer be informed about the evidence concerning a particular referral, any more than a buyer of a pocket calculator needs to second-guess the manufacturer's choice of input suppliers.

In the real world, neither the assumption of independence of demands nor that of full consumer information about quality may hold. More to the point, there appear to be real resource costs of making demands independent and consumers fully informed. These resource costs are of three types. First, resources must be used to evaluate the quality of different providers. Second, the information must be made available to potential consumers. And third, consumers must expend real resources (primarily time) to "process" the information provided. All of these observations suggest that in equilibrium consumers are not likely to be fully informed. Given that information will not be complete, is this industry then different in the sense that public intervention in information provision may be required?

One kind of efficiency-improving public intervention can occur when provision of information itself is not cost effective.[9] If the cost of providing information to all consumers is sufficiently high, it may be cheaper to ban the good or service than to provide information which indicates that it is of lower quality. Some consumers lose when (low) quality levels are banned, but the gain to the rest may be substantial.

If there are costs of getting information to consumers, or if consumers incur a cost in processing it, then it is possible that either producer liability for lower than expected levels of quality or prohibition of certain qualities or quality proxies may be appropriate (C. Colantoni et al.). In medical care, both approaches are used. Providers are liable for negligent behavior which results in adverse outcomes under malpractice law. "Unqualified persons" (usually everyone except a physician) are legally forbidden to render certain medical-care services. The malpractice question does not appear to differ from that of products liability generally, and so I will emphasize the second (prohibition or exclusive licensing) approach.

There is a tradeoff among denying their ideal choice to relatively more knowledgeable persons, saving ignorant ones from their mistakes, and saving on information costs for all. It is surely *possible* that at least some consumers will be made better off if some low quality products are banned, and that the gain to them will exceed the loss to others. Consumer ignorance alone is not sufficient, of course; one needs to show that ignorant consumers are more likely to misestimate the chance of injury from a "low-quality" provider. We are prohibited from saying more by the old problem—second best. While such rules may improve aggregate welfare, it is not necessary that they do so, and one cannot tell a priori.

One way to settle the question is by a cost-benefit type of study. But perhaps some crude beginnings can be made first. While it is true that one does not wish simply to count heads, but rather willingness to pay (Walter Oi), as a rough approximation it does seem reasonable to assert that a good case can be made for banning quality levels which would be almost no one's choice if fully informed, but which would be regarded as decidely inferior by many.

Perhaps surprisingly, there appears to be almost no empirical work designed to answer this question: How heterogeneous are demands or tastes for types of medical care? Nor has there been any investigation, other than Bunker and Brown's study of physicians' families, to indicate what a fully informed consumer would do.

EXCLUSIVE LICENSURE AND POLITICAL CHOICE

In practice, laws typically govern the provider and not (within broad limits) his performance. These laws do more than just certify competence. They restrict the performance of certain actions to people with certain qualifications. One rationale for this policy would involve a kind of regress. Consumers do not have sufficient information to choose medical care on their own, so they hire an expert, the physician, to guide their choices. They do not have sufficient information to choose a physician, so, in effect, they can gain from having the Government hire experts to guide their choices of physicians. If people prefer to have their choices of quality guided or restricted, that is a service which the market can also surely provide. The critical question is whether there is any reason to suppose that public provision, via Government, of this choice of expert, and the restriction on individual choices it implies, is likely to be different from and superior to market alternatives. There are two possible reasons. First, the choice itself may in some sense be "better." Second, limiting choice to a small set of options, even if it is arbitrarily chosen, may improve matters.

To answer the question of whether choice is "better," the following non-transformation theorem on the usefulness of public intention will be useful. *The mere transfer of the locus of choice from the market to the political process does not transform consumers into better judges of quality, nor does it necessarily improve the decisions made.*

Since in a democratic policy the ultimate political choice of experts must rest with the voters, it is not clear how "government" (i.e., political regulation) can improve matters. Second-best reasoning suggests that a set of governmental (or other) experts *could* choose restrictions on quality or information which might make consumers better off than they would have been with no limits on quality or information. But the non-transformation theorem says that if these experts could be chosen by the polity, in the political choice of advice, it is approximately true that they could also be chosen in the market. If consumers in the advice markets would not choose the best experts, it is hard to see why they would be more likely to do so in the political market: It is not obvious why or how the transfer of the locus of choice would lead to better choices. There is, of course, a problem of public goods or non-exclusion in the production of information about qualifications, a point which will be discussed shortly.

The actual level that would be chosen would depend on the preferences of voters and the strength of lobbyists or other special interests. To take the simplest voter model: Suppose voters are to choose a minimum quality level for medical care, suppose their preferences for quality levels are absolute, and suppose that the preferences of the median voter (i.e., the voter with median quality preferences) would be decisive. In equilibrium, all quality levels below the optimal quality of the median voter would be banned.

In a more general model, the choice by any individual of his optimal level of quality obviously depends on the price he pays for different quality levels. But if the relationship of price to quality is being determined in an imperfectly informed market, should one expect a voter to take present prices as an indicator? If he does so, this would lead to possible biases in choice.

One may object that the approval of quality levels in medical care by medical examining boards or other government officials is so far removed from either the concern or the power of an average voter, and so frequently combined with other aspects of an election campaign, that voter choice is irrelevant. There are two alternative models. In one, choice is made ultimately by an elected official. Voters choose a governor, say, who appoints board members. But this just puts the process through another regress, and does not change anything fundamental. Instead of choosing the expert, voters choose a general expert agent who picks specialized experts of all sorts.

The second model is one in which voter preferences do not affect the outcome, but those of special interests do. This is a regulatory capture theory; the analytical problem, in a profession such as health where there are lots of special interests, is to explain why some special interests have captured more than others. Whatever the outcome, there is no reason to expect the choice to be "right" in any welfare sense; quality could be too high or too low, but it would only be an accident for it to be appropriate.

Even if the choice is not necessarily better, there are other important differences between market and political choice. One of the most important ones is the uniform and exclusive characteristic of political choice, compared to the pluralistic nature of market choice. This characteristic represents a mixed blessing. The advantage of political choice, as suggested above, is not that the choice is better, but, rather, that reduction in diversity of sellers, even if it is fairly arbitrary, can save buyers the cost of determining quality. For some this is a gain; for others, it is not.

For example, a person who knew he was ignorant about choosing the type of practitioner to treat an illness might well select an expert whose advice would be: You should always seek treatment from someone with a Doctor of Medicine degree. But a person who is more knowledgeable might sometimes wish to seek treatment from someone with less training. In market choice, both of these individuals could have their preferences satisfied, but in an exclusive licensure political arrangement they could not. If the first person is the one with median preferences, exclusive licensure might well be enacted into law, because it would save the decisive individual the cost of finding out what training a given provider of care had received, even if (as is likely to be true) this cost is small. As usual, majority rule equilibrium could be optimal, but it need not be.

There is indeed a kind of external cost imposed on an individual by the existence of quality levels he would not choose if fully informed. If the quality level exists, he would have to determine, at some cost, whether any given provider was of that quality level or not. If he bans quality levels he would not choose anyway, he suffers no loss in utility and he saves himself the cost of finding out whether a provider is or is not of that quality level.

Can it be desirable to ban once certification is provided? Given that certification occurs, it is hard to believe that the cost of examining a label is more than trivial. There is, however, an incentive for the decisive individual to support exclusive licensure rather than certification. With certification he would have to bear some of the cost, whereas banning a set of non-preferred quality levels is costless to him.

A third kind of difference between market and political choice is that political choice may be able to deal with the public good nature of the information production process in a superior way. Resources are consumed to measure quality levels. Once the information on quality has been produced, the amount of it available to any one individual is not diminished by the use of it by another individual. So exclusion of anyone by a positive price is inefficient, and yet the market cannot supply the information unless a positive price is charged.

The logic of this argument is impeccable, and it perhaps applies more strongly to medical care than to some other goods, since the cost per capita of providing information on a physician may be higher than that of providing information on, say, a dishwasher, both because of the difficulty of evaluation and because dishwashers are branded while physicians are not. Even so, the argument seems of limited relevance because (1) much of the cost of providing information is the private good, distribution of the information, rather than the public good, production of the information, and (2) the market price of information is still likely to be sufficiently low that those to whom information is more than trivially useful will still be willing to buy it. Those who would be excluded would be those for whom the information would not have been of much value anyway; while they could be worse off, the loss in per capita welfare would be small. Finally, there is no reason to suppose that actual governments would choose the ideal amount or type of this public good (information) anyway.

There is a fourth difference which is of importance. The consumer has little experience of his own on the outcomes of services provided by a particular seller. He wishes to obtain such information. Clearly, the lowest cost source of the information is the seller himself; for instance, the physician or hospital would be in the best position to know how many adverse outcomes there were among their patients. The same information could be obtained by an independent survey of their patients, but this would obviously be more costly. Those sellers whose quality is high, relative to their price, would obviously be eager to furnish information, but those whose quality was low relative to price would be unenthusiastic about having that fact made known. One solution in a market arrangement would be to list the fact of refusal to provide information, and that alone might be some testimony, even if mute, to the quality actually provided.[10] The Government does, however, have the legal power or the financial leverage to extract this information from all providers. The legal protection it gives to a physician's records it alone can take away. In this sense, it possesses an advantage over voluntary market arrangements in providing accurate information at low cost.[11]

There are, of course, some private organizations that possess the data needed to generate useful information at low cost. Third-party payers of various types could in principle profile that part of the activity of various providers which is covered by insurance. It is of some interest to speculate why, for example, insurers who are concerned with overuse have not informed their insureds about which physicians or hospitals have unusually high claim rates. Of course, the offended parties might retaliate by refusing to accept assignment, but if that is all the threat that is needed, the value of the information could not have been very great.

To summarize: It is easy to exaggerate the ability of government to deal with imperfect information in a way which is superior to the market. The main advantage it possesses arises from its ability to remove, with sufficient reason, a guarantee of property rights in information that it itself provided at an earlier stage. It also can avoid free rider problems, but this at most would give it a role in certification. The principles involved here appear to be general, and not specific to medical care. With regard to the type of care we are considering, one cannot rule out the possibility that it could be desirable to have more information than there currently is. If this information were made available, then this part of the sector might be further analyzed with the usual tools of economic analysis.

INFORMATION AND INTERRELATED DEMANDS

The preceding discussion looked at the possibility of obtaining information from "outside" sources. I remarked that, for the individually-infrequent types of care, there seems to be little such purchase of information from non-physician sources, although information in the form of referrals is very common. Much of the information we buy about the need for procedures we buy from physicians who may provide us with both the information about a procedure and the procedure itself. Since there clearly *can* be an incentive in such an arrangement to distort information, especially if there is excess capacity in the therapeutic service at the going price, why do consumers buy advice *and* treatment from the same seller?

The reason, as suggested by Michael Darby and Edi Karni, is that it is often cheaper to purchase all types of services from the same provider than from different providers. Once I have purchased diagnosis from a given physician, I can purchase therapy or prescriptive advice from him more cheaply than from another physician who would have to repeat at least some of the diagnostic workup.

In this sense, the diagnosing physician can influence the demand for his or others' services at later stages, and may do so in ways intended to enhance his income. In addition, if a diagnosis is required in order to obtain additional services, he can in principle extract all of the consumer's surplus in his charge for diagnosis. The way in which demands for information and care are related is not yet known, although some work has been done (Mark Pauly (1977), (1975), Dennis Smallwood and K. Smith).

The extent to which this power can be exploited by the physician may, however, be severely limited. The expected loss imposed on the consumer cannot exceed the expected cost advantage of single over multiple providers. In concrete terms, this cost advantage appears to be relatively slight. For example, Eugene McCarthy was able to offer second opinions on surgical procedures at a cost of about $40. This is less than 5 percent of the typical cost for an in-hospital surgical procedure. The expected utility loss, measured in dollars, of unnecessary surgery cannot exceed $40. The perhaps surprising result is that, when the second opinion program was voluntary, and covered by insurance, relatively few persons took advantage of it. Clearly, they expect the loss from unnecessary surgery to be small; whether this belief is true or erroneous is not yet clear. Here again, consumers may be so ignorant that they do not even conceive that their physician's advice is not the most accurate he could give.[12] This could also explain why they do not buy second opinions, although it would surely be relatively cheap just to inform consumers that a second opinion would be useful.

INSURANCE

The incidence of illness is random. This leads to a demand for insurance against medical bills on the part of risk-adverse individuals. There are other goods subject to such randomness in demand; for example, all classes of repair service, for which there also tend to be forms of insurance, either explicit policies or as service contracts. What is truly distinctive about medical care is not the risk or consequent insurance as such, but, rather, the way in which insurance benefits are determined.

The great bulk of health insurance is purchased by reasonably well-informed group purchasers, and premiums are reasonably well equated to risk, the two conditions necessary for an efficient competitive market (tax considerations aside). There are some problems raised by insurer ignorance about the probability of loss, but these adverse selection difficulties do not seem of much quantitative importance. Indeed, most of the concern in public policy with respect to selection is not that health insurers sell insurance (at low rates) to bad risks they cannot identify, but that they refuse to sell insurance (at low rates) to bad risks they *can* identify. The market works, but it leaves a residue of persons unable or unwilling to buy insurance. The only real puzzle here is why longer term health insurance against the possibility of becoming a bad risk—guaranteed renewability without strings attached—is not more common. There is potentially a more serious problem if individual insurers cannot measure the *total* amount of health insurance an individual has bought. Since his losses will be functions of his coverage (moral hazard), premiums cannot be appropriately tailored to risks (Pauly (1974)).

The absence of markets for some risks, much emphasized by Arrow as a reason for inefficiency, is now generally viewed as caused by irreducible moral hazard or transactions-information costs. On a priori grounds, one cannot show that it is amenable to improvement (with the possible exception of the relatively small market for individual insurance).

As noted above, the primary distinguishing characteristic of health insurance is the way in which benefits are paid. Much of medical care is covered by an insurance which does have a unique characteristic; the insurance payment depends, not on the amount of loss, but on the expenditure made to repair the loss. This insurance distorts demand curves, reduces the incentive for search, and reduces the extent of competition. But with suitable translations from gross to net price, these alterations, however much they affect welfare, do not affect the extent of competition more than any other similar price reduction, as long as the differences among insurances are limited to paying different fractions of unlimited total expenditures. Problems do arise when insurance covers full cost or full price (perhaps up to a limit), because then there can be no price competition among sellers at prices below the limit.

If insurance plans can place restrictions on use, then there can be a kind of competition based on the appropriateness of these restrictions and the extent to which they are enforced. In a sense, the argument here about market-generated restrictions on quantity is analogous to the earlier argument about market-generated restrictions on quality. It is the consumer's interest to have his use of care restricted in situations where there is moral hazard, as long as he recoups the savings in lower insurance premiums. Health maintenance organizations are a way of restricting quantity to deal with moral hazard. The consumer gets more than just quantity restriction in an HMO; he also gets group practice (possibly, though not demonstrably, more efficient) and restriction on his choice of providers. The more puzzling question is why other third-party payers have not only been unsuccessful but even uninterested in ways of controlling moral hazard. Does this indicate a failure of competition or an inefficient consequence of competition?

There are some possible reasons why typical third-party insurers have in general been unwilling to control use directly. An insurer who wishes to control use by some form of utilization review or denial of benefits can generally expect to be able to offer his insurance package at lower premiums. Of course, there is a cost; some benefits will not be provided and some bills will not be paid. The essence of the moral hazard-welfare loss argument is that the reduction in premiums from controlling use exceeds the value to the individual of the care that would otherwise have been received. Such a gain can be realized, however, only if insureds of this carrier are able to recoup in lower premiums the full reduction in expenditure that restriction on their behavior implies.

There are two reasons why the insureds may not be able to capture all of these benefits. First, it may be that restrictions imposed on, say, physician or hospital behavior with respect to one set of insureds changes the use, in a quantitative sense, of other insureds. An insurer-sponsored second-opinion program for unnecessary hospitalization may reduce the total cost of hospital care not only to its insureds, who bear the time and inconvenience cost, but also for other insureds, if physicians behave in approximately the same way toward all patients. Certain kinds of reduction in use, such as in routine nursing care, would not even be under the control of the insurer, since such services are not itemized, nor would any reduction in use of such services reduce premiums proportionately.

The second reason is the tax treatment of insurance premiums, especially employer-paid premiums. The implicit costs of reduced use are fully borne by the insureds, but the benefit of premium reductions are shared with the Treasury because offsetting increases in money income are taxed. This implies, not only that the fraction of expense covered by insurance will be too large, as has been pointed out by Martin Feldstein (1973a) and others, but also that efforts to reduce use via regulations or controls will not be carried far enough.

Where these conjectures are true is not currently known, or even investigated. It can hardly be alleged that they represent failures of the competitive system as such. Rather, they arise in large part from tax distortion or from average-cost pricing schemes often followed by non-profit hospitals. The solution might be changes in tax treatment or pricing policies. Another option would be to subsidize those cost control activities which generate external benefits.

DIFFERENCES ON THE SUPPLY SIDE

Most of Arrow's discussion of suppliers is hypothetical in nature: Since it would be desirable that physicians or hospitals not take advantage of the imperfect knowledge of consumers, physicians are "supposed" to follow a higher ethical code, and non-profit hospitals are "supposed" to behave in a less mercenary fashion. Unfortunately, he does not provide any suggestions of ways to tell whether providers are doing what they are supposed to do, or indeed, any explanation of why one should have supposed that they would behave this way in the first place. Here again, but in a more qualified way, he seems to be arguing that since these institutions should, in an (first-bet) optimal state, behave this way, they must be doing so.

In this section I consider briefly the theory that might be constructed to explain the behavior of suppliers of medical care. The behavior of this industry seems different enough to suggest that models different from those of the conventional firm should at least be tried. In line with the normative focus of this paper, however, it is important to note that non-wealth-maximizing behavior of suppliers does not necessarily, or even probably, cause outcomes which are non-optimal.

So in what follows I will present some aspects of possible "different" models of medical-care provider behavior, not only to show why, in a positive sense, behavior might be expected to be different, but also to show that these differences do not necessarily imply inefficiency. I will not provide a full treatment of such models because that will be done by other papers at this conference.[13]

It is widely suggested that physicians are not wealth maximizers. It is plausible to argue that physicians may place lower values than other suppliers on money income relative to leisure and relative to their own evaluations of the quality or accuracy of output they provide.

There are two possible reasons. First, it is likely that these nonpecuniary aspects of work are normal goods. Since physician incomes are relatively high, one might expect these income effects to predominate. Second, physicians are not selected in the same way as other entrepreneurs. A successful owner or manager is likely to be one who has worked hard for the financial rewards that success brings. He is likely to be relatively more responsive to financial incentives than a person selected without regard to his financial responsiveness. Because the limited number of medical school-places are allocated on some basis other than financial responsiveness, and because medical care can be provided only by persons who have completed medical education, it is likely that physicians will be less responsive to financial rewards than would a typical provider in another industry. If entry into medicine were not limited, a good bit of this different behavior might be expected to disappear.

The question which is still of particular interest is the following. Given the present process for selecting and training physicians, does the absence of wealth-maximizing behavior suggest inefficiency? At first, one might suppose that the answer to this question should be yes. Absence of wealth maximization implies the possible absence of cost minimization, and that is obviously inefficient. There is even fairly strong empirical evidence that physicians do choose less than the cost-minimizing amount of non-physician inputs in managing their own practices (Uwe Reinhardt). It is difficult to suppose that this arises from unplanned ignorance by physicians. The easiest explanation is based on the "utility-from inefficiency" gambit—the argument that physicians actually *choose* to be inefficient, because of the subjective cost of supervision and control. They may even choose not to obtain information on ways to perform such supervision, because of the subjective cost of both the information and the supervision.

Is this "inefficiency" inefficient? The answer is that, if the incentives faced by physicians reflect the real tradeoff between inefficiency and supervision cost, it would not be desirable either to induce or to compel physicians to reduce costs and increase their money incomes. This anomalous result is based on the notion that the payment that would have to be made to induce the physician to provide more supervision, or the payment he would be willing to make to avoid supervision, would exceed the cost reduction. Public good aspects of information may suggest a role for government in subsidizing information to physicians on how to organize their practice in more profitable or more efficient ways, but I would regard the hypothesis of government ability to reduce significantly producer ignorance as even less plausible than its ability to reduce consumer ignorance.

There is a second peculiar effect of non-maximizing behavior that comes from the interrelatedness of information content and demand for therapeutic care. It is often suggested that, because the physician can control the content of the advice he provides to patients, the physician who wants to increase his income will generate demand for his own output. It is further suggested that the empirical observation that demand is related, *ceteris paribus,* to the availability of physicians supports this view.

I have argued above that the ability of physicians permanently to shift demand may be severely constrained, and I regard the empirical evidence that demand is shifted to be very weak. Nevertheless, it is important to note that, in theory, observation of an availability effect based on information manipulation may require that physicians *not* be income or wealth maximizers. If a physician mazimizes his income, he will choose that level of informational accuracy that maximizes the price he can get for any quantity from him. If the number of physicians increases, this reduces each physician's share of total quantity demanded at any price, but the maximum price at any given total quantity is not changed. So the observed market demand curve will not shift. One way to get such shifting is to assume that physicians value accuracy, and are only willing to trade off accuracy for income as their incomes get sufficiently low or the reward for inaccuracy gets sufficiently high. The normative implication of this discussion is that control of physician stock, below the free entry level, can be welfare increasing if physicians are not wealth maximizers.[14]

With respect to hospitals, we note that one of the most striking aspects of empirical studies of hospital behavior, dominated by not-for-profit and governmental firms, is that it is almost all consistent with the assumption of profit maximization. Suppliers respond, prices rise, and incomes increase when demand increases. Although there are theories to explain these facts in terms of utility-maximization (Feldstein (1971), Joseph Newhouse), it is also possible to suggest profit-maximizing explanations for hospital behavior (Pauly and Michael Redisch). The nonprofit nature of hospitals may be a distinction that does not make much of a difference. In view of empirical evidence and the need to limit this paper, I will not discuss possible theories of hospital behavior further.

CONCLUSION

This paper has emphasized consumer ignorance as the most important potential difference between medical care and other goods. I argued, however, that for some of medical care there was possibly little actual difference even in the present case, while for another part there *could* be market-like institutions to deal with it. This still leaves a third kind of care, which is by definition rare and unusual. Here some Government regulation may help, although even here its superiority over information provision is a second-best conjecture. The most plausible case for public intervention may be, not in the regulation of quality or of information flow, but in the regulation of sheer numbers of providers, especially physicians, and especially with regard to geographical distribution.

The primary message from theory for research is that more empirical information is needed to go from conjectures to fact, that theory itself cannot take us very far. Research on how well informed consumers are, and how differently they might behave with additional information, and how markets would change in response would be of high priority.

NOTES

1. There is a fourth kind of difference, which they do not list and which will not be discussed here, but which may still be of importance. Medical care is one of those goods and services to which *social concern* attaches. People other than the direct user of care are concerned about the amount that is used. This kind of concern can generate an external effect which calls for public subsidization. It need not, however, imply any difference in the operation of the market once the subsidy has been paid.

2. One qualification: If entry restrictions are removed, it is possible that firms might shrink in size to such an extent that economies of scale would appear.

3. The empirical evidence on how people select providers is skimpy. There is a strong suggestion, however, that not only are friends and relatives used as sources of advice, but especially those friends who have had experience with the provider or type of provider contemplated, and who are regarded as more knowledgeable than the direct consumer. See A. Booth and N. Babchuk.

4. Data for 1973 are used for the percent of total expenditures figures; they have changed little over recent years.

5. It should be noted that definition of the "reasonably well informed" part of total spending should *not* be based on the distinction between physician and patient-generated care. Some patient-generated care may be quite poorly informed, while some care may be suggested by the physician but still be of a sort that the consumer is capable of evaluating.

6. Consider the following example. Suppose there are two producers of a medical service, each one producing a different level of quality. Suppose that, if quality levels and marginal costs were known, all consumers in a world of identical consumers would choose the higher level quality. In the absence of information on price or quality, consumers might be randomly distributed in approximately equal numbers across the two producers. Suppose higher quality costs more, and suppose that price advertising is permitted. Ignorant consumers might now all choose the lower quality producer because his equilibrium price is likely to be lower. Those who formerly used the low quality producer may not lose, but those who switched from the high quality producer may be worse off. It is possible, therefore, that partial information can lead to an outcome in which none are better off and some are worse off.

7. This is a restatement of one of the parts of the well-known "Coase Theorem" (Ronald Coase).

8. An alternative approach which is equivalent in some cases is to consider an entire course of treatment from presenting symptoms through therapy, and to evaluate quality as the outcome of an entire course of treatment.

9. As Victor Goldberg has noted, this makes sense only if the consumer is not fully informed. If he is fully informed, he will make appropriate choices in the market. Public intervention can then only serve to make consumers worse off, as Walter Oi has noted.

10. This also suggests that wholehearted voluntary support for PSRO's which provide useful information is *not likely* to be universal among physicians, especially low-quality ones.

11. It may not be efficient to provide information on outcomes because of its incentive effects. Physicians may select cases in such a way as to improve their outcome measures, if those outcome measures cannot be perfectly adjusted for differences in underlying conditions.

12. Another result provided by McCarthy and E. Widmer suggests that consumers are not this ignorant. They compared a mandatory and a voluntary surgical second opinion program and found that the rate at which the initial recommendation for surgery was not confirmed was much greater for the voluntary program. This implies that patients *knew*, even before the second opinion, which recommendations for surgery were likely to be questionable.

13. See also Feldstein (1973b) and Davis (1972) for surveys.

14. Of course, this ignores the direct effect of numbers of physicians on consumers' own ability to generate information, a point discussed above.

REFERENCES

K. Arrow, "Uncertainty and the Welfare Economics of Medical Care," *Amer. Econ. Rev.*, December 1963, 941-973.

A. Booth and N. Babchuk, "Seeking Health Care from New Resources," *J. Health Social Behavior*, March 1972, 90-99.

J. P. Bunker and B. Brown, "The Physician-Patient as One Informed Consumer of Surgical Services," *New England J. Medicine*, May 1974, 1051-55.

R. H. Coase, "The Problem of Social Cost," *J. Law Econ.* October 1960, 1-44.

C. Colantoni, O. A. Davis, and M. Swaminutham, "Imperfect Consumers and Welfare Comparisons of Policies Concerning Information and Regulation," *Bell J. Econ.*, Autumn 1976, 602-15.

M. Darby and E. Karni, "Free Competition and the Optimal Amount of Fraud," *J. Law Econ.*, April 1973, 67-88.

K. Davis, "Economic Theories of Behavior in Nonprofit Private, Hospitals," *J. of Econ. and Bus.*, Winter 1972, 1-13.

———, *National Health Insurance*, Washington 1975.

M. Feldstein, "The Rising Price of Physicians' Services," *Rev. Econ. Statis.*, May 1970, 121-33.

———, "Hospital Cost Inflation: A Study of Nonprofit Price Dynamics *Amer. Econ. Rev.*, December 1971, 853-72.

———, (1973a), "The Welfare Loss of Excess Health Insurance," *J. Polit. Econ.*, March 1973, 255-80.

———, (1973b), "Econometric Studies in Health Economics," in *Frontiers of Quantitative Economics*, 1973.

A. Flexner, "Medical Education in the U.S. and Canada," *Bulletin No. 4*, Carnegie Foundation for the Advancement of Teaching (1910).

V. Goldberg, "The Economics of Product Safety and Imperfect Information," *Bell J. Econ.*, Autumn 1974, 683-88.

S. Grossman and J. Stiglitz, "Information and Competitive Price Systems," *Amer. Econ. Rev.*, May 1976, 246-253.

E. G. McCarthy, and E. Widmer, "Effect of Screening by Consultants on Recommended Elective Surgical Procedures," *New England J. Medicine*, Dec. 1974, 1331-35.

S. Mushkin, "Towards a Definition of Health Economics," *Public Health Reports*, Sept. 1958, 785-93.

P. Nelson, "Information and Consumer Behavior," *J. Polit. Econ.*, March-April 1970, 311-329.

J. Newhouse, "Toward a Theory of Non-profit Institutions: An Economic Model of a Hospital," *Amer. Econ. Rev.*, June 1970, 64-74.

W. Oi, "The Economics of Product Safety," *Bell J. Econ.*, Spring 1973, 3-28.

M. Pauly, "Over insurance and Public Provision of Insurance: Moral Hazard and Adverse Selection," *Quarterly J. Econ.*, February 1974, 44-62.

———, "The Role of Demand Creation in the Provision of Health Services," paper presented at annual meeting of American Economic Association, December 1975.

———, "Information and the Demand for Medical Care," in J. Hixson and L. Krystaniak, Eds., *Theoretical Studies in Health Economics* (forthcoming, 1977).

———, and M. Redisch, "The Not-for-Profit Hospital as a Physicians' Cooperative," *Amer. Econ. Rev.*, March 1973, 87-99.

U. Reinhardt, "A Production Function for Physicians' Services," *Rev. Econ. Statis.*, February 1972, 55-66.

M. Rothschild, "Models of Market Organization with Imperfect Information," *J. of Polit. Econ.*, November-December 1973, 1283-1308.

S. Salop, "Information and Monopolistic Competition," *Amer. Econ. Rev.*, May 1976, 240-45.

M. Satterthwait, "The Pricing of Physicians Services: A Theoretical Analysis," unpublished paper, Northwestern University, April 1977.

D. Smallwood and K. Smith, "Optical Treatment Decisions, Optimal Fee Schedules, and the Allocation of Medical Resources," Northwestern University, processed, 1976.

2. Uncertainty and the Welfare Economics of Medical Care

KENNETH J. ARROW

Reprinted with permission from *American Economic Review* 53. Copyright © 1963, American Economic Association, 941-973.

I. *Introduction: Scope and Method*

This paper is an exploratory and tentative study of the specific differentia of medical care as the object of normative economics. It is contended here, on the basis of comparison of obvious characteristics of the medical-care industry with the norms of welfare economics, that the special economic problems of medical care can be explained as adaptations to the existence of uncertainty in the incidence of disease and in the efficacy of treatment.

It should be noted that the subject is the *medical-care industry,* not *health.* The causal factors in health are many, and the provision of medical care is only one. Particularly at low levels of income, other commodities such as nutrition, shelter, clothing, and sanitation may be much more significant. It is the complex of services that center about the physician, private and group practice, hospitals, and public health, which I propose to discuss.

The focus of discussion will be on the way the operation of the medical-care industry and the efficacy with which it satisfies the needs of society differ from a norm, if at all. The "norm" that the economist usually uses for the purposes of such comparisons is the operation of a competitive model, that is, the flows of services that would be offered and purchased and the prices that would be paid for them if each individual in the market offered or purchased services at the going prices as if his decisions had no influence over them, and the going prices were such that the amounts of services which were available equalled the total amounts which other individuals were willing to purchase, with no imposed restrictions on supply or demand.

The interest in the competitive model stems partly from its presumed descriptive power and partly from its implications for economic efficiency. In particular, we can state the following well-known proposition (First Optimality Theorem). If a competitive equilibrium

* The author is professor of economics at Stanford University. He wishes to express his thanks for useful comments to F. Bator, R. Dorfman, V. Fuchs, Dr. S. Gilson, R. Kessel, S. Mushkin, and C. R. Rorem. This paper was prepared under the sponsorship of the Ford Foundation as part of a series of papers on the economics of health, education, and welfare.

exists at all, and if all commodities relevant to costs or utilities are in fact priced in the market, then the equilibrium is necessarily *optimal* in the following precise sense (due to V. Pareto): There is no other allocation of resources to services which will make all participants in the market better off.

Both the conditions of this optimality theorem and the definition of optimality call for comment. A definition is just a definition, but when the *definiendum* is a word already in common use with highly favorable connotations, it is clear that we are really trying to be persuasive; we are implicitly recommending the achievement of optimal states.[1] It is reasonable enough to assert that a change in allocation which makes all participants better off is one that certainly should be made; this is a value judgment, not a descriptive proposition, but it is a very weak one. From this it follows that it is not desirable to put up with a non-optimal allocation. But it does not follow that if we are at an allocation which is optimal in the Pareto sense, we should not change to any other. We cannot indeed make a change that does not hurt someone; but we can still desire to change to another allocation if the change makes enough participants better off and by so much that we feel that the injury to others is not enough to offset the benefits. Such interpersonal comparisons are, of course, value judgments. The change, however, by the previous argument ought to be an optimal state; of course there are many possible states, each of which is optimal in the sense here used.

However, a value judgment on the desirability of each possible new distribution of benefits and costs corresponding to each possible reallocation of resources is not, in general, necessary. Judgments about the distribution can be made separately, in one sense, from those about allocation if certain conditions are fulfilled. Before stating the relevant proposition, it is necessary to remark that the competitive equilibrium achieved depends in good measure on the initial distribution of purchasing power, which consists of ownership of assets and skills that command a price on the market. A transfer of assets among individuals will, in general, change the final supplies of goods and services and the prices paid for them. Thus, a transfer of purchasing power from the well to the ill will increase the demand for medical services. This will manifest itself in the short run in an increase in the price of medical services and in the long run in an increase in the amount supplied.

With this in mind, the following statement can be made (Second Optimality Theorem): If there are no increasing returns in production, and if certain other minor conditions are satisfied, then every optimal state is a competitive equilibrium corresponding to some initial distribution of purchasing power. Operationally, the significance of this proposition is that if the conditions of the two optimality theorems are

---

[1] This point has been stressed by I. M. D. Little [19, pp. 71-74]. For the concept of a "persuasive definition," see C. L. Stevenson [27, pp. 210-17].

satisfied, and if the allocation mechanism in the real world satisfies the conditions for a competitive model, then social policy can confine itself to steps taken to alter the distribution of purchasing power. For any given distribution of purchasing power, the market will, under the assumptions made, achieve a competitive equilibrium which is necessarily optimal; and any optimal state is a competitive equilibrium corresponding to some distribution of purchasing power, so that any desired optimal state can be achieved.

The redistribution of purchasing power among individuals most simply takes the form of money: taxes and subsidies. The implications of such a transfer for individual satisfactions are, in general, not known in advance. But we can assume that society can *ex post* judge the distribution of satisfactions and, if deemed unsatisfactory, take steps to correct it by subsequent transfers. Thus, by successive approximations, a most preferred social state can be achieved, with resource allocation being handled by the market and public policy confined to the redistribution of money income.[2]

If, on the contrary, the actual market differs significantly from the competitive model, or if the assumptions of the two optimality theorems are not fulfilled, the separation of allocative and distributional procedures becomes, in most cases, impossible.[3]

The first step then in the analysis of the medical-care market is the comparison between the actual market and the competitive model. The methodology of this comparison has been a recurrent subject of controversy in economics for over a century. Recently, M. Friedman [15] has vigorously argued that the competitive or any other model should be tested solely by its ability to predict. In the context of competition, he comes close to arguing that prices and quantities are the only relevant data. This point of view is valuable in stressing that a certain amount of lack of realism in the assumptions of a model is no argument against its value. But the price-quantity implications of the competitive model for pricing are not easy to derive without major—and, in many cases, impossible—econometric efforts.

In this paper, the institutional organization and the observable mores of the medical profession are included among the data to be used in assessing the competitiveness of the medical-care market. I shall also examine the presence or absence of the preconditions for the equivalence of competitive equilibria and optimal states. The major competi-

---

[2] The separation between allocation and distribution even under the above assumptions has glossed over problems in the execution of any desired redistribution policy; in practice, it is virtually impossible to find a set of taxes and subsidies that will not have an adverse effect on the achievement of an optimal state. But this discussion would take us even further afield than we have already gone.

[3] The basic theorems of welfare economics alluded to so briefly above have been the subject of voluminous literature, but no thoroughly satisfactory statement covering both the theorems themselves and the significance of exceptions to them exists. The positive assertions of welfare economics and their relation to the theory of competitive equilibrium are admirably covered in Koopmans [18]. The best summary of the various ways in which the theorems can fail to hold is probably Bator's [6].

tive preconditions, in the sense used here, are three: the *existence* of competitive equilibrium, the *marketability* of all goods and services relevant to costs and utilities, and *nonincreasing returns*. The first two, as we have seen, insure that competitive equilibrium is necessarily optimal; the third insures that every optimal state is the competitive equilibrium corresponding to some distribution of income.[4] The first and third conditions are interrelated; indeed, nonincreasing returns plus some additional conditions not restrictive in a modern economy imply the existence of a competitive equilibrium, i.e., imply that there will be some set of prices which will clear all markets.[5]

The concept of marketability is somewhat broader than the traditional divergence between private and social costs and benefits. The latter concept refers to cases in which the organization of the market does not require an individual to pay for costs that he imposes on others as the result of his actions or does not permit him to receive compensation for benefits he confers. In the medical field, the obvious example is the spread of communicable diseases. An individual who fails to be immunized not only risks his own health, a disutility which presumably he has weighed against the utility of avoiding the procedure, but also that of others. In an ideal price system, there would be a price which he would have to pay to anyone whose health is endangered, a price sufficiently high so that the others would feel compensated; or, alternatively, there would be a price which would be paid to him by others to induce him to undergo the immunization procedure. Either system would lead to an optimal state, though the distributional implications would be different. It is, of course, not hard to see that such price systems could not, in fact, be practical; to approximate an optimal state it would be necessary to have collective intervention in the form of subsidy or tax or compulsion.

By the absence of marketability for an action which is identifiable, technologically possible, and capable of influencing some individual's welfare, for better or for worse, is meant here the failure of the existing market to provide a means whereby the services can be both offered and demanded upon payment of a price. Nonmarketability may be due to intrinsic technological characteristics of the product which prevent a suitable price from being enforced, as in the case of communicable diseases, or it may be due to social or historical controls, such as those prohibiting an individual from selling himself into slavery. This distinction is, in fact, difficult to make precise, though it is obviously of importance for policy; for the present purposes, it will be sufficient to identify nonmarketability with the observed absence of markets.

The instance of nonmarketability with which we shall be most concerned is that of risk-bearing. The relevance of risk-bearing to medical

---

[4] There are further minor conditions, for which see Koopmans [18, pp. 50-55].

[5] For a more precise statement of the existence conditions, see Koopmans [18, pp. 56-60] or Debreu [12, Ch. 5].

care seems obvious; illness is to a considerable extent an unpredictable phenomenon. The ability to shift the risks of illness to others is worth a price which many are willing to pay. Because of pooling and of superior willingness and ability, others are willing to bear the risks. Nevertheless, as we shall see in greater detail, a great many risks are not covered, and indeed the markets for the services of risk-coverage are poorly developed or nonexistent. Why this should be so is explained in more detail in Section IV.C below; briefly, it is impossible to draw up insurance policies which will sufficiently distinguish among risks, particularly since observation of the results will be incapable of distinguishing between avoidable and unavoidable risks, so that incentives to avoid losses are diluted.

The optimality theorems discussed above are usually presented in the literature as referring only to conditions of certainty, but there is no difficulty in extending them to the case of risks, provided the additional services of risk-bearing are included with other commodities.[6]

However, the variety of possible risks in the world is really staggering. The relevant commodities include, in effect, bets on all possible occurrences in the world which impinge upon utilities. In fact, many of these "commodities," i.e., desired protection against many risks, are simply not available. Thus, a wide class of commodities is nonmarketable, and a basic competitive precondition is not satisfied.[7]

There is a still more subtle consequence of the introduction of risk-bearing considerations. When there is uncertainty, information or knowledge becomes a commodity. Like other commodities, it has a cost of production and a cost of transmission, and so it is naturally not spread out over the entire population but concentrated among those who can profit most from it. (These costs may be measured in time or disutility as well as money.) But the demand for information is difficult to discuss in the rational terms usually employed. The value of information is frequently not known in any meaningful sense to the buyer; if, indeed, he knew enough to measure the value of information, he would know the information itself. But information, in the form of skilled care, is precisely what is being bought from most physicians, and, indeed, from most professionals. The elusive character of information as a commodity suggests that it departs considerably from the usual marketability assumptions about commodities.[8]

---

[6] The theory, in variant forms, seems to have been first worked out by Allais [2], Arrow [5], and Baudier [7]. For further generalization, see Debreu [11] and [12, Ch. 7].

[7] It should also be remarked that in the presence of uncertainty, indivisibilities that are sufficiently small to create little difficulty for the existence and viability of competitive equilibrium may nevertheless give rise to a considerable range of increasing returns because of the operation of the law of large numbers. Since most objects of insurance (lives, fire hazards, etc.) have some element of indivisibility, insurance companies have to be above a certain size. But it is not clear that this effect is sufficiently great to create serious obstacles to the existence and viability of competitive equilibrium in practice.

[8] One form of production of information is research. Not only does the product have unconventional aspects as a commodity, but it is also subject to increasing returns in use, since new ideas, once developed, can be used over and over without being consumed, and

That risk and uncertainty are, in fact, significant elements in medical care hardly needs argument. I will hold that virtually all the special features of this industry, in fact, stem from the prevalence of uncertainty.

The nonexistence of markets for the bearing of some risks in the first instance reduces welfare for those who wish to transfer those risks to others for a certain price, as well as for those who would find it profitable to take on the risk at such prices. But it also reduces the desire to render or consume services which have risky consequences; in technical language, these commodities are complementary to risk-bearing. Conversely, the production and consumption of commodities and services with little risk attached act as substitutes for risk-bearing and are encouraged by market failure there with respect to risk-bearing. Thus the observed commodity pattern will be affected by the nonexistence of other markets.

The failure of one or more of the competitive preconditions has as its most immediate and obvious consequence a reduction in welfare below that obtainable from existing resources and technology, in the sense of a failure to reach an optimal state in the sense of Pareto. But more can be said. I propose here the view that, when the market fails to achieve an optimal state, society will, to some extent at least, recognize the gap, and nonmarket social institutions will arise attempting to bridge it.[9] Certainly this process is not necessarily conscious; nor is it uniformly successful in approaching more closely to optimality when the entire range of consequences is considered. It has always been a favorite activity of economists to point out that actions which on their face achieve a desirable goal may have less obvious consequences, particularly over time, which more than offset the original gains.

But it is contended here that the special structural characteristics of the medical-care market are largely attempts to overcome the lack of optimality due to the nonmarketability of the bearing of suitable risks and the imperfect marketability of information. These compensatory institutional changes, with some reinforcement from usual profit motives, largely explain the observed noncompetitive behavior of the medical-care market, behavior which, in itself, interferes with optimality. The social adjustment towards optimality thus puts obstacles in its own path.

The doctrine that society will seek to achieve optimality by nonmarket means if it cannot achieve them in the market is not novel. Certainly, the government, at least in its economic activities, is usually implicitly or explicitly held to function as the agency which substitutes

---

to difficulties of market control, since the cost of reproduction is usually much less than that of production. Hence, it is not surprising that a free enterprise economy will tend to underinvest in research; see Nelson [21] and Arrow [4].

[9] An important current situation in which normal market relations have had to be greatly modified in the presence of great risks is the production and procurement of modern weapons; see Peck and Scherer [23, pp. 581-82] (I am indebted for this reference to V. Fuchs) and [1, pp. 71-75].

for the market's failure.[10] I am arguing here that in some circumstances other social institutions will step into the optimality gap, and that the medical-care industry, with its variety of special institutions, some ancient, some modern, exemplifies this tendency.

It may be useful to remark here that a good part of the preference for redistribution expressed in government taxation and expenditure policies and private charity can be reinterpreted as desire for insurance. It is noteworthy that virtually nowhere is there a system of subsidies that has as its aim simply an equalization of income. The subsidies or other governmental help go to those who are disadvantaged in life by events the incidence of which is popularly regarded as unpredictable: the blind, dependent children, the medically indigent. Thus, optimality, in a context which includes risk-bearing, includes much that appears to be motivated by distributional value judgments when looked at in a narrower context.[11]

This methodological background gives rise to the following plan for this paper. Section II is a catalogue of stylized generalizations about the medical-care market which differentiate it from the usual commodity markets. In Section III the behavior of the market is compared with that of the competitive model which disregards the fact of uncertainty. In Section IV, the medical-care market is compared, both as to behavior and as to preconditions, with the ideal competitive market that takes account of uncertainty; an attempt will be made to demonstrate that the characteristics outlined in Section II can be explained either as the result of deviations from the competitive preconditions or as attempts to compensate by other institutions for these failures. The discussion is not designed to be definitive, but provocative. In particular, I have been chary about drawing policy inferences; to a considerable extent, they depend on further research, for which the present paper is intended to provide a framework.

II. *A Survey of the Special Characteristics of the Medical-Care Market*[12]

This section will list selectively some characteristics of medical care which distinguish it from the usual commodity of economics textbooks. The list is not exhaustive, and it is not claimed that the characteristics listed are individually unique to this market. But, taken together, they do establish a special place for medical care in economic analysis.

A. *The Nature of Demand*

The most obvious distinguishing characteristics of an individual's demand for medical services is that it is not steady in origin as, for example, for food or clothing, but irregular and unpredictable. Medi-

---

[10] For an explicit statement of this view, see Baumol [8]. But I believe this position is implicit in most discussions of the functions of government.

[11] Since writing the above, I find that Buchanan and Tullock [10, Ch. 13] have argued that all redistribution can be interpreted as "income insurance."

[12] For an illuminating survey to which I am much indebted, see S. Mushkin [20].

cal services, apart from preventive services, afford satisfaction only in the event of illness, a departure from the normal state of affairs. It is hard, indeed, to think of another commodity of significance in the average budget of which this is true. A portion of legal services, devoted to defense in criminal trials or to lawsuits, might fall in this category but the incidence is surely very much lower (and, of course, there are, in fact, strong institutional similarities between the legal and medical-care markets.)[13]

In addition, the demand for medical services is associated, with a considerable probability, with an assault on personal integrity. There is some risk of death and a more considerable risk of impairment of full functioning. In particular, there is a major potential for loss or reduction of earning ability. The risks are not by themselves unique; food is also a necessity, but avoidance of deprivation of food can be guaranteed with sufficient income, where the same cannot be said of avoidance of illness. Illness is, thus, not only risky but a costly risk in itself, apart from the cost of medical care.

B. *Expected Behavior of the Physician*

It is clear from everyday observation that the behavior expected of sellers of medical care is different from that of business men in general. These expectations are relevant because medical care belongs to the category of commodities for which the product and the activity of production are identical. In all such cases, the customer cannot test the product before consuming it, and there is an element of trust in the relation.[14] But the ethically understood restrictions on the activities of a physician are much more severe than on those of, say, a barber. His behavior is supposed to be governed by a concern for the customer's welfare which would not be expected of a salesman. In Talcott Parsons's terms, there is a "collectivity-orientation," which distinguishes medicine and other professions from business, where self-interest on the part of participants is the accepted norm.[15]

A few illustrations will indicate the degree of difference between the behavior expected of physicians and that expected of the typical businessman.[16] (1) Advertising and overt price competition are virtually eliminated among physicians. (2) Advice given by physicians as to further treatment by himself or others is supposed to be completely

---

[13] In governmental demand, military power is an example of a service used only irregularly and unpredictably. Here too, special institutional and professional relations have emerged, though the precise social structure is different for reasons that are not hard to analyze.

[14] Even with material commodities, testing is never so adequate that all elements of implicit trust can be eliminated. Of course, over the long run, experience with the quality of product of a given seller provides a check on the possibility of trust.

[15] See [22, p. 463]. The whole of [22, Ch. 10] is a most illuminating analysis of the social role of medical practice; though Parsons' interest lies in different areas from mine, I must acknowledge here my indebtedness to his work.

[16] I am indebted to Herbert Klarman of Johns Hopkins University for some of the points discussed in this and the following paragraph.

divorced from self-interest. (3) It is at least claimed that treatment is dictated by the objective needs of the case and not limited by financial considerations.[17] While the ethical compulsion is surely not as absolute in fact as it is in theory, we can hardly suppose that it has no influence over resource allocation in this area. Charity treatment in one form or another does exist because of this tradition about human rights to adequate medical care.[18] (4) The physician is relied on as an expert in certifying to the existence of illnesses and injuries for various legal and other purposes. It is socially expected that his concern for the correct conveying of information will, when appropriate, outweigh his desire to please his customers.[19]

Departure from the profit motive is strikingly manifested by the overwhelming predominance of nonprofit over proprietary hospitals.[20] The hospital per se offers services not too different from those of a hotel, and it is certainly not obvious that the profit motive will not lead to a more efficient supply. The explanation may lie either on the supply side or on that of demand. The simplest explanation is that public and private subsidies decrease the cost to the patient in nonprofit hospitals. A second possibility is that the association of profit-making with the supply of medical services arouses suspicion and antagonism on the part of patients and referring physicians, so they do prefer nonprofit institutions. Either explanation implies a preference on the part of some group, whether donors or patients, against the profit motive in the supply of hospital services.[21]

Conformity to collectivity-oriented behavior is especially important since it is a commonplace that the physician-patient relation affects the quality of the medical care product. A pure cash nexus would be in-

---

[17] The belief that the ethics of medicine demands treatment independent of the patient's ability to pay is strongly ingrained. Such a perceptive observer as René Dubos has made the remark that the high cost of anticoagulants restricts their use and may contradict classical medical ethics, as though this were an unprecedented phenomenon. See [13, p. 419]. "A time *may come* when medical ethics will have to be considered in the harsh light of economics" (emphasis added). Of course, this expectation amounts to ignoring the scarcity of medical resources; one has only to have been poor to realize the error. We may confidently assume that price and income do have some consequences for medical expenditures.

[18] A needed piece of research is a study of the exact nature of the variations of medical care received and medical care paid for as income rises. (The relevant income concept also needs study.) For this purpose, some disaggregation is needed; differences in hospital care which are essentially matters of comfort should, in the above view, be much more responsive to income than, e.g., drugs.

[19] This role is enhanced in a socialist society, where the state itself is actively concerned with illness in relation to work; see Field [14, Ch. 9].

[20] About 3 per cent of beds were in proprietary hospitals in 1958, against 30 per cent in voluntary nonprofit, and the remainder in federal, state, and local hospitals; see [26, Chart 4-2, p. 60].

[21] C. R. Rorem has pointed out to me some further factors in this analysis. (1) Given the social intention of helping all patients without regard to immediate ability to pay, economies of scale would dictate a predominance of community-sponsored hospitals. (2) Some proprietary hospitals will tend to control total costs to the patient more closely, including the fees of physicians, who will therefore tend to prefer community-sponsored hospitals.

adequate; if nothing else, the patient expects that the same physician will normally treat him on successive occasions. This expectation is strong enough to persist even in the Soviet Union, where medical care is nominally removed from the market place [14, pp. 194-96]. That purely psychic interactions between physician and patient have effects which are objectively indistinguishable in kind from the effects of medication is evidenced by the use of the placebo as a control in medical experimentation; see Shapiro [25].

C. *Product Uncertainty*

Uncertainty as to the quality of the product is perhaps more intense here than in any other important commodity. Recovery from disease is as unpredictable as is its incidence. In most commodities, the possibility of learning from one's own experience or that of others is strong because there is an adequate number of trials. In the case of severe illness, that is, in general, not true; the uncertainty due to inexperience is added to the intrinsic difficulty of prediction. Further, the amount of uncertainty, measured in terms of utility variability, is certainly much greater for medical care in severe cases than for, say, houses or automobiles, even though these are also expenditures sufficiently infrequent so that there may be considerable residual uncertainty.

Further, there is a special quality to the uncertainty; it is very different on the two sides of the transaction. Because medical knowledge is so complicated, the information possessed by the physician as to the consequences and possibilities of treatment is necessarily very much greater than that of the patient, or at least so it is believed by both parties.[22] Further, both parties are aware of this informational inequality, and their relation is colored by this knowledge.

To avoid misunderstanding, observe that the difference in information relevant here is a difference in information as to the consequence of a purchase of medical care. There is always an inequality of information as to production methods between the producer and the purchaser of any commodity, but in most cases the customer may well have as good or nearly as good an understanding of the utility of the product as the producer.

D. *Supply Conditions*

In competitive theory, the supply of a commodity is governed by the net return from its production compared with the return derivable from the use of the same resources elsewhere. There are several significant departures from this theory in the case of medical care.

Most obviously, entry to the profession is restricted by licensing. Licensing, of course, restricts supply and therefore increases the cost of medical care. It is defended as guaranteeing a minimum of quality.

---

[22] Without trying to assess the present situation, it is clear in retrospect that at some point in the past the actual differential knowledge possessed by physicians may not have been much. But from the economic point of view, it is the subjective belief of both parties, as manifested in their market behavior, that is relevant.

Restriction of entry by licensing occurs in most professions, including barbering and undertaking.

A second feature is perhaps even more remarkable. The cost of medical education today is high and, according to the usual figures, is borne only to a minor extent by the student. Thus, the private benefits to the entering student considerably exceed the costs. (It is, however, possible that research costs, not properly chargeable to education, swell the apparent difference.) This subsidy should, in principle, cause a fall in the price of medical services, which, however, is offset by rationing through limited entry to schools and through elimination of students during the medical-school career. These restrictions basically render superfluous the licensing, except in regard to graduates of foreign schools.

The special role of educational institutions in simultaneously subsidizing and rationing entry is common to all professions requiring advanced training.[23] It is a striking and insufficiently remarked phenomenon that such an important part of resource allocation should be performed by nonprofit-oriented agencies.

Since this last phenomenon goes well beyond the purely medical aspect, we will not dwell on it longer here except to note that the anomaly is most striking in the medical field. Educational costs tend to be far higher there than in any other branch of professional training. While tuition is the same, or only slightly higher, so that the subsidy is much greater, at the same time the earnings of physicians rank highest among professional groups, so there would not at first blush seem to be any necessity for special inducements to enter the profession. Even if we grant that, for reasons unexamined here, there is a social interest in subsidized professional education, it is not clear why the rate of subsidization should differ among professions. One might expect that the tuition of medical students would be higher than that of other students.

The high cost of medical education in the United States is itself a reflection of the quality standards imposed by the American Medical Association since the Flexner Report, and it is, I believe, only since then that the subsidy element in medical education has become significant. Previously, many medical schools paid their way or even yielded a profit.

Another interesting feature of limitation on entry to subsidized education is the extent of individual preferences concerning the social welfare, as manifested by contributions to private universities. But whether support is public or private, the important point is that both

---

[23] The degree of subsidy in different branches of professional education is worthy of a major research effort.

the quality and the quantity of the supply of medical care are being strongly influenced by social nonmarket forces.[24, 25]

One striking consequence of the control of quality is the restriction on the range offered. If many qualities of a commodity are possible, it would usually happen in a competitive market that many qualities will be offered on the market, at suitably varying prices, to appeal to different tastes and incomes. Both the licensing laws and the standards of medical-school training have limited the possibilities of alternative qualities of medical care. The declining ratio of physicians to total employees in the medical-care industry shows that substitution of less trained personnel, technicians, and the like, is not prevented completely, but the central role of the highly trained physician is not affected at all.[26]

E. *Pricing Practices*

The unusual pricing practices and attitudes of the medical profession are well known: extensive price discrimination by income (with an extreme of zero prices for sufficiently indigent patients) and, formerly, a strong insistence on fee for services as against such alternatives as prepayment.

The opposition to prepayment is closely related to an even stronger opposition to closed-panel practice (contractual arrangements which bind the patient to a particular group of physicians). Again these attitudes seem to differentiate professions from business. Prepayment and closed-panel plans are virtually nonexistent in the legal profession. In ordinary business, on the other hand, there exists a wide variety of exclusive service contracts involving sharing of risks; it is assumed that competition will select those which satisfy needs best.[27]

The problems of implicit and explicit price-fixing should also be mentioned. Price competition is frowned on. Arrangements of this type are not uncommon in service industries, and they have not been subjected to antitrust action. How important this is is hard to assess. It has been pointed out many times that the apparent rigidity of so-called administered prices considerably understates the actual flexibility. Here, too, if physicians find themselves with unoccupied time, rates are likely to go down, openly or covertly; if there is insufficient time for

---

[24] Strictly speaking, there are four variables in the market for physicians: price, quality of entering students, quality of education, and quantity. The basic market forces, demand for medical services and supply of entering students, determine two relations among the four variables. Hence, if the nonmarket forces determine the last two, market forces will determine price and quality of entrants.

[25] The supply of Ph.D.'s is similarly governed, but there are other conditions in the market which are much different, especially on the demand side.

[26] Today only the Soviet Union offers an alternative lower level of medical personnel, the feldshers, who practice primarily in the rural districts (the institution dates back to the 18th century). According to Field [14, pp. 98-100, 132-33], there is clear evidence of strain in the relations between physicians and feldshers, but it is not certain that the feldshers will gradually disappear as physicians grow in numbers.

[27] The law does impose some limits on risk-shifting in contracts, for example, its general refusal to honor exculpatory clauses.

the demand, rates will surely rise. The "ethics" of price competition may decrease the flexibility of price responses, but probably that is all.

III. *Comparisons with the Competitive Model under Certainty*

A. *Nonmarketable Commodities*

As already noted, the diffusion of communicable diseases provides an obvious example of nonmarket interactions. But from a theoretical viewpoint, the issues are well understood, and there is little point in expanding on this theme. (This should not be interpreted as minimizing the contribution of public health to welfare; there is every reason to suppose that it is considerably more important than all other aspects of medical care.)

Beyond this special area there is a more general interdependence, the concern of individuals for the health of others. The economic manifestations of this taste are to be found in individual donations to hospitals and to medical education, as well as in the widely accepted responsibilities of government in this area. The taste for improving the health of others appears to be stronger than for improving other aspects of their welfare.[28]

In interdependencies generated by concern for the welfare of others there is always a theoretical case for collective action if each participant derives satisfaction from the contributions of all.

B. *Increasing Returns*

Problems associated with increasing returns play some role in allocation of resources in the medical field, particularly in areas of low density or low income. Hospitals show increasing returns up to a point; specialists and some medical equipment constitute significant indivisibilities. In many parts of the world the individual physician may be a large unit relative to demand. In such cases it can be socially desirable to subsidize the appropriate medical-care unit. The appropriate mode of analysis is much the same as for water-resource projects. Increasing returns are hardly apt to be a significant problem in general practice in large cities in the United States, and improved transportation to some extent reduces their importance elsewhere.

C. *Entry*

The most striking departure from competitive behavior is restriction on entry to the field, as discussed in II.D above. Friedman and Kuznets, in a detailed examination of the pre-World War II data, have

---

[28] There may be an identification problem in this observation. If the failure of the market system is, or appears to be, greater in medical care than in, say, food an individual otherwise equally concerned about the two aspects of others' welfare may prefer to help in the first.

argued that the higher income of physicians could be attributed to this restriction.[29]

There is some evidence that the demand for admission to medical school has dropped (as indicated by the number of applicants per place and the quality of those admitted), so that the number of medical-school places is not as significant a barrier to entry as in the early 1950's [28, pp. 14-15]. But it certainly has operated over the past and it is still operating to a considerable extent today. It has, of course, constituted a direct and unsubtle restriction on the supply of medical care.

There are several considerations that must be added to help evaluate the importance of entry restrictions: (1) Additional entrants would be, in general, of lower quality; hence, the addition to the supply of medical care, properly adjusted for quality, is less than purely quantitative calculations would show.[30] (2) To achieve genuinely competitive conditions, it would be necessary not only to remove numerical restrictions on entry but also to remove the subsidy in medical education. Like any other producer, the physician should bear all the costs of production, including, in this case, education.[31] It is not so clear that this change would not keep even unrestricted entry down below the present level. (3) To some extent, the effect of making tuition carry the full cost of education will be to create too few entrants, rather than too many. Given the imperfections of the capital market, loans for this purpose to those who do not have the cash are difficult to obtain. The lender really has no security. The obvious answer is some form of insured loans, as has frequently been argued; not too much ingenuity would be needed to create a credit system for medical (and other branches of higher) education. Under these conditions the cost would still constitute a deterrent, but one to be compared with the high future incomes to be obtained.

If entry were governed by ideal competitive conditions, it may be that the quantity on balance would be increased, though this conclusion is not obvious. The average quality would probably fall, even under an ideal credit system, since subsidy plus selected entry draw some highly qualified individuals who would otherwise get into other fields. The decline in quality is not an over-all social loss, since it is accompanied by increase in quality in other fields of endeavor; indeed,

---

[29] See [16, pp. 118-37]. The calculations involve many assumptions and must be regarded as tenuous; see the comments by C. Reinold Noyes in [16, pp. 407-10].

[30] It might be argued that the existence of racial discrimination in entrance has meant that some of the rejected applicants are superior to some accepted. However, there is no necessary connection between an increase in the number of entrants and a reduction in racial discrimination; so long as there is excess demand for entry, discrimination can continue unabated and new entrants will be inferior to those previously accepted.

[31] One problem here is that the tax laws do not permit depreciation of professional education, so that there is a discrimination against this form of investment.

if demands accurately reflected utilities, there would be a net social gain through a switch to competitive entry.[32]

There is a second aspect of entry in which the contrast with competitive behavior is, in many respects, even sharper. It is the exclusion of many imperfect substitutes for physicians. The licensing laws, though they do not effectively limit the number of physicians, do exclude all others from engaging in any one of the activities known as medical practice. As a result, costly physician time may be employed at specific tasks for which only a small fraction of their training is needed, and which could be performed by others less well trained and therefore less expensive. One might expect immunization centers, privately operated, but not necessarily requiring the services of doctors.

In the competitive model without uncertainty, consumers are presumed to be able to distinguish qualities of the commodities they buy. Under this hypothesis, licensing would be, at best, superfluous and exclude those from whom consumers would not buy anyway; but it might exclude too many.

D. *Pricing*

The pricing practices of the medical industry (see II.E above) depart sharply from the competitive norm. As Kessel [17] has pointed out with great vigor, not only is price discrimination incompatible with the competitive model, but its preservation in the face of the large number of physicians is equivalent to a collective monopoly. In the past, the opposition to prepayment plans has taken distinctly coercive forms, certainly transcending market pressures, to say the least.

Kessel has argued that price discrimination is designed to maximize profits along the classic lines of discriminating monopoly and that organized medical opposition to prepayment was motivated by the desire to protect these profits. In principle, prepayment schemes are compatible with discrimination, but in practice they do not usually discriminate. I do not believe the evidence that the actual scale of discrimination is profit-maximizing is convincing. In particular, note that for any monopoly, discriminating or otherwise, the elasticity of demand in each market at the point of maximum profits is greater than one. But it is almost surely true for medical care that the price elasticity of demand for all income levels is less than one. That price discrimination by income is not completely profit-maximizing is obvious in the extreme case of charity; Kessel argues that this represents an appeasement of public opinion. But this already shows the incompleteness of the model and suggests the relevance and importance of social and ethical factors.

Certainly one important part of the opposition to prepayment was its close relation to closed-panel plans. Prepayment is a form of insurance, and naturally the individual physician did not wish to assume the

---

[32] To anticipate later discussion, this condition is not necessarily fulfilled. When it comes to quality choices, the market may be inaccurate.

risks. Pooling was intrinsically involved, and this strongly motivates, as we shall discuss further in Section IV below, control over prices and benefits. The simplest administrative form is the closed panel; physicians involved are, in effect, the insuring agent. From this point of view, Blue Cross solved the prepayment problem by universalizing the closed panel.

The case that price discrimination by income is a form of profit maximization which was zealously defended by opposition to fees for service seems far from proven. But it remains true that this price discrimination, for whatever cause, is a source of nonoptimality. Hypothetically, it means everyone would be better off if prices were made equal for all, and the rich compensated the poor for the changes in the relative positions. The importance of this welfare loss depends on the actual amount of discrimination and on the elasticities of demand for medical services by the different income groups. If the discussion is simplified by considering only two income levels, rich and poor, and if the elasticity of demand by either one is zero, then no reallocation of medical services will take place and the initial situation is optimal. The only effect of a change in price will be the redistribution of income as between the medical profession and the group with the zero elasticity of demand. With low elasticities of demand, the gain will be small. To illustrate, suppose the price of medical care to the rich is double that to the poor, the medical expenditures by the rich are 20 per cent of those by the poor, and the elasticity of demand for both classes is .5; then the net social gain due to the abolition of discrimination is slightly over 1 per cent of previous medical expenditures.[33]

---

[33] It is assumed that there are two classes, rich and poor; the price of medical services to the rich is twice that to the poor, medical expenditures by the rich are 20 per cent of those by the poor, and the elasticity of demand for medical services is .5 for both classes. Let us choose our quantity and monetary units so that the quantity of medical services consumed by the poor and the price they pay are both 1. Then the rich purchase .1 units of medical services at a price of 2. Given the assumption about the elasticities of demand, the demand function of the rich is $D_R(p) = .14\ p^{-.5}$ and that of the poor is $D_P(p) = p^{-.5}$. The supply of medical services is assumed fixed and therefore must equal 1.1. If price discrimination were abolished, the equilibrium price, $\bar{p}$, must satisfy the relation,

$$D_R(\bar{p}) + D_P(\bar{p}) = 1.1,$$

and therefore $\bar{p} = 1.07$. The quantities of medical care purchased by the rich and poor, respectively, would be $D_R(\bar{p}) = .135$ and $D_P(\bar{p}) = .965$.

The inverse demand functions, the price to be paid corresponding to any given quantity are $d_R(q) = .02/q^2$, and $d_P(q) = 1/q^2$. Therefore, the consumers' surplus to the rich generated by the change is:

(1) $$\int_{.1}^{.135} (.02/q^2)dq - \bar{p}(.135 - .1),$$

and similarly the loss in consumers' surplus by the poor is:

(2) $$\int_{.965}^{1} (1/q^2)dq - \bar{p}(1 - .965)$$

If (2) is subtracted from (1), the second terms cancel, and the aggregate increase in consumers' surplus is .0156, or a little over 1 per cent of the initial expenditures.

The issues involved in the opposition to prepayment, the other major anomaly in medical pricing, are not meaningful in the world of certainty and will be discussed below.

IV. *Comparison with the Ideal Competitive Model under Uncertainty*
A. *Introduction*

In this section we will compare the operations of the actual medical-care market with those of an ideal system in which not only the usual commodities and services but also insurance policies against all conceivable risks are available.[34] Departures consist for the most part of insurance policies that might conceivably be written, but are in fact not. Whether these potential commodities are nonmarketable, or, merely because of some imperfection in the market, are not actually marketed, is a somewhat fine point.

To recall what has already been said in Section I, there are two kinds of risks involved in medical care: the risk of becoming ill, and the risk of total or incomplete or delayed recovery. The loss due to illness is only partially the cost of medical care. It also consists of discomfort and loss of productive time during illness, and, in more serious cases, death or prolonged deprivation of normal function. From the point of view of the welfare economics of uncertainty, both losses are risks against which individuals would like to insure. The nonexistence of suitable insurance policies for either risk implies a loss of welfare.

B. *The Theory of Ideal Insurance*

In this section, the basic principles of an optimal regime for risk-bearing will be presented. For illustration, reference will usually be made to the case of insurance against cost in medical care. The principles are equally applicable to any of the risks. There is no single source to which the reader can be easily referred, though I think the principles are at least reasonably well understood.

As a basis for the analysis, the assumption is made that each individual acts so as to maximize the expected value of a utility function. If we think of utility as attached to income, then the costs of medical care act as a random deduction from this income, and it is the expected value of the utility of income after medical costs that we are concerned with. (Income after medical costs is the ability to spend money on other objects which give satisfaction. We presuppose that illness is not a source of satisfaction in itself; to the extent that it is a source of dissatisfaction, the illness should enter into the utility function as a separate variable.) The expected-utility hypothesis, due originally to Daniel Bernoulli (1738), is plausible and is the most analytically man-

---

[34] A striking illustration of the desire for security in medical care is provided by the expressed preferences of *émigrés* from the Soviet Union as between Soviet medical practice and German or American practice; see Field [14, Ch. 12]. Those in Germany preferred the German system to the Soviet, but those in the United States preferred (in a ratio of 3 to 1) the Soviet system. The reasons given boil down to the certainty of medical care, independent of income or health fluctuations.

ageable of all hypotheses that have been proposed to explain behavior under uncertainty. In any case, the results to follow probably would not be significantly affected by moving to another mode of analysis.

It is further assumed that individuals are normally risk-averters. In utility terms, this means that they have a diminishing marginal utility of income. This assumption may reasonably be taken to hold for most of the significant affairs of life for a majority of people, but the presence of gambling provides some difficulty in the full application of this view. It follows from the assumption of risk aversion that if an individual is given a choice between a probability distribution of income, with a given mean m, and the certainty of the income m, he would prefer the latter. Suppose, therefore, an agency, a large insurance company plan, or the government, stands ready to offer insurance against medical costs on an actuarially fair basis; that is, if the costs of medical care are a random variable with mean m, the company will charge a premium m, and agree to indemnify the individual for all medical costs. Under these circumstances, the individual will certainly prefer to take out a policy and will have a welfare gain thereby.

Will this be a social gain? Obviously yes, if the insurance agent is suffering no social loss. Under the assumption that medical risks on different individuals are basically independent, the pooling of them reduces the risk involved to the insurer to relatively small proportions. In the limit, the welfare loss, even assuming risk aversion on the part of the insurer, would vanish and there is a net social gain which may be of quite substantial magnitude. In fact, of course, the pooling of risks does not go to the limit; there is only a finite number of them and there may be some interdependence among the risks due to epidemics and the like. But then a premium, perhaps slightly above the actuarial level, would be sufficient to offset this welfare loss. From the point of view of the individual, since he has a strict preference for the actuarially fair policy over assuming the risks himself, he will still have a preference for an actuarially unfair policy, provided, of course, that it is not too unfair.

In addition to a residual degree of risk aversion by insurers, there are other reasons for the loading of the premium (i.e., an excess of premium over the actuarial value). Insurance involves administrative costs. Also, because of the irregularity of payments there is likely to be a cost of capital tied up. Suppose, to take a simple case, the insurance company is not willing to sell any insurance policy that a consumer wants but will charge a fixed-percentage loading above the actuarial value for its premium. Then it can be shown that the most preferred policy from the point of view of an individual is a coverage with a deductible amount; that is, the insurance policy provides 100 per cent coverage for all medical costs in excess of some fixed-dollar limit. If, however, the insurance company has some degree of risk aversion, its loading may also depend on the degree of uncertainty of the risk. In that case, the Pareto optimal policy will involve some element of co-insurance, i.e., the coverage for costs over the minimum limit will be some fraction less than 100 per cent (for proofs of these statements, see Appendix).

These results can also be applied to the hypothetical concept of insurance against failure to recover from illness. For simplicity, let us assume that the cost of failure to recover is regarded purely as a money cost, either simply productive opportunities foregone or, more generally, the money equivalent of all dissatisfactions. Suppose further that, given that a person is ill, the expected value of medical care is greater than its cost; that is, the expected money value attributable to recovery with medical help is greater than resources devoted to medical help. However, the recovery, though on the average beneficial, is uncertain; in the absence of insurance a risk-averter may well prefer not to take a chance on further impoverishment by buying medical care. A suitable insurance policy would, however, mean that he paid nothing if he doesn't benefit; since the expected value is greater than the cost, there would be a net social gain.[35]

C. *Problems of Insurance*

1. *The moral hazard*. The welfare case for insurance policies of all sorts is overwhelming. It follows that the government should undertake insurance in those cases where this market, for whatever reason, has failed to emerge. Nevertheless, there are a number of significant practical limitations on the use of insurance. It is important to understand them, though I do not believe that they alter the case for the creation of a much wider class of insurance policies than now exists.

One of the limits which has been much stressed in insurance literature is the effect of insurance on incentives. What is desired in the case of insurance is that the event against which insurance is taken be out of the control of the individual. Unfortunately, in real life this separation can never be made perfectly. The outbreak of fire in one's house or business may be largely uncontrollable by the individual, but the probability of fire is somewhat influenced by carelessness, and of course arson is a possibility, if an extreme one. Similarly, in medical policies the cost of medical care is not completely determined by the illness suffered by the individual but depends on the choice of a doctor and his willingness to use medical services. It is frequently observed that widespread medical insurance increases the demand for medical care. Coinsurance provisions have been introduced into many major medical policies to meet this contingency as well as the risk aversion of the insurance companies.

To some extent the professional relationship between physician and patient limits the normal hazard in various forms of medical insurance. By certifying to the necessity of given treatment or the lack thereof, the physician acts as a controlling agent on behalf of the insurance companies. Needless to say, it is a far from perfect check; the phy-

---

[35] It is a popular belief that the Chinese, at one time, paid their physicians when well but not when sick.

sicians themselves are not under any control and it may be convenient for them or pleasing to their patients to prescribe more expensive medication, private nurses, more frequent treatments, and other marginal variations of care. It is probably true that hospitalization and surgery are more under the casual inspection of others than is general practice and therefore less subject to moral hazard; this may be one reason why insurance policies in those fields have been more widespread.

2. *Alternative methods of insurance payment.* It is interesting that no less than three different methods of coverage of the costs of medical care have arisen: prepayment, indemnities according to a fixed schedule, and insurance against costs, whatever they may be. In prepayment plans, insurance in effect is paid in kind—that is, directly in medical services. The other two forms both involve cash payments to the beneficiary, but in the one case the amounts to be paid involving a medical contingency are fixed in advance, while in the other the insurance carrier pays all the costs, whatever they may be, subject, of course, to provisions like deductibles and coinsurance.

In hypothetically perfect markets these three forms of insurance would be equivalent. The indemnities stipulated would, in fact, equal the market price of the services, so that value to the insured would be the same if he were to be paid the fixed sum or the market price or were given the services free. In fact, of course, insurance against full costs and prepayment plans both offer insurance against uncertainty as to the price of medical services, in addition to uncertainty about their needs. Further, by their mode of compensation to the physician, prepayment plans are inevitably bound up with closed panels so that the freedom of choice of the physician by the patient is less than it would be under a scheme more strictly confined to the provision of insurance. These remarks are tentative, and the question of coexistence of the different schemes should be a fruitful subject for investigation.

3. *Third-party control over payments.* The moral hazard in physicians' control noted in paragraph 1 above shows itself in those insurance schemes where the physician has the greatest control, namely, major medical insurance. Here there has been a marked rise in expenditures over time. In prepayment plans, where the insurance and medical service are supplied by the same group, the incentive to keep medical costs to a minimum is strongest. In plans of the Blue Cross group, there has developed a conflict of interest between the insurance carrier and the medical-service supplier, in this case particularly the hospital.

The need for third-party control is reinforced by another aspect of the moral hazard. Insurance removes the incentive on the part of individuals, patients, and physicians to shop around for better prices for hospitalization and surgical care. The market forces, therefore, tend to be replaced by direct institutional control.

4. *Administrative costs.* The pure theory of insurance sketched in Section B above omits one very important consideration: the costs of operating an insurance company. There are several types of operating

costs, but one of the most important categories includes commissions and acquisition costs, selling costs in usual economic terminology. Not only does this mean that insurance policies must be sold for considerably more than their actuarial value, but it also means there is a great differential among different types of insurance. It is very striking to observe that among health insurance policies of insurance companies in 1958, expenses of one sort or another constitute 51.6 per cent of total premium income for individual policies, and only 9.5 per cent for group policies [26, Table 14-1, p. 272]. This striking differential would seem to imply enormous economies of scale in the provision of insurance, quite apart from the coverage of the risks themselves. Obviously, this provides a very strong argument for widespread plans, including, in particular, compulsory ones.

5. *Predictability and insurance.* Clearly, from the risk-aversion point of view, insurance is more valuable, the greater the uncertainty in the risk being insured against. This is usually used as an argument for putting greater emphasis on insurance against hospitalization and surgery than other forms of medical care. The empirical assumption has been challenged by O. W. Anderson and others [3, pp. 53-54], who asserted that out-of-hospital expenses were equally as unpredictable as in-hospital costs. What was in fact shown was that the probability of costs exceeding $200 is about the same for the two categories, but this is not, of course, a correct measure of predictability, and a quick glance at the supporting evidence shows that in relation to the average cost the variability is much lower for ordinary medical expenses. Thus, for the city of Birmingham, the mean expenditure on surgery was $7, as opposed to $20 for other medical expenses, but of those who paid something for surgery the average bill was $99, as against $36 for those with some ordinary medical cost. Eighty-two per cent of those interviewed had no surgery, and only 20 per cent had no ordinary medical expenses [3, Tables A-13, A-18, and A-19 on pp. 72, 77, and 79, respectively].

The issue of predictability also has bearing on the merits of insurance against chronic illness or maternity. On a lifetime insurance basis, insurance against chronic illness makes sense, since this is both highly unpredictable and highly significant in costs. Among people who already have chronic illness, or symptoms which reliably indicate it, insurance in the strict sense is probably pointless.

6. *Pooling of unequal risks.* Hypothetically, insurance requires for its full social benefit a maximum possible discrimination of risks. Those in groups of higher incidences of illness should pay higher premiums. In fact, however, there is a tendency to equalize, rather than to differentiate, premiums, especially in the Blue Cross and similar widespread schemes. This constitutes, in effect, a redistribution of income from those with a low propensity to illness to those with a high propensity. The equalization, of course, could not in fact be carried through if the market were genuinely competitive. Under those circumsances, insurance plans could arise which charged lower premiums to preferred

risks and draw them off, leaving the plan which does not discriminate among risks with only an adverse selection of them.

As we have already seen in the case of income redistribution, some of this may be thought of as insurance with a longer time perspective. If a plan guarantees to everybody a premium that corresponds to total experience but not to experience as it might be segregated by smaller subgroups, everybody is, in effect, insured against a change in his basic state of health which would lead to a reclassification. This corresponds precisely to the use of a level premium in life insurance instead of a premium varying by age, as would be the case for term insurance.

7. *Gaps and coverage.* We may briefly note that, at any rate to date, insurances against the cost of medical care are far from universal. Certain groups—the unemployed, the institutionalized, and the aged—are almost completely uncovered. Of total expenditures, between one-fifth and one-fourth are covered by insurance. It should be noted, however, that over half of all hospital expenses and about 35 per cent of the medical payments of those with bills of $1,000 a year and over, are included [26, p. 376]. Thus, the coverage on the more variable parts of medical expenditure is somewhat better than the over-all figures would indicate, but it must be assumed that the insurance mechanism is still very far from achieving the full coverage of which it is capable.

D. *Uncertainty of Effects of Treatment*

1. There are really two major aspects of uncertainty for an individual already suffering from an illness. He is uncertain about the effectiveness of medical treatment, and his uncertainty may be quite different from that of his physician, based on the presumably quite different medical knowledges.

2. *Ideal insurance.* This will necessarily involve insurance against a failure to benefit from medical care, whether through recovery, relief of pain, or arrest of further deterioration. One form would be a system in which the payment to the physician is made in accordance with the degree of benefit. Since this would involve transferring the risks from the patient to the physician, who might certainly have an aversion to bearing them, there is room for insurance carriers to pool the risks, either by contract with physicians or by contract with the potential patients. Under ideal insurance, medical care will always be undertaken in any case in which the expected utility, taking account of the probabilities, exceeds the expected medical cost. This prescription would lead to an economic optimum. If we think of the failure to recover mainly in terms of lost working time, then this policy would, in fact, maximize economic welfare as ordinarily measured.

3. *The concepts of trust and delegation.* In the absence of ideal insurance, there arise institutions which offer some sort of substitute guarantees. Under ideal insurance the patient would actually have no concern with the informational inequality between himself and the physician, since he would only be paying by results anyway, and his utility position would in fact be thoroughly guaranteed. In its absence

he wants to have some guarantee that at least the physician is using his knowledge to the best advantage. This leads to the setting up of a relationship of trust and confidence, one which the physician has a social obligation to live up to. Since the patient does not, at least in his belief, know as much as the physician, he cannot completely enforce standards of care. In part, he replaces direct observation by generalized belief in the ability of the physician.[36] To put it another way, the social obligation for best practice is part of the commodity the physician sells, even though it is a part that is not subject to thorough inspection by the buyer.

One consequence of such trust relations is that the physician cannot act, or at least appear to act, as if he is maximizing his income at every moment of time. As a signal to the buyer of his intentions to act as thoroughly in the buyer's behalf as possible, the physician avoids the obvious stigmata of profit-maximizing. Purely arms-length bargaining behavior would be incompatible, not logically, but surely psychologically, with the trust relations. From these special relations come the various forms of ethical behavior discussed above, and so also, I suggest, the relative unimportance of profit-making in hospitals. The very word, "profit," is a signal that denies the trust relations.

Price discrimination and its extreme, free treatment for the indigent, also follow. If the obligation of the physician is understood to be first of all to the welfare of the patient, then in particular it takes precedence over financial difficulties.

As a second consequence of informational inequality between physician and patient and the lack of insurance of a suitable type, the patient must delegate to the physician much of his freedom of choice. He does not have the knowledge to make decisions on treatment, referral, or hospitalization. To justify this delegation, the physician finds himself somewhat limited, just as any agent would in similar circumstances. The safest course to take to avoid not being a true agent is to give the socially prescribed "best" treatment of the day. Compromise in quality, even for the purpose of saving the patient money, is to risk an imputation of failure to live up to the social bond.

The special trust relation of physicians (and allied occuptions, such as priests) extends to third parties so that the certifications of physicians as to illness and injury are accepted as especially reliable (see Section II.B above). The social value to all concerned of such presumptively reliable sources of information is obvious.

Notice the general principle here. Because there are barriers to the information flow and because there is no market in which the risks involved can be insured, coordination of purchase and sales must take place through convergent expectations, but these are greatly assisted by having clear and prominent signals, and these, in turn, force pat-

---

[36] Francis Bator points out to me that some protection can be achieved, at a price, by securing additional opinions.

terns of behavior which are not in themselves logical necessities for optimality.[37]

4. *Licensing and educational standards*. Delegation and trust are the social institutions designed to obviate the problem of informational inequality. The general uncertainty about the prospects of medical treatment is socially handled by rigid entry requirements. These are designed to reduce the uncertainty in the mind of the consumer as to the quality of product insofar as this is possible.[38] I think this explanation, which is perhaps the naive one, is much more tenable than any idea of a monopoly seeking to increase incomes. No doubt restriction on entry is desirable from the point of view of the existing physicians, but the public pressure needed to achieve the restriction must come from deeper causes.

The social demand for guaranteed quality can be met in more than one way, however. At least three attitudes can be taken by the state or other social institutions toward entry into an occupation or toward the production of commodities in general; examples of all three types exist. (1) The occupation can be licensed, nonqualified entrants being simply excluded. The licensing may be more complex than it is in medicine; individuals could be licensed for some, but not all, medical activities, for example. Indeed, the present all-or-none approach could be criticized as being insufficient with regard to complicated specialist treatment, as well as excessive with regard to minor medical skills. Graded licensing may, however, be much harder to enforce. Controls could be exercised analogous to those for foods; they can be excluded as being dangerous, or they can be permitted for animals but not for humans. (2) The state or other agency can certify or label, without compulsory exclusion. The category of Certified Psychologist is now under active discussion; canned goods are graded. Certification can be done by nongovernmental agencies, as in the medical-board examinations for specialists. (3) Nothing at all may be done; consumers make their own choices.

The choice among these alternatives in any given case depends on the degree of difficulty consumers have in making the choice unaided, and on the consequences of errors of judgment. It is the general social consensus, clearly, that the *laissez-faire* solution for medicine is intolerable. The certification proposal never seems to have been discussed seriously. It is beyond the scope of this paper to discuss these proposals in detail. I wish simply to point out that they should be judged in terms of the ability to relieve the uncertainty of the patient in regard to the quality of the commodity he is purchasing, and that entry restrictions are the consequences of an apparent inability to devise a system in which the

---

[37] The situation is very reminiscent of the crucial role of the focal point in Schelling's theory of tacit games, in which two parties have to find a common course of action without being able to communicate; see [24, esp. pp. 225 ff.].

[38] How well they achieve this end is another matter. R. Kessel points out to me that they merely guarantee training, not continued good performance as medical technology changes.

risks of gaps in medical knowledge and skill are borne primarily by the patient, not the physician.

Postscript

I wish to repeat here what has been suggested above in several places: that the failure of the market to insure against uncertainties has created many social institutions in which the usual assumptions of the market are to some extent contradicted. The medical profession is only one example, though in many respects an extreme one. All professions share some of the same properties. The economic importance of personal and especially family relationships, though declining, is by no means trivial in the most advanced economies; it is based on non-market relations that create guarantees of behavior which would otherwise be afflicted with excessive uncertainty. Many other examples can be given. The logic and limitations of ideal competitive behavior under uncertainty force us to recognize the incomplete description of reality supplied by the impersonal price system.

REFERENCES

1. A. A. ALCHIAN, K. J. ARROW, AND W. M. CAPRON, *An Economic Analysis of the Market for Scientists and Engineers*, RAND RM-2190-RC. Santa Monica 1958.
2. M. ALLAIS, "Généralisation des théories de l'équilibre économique général et du rendement social au cas du risque," in Centre National de la Recherche Scientifique, *Econometrie*, Paris 1953, pp. 1-20.
3. O. W. ANDERSON AND STAFF OF THE NATIONAL OPINION RESEARCH CENTER, *Voluntary Health Insurance in Two Cities.* Cambridge, Mass. 1957.
4. K. J. ARROW, "Economic Welfare and the Allocation of Resources for Invention," in Nat. Bur. Econ. Research, *The Role and Direction of Inventive Activity: Economic and Social Factors*, Princeton 1962, pp. 609-25.
5. ———, "Les rôle des valeurs boursières pour la répartition la meilleure des risques," in Centre National de la Recherche Scientifique, *Econometrie*, Paris 1953, pp. 41-46.
6. F. M. BATOR, "The Anatomy of Market Failure," *Quart. Jour. Econ.* Aug. 1958, *72*, 351-79.
7. E. BAUDIER, "L'introduction du temps dans la théorie de l'équilibre général," *Les Cahiers Economiques*, Dec. 1959, 9-16.
8. W. J. BAUMOL, *Welfare Economics and the Theory of the State.* Cambridge, Mass. 1952.
9. K. BORCH, "The Safety Loading of Reinsurance Premiums," *Skandinavisk Aktuariehdskrift*, 1960, pp. 163-84.
10. J. M. BUCHANAN AND G. TULLOCK, *The Calculus of Consent.* Ann Arbor 1962.
11. G. DEBREU, "Une économique de l'incertain," *Economie Appliquée*, 1960, *13*, 111-16.
12. ———, *Theory of Values.* New York 1959.
13. R. DUBOS, "Medical Utopias," *Daedalus*, 1959, *88*, 410-24.

14. M. G. FIELD, *Doctor and Patient in Soviet Russia.* Cambridge, Mass. 1957.
15. MILTON FRIEDMAN, "The Methodology of Positive Economics," in *Essays in Positive Economics,* Chicago 1953, pp. 3-43.
16. —— AND S. S. KUZNETS, *Income from Independent Professional Practice.* Nat. Bur. Econ. Research, New York 1945.
17. R. A. KESSEL, "Price Discrimination in Medicine," *Jour. Law and Econ.,* 1958, *1,* 20-53.
18. T. C. KOOPMANS, "Allocation of Resources and the Price System," in *Three Essays on the State of Economic Science,* New York 1957, pp. 1-120.
19. I. M. D. LITTLE, *A Critique of Welfare Economics.* Oxford 1950.
20. SELMA MUSHKIN, "Towards a Definition of Health Economics," *Public Health Reports,* 1958, *73,* 785-93.
21. R. R. NELSON, "The Simple Economics of Basic Scientific Research," *Jour. Pol. Econ.,* June 1959, *67,* 297-306.
22. T. PARSONS, *The Social System.* Glencoe 1951.
23. M. J. PECK AND F. M. SCHERER, *The Weapons Acquisition Process: An Economic Analysis.* Div. of Research, Graduate School of Business, Harvard University, Boston 1962.
24. T. C. SCHELLING, *The Strategy of Conflict.* Cambridge, Mass. 1960.
25. A. K. SHAPIRO, "A Contribution to a History of the Placebo Effect," *Behavioral Science,* 1960, *5,* 109-35.
26. H. M. SOMERS AND A. R. SOMERS, *Doctors, Patients, and Health Insurance.* The Brookings Institution, Washington 1961.
27. C. L. STEVENSON, *Ethics and Language.* New Haven 1945.
28. U. S. DEPARTMENT OF HEALTH, EDUCATION AND WELFARE, *Physicians for a Growing America,* Public Health Service Publication No. 709, Oct. 1959.

APPENDIX

On Optimal Insurance Policies

The two propositions about the nature of optimal insurance policies asserted in Section IV.B above will be proved here.

Proposition 1. If an insurance company is willing to offer any insurance policy against loss desired by the buyer at a premium which depends only on the policy's actuarial value, then the policy chosen by a risk-averting buyer will take the form of 100 per cent coverage above a deductible minimum.

Note: The premium will, in general, exceed the actuarial value; it is only required that two policies with the same actuarial value will be offered by the company for the same premium.

Proof: Let W be the initial wealth of the individual, X his loss, a random variable, $I(X)$ the amount of insurance paid if loss X occurs, P the premium, and $Y(X)$ the wealth of the individual after paying the premium, incurring the loss, and receiving the insurance benefit.

$$(1) \qquad Y(X) = W - P - X + I(X).$$

The individual values alternative policies by the expected utility of his final wealth position, $Y(X)$. Let $U(y)$ be the utility of final wealth, y; then his aim is to maximize,

(2) $$E\{U[Y(X)]\},$$

where the symbol, E, denotes mathematical expectation.

An insurance payment is necessarily nonnegative, so the insurance policy must satisfy the condition,

(3) $$I(X) \geq 0 \quad \text{for all} \quad X.$$

If a policy is optimal, it must in particular be better in the sense of the criterion (2), than any other policy with the same actuarial expectation, $E[I(X)]$. Consider a policy that pays some positive amount of insurance at one level of loss, say X_1, but which permits the final wealth at some other loss level, say X_2, to be lower than that corresponding to X_1. Then, it is intuitively obvious that a risk-averter would prefer an alternative policy with the same actuarial value which would offer slightly less protection for losses in the neighborhood of X_1 and slightly higher protection for those in the neighborhood of X_2, since risk aversion implies that the marginal utility of $Y(X)$ is greater when $Y(X)$ is smaller: hence, the original policy cannot be optimal.

To prove this formally, let $I_1(X)$ be the original policy, with $I_1(X) > 0$ and $Y_1(X_1) > Y_2(X_2)$, where $Y_1(X)$ is defined in terms of $I_1(X)$ by (I). Choose δ sufficiently small so that,

(4) $I_1(X) > 0 \quad \text{for} \quad X_1 \leq X \leq X_1 + \delta,$

(5) $Y_1(X') < Y_1(X) \quad \text{for} \quad X_2 \leq X' \leq X_2 + \delta, \quad X_1 \leq X \leq X_1 + \delta.$

(This choice of δ is possible if the functions $I_1(X)$, $Y_1(X)$ are continuous; this can be proved to be true for the optimal policy, and therefore we need only consider this case.)

Let π_1 be the probability that the loss, X, lies in the interval $\langle X_1, X_1 + \delta \rangle$, π_2 the probability that X lies in the interval $\langle X_2, X_2 + \delta \rangle$. From (4) and (5) we can choose $\epsilon > 0$ and sufficiently small so that,

(6) $I_1(X) - \pi_2\epsilon \geq 0 \quad \text{for} \quad X_1 \leq X \leq X_1 + \delta,$

(7) $Y_1(X') + \pi_1\epsilon < Y_1(X) - \pi_2\epsilon$

$$\text{for} \quad X_2 \leq X' \leq X_2 + \delta, \quad X_1 \leq X \leq X_1 + \delta.$$

Now define a new insurance policy, $I_2(X)$, which is the same as $I_1(X)$ except that it is smaller by $\pi_2\epsilon$ in the interval from X_1 to $X_1 + \delta$ and larger by $\pi_1\epsilon$ in the interval from X_2 to $X_2 + \delta$. From (6), $I_2(X) \geq 0$ everywhere, so that (3) is satisfied. We will show that $E[I_1(X)] = E[I_2(X)]$ and that $I_2(X)$ yields the higher expected utility, so that $I_1(X)$ is not optimal.

Note that $I_2(X) - I_1(X)$ equals $-\pi_2\epsilon$ for $X_1 \leq X \leq X_1 + \delta$, $\pi_1\epsilon$ for $X_2 \leq X \leq X_2 + \delta$, and 0 elsewhere. Let $\phi(X)$ be the density of the random variable X. Then,

$$E[I_2(X) - I_1(X)] = \int_{X_1}^{X_1+\delta} [I_2(X) - I_1(X)]\phi(X)dX$$

$$+ \int_{X_2}^{X_2+\delta} [I_2(X) - I_1(X)]dX$$

$$= (-\pi_2\epsilon) \int_{X_1}^{X_1+\delta} \phi(X)dX + (\pi_1\epsilon) \int_{X_2}^{X_2+\delta} \phi(X)dX$$

$$= -(\pi_2\epsilon)\pi_1 + (\pi_1\epsilon)\pi_2 = 0,$$

so that the two policies have the same actuarial value and, by assumption, the same premium.

Define $Y_2(X)$ in terms of $I_2(X)$ by (1). Then $Y_2(X) - Y_1(X) = I_2(X) - I_1(X)$. From (7),

(8) $Y_1(X') < Y_2(X') < Y_2(X) < Y_1(X)$

$$\text{for} \quad X_2 \leq X' \leq X_2 + \delta, \quad X_1 \leq X \leq X_1 + \delta.$$

Since $Y_1(X) - Y_2(X) = 0$ outside the intervals $\langle X_1, X_1 + \delta \rangle$, $\langle X_2, X_2 + \delta \rangle$, we can write,

(9) $\displaystyle E\{U[Y_2(X)] - U[Y_1(X)]\} = \int_{X_1}^{X_1+\delta} \{U[Y_2(X)] - U[Y_1(X)]\}\phi(X)dX$

$$+ \int_{X_2}^{X_2+\delta} \{U[Y_2(X)] - U[Y_1(X)]\}\phi(X)dX.$$

By the Mean Value Theorem, for any given value of X,

(10) $U[Y_2(X)] - U[Y_1(X)] = U'[Y(X)][Y_2(X) - Y_1(X)]$

$$= U'[Y(X)][I_2(X) - I_1(X)],$$

where $Y(X)$ lies between $Y_1(X)$ and $Y_2(X)$. From (8),

$$Y(X') < Y(X) \quad \text{for} \quad X_2 \leq X' \leq X_2 + \delta, \quad X_1 \leq X \leq X_1 + \delta,$$

and, since $U'(y)$ is a diminishing function of y for a risk-averter,

$$U'[Y(X')] > U'[Y(X)]$$

or, equivalently, for some number u,

(11)
$$U'[Y(X')] > u \quad \text{for} \quad X_2 \leq X' \leq X_2 + \delta,$$
$$U'[Y(X)] < u \quad \text{for} \quad X_1 \leq X \leq X_1 + \delta.$$

Now substitute (10) into (9),

$$E\{U[Y_2(X)] - U[Y_1(X)]\} = -\pi_2\epsilon \int_{X_1}^{X_1+\delta} U'[Y(X)]\phi(X)dX$$

$$+ \pi_1\epsilon \int_{X_2}^{X_2+\delta} U'[Y(X)]\phi(X)dX.$$

From (11), it follows that,

$$E\{U[Y_2(X)] - U[Y_1(X)]\} > -\pi_2\epsilon u\pi_1 + \pi_1\epsilon u\pi_2 = 0,$$

so that the second policy is preferred.

It has thus been shown that a policy cannot be optimal if, for some X_1 and X_2, $I(X_1) > 0$, $Y(X_1) > Y(X_2)$. This may be put in a different form: Let Y_{min} be the minimum value taken on by $Y(X)$ under the optimal policy; then we must have $I(X) = 0$ if $Y(X) > Y_{min}$. In other words, a minimum final wealth level is set; if the loss would not bring wealth below this level, no benefit is paid, but if it would, then the benefit is sufficient to bring up the final wealth position to the stipulated minimum. This is, of course, precisely a description of 100 per cent coverage for loss above a deductible.

We turn to the second proposition. It is now supposed that the insurance company, as well as the insured, is a risk-averter; however, there are no administrative or other costs to be covered beyond protection against loss.

Proposition 2. If the insured and the insurer are both risk-averters and there are no costs other than coverage of losses, then any nontrivial Pareto-optimal policy, $I(X)$, as a function of the loss, X, must have the property, $0 < dI/dX < 1$.

That is, any increment in loss will be partly but not wholly compensated by the insurance company; this type of provision is known as coinsurance. Proposition 2 is due to Borch [9, Sec. 2]; we give here a somewhat simpler proof.

Proof: Let $U(y)$ be the utility function of the insured, $V(z)$ that of the insurer. Let W_0 and W_1 be the initial wealths of the two, respectively. In this case, we let $I(X)$ be the insurance benefits less the premium; for the present purpose, this is the only significant magnitude (since the premium is independent of X, this definition does not change the value of dI/dX). The final wealth positions of the insured and insurer are:

$$
\begin{aligned}
Y(X) &= W_0 - X + I(X), \\
Z(X) &= W_1 - I(X),
\end{aligned}
\tag{12}
$$

respectively. Any given insurance policy then defines expected utilities, $u = E\{U[Y(X)]\}$ and $v = E\{V[Z(X)]\}$, for the insured and insurer, respectively. If we plot all points (u, v) obtained by considering all possible insurance policies, the resulting expected-utility-possibility set has a boundary that is convex to the northeast. To see this, let $I_1(X)$ and $I_2(X)$ be any two policies, and let (u_1, v_1) and (u_2, v_2) be the corresponding points in the two-dimensional expected-utility-possibility set. Let a third insurance policy, $I(X)$, be defined as the average of the two given ones,

$$ I(X) = (\tfrac{1}{2})I_1(X) + (\tfrac{1}{2})I_2(X), $$

for each X. Then, if $Y(X)$, $Y_1(X)$, and $Y_2(X)$ are the final wealth positions of the insured, and $Z(X)$, $Z_1(X)$, and $Z_2(X)$ those of the insurer for each of the three policies, $I(X)$, $I_1(X)$, and $I_2(X)$, respectively,

$$
\begin{aligned}
Y(X) &= (\tfrac{1}{2})Y_1(X) + (\tfrac{1}{2})Y_2(X), \\
Z(X) &= (\tfrac{1}{2})Z_1(X) + (\tfrac{1}{2})Z_2(X),
\end{aligned}
$$

and, because both parties have diminishing marginal utility,

$$
\begin{aligned}
U[Y(X)] &\geq (\tfrac{1}{2})U[Y_1(X)] + (\tfrac{1}{2})U[Y_2(X)], \\
V[Z(X)] &\geq (\tfrac{1}{2})V[Z_1(X)] + (\tfrac{1}{2})V[Z_2(X)].
\end{aligned}
$$

Since these statements hold for all X, they also hold when expectations are taken. Hence, there is a point (u, v) in the expected-utility-possibility set for which $u \geq (\tfrac{1}{2})u_1 + (\tfrac{1}{2})u_2$, $v \geq (\tfrac{1}{2})v_1 + (\tfrac{1}{2})v_2$. Since this statement holds for every pair of points (u_1, y_1) and (u_2, v_2) in the expected-utility-possibility set, and in particular for pairs of points on the northeast boundary, it follows that the boundary must be convex to the northeast.

From this, in turn, it follows that any given Pareto-optimal point (i.e., any point on the northeast boundary) can be obtained by maximizing a linear function, $\alpha u + \beta v$, with suitably chosen α and β nonnegative and at least one positive, over the expected-utility-possibility set. In other words, a Pareto-optimal insurance policy, $I(X)$, is one which maximizes,

$$ \alpha E\{U[Y(X)]\} + \beta E\{V[Z(X)]\} = E\{\alpha U[Y(X)] + \beta V[Z(X)]\}, $$

for some $\alpha \geq 0$, $\beta \geq 0$, $\alpha > 0$ or $\beta > 0$. To maximize this expectation, it is obviously sufficient to maximize:

$$ \alpha U[Y(X)] + \beta V[Z(X)], \tag{13} $$

with respect to $I(X)$, for each X. Since, for given X, it follows from (12) that,

$$dY(X)/dI(X) = 1, \qquad dZ(X)/dI(X) = -1,$$

it follows by differentiation of (13) that $I(X)$ is the solution of the equation,

(14) $\qquad\qquad \alpha U'[Y(X)] - \beta V'[Z(X)] = 0.$

The cases $\alpha = 0$ or $\beta = 0$ lead to obvious trivialities (one party simply hands over all his wealth to the other), so we assume $\alpha > 0, \beta > 0$. Now differentiate (14) with respect to X and use the relations, derived from (12),

$$dY/dX = (dI/dX) - 1, \qquad dZ/dX = -(dI/dX).$$

$$\alpha U''[Y(X)][(dI/dX) - 1] + \beta V''[Z(X)](dI/dX) = 0,$$

or

$$dI/dX = \alpha U''[Y(X)]/\{\alpha U''[Y(X)] + \beta V''[Z(X)]\}.$$

Since $U''[Y(X)] < 0$, $V''[Z(X)] < 0$ by the hypothesis that both parties are risk-averters, Proposition 2 follows.

3. Value for Money in Health Services

BRIAN ABEL-SMITH

Reprinted with permission from *Social Security Bulletin* 37, Social Security Administration, 1974, 17-28.

There are now so many innovative experiments, so many varying solutions to the problem of rising costs, and so many different plans for health insurance that it is not easy to discuss in some 50 minutes—in a country not your own—a question of such bewildering complexity as how to get value for money in health services. What is quality? Whose money? What ultimately are health services?

I can only discuss the subject by greatly simplifying the issues. Moreover, there is one great simplification I must make. I must ignore your political realities, simply because I am in no position to judge what they are or will be.

ATTITUDES TOWARD PROVISION OF HEALTH SERVICES

Some 20 years ago, on an early visit to Washington, it seemed to me that compulsory health insurance was not on the map, Government planning of hospitals seemed little more than a dream, and Government price controls unthinkable. It was before your language or at least your alphabet had been embellished by such concepts as PPBS or PSRO or HMO. Health insurance was voluntary in the curious sense in which the term is used over here, though vast numbers of individuals were forced to buy it or have it bought for them as a consequence of the jobs they had taken. Health insurance was and still often is heavily restricted by co-payment, coinsurance, and deductibles—by what we in England simply call charges.

There is now more of a demand that people should have health insurance though not necessarily health care as a right—a distinction to which I attach great importance. There is somewhat less concern about what I used to see curiously described as the moral hazard of the insured. (Is it immoral to want more health services?) How many of us are such chronic hypochondriacs that we are likely to camp out on our physician's doorstep, take our vacations in hospitals, or beg for prescriptions we can fill? Or are we worried that people may make hats out of gauze and suture? Is this immorality or a special form of sickness?

Now more attention is paid to the incentives and moral hazards facing the unregulated provider. It is increasingly accepted that it is the physician who authorizes the use of most of a nation's resources. While it is the patient who presents himself to the physician, it is the physician who terminates the interview, suggests a further consultation, writes the prescription, orders the diagnostic tests, arranges the hospital admission, recommends the surgery, and authorizes the hospital discharge. In an unregulated system there is a moral conflict for the physician between what is best for him and what is best for his patient.

There is less faith now in the combination of consumer demand and competitive free enterprise as mechanisms for controlling cost and promoting quality. Perhaps it is Medicare that brought home to the more straightlaced economists that the market for health services is no ordinary market. Does the consumer make a free choice between purchasing medical care or purchasing a new automobile when he is told the serious consequences of not having surgery or lies unconscious at the emergency-room door? As Professor Berki put it, "Medical care is not a good: it is a least bad."[1]

Increasingly it is accepted that, while the ordinary consumer can judge standards of amenity and levels of care, he can seldom judge the quality of medical intervention either before or after he has received it. Few of us challenge the recommendations made by our physician when they are made, though over here they are not infrequently challenged afterwards in the courts. We place ourselves in his hands to provide us with what he thinks we need and to make purchases for us in the health market. All over the world, the physician is not only a provider but a purchasing agent or rationer of resources on a vast scale, whether he recognizes this role or not.

Is the physician trained and motivated to get value for money in the use of the resources he authorizes for his patients? If not, does the market for health services have other forces working within it and do they lead to higher quality or to lower quality, to waste or economy? Do the invisible forces of the market ensure that what the consumer hopes to get is available where he wants to get it? When market forces fail to promote economy, quality, and equitable distribution, how have the governments of other countries—particularly European countries—intervened to regulate the health market to correct this situation and with what effect?

NATURE OF FREE HEALTH MARKET

There are five fundamental propositions about a free health market that I believe to be true. I acknowledge that not all of them can be supported by scientifically valid proof. Indeed, all sorts of hangups stop us from introducing the carefully designed experiments that could give us this proof.

My first proposition is far from original, nor is it accepted by all observers: Within limits the supply of hospital beds generates the demand for them. Milton Roemer is credited with formulating this proposition,[2] but in more and more countries it has come independently to be accepted. When the money barrier is removed, the need for hospital beds is not the same as the demand for hospital beds. It is, of course, very difficult to establish the need for hospital beds, and I will return to this subject later.

My second proposition is that unregulated competition in a free health care market can lead to a loss of quality in a number of different respects: it can lead to unnecessary surgery; it can lead to excessive prescribing of effective drugs, of ineffective drugs, and of dangerous drugs; it can lead to suboptimal skill and performance. An excess of specialists means a lower average experience in specialist work. A part-time heart surgeon who only occasionally uses this particular skill will function less well than a heart surgeon who regularly uses this skill. The operating team that is only occasionally called together will function less well than the team that works together regularly. The more cases a specialist sees in his specialty the more skill he will acquire in distinguishing them and treating them accordingly.

My third proposition is that the free forces of the market under an unregulated fee-for-service payment system do not secure an even geographical distribution of physicians. Again within limits, physicians can enter communities already generously supplied with physicians and make a living—particularly if they come with specialist qualifications. Doctors can make work for themselves when they are plentiful. Economic forces alone are not sufficient to attract doctors to work in areas where they are not otherwise inclined to want to work.

Fourth, the physician is trained to buy the best rather than find the best buy. After training he is exposed to conflicts between his conscience and his pocket and conflicts between the interests of his paymaster and those of competing commercial interests. His doormat is piled high with drug firm literature, and his doorstep is shaded by drug house detail men. Over his shoulder looms the risk of malpractice litigation. His hospital, rather than any other, is his preferred workshop. Nearly all his decisions are of financial consequence to him as well as to his patient or the third party paying the patient's bill.

My fifth proposition is that where the physician is not cost-conscious and the patient acts on his advice there is no pressure on those from whom he purchases to be cost-conscious either. The drug market is carved up by patients and branding: competition is by product and not by price. Unless they are regulated, nonprofit hospitals enjoy what almost amounts to the arbitrary taxing powers of medieval princes. They use these powers to finance the twentieth-century palaces that dominate both cities and suburbs—palaces with almost the same proportion of underoccupied bedrooms and a much higher proportion of underoccupied powder rooms.

HEALTH CARE EXPENDITURES AND GROSS NATIONAL PRODUCT

National income accounting was not employed by medieval monarchs so we do not know what proportion of GNP was used in constructing and running their palaces. We do know what countries are spending on their health services though each country defines them in a slightly different way.

Some years ago I analyzed international trends in health expenditure in the 1950's and concluded that most developed countries seemed to be transferring an additional 1-2 percent of GNP to health services in a 10-year period.[3] This trend has continued in the sixties as Joseph Simanis[4] and others have shown. By the end of the sixties the United States, Canada, and Sweden were all spending 7 percent or more of their resources on health services. If present trends continue, several countries will be spending a tenth of their resources on health services before the end of this century. Nor is this only in prospect for Sweden or North America. Projections for Australia indicate that medical expenditures will reach 12 percent of GNP in 25 years' time.[5] Projections for France show medical expenditure as 11-13 percent of GNP by 1985.[6]

EFFECTIVENESS OF HEALTH CARE EXPENDITURES

What are we likely to get for all this money? What indeed are we getting for what is being spent now? Is this money spent to provide maximum health care out of the health dollar? Here we have to admit the ambivalence of our societies. We worship speedy transport at the price of vast carnage and maiming on our roads. We tolerate poverty and slums and all the health risks that they generate. We tolerate industries that pollute land, sea, and air and maim or disease their workers. We encourage sedentary work, stress, and striving as if they were proved to be the inevitable price of economic progress. We put little emphasis on safety in the construction of our automobiles or the design of our industrial processes. We do little to promote or facilitate vigorous exercise to control our coronaries. We are reluctant to redistribute income or ensure adequate standards of housing. We do not ban cigarette smoking to protect our hearts and lungs. We do not provide free prophylactics to protect the promiscuous from venereal disease. We look to the health services to cure us whatever we do to ourselves.

While much more could be done at little cost to prevent ill health in ways known to be effective, much is done in the cause of curing ill health that is of questionable effectiveness, known to be ineffective, or known to be unnecessary and dangerous. For some time, many countries have been trying to remove from the market that vast range of pharmaceutical products which are known to be ineffective or for which manufacturers' claims of effectiveness are not substantiated. In addition, many effective drugs are overused. I am not just referring here to the staggering use of sleeping pills, tranquilizers, and antidepressants but to such classic problems as the overuse of chloromycetin. I am referring also to excessive surgery — and all surgery has risks attached to it. It is a matter of concern when without good cause so many people lose their appendixes, their wombs, or their tonsils.

Many expensive innovations in medical care come to be generally used before there is robust evidence that they really work. And once they are in general use it is regarded as unethical to evaluate them. It is, moreover, risky for the physician in terms of possible litigation. In making such bold statements about medicine, I am relying on the evidence accumulated by Dr. Archie Cochrane, President of our Faculty of Community Medicine.[7] His book should be compulsory reading for all those sociologists, economists, operations researchers, systems analysts, and futurologists who are now applying their skills to the health industry. Too often it is assumed that hospitals and physicians have not only uniform outputs but outputs of the same quality and outputs that are wholly beneficial. Such assumptions open the door to sophisticated yet irrelevant regression analysis but not to enlightenment or wise policy formation.

Dr. Cochrane quotes the results of a random-controlled trial in Bristol which "do not suggest that there is any medical gain in admission to hospital compared with treatment at home," for ischemic heart disease. He also quotes trials showing that insulin treatment is no better than diet alone in treating mature diabetics, that iron does not cure the classical symptoms of anemia at certain hemoglobin levels, and that ergotamine tartrate does not help newly diagnosed cases of migraine. As no random controlled trials have ever been carried out to evaluate them, he casts doubt on the value of surgery for carcinoma of the lung, cytological screening tests for the prevention of cervical carcinoma, and dietetic therapy for phenylketonuria.

Technical Innovations and Developments

Ultimately, we are concerned with health rather than health insurance. Problems of quality are not solved by removing the money barrier and pumping in resources to ensure that what the individual physician demands is supplied. Nor indeed are the problems of distributions solved. Ultimately, society must be concerned about the quality of medical practice, and this is not just a question of the money incentives on the doctor or even of commercial interests attempting to distort the physician's judgment. We know that the physician can quickly become out of date after he has left medical school. What is even more challenging is that leading physicians can come to accept as advances expensive technical innovations which no individual physican can evaluate from day-to-day practice.

What mechanisms do we need to prevent whole societies from spending vast sums of money on innovations of unproved value? How can we reconcile the need for such mechanisms with such cherished notions as clinical freedom and the free practice of medicine?

At the very least, we need to ensure that new and expensive developments are not widely adopted until proper control trials have been conducted to establish their usefulness. Your society and many other societies accept this in principle in the case of new drug products. You require evidence that a preparation is effective and of acceptable safety before it can be marketed. Why is not similar proof required for such innovations as coronary care units?

I have already mentioned the difficulty you are having in getting old, ineffective drug products removed from the market. But marketing control does not deal with the wider and no less dangerous problem of the inappropriate use of drugs. What would puzzle an observer from another planet is our attitude toward the education of the physician. After his initial education we allow him to be exposed to a course of education by competing commercial interests that costs much more over the professional's life in practice than his original education. Surely advertising by commercial interests should be wholly replaced by noncommercial continuing education. Such education would be wider, much more cost effective, and fundamental to the promotion of quality of care in an era of rapid technological change.

Drug Prices

Action is surely needed to control the prices paid for drugs in view of the vast profits that emerge from patents, branding, and other market imperfections. Of course we want to encourage research and of course successful innovators deserve rewards. But should the innovators themselves decide within wide limits the scale of their rewards? The scale of the problem can be reduced by the wider use of generics, by the restriction of proprietary rights to brand, by rights for pharmacists to substitute, and by reduction in patent life. But should prices as a whole be subject to regulation—not only those charged by suppliers but those charged by chemists? Many European countries—not least Britain—have had considerable success in this field.

In Britain, prices for National Health Service drugs are centrally negotiated against a background of legislative sanctions and the markups of pharmacies are also centrally negotiated. As a result, pharmaceuticals cost less in Britain than in virtually all other developed Western nations. In Sweden and Denmark, import controls are used to control both the effectiveness and the price of drugs. Medical committees decide what can be allowed in taking account both of effectiveness and price.

At first sight it seems that what society wants is the provision of all those curative actions and preventive actions that are effective at the lowest costs at which they can be provided. This is to take a mechanistic and narrow view of medicine. We also need placebos that are no more expensive than is necessary to achieve their purpose. Last but not least, we need care both when we are being treated and when cure is not in prospect. It is a paradox of so many medical systems that so much is spent on ineffective cure and so little to promote standards of care. Indeed, in fee-for-service health insurance, care is underrewarded.

PATHS TO INTERVENTION

I have explained why I believe it to be necessary for societies at least to regulate if not to plan or even control the provision of their health services. There are, it seems to me, three paths to intervention. The first is the regulation of services that are delivered. The second is the planning of the system of delivery. The third is action to change the behavior of those who control the system. All three approaches can be applied simultaneously, or different approaches can be applied to different parts of the system.

Regulation

Regulation is the road down which you seem to be moving at an accelerating pace. Indeed, outside observers like myself cannot keep pace with the number of different regulating agencies. Of course, I have long been familiar with what I call the persuasive type of regulation which underlays the Hill-Burton Act, accreditation, and peer review. Now I must try to understand the potentially more restrictive if not punitive regulation of the payment systems under Medicare and Medicaid. I must understand your cost control regulations, your certificates of need, and the potentiality of PSRO (Professional Standards and Review Organizations).

Post-Event Regulation

The general drift of policy is towards the control of the construction of facilities and the evaluation of services after they have been delivered. Post-event controls are, of course, widely used in many European systems of health insurance. But in general they are only used to police extremes by examining patterns of resource use that are far above average—excessive consultations, prescribing, diagnostic tests, and medical acts. Physicians or administrators may pick out the doctors who seem to generate high costs, but any disciplinary action is normally taken by local committees of doctors who examine very carefully the circumstances of the patients.

Perhaps the most ingenious solution is that of Germany where doctors are paid from a local fund established by the income of the health insurance system. If services increase then every doctor may only be paid 90 percent or 80 percent of his fees. This places the responsibility on the local medical association to deal with those of their colleagues who are making excessive demands on the fund. Normally, the purpose of some systems of regulations is not so much to catch the offender but to discourage others from committing such offenses.

(An alternative system of regulation, used to some extent in Europe, is to require prior approval before some procedures are undertaken. But this also requires duplication of the diagnostic work and anyway can only be used for nonurgent needs for medical care such as dentistry and "cold" surgery.)

In the United States, however, you seem to be going further towards a more compre-hensive effort to keep costs down and control budgets and prices. If such systems are used to do more than punish the worst offenders, they could themselves become very costly. While computers can be programmed to pick up cases that need examination—and this is not inexpensive—the process of examination virtually involves a dummy run of the diagnosis and treatment, a still greater duplication of professional work.

Moreover, world experience has shown, as the United States experience is also beginning to show, the paradox underlying attempts to preserve the free and independent practice of medicine. At first sight, fee-for-service payment enables private free-market medicine to be readily combined with health insurance. In practice, it is not long before interference with medical practice becomes much greater than occurs or needs to occur when physicians are salaried employees in government service. Physicians are made answerable for each of their acts. Because there are incentives for abuse, restrictive and punitive safeguards are established to prevent abuse from occurring. Sometimes the punishment falls on the physician, but sometimes it falls on the patient.

The most important risks attached to this type of evaluation of medical acts is that the values hidden beneath the system of evaluation may be not just inappropriate but positively harmful. Carried to their logical conclusion they imply a false standardization of patients' needs and of patients' social situations. For example, at first sight it would seem possible to detect statistically unnecessary or inappropriate use of hospital beds. But what is appropriate for a particular patient depends on the alternatives available for the patient. Post-event regulation can only operate on what is available to be used. It cannot alter supply. It cannot create alternatives to hospital care that do not exist. The regulation system may induce the physician to chop 2 days off Mrs. Jones' stay in the hospital. What value is this if Mrs. Jones cannot obtain proper care after her discharge and has to be readmitted? What is wrong is to apply to human beings systems of cost control appropriate for securing the most economical production of battery hens.

Certificate-of-Need Regulation

Quite separate from post-event regulation, you are gradually evolving towards what is, in my view, often incorrectly called certificate-of-need regulation. Often it is not a certificate-of-need but a certificate-of-demand. This depends on whether the aim is to restrict the number of beds to those that seem to be demanded or to those that are calculated to be needed according to some criterion. In the long run, this could have more impact on the system. It is not enough, however, to be able to refuse permission without having any authority to initiate action either to build more beds when they are needed or to develop alternative patterns of care that would make more beds unnecessary.

What are in effect certificate-of-need regulations are now widely used in Europe—not only in Britain and Scandinavia, but in continental Europe. There has been a burst of legislation in the last decade that has attracted little attention over here: The French law of December 31, 1970; the Dutch law of March 25, 1971; the Belgian law of December 23, 1963; and the German law of June 29, 1972. The general tendency in Europe now is to look more at the number of beds needed rather than at the number currently demanded. The switch from demand to need implies mechanisms for providing alternative ways of meeting demands.

Restriction by Area

One use of regulation that would at present be unacceptable in the United States but is found in several European countries is restriction on the number of doctors who can practice in a particular area. In Britain, Finland, and Sweden there is tight control of the number of posts in particular specialties in hospitals in each area and this controls the vast majority of specialist work. Medical establishments are laid down centrally for each hospital—not only in total but in each specialty. Britain goes further and designates certain areas as "overdoctored" for general practice. Only in special circumstances can a doctor enter general practice under the national health service in an overdoctored area. But, again, supply restrictions can only be operated in the context of the way medicine is practiced. The supply of doctors required for a community depends on the number and qualifications of staff working with them and thus what can be safely delegated to them.

Planned and Structured System

It is because of all these limitations of action to regulate events or to control the quantity of supply that some countries are going further and attempting to control the character of the supply—in other words, to change the system. Attempts are being made in more and more countries in Europe to push both hospitals and primary care into a planned and structured system, as well as to change incentives for those in the health care system.

Structuring of Hospital System

There have been two main reasons for planning a structured hospital system. First has been the desire to eliminate the provision of the rarer specialties in small, costly, and inefficient units within most general hospitals by concentrating them in designated regional hospitals. The second has been the desire to prevent the use of the general acute hospital with its expensive facilities by those who do not need these facilities and can be treated in smaller community hospitals nearer their homes. The purpose of all this planning is not so much to save money but to promote quality of care.

In Britain the desire to plan hospitals on a regional basis was one of the reasons for taking hospitals away from local government and non-profit bodies when the National Health Service was established in 1948. The location of the rarer specialties is now planned on a regional basis in Britain by ad hoc public authorities, and we are currently rethinking the precise role of small community hospitals within our hospital structure. In Sweden, regional hospitals are currently being developed that will alone provide the rarer specialties. The location of these hospitals has been carefully chosen to minimize travel time and travel costs for patients.

If it should be thought that this type of planning would be tolerable only in countries with socialist governments, I should add that regional planning is also being imposed in both Germany and France. In Germany, the Central Government requires the counties (lander) to collaborate with the hospital associations and health insurance agencies to produce regional plans. Public money for depreciation or construction is denied to any hospital project that does not fit in with the regional plan.

France is now divided into 21 regions for hospital planning purposes. A commission for each region is appointed by the Central Government to plan hospital construction needs. No new hospital—public or private—can be built without the authorization of the Ministry. In each region, one or two regional teaching hospitals are the sole providers of the rarer specialties. Under the Law of 1970, public and private hospitals are being formed into districts that are intended to have a common management eventually. This law is designed to do for French hospitals what was done for British hospitals by the Act establishing the National Health Service.

Structural change in Europe has not been confined to the hospitals, however. In Britain, Finland, and Sweden there has been a rapid development of health centers in which doctors provide a full range of curative and preventive services and work with related staff in premises owned by public authorities. In Finland, the system is most developed, and general practitioners who used to be paid under fee-for-service are now paid by salary though they are allowed to see private patients after they have done their designated hours for health insurance. In Sweden, the vast majority of doctors in clinic practice are now salaried. In Britain, more than half the remuneration of general practitioners comes in the form of payments that are akin to salaries—initial practice allowances, seniority payments, and other payments that vary neither with the number of services nor with the number of patients for which the doctor accepts responsibility. Moreover, home nurses and public health nurses increasingly work from doctors' premises—both those that are owned by the practitioner and those that are not—and each practitioner can in addition be reimbursed for two-thirds of the salary of two ancillary workers.

The provincial government of Manitoba (Canada) is planning "a controlled and substantial experiment in community health centers." Many of you may also have read the Hastings Report on health centers for Canada as a whole. Similarly, Australia is making experiments with community health centers. Thus in more and more countries it has been accepted that the use of hospitals depends upon the extent and coordination of provisions outside the hospital. This idea has also been accepted in the United States in the context of proposals for health maintenance organizations (HMOs). But what is critical is that these countries are trying to plan ways of providing quality community care services, not just to save hospital costs.

In many countries of Europe, thinking goes still wider. It is believed that the use of hospitals depends not only on action by health-oriented staff but by a whole range of social services that support the family and provide substitutes for care by the family.

It is also believed that, for certain patients, services can be developed to provide a higher quality of care in the home than can be provided in any type of institution.

According to this view the number of hospital beds needed depends not just on the number of people who could be treated or cared for in hospital but on the number who should be in hospital. It is believed that the hospital should not be overused, not only because it is so costly but because it is dangerous: in all hospitals there is a considerable risk of cross-infection. Unnecessary admission to a hospital may make the patient sicker and also make him think that he is sicker than he is. Moreover, the artificial community contacts of hospital visiting are no substitute for living in the community. The patient's involvement with the community is seen as part of the quality of patient care.

Thus the need for hospital beds depends on what alternative arrangements are available for the care of the patient. This depends in part on how far relatives and others are prepared to care for the sick at home and on the services provided to assist them to do so. Are doctors, nurses, occupational therapists, physiotherapists, and others available to provide services in the home? Are there staff to help with cleaning and cooking, or can meals be delivered to the home? Are there neighbors or paid staff available to look after the patient while relatives go out in the evening or go away for holidays? Are there nursing homes for a patient while relatives are away for any reason or unable temporarily to provide care?

Much also depends on the suitability of the home for the care of the short-term or long-term sick. Can ground-floor accommodation be made available with convenient bathing and toilet facilities? Can the home be adapted by installing hoists, rails, and ramps and by widening doorways to take wheelchairs? Nor is care in hospital the only alternative to care at home. People who need care—those, for example, who are mentally handicapped or suffering from depression or senility—can be boarded out with people paid to look after them in their homes or housed in flatlets or grouped housing where a warden can keep an eye on them and provide support and services. Alternatively, they can be cared for in hostels. The hospital is therefore seen as at one extreme end of a variety of care institutions and should be used for tasks that cannot be done elsewhere or that only the hospital can do at reasonable cost.

Much will depend on who pays for what when the choice is made between care at home and care elsewhere—on the incentives for those who decide or influence the decision. Much also will depend on relative costs wherever they fall. Much will depend on the preferences and attitudes of both the patient and the relatives and on who interprets them. Ultimately a choice must be made after assessing the burdens, calculating the costs, and weighing the risks. Do physicians in the United States see it as their task to present these choices? Are these choices available? Are there agencies to make them available?

In terms of the fundamental values of medicine, or at least my values of medicine, it becomes artificial to attempt to draw hard and fast lines between health care and social care. Some people clearly need health services, others only need social services, but many need both. Requirements may often shift radically on a day-to-day basis. Yet in many countries of the world the pattern of services and the financing of services—particularly health insurance—is based on three unstated assumptions: That health institutions and social services can be clearly delineated, that preventive medicine can or should be separated from curative medicine, and that cure rather than care is the overwhelming need of Western nations. There is an unwillingness to accept the fact that for many the prospects of cure are limited and that, with an aging population, the quality of care and support is the most important requirement for the chronic sick and disabled.

Structuring of Primary Care

The key to the proper use of hospital beds is not more and more regulation through hospital records but a strong and organized system of primary care closely coordinated into a wide range of related services. The essence of primary care is continuity of relationship so that knowledge is acquired of each patient's medical history and family setting, and possibly his occupational setting—all of which may be relevant for the patient's health care and for helping to assess where that care can most appropriately be provided.

The role and training of the primary doctor or general practitioner has been hotly debated over the past few decades. Some have argued that much of what a general practitioner does could be done by someone with less training. But extensive education and training are needed to decide when specialist care is required and from what specialty, to advise on the practicability of care outside hospital, and in general to assess what services are needed and see that they are provided. In particular, a physician is needed to select and mobilize a package of services for care at home. Without authoritative leadership, the alternative of care at home will go by default. Thus I believe that general practitioners need every bit as much training as is needed for any specialty and they also need staff working closely with them to whom particular tasks can be delegated.

First of all, a primary doctor needs nursing staff to assist him in his consulting room and also to visit his patients in their homes — not just to provide nursing services but to assess when further visits from the physician may be required and to train relatives to provide simple nursing care when the nurse is not present. Second, he needs staff to help him with preventive work and discover patients who may need services but are not receiving them. Third, he needs a supporting staff to arrange, on his behalf,

for whatever further services a patient may require.

This managerial work in primary care, like other managerial work, does not lend itself to fee-for-service payment. For the services that are of critical importance to patient care are communication with others on behalf of the patient—explaining the patient's needs to the occupational therapist or physiotherapist, discussing the case on the telephone with the specialist, and explaining why priority should be given in the assignment of domestic help. Whether these tasks are actually done by the doctor himself or by his staff, they are not tasks for which standard payments can satisfactorily be made. Fee-for-service payment encourages the doctor to see his role in terms of tasks that bring reward—the consultation, the diagnostic test, the treatment procedure. The task of arranging for the home care of the patient may be much more time consuming—time for which a fee schedule cannot appropriately provide.

Moreover, the concept of social care does not fit happily with fee-for-service payment. Here the task of the physician is not to deliver procedures but deliver emotional support—to comfort the dying, to prepare women for widowhood, to teach people how to live with a disability, to accept the consequences of aging, and to give comfort to distressed relatives. These were tasks that, in an earlier age, we looked to the church to provide. Some still look to the church; others expect these services from their physician. Can we program our cost-regulatory computers to accept fee claims for tender loving care? Or must the physician provide it free and at the sacrifice of time that could be spent in services for which he could readily claim? The fundamental question is whether it is the task of the physician simply to perform medical acts or to deliver comprehensive health care.

Nor does the concept of heading a domiciliary team readily fit with private practice. In many countries, home nursing is underdeveloped and when it exists it is a service wholly separate from the doctor. The home nurse is expected to communicate with the doctor in writing or by telephone, yet the doctor may not know the nurse personally. The nature of home nursing is such that unless the patient has a whole-time nurse, the nurse is unlikely to be present when the doctor happens to visit. In the hospital setting the nurse makes it her business to be present when the doctor visits, and mutual confidence and effective teamwork are encouraged by these regular meetings. Similarly, it is much more satisfactory for home nurses to work with a particular doctor or practice to ease communication and simplify the task of seeing that patients who need nursing help receive it rapidly. But the nurse needs an office from which to work. If she goes on holiday or is sick, a replacement must be found quickly. These problems are more readily solved if both doctor and nurse are part of a wider organization that provides accommodation and pays for all expenses.

Working toward Economy and Quality

For all these reasons I advocate a structured system of hospitals and of primary care as mechanisms for promoting economy and quality in the wide sense that I have indicated. A system of organization may or may not work as it is designed to work, however. How is it possible to generate incentives for economy and incentives for quality? Economy can be imposed by limiting budgets and scrutinizing bills, but, if each hospital is given a separate budget, incentives can be distorted. The hospital can curtail its costs by treating fewer patients, admitting less severe cases, or treating cases less intensively. A reduction in length of stay and more admissions to maintain occupancy would generate greater costs than the annual budget could cover. Indeed, no hospital may be able to attain maximum efficiency because its budget is insufficient for it to do so. Thus it is preferable to have one

budget for all hospitals serving a defined population. But separate budgets for hospital and nonhospital purposes obstruct the process of finding the appropriate balance between hospital and nonhospital services. It is for this among other reasons that the British National Health Service has been reorganized to provide one regional budget out of which comprehensive health services are financed.

HMOs as Answer

The same type of thinking underlies the concept of the HMOs, though the scope of HMO services is much narrower. HMOs are currently seen as the American answer to value for money in medicine. Yet surely much must depend on how they are operated and who controls them. Here I would like to raise some questions about HMO proposals that I think many other European observers might ask.

Are competing HMOs to have their own hospitals in the same area? If so, would that not either result in the uneconomic duplication of facilities or else generate greater travel costs for hospital users? If HMOs are competitive, could not this lead to an undesirable emphasis on amenity and convenience at the expense of economies in those services, the importance of which patients are not aware?

If the services offered by different HMOs are available at varying prices, might not the better-off choose the more expensive contracts on the assumption that they *must* be purchasing better services? Will such choices frustrate the pressures for economy that competition is expected to generate? If organizations are allowed to select their members, premiums will presumably become risk-rated. Will high-risk users be forced to pay high premiums or find their health services elsewhere?

Would not competition between organizations lead to competition for scarce resources so that geographical distribution of health services could become even worse than at present? This seems more likely to happen if doctors shared all or part of the profits of HMOs. Moreover, would it not place too heavy a strain on medical ethics if doctors were placed in such a position that every dollar of expenditure they authorized for patients affected, dollar for dollar, their own remuneration?

Most of these problems would be avoided if only one organization were responsible for providing health services for all in a region of some 1–2 million people. I realize that this involves the removal of certain aspects of choice to which so much importance is attached over here, even though it is acknowledged that the user is not well-equipped to exercise such choices. It also involves entrusting one monopoly organization with substantial power. Even if choice were sacrificed, there would still be the risk that resources might be heavily concentrated in the richer areas and in areas where professional people prefer to practice—unless manpower ceilings were set for each region for different categories of scarce personnel. Health insurance can provide money, but it cannot ensure that there are doctors, dentists, nurses, and other health manpower wherever that money is spent.

Regional Budgeting

I personally believe that regional budgeting accompanied by regional planning and central control of posts for scarce personnel provides the best available answer to the problem of creating a setting where quality, economy, and equity can be promoted. Those who control the budget are thus forced to make choices in the use of that budget between hospital care and out-of-hospital care; between finding those who need but do not demand and those for whom demands are made, some of them unnecessary or of low priority; between the prevention of ill health and the cure of ill health; between standards of amenity and care and valiant efforts to cure or keep alive that have no serious prospects of success; and

between high standards of care for those who can appreciate it and technical survival for those who cannot.

New Incentives for Decision Makers

Who should make these choices? In the last analysis, whose values should prevail? How can an effective working relationship be established between representatives of patients, representatives of those who bear the costs, and health professionals? How can lay representatives be found with the judgment to know where it is proper to overrule professional opinion in establishing broad priorities and when professional opinion should always prevail?

Information System

At the very least, we need more information about levels of health in different social and occupational groups, the activities of health professionals, and the results of those activities. Despite the vast resources devoted to health services, extremely little information is currently available that relates the use of health resources to health benefits in any sense. While some doctor may come to know of a patient's death, disability, or recovery, he may not know who took the critical decision in the patient's management. While death and recorded causes of death are carefully registered, this information is not systematically related to past patient management or to the use of health resources on the care of that patient. Rarely is the clinician able to compare his performance with that of his colleagues in a systematic way, standardized for diagnosis, severity, age, and other variables. New treatment procedures are still often introduced before their value has been meticulously evaluated.

What is needed is a system of information that shows those who make professional decisions, the results of those decisions, and the resources used to achieve these results. This information should also be available for independent professional review. This seems to me the constructive use of computerized information systems rather than the examination of medical acts against medians and means. A number of people have been working on this type of problem over here as well as in Britain[8] and elsewhere.

Responsibility of Health Care Workers

Better information will not necessarily be enough to change behavior or improve the quality of decisionmaking so that unnecessary costs are avoided and quality care in its widest sense promoted. Thus, ultimately, we must look not just at the financial incentives on those who operate our health services, but at their ethos, their commitment, and at what gives them satisfaction in their job. Here I am thinking not only of physicians and dentists or administrators and managers but of nurses, social workers, and paramedical workers. We will not get value for money in health care until health professionals see it as part of their responsibility to see that we do.

This has major implications for the original education and continuing education of those working in our health services. It has major implications for the selection of those

who are educated and trained and for those who provide that education and training. The health professionals must accept their responsibility for using health resources effectively and efficiently or the immense power we currently give to the health professions may be challenged and part of it transferred to others. This would, in my view, be the wrong solution.

CONCLUSION

The central questions are not so much of value in its narrow sense but of social value in its widest sense. We are not just concerned with the justifiability of medical acts and the price tag they should carry. Nor are we simply concerned with the technical quality of the services rendered by teams of professionals. We are concerned with equity in the distribution of health resources, with their deployment in the promotion of health, and with the integration of health and social care. Value for money in this last sense cannot be achieved by fragmented providers or pluralistic financing agencies. Somehow a socially responsive organization is needed that can mobilize the resources needed to promote these values.

NOTES

1. Sylvester E. Berki, *Hospital Economics*, Lexington Books, 1972, p. 131.

2. Milton I. Roemer, "Bed Supply and Hospital Utilization: A Natural Experiment," *Hospitals* (American Hospital Association), Vol. 35, No. 21, 1961.

3. Brian Abel-Smith, *An International Study of Health Expenditure*, World Health Organization, 1957, p. 92.

4. Joseph G. Simanis, "Medical Care Expenditures," *Social Security Bulletin*, March 1973.

5. Ministry for Social Security, *The Australian Health Insurance Program*, Canberra, 1973, p. 2.

6. P. Comillot and P. Bonamour, "France," in *Health Services Prospects: An International Survey*, Nuffield Provincial Hospitals Trust, 1973, p. 75.

7. A. L. Cochrane, *Effectiveness and Efficiency* (Rock Carling Fellowship, 1971), Nuffield Provincial Hospitals Trust, 1972.

8. See, for example, B. Abel-Smith et al., *Accounting for Health*, King Edward Health Fund, London, 1973.

4. Economics, Health and Post-Industrial Society

VICTOR R. FUCHS

Reprinted from *The Milbank Memorial Fund Quarterly/Health and Society* 57. Copyright © 1979, Milbank Memorial Fund, 153-182.

Two hundred years ago the industrial revolution was figuratively and literally beginning to pick up steam. In a few Western countries agricultural advances, which came faster than population growth, enabled some men and women to escape from grinding poverty. Life for most, however, was still "nasty, brutish, and short." Infant mortality rates of 200 or 300 per 1000 births were the rule, and life expectancy in Western Europe was not very different from what it had been under the Romans. The great majority of men and women worked on farms, producing barely enough to feed themselves plus a small surplus for the relatively few workers engaged in the production of other goods and services. Widows and orphans, the sick, the elderly, and the destitute relied primarily on family and church for help in their time of need.

Agriculture continued to dominate employment for another century; as recently as 1877, half the United States labor force was still engaged in farming. Then, very quickly, in less than "thirty minutes" if we think of recorded history as a "day," most of the countries of Western Europe and North America became industrialized. But the process of economic development did not stop with industrialization. As Colin Clark noted so accurately in 1940: "The most important concomitant of economic progress is the movement of labor from agriculture to manufacture, and from manufacture to commerce and services." By 1957, the United States had become the world's first "service economy"—that is, the first nation in which more than half of the labor force was engaged in producing services rather than goods.

Today, many Western societies can be described as "post-industrial" (Bell, 1973). Such societies are characterized by a variety

*This paper is based on The E. S. Woodward Lectures in Economics delivered at The University of British Columbia, Vancouver on November 1-2, 1978. Copyright 1978, The University of British Columbia.

of special features—affluence, urbanization, infant mortality rates of 10 to 15 per 1000, high female labor force participation, low fertility, decreased importance of family and traditional religions, increased importance of the state, long life expectancy, and, of course, a substantial change in the locus of economic activity. The hospital, the classroom, and the shopping center have replaced the coal mine, the steel mill, and the assembly line as the major work sites of modern society. "Industrial man" has been succeeded by "post-industrial person," but the import of this transformation for society has not yet been fully analyzed.

In these lectures I shall focus on one of the largest and fastest growing industries in post-industrial society—medical care—and on a range of problems specifically related to medicine and health. I will use the discipline of economics to provide some insights concerning these problems, and will also attempt to use the health field to illuminate more general problems of post-industrial society. In this last respect I wish to ally myself with the first Woodward Lecturer, H. Scott Gordon, who wrote in 1971: "I have never regarded economics as a discipline that is inherently narrow." At the same time, I am aware of the limits of economics—both those limits that stem from shortcomings in current theoretical and empirical knowledge and those limits that are inherent in any science of man.

For instance, it should be clear that economics alone does not, indeed should not, tell us whether it is better to devote resources to extending the life of an 80-year-old man with terminal cancer or to reducing the risk of birth defects in a population of newborns. What economics does do is help us arrange the relevant information in a systematic way and make explicit the choices that individuals and society face. Therein lies much of its unpopularity. Economics earns the label "the dismal science" because it constantly reminds us that we have been turned out of the Garden of Eden. Many persons prefer to pretend that choices do not have to be made; many like to believe that they are not being made at present.

These lectures will not offer that kind of comfort or reassurance; neither will they supply simple answers to the major policy issues of the day. They are, rather, one man's attempt to report some key findings from more than a decade of research in health economics, and to offer some generalizations from these findings. I am aware, and you are forewarned, that such generalizations, based on only one aspect of society, must necessarily be speculative.

Lecture I: The Determinants of Health

In this first lecture I will review some major results concerning the determinants of health, especially the roles played by medical care, income, and education. We will see that changes in health are much more dependent on non-medical factors than on the quantity of medical care. Nevertheless, medical care has become one of the largest industries in modern society. The second part of this lecture discusses some of the reasons for this rapid growth.

Medical Care

One of the first things economics does is to sensitize us to the distinction between *inputs* and *outputs*—that is, in the present context, to the difference between *medical care* and *health*. This perspective can be found in the wise observations of René Dubos and has been ably articulated in Canada by Marc Lalonde (Dubos, 1959; Lalonde, 1974). It remained for economists, however, to develop the matter systematically and quantitatively in multivariate analyses that examine the effect on health of medical inputs, income, education, and other variables.

The basic finding is: when the state of medical science and other health-determining variables are held constant, the marginal contribution of medical care to health is very small in modern nations. Those who advocate ever more physicians, nurses, hospitals, and the like are either mistaken or have in mind objectives other than the improvement of the health of the population. The earliest studies that reported this conclusion were greeted with skepticism in some quarters because the analyses typically relied on mortality as the measure of health. Mortality, it was said, is a rather crude index of health. It was suggested that more sophisticated measures would reveal the favorable effects of greater numbers of physicians, nurses, and hospital beds. A recent Rand study, however, based on six sensitive indicators of ill health (elevated cholesterol levels, varicose veins, high blood pressure, abnormal chest X-ray, abnormal electrocardiogram, and an unfavorable periodontal index) provides striking confirmation of the results based on mortality (Newhouse and Friedlander, 1977). Variations in the amount of health resources available across 39 metropolitan areas of the United States had no systematic effect on these health measures taken alone or in linear combination.

Examples of the distinction between medical care and health can be drawn from many countries other than the United States. In Great Britain, for instance, the National Health Service (NHS) has undoubtedly served to sharply reduce class differences in access to medical care, but the traditionally large class differentials in infant mortality and life expectancy are no smaller after three decades of the NHS. Also, despite free access to medical care, time lost from work because of sickness has actually increased greatly in Britain in recent decades. The number of sick days depends on many factors in addition to health, but these data hardly support the notion that there has been a large payoff from the NHS in that area (Townsend, 1974). The discrepancy between health and medical care is even sharper in the USSR. In recent years there apparently has been a deterioration in health as measured either by infant mortality or life expectancy, even though the Soviet medical care system is said to have expanded (Davis and Feshbach, 1978).

There are several reasons why an increase in medical resources, given a reasonable quantity as a base, does not have much effect on health. First, if physicians are scarce, they tend to concentrate on those patients for whom their attention is likely to make the most difference. As doctors become more plentiful, they naturally tend to spend more time on patients less in need of attention. Second, patients also alter their behavior, depending upon how easy or difficult it is to get to see a physician. When physicians are more numerous, patients tend to seek attention for more trivial conditions. Third, many of the most effective interventions, such as vaccinations or treatment of bacterial infections, require only modest amounts of resources. Quite often, one "shot" goes a long way. On the other hand, the long-term benefits of some of the most expensive procedures, such as open-heart surgery or organ transplants, are still in doubt. Fourth, there is the problem of "iatrogenic disease"—illness that arises as a result of medical care. Because medical and surgical interventions are more powerful than ever before, they carry with them greater risk. Sometimes too much care, or the wrong care, can be more deleterious to health than no care at all. Finally, it is abundantly clear that factors other than medical care (e.g., genes, environment, life-style) play crucial roles in many of the most important health problems.

Income and Inequality

For most of man's history, income has been the primary determinant of health and life expectancy—the major explanation for differences in health among nations and among groups within a nation. A strong income effect is still observed in the less-developed nations, but in the United States the relation between income and life expectancy has tended to disappear. This is true when health is measured by mortality, or by indicators such as high blood pressure, varicose veins, elevated cholesterol levels, and abnormal X-rays or cardiograms, or by subjective evaluation of health status. Other things equal, there is no longer a clearly discernible effect of income on health except at the deepest levels of poverty. I regard the disappearance of the income effect as an important aspect of post-industrial society, but the fact is not widely known, and the implications are rarely discussed. To realize one such implication, consider how attitudes toward economic growth might differ, depending upon whether further growth was or was not expected to reduce mortality

The favorable effect of economic growth and technological change on *average* life expectancy is well known. Less appreciated is the extent to which growth has also reduced *inequality* in life expectancy across individuals and groups. The principal reason for the reduction is that general economic growth, even if unaccompanied by any reduction in income inequality, has more favorable effects on the health of the very poor than on those who have already reached a level of living well above subsistence. A second reason is that many effective medical discoveries of the past half-century, such as antibiotics, have been relatively low in cost and widely available.

Consider the following statistics taken from U.S. life tables for the white population. At the turn of this century, given the age-specific death rates then prevailing, one-fourth of a newborn cohort of males would die before the age of 23. On the other hand, one-fourth could expect to live beyond the age of 72. In other words, the variation in life expectancy was great. One simple measure of variation is the interquartile ratio—i.e., the difference between the age of death at the third quartile and at the first quartile divided by the median age at death. For white males in 1900, this variation was 86% $[(72 - 23) \div 57]$, but by 1975 it had fallen to 26%. This large reduction is attributable in part to drastic declines in infant and child mortality, but even if one looks at years of life remaining at age 20, the interquartile ratio fell from 59% to 35% between 1900 and 1975. White females experienced a similar decline in variation in life expectancy. Furthermore, nearly all of the decline occurred before the advent of Medicare and Medicaid.

Not only has the distribution of life expectancy become much more nearly equal within the white population, but the difference between white and non-white life expectancy has also been reduced substantially in this century. In 1900, life expectancy for whites was 47% higher than for non-whites. In 1975, the differential was 8%! The overall reduction in inequality of life expectancy bears a strong relationship to reduction in inequality by income class. In 1900, those with short life expectancy were disproportionately from the lower half of the income distribution. Now, with the correlation between income and life expectancy much weaker, we can say that with respect to the most precious good of all, life itself, the United States is approaching an egalitarian distribution.

Education

Despite the general trend toward equality in life expectancy, there is one factor—education—that consistently appears as a significant correlate of good health. The same research by health economists that reveals the small marginal contributions of medical care and of income to health reports a strong positive relation between health and years of schooling. In the United States, regardless of the way health is measured (e.g., mortality, morbidity, symptoms, or subjective evaluation), and regardless of the unit of observation (e.g., individuals, city or state averages), years of schooling usually emerges as the most powerful correlate of good health. Michael Grossman, an economist who has done extensive research on this question, has tended to interpret this relationship as evidence that schooling increases the individual's efficiency in producing health, although he recognizes that some causality may run from better health to more schooling (Grossman, 1976). The way schooling contributes to efficiency in producing health has never been made explicit, but

Grossman has speculated that persons with more education might choose healthier diets, be more aware of health risks, obtain healthier occupations, and use medical care more wisely.

I accept the "efficiency" hypothesis, but I think that it explains only a part of the correlation. One reason for my skepticism is that Grossman did not find any favorable effect of IQ on health, holding constant schooling and other variables. If more years of schooling increases efficiency in producing health, it seems that a higher IQ ought to work in the same direction. Furthermore, recent research on surgical utilization casts doubt on the proposition that the better educated individuals use medical care differently than do the less educated. While the probability of surgery is much lower for the highly educated than for the rest of the U.S. population, a new study by Louis Garrison (1978) shows that the highly educated who do undergo surgery enter the hospital at the same stage of disease as do the less educated. He also finds that the better educated patients choose the same kinds of physicians, have about the same length of stay, and, apart from the fact that their general health is a little better than average, have about the same outcomes from surgery. Thus, at least in the context of in-hospital surgery, there is little support for the "efficiency" effect in the use of medical care.

The most plausible explanation for the lower surgery rates of the highly educated is that they have less need for surgery, i.e., they are in better health. The question remains, Why? One explanation that I favor is that both schooling and health are manifestations of differences among individuals in the willingness and/or ability to invest in human capital. Both schooling and health-related activities involve incurring current costs for the sake of future benefits, and it seems quite clear that individuals differ in the "rate of return" that will induce them (or their parents) to undertake such investments. There are numerous possible reasons for such differences. For instance, some individuals have much better access to capital than do others. Even holding access to capital constant, individuals differ in their skills of self-control and in their ability to visualize the future.

Recent preliminary research gives modest support for this view. A colleague and I surveyed a group of young adults to ascertain their rate of time discount, measured by the extra money they would require to wait for a money award in the future rather than collecting a smaller sum in the present. My colleague was interested in the pattern of the rates, i.e., how they changed with length of time involved, the size of the award, etc. I added a few questions about the respondents' health and then looked at the relation between health and discount rate across individuals. I found a strong, statistically significant, negative correlation between the rate of discount and the subjective assessment of health. For the 25% of the sample with the lowest discount rates, the probability of being in excellent health was 63%; for the quarter with the highest rates, the probability was only 32%.

Some recent statistics from England seem to provide additional support for my view of the correlation between health and schooling. A study of cigarette smoking revealed that among men in social class I (highly educated) the proportion who smoked fell almost by half between 1958 and 1975. In contrast, among men in social class V (poorly educated) the proportion scarcely changed. It seems unlikely that this difference in behavior arises primarily because the men in class V have not heard about the dangers of smoking or do not understand the implications for health. It is more likely that they are unwilling (or unable) to give up a present pleasure for a distant and uncertain benefit. I suspect that if one compared these two groups of men with regard to other aspects of behavior that involve explicit or implicit rates of time discount (e.g., saving, buying on credit), one would find similar differences.

Progress in Medical Science

This discussion of the determinants of health should not close without some consideration of the effects of progress in medical science. Economics not only cautions us to distinguish between inputs and outputs but also calls attention to the distinction between the marginal product of an additional unit of input, holding constant the production function, and the shift of that function through technological progress. In the first instance, we ask what will be the effects on health of an increase in the quantity of physicians, nurses, and hospitals, assuming no change in the way care is delivered. In the second, we ask what will be the effects on health of an advance in medical science, assuming no change in the quantity of physicians, nurses, and hospitals.

With respect to the latter question, it seems to me that the "medical care doesn't matter" argument is overstated by some writers. To be sure, medical progress was slow until well into the twentieth century, but from about 1935 to about 1955, a period which marked the introduction of anti-infectious drugs, major improvements in health were recorded in all industrial nations. The decreases in mortality were far greater than could be attributed to general economic advance, increases in the *quantity* of medical care, or similar changes.

The only reasonable explanation, in my view, is that advances in medical knowledge changed the structural relations governing the production of health. In a study of changes in infant mortality in 15 Western nations between 1937 and 1965, for instance, I estimated that the change in structure accounted for at least half of the large decline in infant mortality over that period (Fuchs, 1974).

The application of medical and public health knowledge also improved health in the less developed countries, and at unprecedented speed. In a sample of 16 less developed countries studied by demographer Sam Preston, life expectancy was only 39 years in

1940, but rose to 60 years by 1970 (Preston, 1979). He and I estimated that about two-thirds of the increase was attributable to better health technology and similar structural changes and only one-third to a rise in per capita income. By contrast, in the United States the same change in life expectancy—from 39 to 60 years—required three-quarters of a century, from 1855 to 1930, because health technology was developing so slowly at that time.

It remains true that advances in medical science do not come at a steady or predictable pace. During the 1960s many "breakthroughs" were hailed, and expenditures for medical care rose appreciably, but the favorable consequences for health were quite limited. In recent years, however, U.S. death rates, especially from heart disease, have decreased rapidly. For men and women at most ages, the probability of death from arteriosclerotic heart disease in 1975 was 20% to 25% lower than in 1968. Analysts who are technologically inclined attribute most of this large decrease to better control of hypertension, special coronary care units in hospitals, open-heart surgery, and similar medical innovations. Some observers are more prone to credit changes in diet, smoking, exercise, and other aspects of personal behavior. We do not know the true explanation; I suspect that there is some validity to both points of view.

The Growth of Medical Care

While the pace of medical advance has been highly uneven, the growth of expenditures for medical care has been unrelenting. For at least the past three decades (and probably for much longer) the share of gross national product (GNP) devoted to medical care has steadily increased in the United States and many other countries. Today, in every post-industrial society, health care absorbs a substantial portion of the nation's resources; in several, the share devoted to health is rapidly approaching 10%. In the remainder of this lecture I will consider several possible explanations for the rapid growth of health care as an industry. In so doing, I will make a few remarks regarding the growth of services in general, and I will offer some speculations concerning medical care as a substitute for family and religion.

Income and Productivity

One popular, but I believe exaggerated, explanation for the relative growth of service employment is the growth of per capita income. With respect to health care, higher income is clearly not a *direct* causal factor. Precise estimates of the income elasticity of the demand for health care differ, but almost all investigators agree that it is well below unity—i.e., people behave as if health care is a "necessity." It follows, therefore, that the direct effect of a rise in per capita income should be a *decrease* in health care's share of real GNP. Some services other than health may be considered as "luxuries," i.e., they have income elasticities greater than one, but it is interesting to note that according to the U.S. national income accounts there has been only a small increase in the service sector's share of gross product measured in *constant dollars* (Fuchs, 1978). To be specific, during the past 30 years, while service employment was growing from 46% to 61% of total employment, the share of real output (1972 dollars) originating in the service sector changed only from 51% to 56%. If services had the high income elasticity of demand that is often ascribed to them, the growth of service output would surely have been more rapid.

The differential trends in employment and real output are the result of a relatively slow growth of output per worker in services. In this respect, health care has been no exception. Labor input per patient, especially in hospitals, has grown at an extremely rapid rate. In 1976, there were 304 full-time equivalent employees per 100 patients in the U.S. short-term hospitals compared with 178 per 100 patients in 1950.

Taken at face value, these data suggest that there has been a *decrease* in productivity, but that is highly problematical. The character of hospital *activity* has changed greatly since 1950. Each patient now has many more laboratory and X-ray tests, more complex surgery is performed, and new treatment approaches, such as intensive care units, have proliferated. I use the word "activity" rather than "output" deliberately, because we are far from knowing how much this increased activity has resulted in better health. Some changes in medical technology, such as the anti-infectious drugs mentioned previously, have clearly raised productivity enormously, but the only thing we know with certainty about some of the other technological changes is that they have greatly raised expenditures.

One reason why it is so difficult to measure productivity in medical care is that the consumer is an integral part of the production process. Health depends not only on how efficiently the physicians and nurses work, but also on what the patient does. Similar problems arise in attempts to measure change in real output and productivity in education, social services, police protection, entertainment, and many other service industries. As more and more of the work force becomes employed in industries whose output cannot be accurately measured, the "real" GNP will become increasingly unreliable as the measure of the welfare of society. We will probably be forced to abandon faith in a single summary index for measuring long-term changes or for international comparisons. Instead, welfare comparisons will be sought through mortality and morbidity indexes, crime rates, reading ability, and other more direct indicators of well-being.

The rapid growth of medical technology—the vast expansion in the character and scope of interventions that physicians can undertake—has been a major factor in the growth of health expenditures in recent decades. Familiar examples include renal dialysis, open-heart surgery, organ transplants, and high-energy cancer treatments. These innovations, attributable in large part to the investment in medical research of the past quarter-century, may or may not make major contributions to improved health, but relative ineffectiveness does not deter their use.

In the past I have referred to the proclivity of physicians to employ new technologies simply because they exist as the "technological imperative" (Fuchs, 1968). Recent economic research, however, provides a different explanation for the emphasis on expensive treatments that yield little in lives saved, while preventive activities with high potential yield per dollar of expenditures are denied resources. Such behavior may be fully consistent with consumer sovereignty (i.e., willingness to pay) even in a population with uniform incomes and preferences. The reason is that the amount most people are willing to pay for a given reduction in the probability of death is positively related to the *level* of the probability. Thus, a person facing almost certain death would usually be willing to pay a great deal for even a small increase in the chance of survival; that same person, facing a low probability of death, would not pay nearly as much for the same increase in survival probability. If one infers the "value of life" from the amount the person is willing to pay for the change in the probability of survival, it is clear that the value of life varies for the same individual, depending upon the circumstances.

Imagine, if you will, a cancer treatment program that costs $1 million per life saved, and another program to lower the probability of getting cancer that costs only $500,000 per life saved. People might be more willing to pay for the *treatment,* if sick, than to pay for the *prevention,* if well. This behavior is not necessarily "irrational," nor need it be the result of some "death-denying" psychological quirk. We do not think it odd that a thirsty man will pay a large amount for a small drink of water if there is very little available, but is not willing to pay much for a drink when water is plentiful and he is not particularly thirsty.

The medical profession has been frequently criticized for failing to allocate resources so as to maximize the number of lives saved, but some of this criticism may be unjustified—at least in the sense that the emphasis on heroic efforts in life-threatening situations at the expense of preventive measures may be a reasonable response to consumer preferences. If we seek a health care system that does what people want it to do (regardless of whether that preference is expressed in the market or through political processes), we should expect considerable inequality at the margin in costs per life saved. To the extent that we deem this an undesirable outcome, the way to guard against it is to rule out the *possibility* of relatively high-cost interventions. If the intervention is unknown, society may, in some sense, be better off. For instance, suppose the very expensive cancer treatment did not exist. People might be more likely to avail themselves of the cancer prevention program. Perhaps even more to the point, suppose a project to develop a cancer treatment with the characteristics described above was being considered. It could be socially advantageous *not* to support the research, even though, once completed, the results would be used.

Government, Family, and Religion

The growth of government, the decline in importance of the family, and the weakening of traditional religion are three closely related factors that I believe have also contributed substantially to the growth of the health care industry. The growing importance of government will be discussed in some detail in the next lecture. At this point I want to call attention to the fact that subsidization of health care by government induces additional demand. Nearly all health economists believe that the *price* elasticity of demand for care is smaller than one, but none believes that it is zero. It follows, therefore, that a reduction in the price of care at the point of decision through public (or private) insurance increases the quantity demanded. To get some feel for the possible magnitude of this effect, let us assume that the total price (including money, time, and psychic costs) of care has been reduced by one-half as a result of government intervention, and let us also assume that the price elasticity of demand is −0.5. If nothing else changed, the increase in quantity demanded would be two-fifths. A decline in price of three-fourths with an elasticity of −0.28 would produce approximately the same change.[1] These examples suggest that the government's effect on price has probably been a major factor in increased utilization.

The effects of the decline of the family and of traditional religion are more difficult to quantify, but I offer a few examples to convey the flavor of the argument. Consider nursing homes. In the United States they are by far the fastest growing component of the health care sector; their share of total spending climbed from less than 2% in 1960 to almost 8% in 1977. Nursing home expenditures now exceed spending for drugs or for dentists' services; the only larger categories are hospitals and physicians' services. But what is a nursing home and what services does it provide? I would argue that it provides very little that was not provided in the past at home by the family. Indeed, in some cases it does not provide as much.

To be sure, the growth of nursing homes is attributable in part to growth in the relative number of the aged. But more important, in my opinion, is the growth in female labor force participation and the mobility of the population. Elderly widows comprise the bulk of the nursing home population, and there has been tremendous increase in the percentage of widows 65 and over who live alone. In 1950 that

---

[1]The change in quantity is equal to the product of the change in price and the elasticity of demand, where the changes between period 1 and period 2 are measured as percentages according to the following formula: $(2 - 1) \div (2 + 1) \div 2$.

figure was 25%; in 1976 it was 65%. True enough, rising income makes living alone possible and helps pay for nursing home care; however, a considerable amount of what we think of as an *increase* in health care is not an increase at all, but rather a substitute for care that was formerly provided within the family.

The same may be said about the growth of child care and many other services. Contrary to the assumption underlying the national income accounts, these services do not represent a completely new addition to the nation's output; they are in part simply a transfer from home production to the exchange economy. The rise of female labor force participation and the growth of service employment are bound together in a nexus of mutual reinforcement. Each is both cause and consequence of the other.

Not only does purchased medical care in part take the place of the family, but I believe that it is also frequently a modern substitute for religion. This is most obvious in the case of mental illness, and the similarity between psychiatry and religion has been frequently discussed. It needs to be emphasized, however, that many visits to physicians who are not psychiatrists are undertaken for reasons other than specific diagnostic or therapeutic intervention. The patient may be seeking sympathy, or reassurance, or help in facing death (his own or that of someone close to him). The patient may want to unburden himself to an authority figure who will keep his secrets confidential. There may be a desire to find someone to assume responsibility for a difficult decision, or there may be a need for validation of a course of action already decided upon. The ability to state "The doctor says I should (or shouldn't) do this" often is worth a great deal.

In an earlier day, priests, ministers, and rabbis met many of these demands. For some persons they still do, but today many find a white coat more reassuring than a black one, a medical center more impressive than a cathedral. One striking change is in the customary site of death. In an earlier day dying was usually a private affair, attended by family and friends, and legitimized by priest or shaman or witch doctor. Today, in most Western nations, more than half of all deaths occur in hospitals. The physician is now our chief ambassador to death.

The analogy I have drawn between medical care and religion may be regarded as disparagement of care by those who share Marx's opinion of religion as the "opium of the people." But it is well to remember that in the very same passage Marx also called religion the "heart of a heartless world . . . the spirit of spiritless conditions." Despite the many criticisms that can be raised about medicine today—its high cost, its preoccupation with technology, its fragmentation into specialties and subspecialties—the truth is that for many people it is the "heart of a heartless world . . . the spirit of spiritless conditions."

Lecture II: The Growth of Government

In the previous lecture I presented an economist's view of the determinants of health and discussed the growth of medical care into one of the largest industries in modern society. In this lecture I will consider the tremendous expansion of government in the health field, and will use health as a test case to appraise Right-wing and Left-wing approaches to economic policy. Finally, I will articulate my own values and judgments, bearing in mind the focus of the Woodward Lecture series on economic freedom and contemporary economic problems.

The extension of the scope of government in the health field, like the extension of government in many other aspects of post-industrial society, is too obvious to require elaboration. I shall, therefore, move immediately to a consideration of possible explanations.

One likely reason is the ever-increasing complexity of modern life. Consumers are now faced with a bewildering array of goods and services and they feel a great need for information about them. There can be significant economies of scale in the provision of information about the quality of beef, the purity of drugs, and the safety of airlines; thus, it may be more efficient to have a single agency, the government, provide that information.

Many observers also believe that urbanization and the growth of population and income have increased the importance of *externalities,* so that there is legitimate scope for the government to do more than simply provide information. An externality in health exists if Brown's consumption or other actions have favorable (or unfavorable) effects on Smith's health, but these effects are not reflected in the prices Brown faces and there is no feasible way for Brown and Smith to make a private arrangement that would cause Brown to take these effects into account.

Familiar examples in this category include vaccinations (positive externality) and air pollution (negative externality). When externalities exist, the solution most economists prefer is to use subsidies or taxes to bring private costs (or benefits) into line with social costs (or benefits). Direct regulation that compels or forbids certain activities outright should generally be avoided unless the costs of administering the subsidies or taxes are unreasonably high.

A special kind of externality discussed by Calabresi and Bobbitt (1978) in their recent book *Tragic Choices* concerns society's unwillingness to "see" some of its members (typically the very poor) take unusual risks or pursue degrading activities. An example is the inhibition to the sale of kidneys or other organs by living donors. Calabresi and Bobbitt refer to society's unwillingness to countenance behavior that is an "affront to values" as a "moralism." Is it really "moral," however, to force an already disadvantaged person to be more disadvantaged by denying him the opportunity to do that

which he thinks it is to his advantage to do? It seems to me that in-
hibitions of this character might more accurately be described as
"estheticisms"; that is, they are really matters of taste. The importance of taste and social conventions in these matters is nicely illustrated by the fact that society readily permits individuals to work
in coal mines and to pursue other activities that are far more
dangerous to health than is the absence of one kidney.

Or consider public policy with respect to abortions. At one time
most governments forbade them. More recently we have seen
governments encourage abortion through subsidies. Someday
governments may compel an abortion rather than allow the birth of
a horribly deformed child, either because the public does not want to
have to support the child, or simply because it upsets people to see or
hear about the child. In each case the majority in society uses
government to influence the behavior of others, always in the name
of "morality," but probably because such behavior affects the majority through tangible or psychological externalities. One can
speculate that such psychological externalities have grown in importance with urbanization, affluence, and, especially, more rapid,
widespread, and vivid communications.

A pure libertarian, confronted with these alternative governmental policies toward abortion, would say: "A plague on *all* your
houses." The libertarian position is that the government should not
forbid abortions, should not subsidize them, should not compel
them—in short, should do nothing to interfere with the right of the
individual to do as he or she pleases—unless the action harms
someone else. Ah, there's the rub. What constitutes harm? The libertarian would not allow murder, robbery, or rape. Many libertarians
would go along with economically sound measures to deal with air
pollution. But what if I find abortion, or prostitutes soliciting on the
street, more offensive than air pollution, and most voters feel as I
do? The distinction between physiological and psychological harm is
rather fragile; the head is connected to the body, and we now know
that there are important interchanges between the psyche and the
soma. This discussion illustrates the importance of widely shared
values for the smooth functioning of a democratic society. As
Tawney (1926) has written: "The condition of effective action in a
complex civilization is cooperation. And the condition of cooperation is agreement, both to ends to which effort should be applied, and
the criteria by which its success is to be judged."

In post-industrial society, governments clearly go far beyond
providing information or dealing with obvious externalities. In the
United States, especially, the government, in the name of health and
safety, now undertakes detailed regulation and control of thousands
of products and activities. One possible reason for the proliferation
of government interventions is that they serve as a form of "pre-
commitment" concerning certain kinds of behavior. In other words,
Smith may vote for laws that force persons in Brown's circumstances to behave in ways contrary to Brown's preference in order to

pre-commit himself (Smith) if his circumstances should change to those of Brown. Smith, then, might think that if he were to become poor he would be tempted to sell a kidney. He might therefore now vote to make such sales illegal in order to prevent himself from ever taking such action.

I believe that health insurance can in part be regarded as a form of pre-commitment; the insured is pre-committing himself or herself to disregard price in making decisions about the utilization of care. Economists have had a great deal of difficulty explaining the popularity of "first dollar" coverage in health insurance policies. It is easy to see why risk-averse individuals might want to insure against large medical bills, but why would they want to bear the administrative costs and the excess utilization costs associated with insurance for small bills that they could pay out of their normal income? One possible answer is that they do not want money costs to influence their decisions about the utilization of care. *Compulsory* health insurance can be viewed as pre-commitment to buy insurance regardless of changes in income or other circumstances.

Conventional economic analysis regards "pre-commitment" as irrational; why should anyone ever want to gratuitously restrict his options? Economist Richard Thaler has suggested an answer: "pre-commitment" may be a rational strategy for dealing with problems of self-control (Shefrin and Thaler, 1977). Such problems can arise when there is tension between alternative behaviors that have very different implications for our welfare in the short and long run. For instance, in the short run I may get pleasure from smoking or from spending, but I also know that in the long run I will suffer from the effects of smoking or from a lack of savings. I may pre-commit myself by taking a job where smoking is prohibited, and I may join a Christmas Club.

The financial field offers numerous examples of pre-commitment strategies including front-end loaded life insurance policies and mutual fund plans, passbook loans, and prepayment of real estate taxes to banks. Even installment buying has a pre-commitment aspect as evidenced by the many consumers who pay high consumer loan interest rates while maintaining low-yielding savings accounts.

Government regulation may also be a strategy to reduce the opportunity to make decisions that turn out badly. Consider airline safety. Instead of the current practice of setting a single standard of safety, the government could merely provide information about the safety standards adhered to by different airlines and let individuals choose among airlines on the basis of safety, price, and so on. There are costs associated with making airlines safer; one could imagine consumers being offered a choice between a high price/high safety airline and a low price/low safety line. Conventional economics tells us that the larger the range of choice, the greater is consumer welfare. But many (perhaps most) people would not like to make this kind of choice; they prefer to have the Federal Aviation Authority set a single minimum "safe" standard which all scheduled airlines must meet. In so doing, they seek to minimize the regret or guilt that they might experience if there is a crash.

There has been some discussion in economics about the "costs" of decision-making, but these costs have generally been assumed to be experienced in the process of *making* the decision, i.e., acquiring the information and taking time to think about alternatives. Having the government set a single safety standard clearly reduces those costs. The point at issue here, however, is that there are psychic costs associated with having *made* a decision that turns out badly, and individuals may very well opt for government regulations that preclude such decisions.

The growth of government can also be viewed as a substitute for family or church as the principal institution assisting individuals who experience economic or social misfortune. Private insurance could conceivably do the same job, but problems of "free riders" (those who don't buy insurance and then need help anyway), adverse selection (the tendency for the poorer risks to buy the insurance), or excessive sales and administrative costs may make universal, compulsory programs the more sensible way to proceed. Moreover, a principal thrust of many government programs is to combine insurance with *redistribution*. Indeed, I believe that an unrelenting pressure for a more egalitarian society is one of the most important explanations for the growth of government in health and other areas.

The conditions of modern life seem to compel a more equal sharing of material goods and political power. In *Equality and Efficiency: The Big Tradeoff*, Arthur Okun (1975) assumes that this occurs because people have a "preference" for equality. Perhaps some do, but it is also possible that many who have power and goods would rather not share them; their ability to maintain inequality, however, may vary with circumstances. It seems to me that, the more affluent and the more complex a society becomes, the more it depends on the willing, cooperative, conscientious efforts of the people who work in that society and the more difficult it is to obtain satisfactory effort through the use of force.

When the main task at hand consisted of hauling large blocks of stone from the river to the pyramid, it was a relatively simple matter to rope a dozen slaves together and use a whip and the threat of starvation to secure compliance. In feudal societies, the predominantly agricultural work force was kept in line despite huge inequalities in income through force, the need for protection, the limited mobility of the poor, and through the promise of Heaven and the threat of Hell. But when a nation's workers are airplane mechanics, teachers, and operating-room nurses, for example, it is clear that such techniques will not do. A few dissatisfied air-traffic controllers can change the pace of a continent. Even such low-paid work as the changing of tires in a tire store involves considerable potential for danger and disruption. It would be very expensive to check every bolt on every wheel, but the management lives in fear that a few carelessly tightened bolts will allow a wheel to fall off and result in a million-dollar damage suit against the company. Furthermore, in the affluent post-industrial society virtually all persons live above a subsistence level—and will be maintained at above subsistence whether they work or not.

The problem of getting everyone to "go along" is compounded by the declining force of religion, nationalism, and other traditional control structures. Calls to serve "God and Country" do not meet with as enthusiastic a response as they once did, whether that service is military or some onerous and not particularly rewarding civilian task. A weakening of hierarchical structures is evident wherever we look—in the family, in the church, in the school, in the workplace. Romantics of the Right yearn for a return to the "good old days," but such yearning is not likely to avail much against economic growth and technological change. As Norman Macrae (1976) has so aptly noted in *America's Third Century*:

> It is pointless to say . . . that society must therefore return to being ruled by the old conventions, religious restrictions, craven obedience to the convenience of the boss at work. Individuals will not accept these restrictions now they see that wealth and the birth control pill and transport technology make them no longer necessary. . . .

The preoccupation with equality, or the *appearance* of equality, is evident in many discussions about health. With respect to the British National Health Service, for instance, economists John and Sylvia Jewkes (1963) have argued that: "The driving force behind [its] creation . . . was not the search for efficiency or for profitable social investment. It was something quite different: it was a surging national desire to share something equally." As noted in my first lecture, the results of the NHS seem consistent with that view.

Or think of the buckets of ink that have been spilled over regional inequality in the physician/population ratio in Canada, the United States, and most other countries. In the United States, at least, this interminable discussion has proceeded without any evidence that health is adversely affected by a low physician/population ratio. Indeed, in the United States one cannot even show that the number of physician visits per capita is significantly lower in areas that have been identified as "medically underserved." Moreover, the oft-heard argument that an overall increase in the number of physicians will result in a reduction in regional inequality seems to be without empirical foundation.

The more one examines this issue the more puzzling it appears. Nearly everyone says regional inequality in physician supply is bad, but no one quite explains why. Nearly everyone says it should be reduced, but not much is done about reducing it. In California, for a long while we had the spectacle of the state's political leaders voicing loud complaints about how difficult it was to get physicians to settle in rural areas, at the same time setting fee schedules for MediCal (Medicaid) patients that reimbursed rural physicians at a lower rate than their urban counterparts. In my view, national health insurance and other governmental interventions in health are best viewed as political acts undertaken for political and social objectives relatively unrelated to the health of the population. This seems to be an inescapable conclusion from the evidence now available.

The discussion of the proper role of government in society is central to the debate between the ideologues of the Right and the Left, a debate that seems to me to capture a degree of attention far in excess of the merits of the theories propounded by either side. The positions of the arch conservatives and the radicals are usually clear-cut and often provocative. In my judgment, however, they are ultimately unsatisfactory either as analyses of how we have come to our present position or as prescriptions for where we ought to go from here. I shall try to illustrate my proposition with references to health and medical care, but I believe the same critique is valid in a more general framework.

I begin with the Right. And I admit at the outset that some of its favorite themes seem to have considerable value. For one thing, it is the Right that regularly reminds us of the efficiency of a *decentralized* price system as a mechanism for allocating scarce resources. Frankly, it is a shame that we need to be reminded of this—surely, theory and experience combine to teach us that the alternative (some sort of centralized control) will usually be much less efficient.

Second, we should be indebted to the Right for reminding us, in the words of a Milton Friedman lecture title, of "the fragility of freedom." Accustomed as we are to freedom of speech, press, religion, and more, we are too prone to take them for granted—to imagine that they are the normal and expected state of affairs—rather than, as any comprehensive view of past or contemporary societies reveals, a precious exception. When conservatives insist that there are important complementarities between property rights and human rights, we ignore them at our peril.

So much for their good points; where does the Right go wrong? One big problem is that the Right, with the notable exception of Joseph Schumpeter (1942), seems to lack any plausible view of the historical development of society. This is nicely illustrated if one looks at the Right's analysis of the growth of national health insurance around the world.

How does the Right deal with such a phenomenon? The first response (and often the last) is to castigate it as one more deplorable trend toward socialism. When pressed for an explanation of the trend, the Right offers two types of theories. First, there is the "people are stupid" explanation. The same people who are supposedly so knowledgeable when running businesses or choosing occupations or spending money are presumed foolish, irrational, or worse when they must make choices about government policy. This is not very convincing. If there is some widespread behavior that we do not understand, let's not automatically attribute it to the other fellow's ignorance or irrationality.

Not all conservatives subscribe to the "people are stupid" theory. A substantial number try to explain the growth of national health insurance and similar (in their view) misguided legislation as the triumph of special interests over the general public interest. The research strategy is to identify the special groups that gain from policies that seem to result in a general welfare loss (and many economists believe national health insurance fits that category because it encourages excessive utilization). A second task is to figure out how the special groups are able to assert and maintain their interest over that of the majority. Sometimes this strategy is useful, but with respect to the growth of national health insurance, it has not been notably successful. Indeed, in the United States, one special interest group that has benefited greatly from Medicare and Medicaid has been the physicians, and they were in the forefront of the groups that opposed such legislation.

What the Right apparently cannot accept, but neither can it refute, is the hypothesis that national health insurance comes to developed countries not out of ignorance, not out of irrationality, not at the behest of narrowly defined special interest groups, but because most of the people want it, because it meets certain needs better than alternative forms of organization. That these needs are often political, social, and psychological rather than physiological is one of the principal themes of these lectures.

Another problem with the Right is its failure to apply its own economic reasoning to institutions and to goals. For instance, granted that the market is an efficient institution for allocating most goods and services, the extension of the market mechanism to all aspects of human society at the expense of other institutions such as the family may well run into diminishing returns. For the market to be most effective it needs complementary inputs from other institutions, just as capital needs labor and land.

Or consider the Right's preoccupation with the goal of freedom. It is easy to agree that certain basic freedoms of thought and expression are essential to a good society, but more difficult to accept George Stigler's position that freedom should always dominate other goals. He writes (1958 and 1975; italics mine): "The supreme goal of the Western world is the development of the individual: the creation for the individual of a *maximum* area of personal freedom, and with this a corresponding area of personal responsibility." It seems to me odd that an economist would want to maximize personal freedom or any other single goal rather than to find an optimum balance among various goals. Surely, the law of decreasing marginal utility must apply to freedom as well as to other goals, and one suspects that there is increasing marginal disutility to the personal responsibility that Stigler notes is a corollary of freedom. It is reasonable to suppose that there is some *combination* of freedom and responsibility that is optimal, although that optimum probably varies among individuals, depending on their ability to benefit from freedom and to handle responsibility.

Let us turn now to the Left. And let us again begin on a positive note. We should be grateful to the Left for two reasons. First, it reminds us that a decentralized price system isn't *always* the best way to allocate scarce resources. There are things such as externalities and transaction costs that may mean that some allocation problems are better handled by institutions other than the market.

More important, the Left at its best makes a contribution by keeping before us a vision of a just society. Like the prophets of old, it scolds, it warns, it preaches. And so it should. The Left reaffirms in secular form the ancient cry for justice. The big problem with the Left is not its inability to identify important problems. It is its analysis of the causes and its proposed solutions that must give one pause. Who among us would not like to see a world free of war, poverty, racism, sexism, and ignorance? Or, to narrow it down to the field of health, who among us does not think that health is better than illness, life better than death? But to state worthwhile goals is one thing; to have some good ideas about how to reach them is another.

Consider Leftist critiques of health and medical care. First, there is the naive reformist position, typified by, say, John Kenneth Galbraith (1958). According to this view, the problem is one of insufficient public funds. If only we had more hospitals, more physicians, more medical schools, and so on, the problem would be solved. This at a time when, in the United States, there is excess hospital capacity in every major metropolitan area, when general surgeons are carrying what they themselves agree is only 40% of a reasonable workload (and there is widespread suspicion that many of the operations should not be done), and when iatrogenic illness (arising out of the medical care process itself) is a major problem! That so many on the Left can still believe so many shibboleths is a tribute to the triumph of ideology over analysis.

There is another type of Leftist critique, however, which is slightly more sophisticated and far more radical. Far from simply prescribing "more medical care," these Leftist critics argue that the "system" is at fault. The trouble, we are told, is that providers are oriented to profits rather than to health, that if only we made the system more "democratic," placed public health at top priority, put physicians on salaries, and so on, all would be well. Would it? Right now in the United States about 95% of the hospital industry is in the hands of nonprofit organizations, either public or private, yet the escalation in costs in these hospitals has been tremendous, and the emphasis on complex, esoteric technology great. When we look at other systems with other forms of organization and reimbursement, such as in England or Russia, do we see more emphasis on preventive medicine, more action on environmental health problems, more consumer control of the medical care process? The answer is overwhelmingly negative. Indeed, even in China and Cuba, which have done some fine things in delivering simple but effective medical care to the general population, a basic health problem like cigarette smoking is left virtually untouched. Some say this is because certain Communist leaders are avid smokers, or because tobacco is an important crop. Whatever the reason, it is a strange way for these governments to fulfill their self-proclaimed responsibility for the health of the people.

Because the Left is so eager to attribute the problems of the world to capitalism, it ignores some basic observations about human behavior. Most of the health problems that it identifies existed before capitalism and persist in non-capitalist countries. Many problems arise from the conflict between health and other goals, rather than from the evil or selfish intent of physicians. Personal behavior and genetic endowment are far more important to health than is medical care—whatever the system. Even when medical care is relevant, health is rarely something one person can *give* to another. It comes, if at all, from the efforts of physician and patient working together, often in the face of uncertainty and fear.

One of the strongest generalizations warranted by a comparative study of medical care in modern nations is the inability of planning agencies, insurance funds, hospital boards, and other lay authorities to completely control the medical profession. In country after country, the introduction of national health insurance was marked by significant concessions to physicians with respect to methods and levels of reimbursement, procedures for reviewing the quantity and quality of care, geographical and specialty choice, and control over allied (competing?) professions.

What's the problem? In part, the power of physicians derives from their ability to withhold what is sometimes an essential service. A strike by physicians may not be as threatening as one by coal miners in winter, or bartenders on New Year's Eve, but it is not negligible. Emigration by physicians is a more distant, but probably more effective, threat against unacceptable pressure. Because medical skills are more easily transferred from one country to another than are those of most other professions, and because physicians earn a high income, their return to migration is large relative to costs.

In my opinion, more subtle factors are also at work. The effectiveness of medical care depends in considerable measure on a bond of mutual confidence between physician and patient. Too much external control can break that bond. Moreover, physicians, like priests or magicians, can fill their roles effectively only if set apart from the common run of mankind. A medical profession that was completely subservient to lay authority would be, in several respects, a less effective profession. This is not to say that fee-for-service reimbursement never leads to over-utilization, or that licensure laws are completely in the public interest, or that present institutional arrangements are ideal. It is to say that many of the most difficult problems of health and medical care transcend particular forms of economic and political organization—a conclusion that the Left leaves out.

Concluding Remarks

These lectures are drawing to a close. The time has come for me to restate my own conclusions and value judgments as clearly as possible. What speculative generalizations do I draw from a broad economic study of health and medical care in modern society? First, I am impressed by the widespread confusion between process and product, the tendency to identify medical care with health, even though the connection is a fairly limited one. I wonder if that same confusion does not exist in other aspects of society, for example, schooling vis-à-vis wisdom, litigation vis-à-vis justice, or police activity vis-à-vis public safety? In the case of medical care and national health insurance, it seems clear to me that institutions often serve purposes other than those that are explicitly articulated. From the health insurance of Bismarck's administration to the Professional Standards Review Organizations of Nixon's, we can see sharp differences between the stated and the actual intent of health legislation.

The growth of big government in modern society stands as a major challenge for social analysis. My reading of its role in health and medical care leads me to emphasize two factors—the decline of other institutions and the pressure for a more egalitarian society. It seems clear to me that the success of the market system in the Western world was attributable in no small measure to the existence of strong non-market institutions such as the family and religion. The fruits of the market system—science, technology, urbanization, affluence—are undermining these institutions, which were the foundations of the social order. Human beings need more than an abundance of material goods. They need a sense of purpose in life—secure relationships with other human beings—something or someone to believe in. With the decline of the family and of religion, the inability of the market system to meet such needs becomes obvious, and the state rushes in to fill the vacuum. But it does so imperfectly because it is so large and so impersonal.

The affluence and complexity of modern life also contribute to the pressure for more equality, and government is now the chief institution for undertaking redistributive functions. This is not to suggest that the pressure for equality is always met quickly and fully. On the contrary, much legislation is designed to give symbolic recognition of the ideal of equality, but does not involve significant redistribution. This is not necessarily to be condemned; a preoccupation with equality and the neglect of other goals can be socially harmful. It is useful to recall Lord Acton's comment on the French Revolution (1907): "The finest opportunity ever given to the world was thrown away because the passion for equality made vain the hope of freedom."

For all its weakness, the family is probably still the greatest single barrier to equality in post-industrial society. As long as mothers and fathers pass on to their offspring their own particular genetic endowment, their own special heritage and values, attempts to achieve complete equality will be frustrated. At some point we shall have to ask whether that last increment of equality is worth the loss of so valuable an institution as the family—one that can stand as a refuge from impersonal markets and authoritarian government.

Government also grows because the majority frequently sees no feasible alternative for dealing with the complexity and interdependence of modern life. Thus, it seems to me that the fulminations of the Right against the ever-increasing role of government are often misdirected. The constant assertions that this or that regulation or subsidy is irrational and inefficient often fall on deaf ears because the majority doesn't see it that way. As I have tried to show with illustrations from health, some individual governmental interventions can perhaps be justified economically—because of economies of scale, or because of externalities (tangible or psychological), or as precommitment strategies, or as techniques for shifting responsibility, or as redistributive mechanisms introduced to buy social tranquility. The point that I think needs emphasis is that the cumulative impact of the growth of government is to weaken (and ultimately destroy) other useful institutions such as the market, family, and private associations of a religious, fraternal, and philanthropic character. Thus, we should be wary of the constant expansion of government, and especially centralized government, not only because any particular proposed expansion is "inefficient"—it may well pass a comprehensive cost-benefit test for a majority of the population—but because there are other goals besides efficiency.

For me the key word is *balance*, both in the goals that we set and in the institutions that we nourish in order to pursue these goals. I value freedom *and* justice *and* efficiency, and economics tells me that I may have to give up a little of one goal to insure the partial achievement of others. Moreover, I believe the best way to seek multiple goals is through a multiplicity of institutions—the market, government, the family, and others. No single institution is superior for all goals. Also, diversification, be it of institutions, genes, or security holdings, is the best assurance of stability and survival in the face of an uncertain future. Above all, we must avoid concentration of power. In the spirit of the lowered aspirations of our time, I conclude that, although diffusion of power may keep us from reaching Utopia, it also limits the harm that may befall us.

References

Lord Acton. 1907. History of Freedom in Christianity. In Figgis, J. N., and Laurence, R. V., eds., *History of Freedom and Other Essays.* p. 57. (Reprinted in 1971 by Arno Publishers, New York.)

Bell, D. 1973. *The Coming of Post-Industrial Society.* New York: Basic Books, Inc.

Calabresi, G. C., and Bobbitt, P. 1978. *Tragic Choices.* New York: W. W. Norton.

Clark, C. 1940. *The Conditions of Economic Progress.* London: Macmillan.

Davis, C., and Feshbach, M. 1978. Life Expectancy in the Soviet Union. *The Wall Street Journal* (June 20).

Dubos, R. 1959. *The Mirage of Health.* New York: Harper.

Fuchs, V. R. 1968. The Growing Demand for Medical Care. *The New England Journal of Medicine* 279 (July 25): 190–195.

_____. 1974. Some Economic Aspects of Mortality in Developed Countries. In Perlman, M., ed., *The Economics of Health and Medical Care.* Proceedings of a Conference Held by the International Economic Association at Tokyo. pp. 174–193. London: Macmillan.

_____. 1978. The Service Industries and U.S. Economic Growth Since World War II. In Backman, J, ed., *Economic Growth or Stagnation?* Indianapolis, Ind.: Bobbs-Merrill.

Galbraith, J. K. 1958. *The Affluent Society.* Boston, Mass.: Houghton Mifflin Co.

Garrison, L. 1978. Studies in the Economics of Surgery. Unpublished Ph.D. Thesis, Stanford University, Stanford, Calif.

Gordon, H. S. 1971. Social Institutions, Change and Progress. *The E. S. Woodward Lectures in Economics.* p. ix. Vancouver, B.C., Canada: University of British Columbia.

Grossman, M. 1976. The Correlation between Health and Schooling. In Terleckyj, N. E., ed., *Household Production and Consumption.* pp. 147–223. National Bureau of Economic Research. Vol. 40, Studies in Income and Wealth. New York: Columbia University Press.

Jewkes, J., and Jewkes, S. 1963. *Value for Money in Medicine.* Oxford, England: Blackwell.

Lalonde, M. 1974. *A New Perspective on the Health of Canadians.* Ottawa, Ontario, Canada: Government of Canada.

Macrae, N. 1976. *America's Third Century,* p. 90. New York: Harcourt Brace Jovanovich.

Newhouse, J. P., and Friedlander, M. J. 1977. *The Relationship between Medical Resources and Measures of Health: Some Additional Evidence.* Rand Corporation Document R-2066-HEW (May). Santa Monica, Calif.: The Rand Corporation.

Okun, M. 1975. *Equality and Efficiency, the Big Tradeoff.* Washington, D.C.: The Brookings Institution.

Preston, S. H. 1979 (forthcoming). Causes and Consequences of Mortality Declines in Less Developed Countries During the Twentieth Century. In Easterlin, R., ed., *Population and Economic Change in Developing Countries.* New York: National Bureau of Economic Research. Chicago, Ill.: University of Chicago Press.

Schumpeter, J. S. 1942. *Capitalism, Socialism and Democracy.* New York: Harper and Brothers.

Shefrin, H. M., and Thaler, R. 1977. An Economic Theory of Self-Control. Working Paper 208. New York: National Bureau of Economic Research.

Stigler, G. J. 1958 and 1975. The Goals of Economic Policy. First published as a pamphlet by the University of Chicago Law School, March, 1958. Printed in the *Journal of Business:* 169 (July), 1958. Reprinted in *The Journal of Law and Economics* 18 (2) (October): 283–292, 1975.

Tawney, R. H. 1926. *Religion and the Rise of Capitalism*. New York: Harcourt Brace and Company.

Townsend, P. 1974. Inequality and the Health Service. *The Lancet* (June 15): 1179 ff.

SECTION II

CONSUMPTION

5. The Concept of Need for Health Services

KENNETH E. BOULDING

Reprinted from *The Milbank Memorial Fund Quarterly/Health and Society* 44. Copyright © 1966, Milbank Memorial Fund 202-221.

The concept of need is often looked upon rather unfavorably by economists, in contrast with the concept of demand. Both, however, have their own strengths and weaknesses. The need concept is criticized as being too mechanical, as denying the autonomy and individuality of the human person, and as implying that the human being is a machine which "needs" fuel in the shape of food, engine dope in the shape of medicine, and spare parts provided by the surgeon. Even if the need concept is expanded to include psychological and emotional needs, the end result would seem to be a wire run into the pleasure center of the brain which could provide a life of unlimited and meaningless ecstasy. Demand, by contrast, implies autonomy of the individual, choice, and a tailoring of inputs of all kinds to individual preferences. Only the slave has needs; the free man has demands.

In spite of the economist's uneasiness about it, a considerable demand exists for the concept of need. As even the most liberal of economists cannot deny the right of a demand to call forth a supply, the development and elaboration of concepts of need can hardly be denied. The demand, however, may be for a number of different concepts, and a single concept will not serve the purpose. The demands for this concept are quite varied, and the supply must be correspondingly differentiated. No single concept of need exists, and especially no single concept of need for health services.

One demand for a concept of need arises because the concept of demand itself has serious weaknesses and limitations. It assumes away, for instance, a serious epistemological problem. The very idea of autonomous choice implies first that the chooser knows the real alternatives which are open to him, and second that he makes the choice according to value criteria or a utility function which he will not later regret. Both the image of the field of choice and the utility function have a learning problem which, by and large, economists have neglected. This problem is particularly acute in the case of medical care, where the demander is usually a layman faced with professional suppliers who know very much more than he does. The demand for medical care, indeed, is primarily a demand for knowledge or at least the results of knowledge. In the case of ordinary commodities the knowledge that is required is fairly easily available and the market itself is a learning process. If one buys something he does not like he will not buy it again. In the case of medical care, however, as in the case of certain other commodities such as automobiles, the learning process can easily be fatal, in which case it is not a learning process at all. In any case the experience of the market cannot teach people what they have to know in regard to the choices they have to make, or even what preference functions they should use in evaluating these choices.

The concept of need which emerges from the criticism of demand is that of professional choice. It is implied to some extent in the very idea of the patient or the client, and it is expressed in the aphorism that doctor (or father, or lawyer, or preacher, or president) knows best. One's demand for medical care is what he wants; his need for medical care is what the doctor thinks he ought to have. The demand for medical care leads to the proliferation of drug stores, patent medicines, osteopaths, chiropractors and faith healers.

That is the market for medical care and it is a large one. It spills over into the medical profession itself, in private practice and the reputation of particular doctors and surgeons, in the prestige of Harley Street and its equivalents in many cities, and it includes both the medicine cabinet in the bathroom and the psychiatrist's couch. It can be thought of as an "industry" or segment of the economy; it is subject to the general principles of the price system, in the sense that wherever a demand is sufficient to make a supply profitable it will arise, even though this principle has to be limited also by the power of the ingenious supplier to create his own demand.

In contrast with the market in medical care, an increasingly professionalized, socialized, organized structure satisfies what the professional conceives of as needs. The periodic medical examinations in corporations and universities, the veterans' hospitals, the school doctor, public health, the professional public provision of clean water and sewage disposal—all this represents a professionalized sector of the economy, characterized by professions which set their own standards of what they ought to do and which are financed by taxation or near-taxation. Among these are Blue Cross and other health insurance plans, Medicare, or even private clinics supported by monthly assessments. Here the activity originates from the profession rather than from the client, from the supplier rather than from the demander. In its extreme form it takes on the flavor of, "What you need is what I as your professional advisor have to give you; what you want is quite irrelevant."

The idea of professional need always rests on some definition of homeostasis or state maintenance of the client, his property or his environment. The professional defines a certain state of his client and his related systems as a state of "health" which he has a professional interest in maintaining. The course of operations of any system, however, involves consumption. That is, the state of the client and his environment change in some way and become "worse," or diverge in a downward direction from the ideal. The ideal in this case is the professional's ideal, that is, his impression of what state should be maintained. The maintenance of a state, however, requires certain inputs to replace what has been lost by consumption. It may also require the professional handling of certain outputs, such as excreta, which must be removed and disposed of if the organism or organization is to continue to maintain its state of activity. A very fundamental principle in nature implies that any state of activity can only be maintained by a throughput involving both inputs and outputs. In part that may be because inputs come in packages in practice, only part of which can be utilized, and what is not utilized must therefore be excreted as output. Even more fundamental reasons, however, dictate the presence of output in the form of excreta, whether gases from automobile exhaust, carbon dioxide given off in breathing or waste products of the digestive process. The transformation of chemical into mechanical energy, on which all organization seems to depend almost universally, seems to require an input of oxygen and an output of an oxide.

This suggests that certain minimum mechanical, chemical, biological, physiological, even economic and sociological requirements exist for the functioning of any organism or organization. That in turn suggests that the concept of professional need can be broken down into two further problems; one the problem of what might be called homeostatic need. That is, what is actually required to maintain a given system in operation. The other is the problem of perception or knowledge of homeostatic need. That is, can the system itself be trusted to maintain the inputs and outputs necessary to satisfy homeostatic need, or is a professional required with a wider body of knowledge who can perceive and prescribe the homeostatic needs? Homeostatic needs can be divided into two categories, those which can be taken care of by the organism itself and those which require a professional decision.

These categories can be illustrated by pointing to certain undignified analogies between the human being as an organization and an item of material capital such as an automobile. Both require inputs of air if they are to function, and the air must be reasonably pure, though usually only automobiles are provided with air filters. Each of them pollutes the air they breathe with the byproducts of combustion, and unless fresh air can be constantly supplied continued operation will become impossible. Both the man and the automobile require food; carbohydrates, proteins and fats in the case of the human, gasoline and oil in the case of the automobile. A certain parallel can even be drawn between the vitamins of the human and the various additives of gasoline. The parallel is particularly striking in Scandinavian countries where automobiles are "buttered," not greased. Food input is usually administered on a fairly nonprofessional basis. The automobile owner buys gas for his car in very much the same way as he buys food for himself, with a certain amount of professional advice but not much professional interference. In the course of operation of the system, internal stocks of food are used up fairly continuously and they have to be replaced at intervals. The auto-

mobile takes its dinner at the gas station, which is a kind of automobile restaurant.

The input of food and of fuel and the output of its waste products are not, however, sufficient. In the course of operation, both of the automobile and of the human, wear and tear occur. Consequently, not only are gas stations, restaurants and food stores needed, but also garages and hospitals. At this level need becomes professionalized. The greasing every thousand miles or the annual physical examination may be fairly routine, though at this point one begins to think of medical care for either automobile or man rather than simple fueling and feeding. The professional need is most apparent in breakdown, that is, when the subject simply refuses to function even when fueled and fed. Then the car goes to the garage, where mechanics perform operations on it, and the human goes to the hospital where surgeons perform operations on him. The atmosphere of the garage, indeed, is curiously like that of the hospital. The garage is permeated by the same air of professional importance, the same feeling that the customer is rather in the way, the same rather offhand bedside manner, the same assumption that the customer or the patient is, professionally speaking, an ignoramus, if not a fool. In fact, the principal difference between the garage and the hospital seems to be that the hospital is cleaner and more expensive. The concept of professional need appears in the helplessness of the customer. All he knows is that he hears a funny noise in the gear box or has a pain in his stomach. Once he puts himself into the hands of the professional, demand disappears and no substitute exists for trust in the professional's concept of need.

The difficulty with homeostasis as the basis for a concept of need is that homeostasis is never really successful. No matter what occurs in the way of inputs, virtually all known organisms and organizations exhibit the phenomenon of aging, which is closely related to the phenomenon of growth. Aging is common both to machines and to biological organisms, and it might almost be defined as that adverse change in state of the organism which no known input can remedy. In biological organisms, growth is actually rather similar. It can be thought of, indeed, as a kind of negative aging. The inputs of the growing child have to be sufficient not only to provide for replacement, but also to provide for growth. Growth, however, is almost as unpreventable as aging. Mechanical organizations such as the automobile are not generally subject to growth. They are more like the moth or the butterfly in that they emerge fully grown from the chrysalis of the factory, and henceforth are subject only to aging. Up to now very little is known about aging, at least in the case of the biological organism. It can perhaps be hastened by certain inputs or outputs or by certain deficiencies in input, which is also true of the automobile. In both cases, a life of hard work and poor nutrition results in premature aging. Up to now, at any rate, any inputs which would postpone the aging process beyond the allotted span have not been discovered. If they are, as seems not impossible, at least in the next 100 years, the human race will probably be faced with the greatest crisis of its history, for no existing human institution would survive in its present form the extension of active human life even to 200 years.[1]

Aging introduces a very tricky problem into the concept of need for maintenance, which is difficult enough even in the case of the machine, more difficult in the case of the horse, and a problem of excruciating delicacy in the case of the human being. The problem with the machine is at what point in its history it should be scrapped. The formal answer to this is fairly easy: a machine should be scrapped when its present value as a functioning apparatus, derived by discounting the future costs and benefits to be allocated to it, has fallen just below the net value of a possible replacement. The net value is defined as the present discounted value of future benefits less that of all future and installment costs of the replacement plus the scrap value of the machine which is replaced. With no technical progress and if the machine is replaced by one exactly like it when new, the main factor determining the age at which it will be replaced is the increase in the maintenance cost and perhaps a decrease in its output as it gets older. Where technical change occurs a machine may be scrapped because of obsolescence, that is, because of a rise in the net value of what might replace it.

A machine is generally regarded as having no value in itself, that is, its value is purely instrumental; hence the owner feels no qualms about scrapping it if he feels such action is necessary. Even horses, however, when they can no longer fulfill their economic function, are sometimes put out to pasture in honorable retirement at some cost to their owners. In the case of the human being, the problem of the person himself becomes very acute, because persons cannot be regarded as purely instrumental. That is, they are not merely good for something else, they are good in themselves. They are, in other words, something *for which* other things are good. Whereas the death of a machine is determined mainly by economic forces, this principle is quite inapplicable to persons, where, in theory at any rate, the person supposedly possesses a positive value even up to the moment of death, and death, therefore, is always regarded as a loss. When death occurred mainly in childhood or middle life, this principle could evoke no criticism. As medical science, however, has successively eliminated the causes of early death, the fiction that death is always an "act of God" is increasingly difficult to maintain.

At this point the concept of professional need for medical care becomes most difficult. Should the medical profession devote a relatively large proportion of its resources, as it does now, in keeping miserable and senile elderly people alive, when their capital value even to themselves has become negative? Men, even physicians, have a reasonable aversion to playing God and to introducing a nonrandom element in what has hitherto been sanctified as random. The only solution may be to substitute an artificially random process for the natural randomness by which death came in the past. If death could be arranged by drawing a random number, perhaps by hiding one euthanasia pill in the nursing home diet each week, the Godlike power of the medical man might be laid on the shoulders of Chance, and death might be restored to its former dignity.

A proposal such as the above will seem deeply shocking to many people, and indeed, is put forward only in the form of a most tentative question, intended merely to illustrate a problem which is likely to be more and more prevalent. One principle in the spirit of the Hippocratic Oath to be argued for very strongly is that the person himself must decide at what point death or the chance of death is preferred to life, and no one else should have the right to make this decision for him. At this point, surely, demand must take precedence of need, and the autonomy of the patient be reasserted. Even at the moment of making this assertion, however, and nailing it to the masthead, realistic doubts arise. At what point, for instance, do people become incapable of making decisions for themselves? That is a question of immediate practical importance for the medical profession, for even if they do not have the power at the moment of consigning people to eternity, they do have the power of consigning them to what is often the living death of the mental hospital, and the moral problems of the latter are surely of the same order of magnitude as those of the former. Nevertheless, people do become incompetent and incapable of managing their own affairs. Society has decided that mental hospitals must exist, and along with them the machinery for committing people to them. Who is better able to estimate hat professional need than the medical profession, especially when its decisions are mediated through the apparatus of the law? One sobering thought, however, is that a person virtually ceases to be

a legal person when he ceases to have demands and has only needs.

Some of the above problems may well reflect a lag in society in the development of a professional sense of what the needs of the incompetent and the aged in fact ought to be. A marked shift has taken place in the care of the aged, from the family into hospitals and nursing homes. Even two generations ago most people died in their own beds in the bosom of their families, amid the consolations of religion and the ministrations of a beloved family physician. Such, at least, is the idyllic picture; the reality was probably more disagreeable. Nevertheless, of the people who die of old age today, most die in nursing homes, old people's homes, and hospitals, away from the comforts of the familiar and the ministrations of kin. No great deal of thought has been devoted to the needs of the departing, and none at all to the need for death. Death, however, is a medical matter. It is certainly part of the need for medical care, if such exists, and it deserves to receive a great deal more care and attention than it has in the past. That is not to suggest that the medical profession should abandon its concern for the needs of the incompetent, the aged and the dying; rather that more attention be given to this problem, both in medical research, so that vigor and physical well-being can be prolonged until the end, and in social and moral research that can devise economic, financial, architectural and social institutions which will give dignity and serenity to the last years of life and will not deprive its end of the majesty which is due it.

At the other end of human life, the increasing control, which the biological sciences seem to be opening up in genetics, presents even more difficult problems in regard to the need for medical activity. If the rights of the living and the dying are hard to determine, the rights of the unborn are an even more difficult problem. The whole problem of population control, in fact, in regard to both quantity and quality, is moving more and more onto the shoulders of the health sciences, and it is a problem for which they cannot escape responsibility. In the last 15 years, the spectacular decline in infant mortality which followed the introduction of malaria control in the tropics has created social problems which seem to be virtually insoluble in the next 15 to 20 years.

One must think here in terms of the homeostasis, not merely of the individual, but of a whole society. When, as a result of the introduction of certain public health measures, a society which previously was in approximate demographic equilibrium, with high birth rates and high death rates, suddenly finds the death rates drastically reduced while the birth rates continue high, an enormous long-run social disequilibrium is created which may have quite unforeseen consequences, both for good and for ill. Many societies in the tropics are now increasing in population at unprecedented rates—between three and four per cent per annum—and this in itself places an enormous burden on the poor society which is anxious for development. When the population doubles every 20 years a whole new country must be built, and the whole physical apparatus of a society doubled in a relatively short space of time, even if per capita capital is not to decline. If the country is already fairly thickly populated, with no unused land areas of any magnitude, the sheer problem of doubling the food supply in 20 years is almost insoluble, and a slow and deadly reduction in nutritive levels can easily follow.

Add to this gloomy picture the fact that in these countries most of the working force was born before the great decline in infant mortality and hence is small. That small working force has to support an enormous number of children and young people—in many of these countries more than half the population is now under the age of 18. Furthermore, very large teenage generations now exist which cannot be absorbed in the traditional structure, especially of the village society, and are forced to migrate to the towns. The towns, because of the phenom-

enon of what has been called the "rural push," are growing much faster than the population itself, some of them as much as 15 per cent annually which means doubling every five years. Under these circumstances providing housing and municipal services is impossible, and enormous slums and shack towns spread over the landscape like a blight. These circumstances dictate an extremely pessimistic forecast for the next 25 years for many of these countries. On the other hand, if a massive campaign for birth reduction takes place now, so that birth rates could be halved in five or ten years, then the next generation will be a large labor force able to cope with the smaller numbers of children and that will be the moment when these countries may be able to make the leap into the modern world. In the absence of substantial reduction in birth rates, however, the outlook is bleak indeed. Enormous famines, disastrous internal strife and even total civil breakdown may be expected. All this may well be the result of the World Health Organization's malaria eradication campaign in the years around 1950.

On the other side of the picture, without a substantial increase in the expectation of life, and particularly without the elimination of mortality in the productive years, economic development is also very difficult. An essential step toward the modern world is the introduction of modern medicine and the elimination of the appalling waste of human knowledge and human capital which occurs in countries where human life expectancy is little more than 30 years. The ideal situation would be a sharp reduction in the death rate and an equally sharp reduction in the birth rate, so that the demographic equilibrium was not unduly disturbed. Even if this happy result were unobtainable, a certain disturbance of the demographic equilibrium is entirely desirable in the interest of development, and a public health campaign is at least a start in disturbing the low-level equilibrium of a traditional society.

These problems present great difficulties, even for social scientists, and up to now at any rate the medical sciences have been extraordinarily lax in attending to them. Medicine has considered health mainly in terms of inputs to an individual, not to a society. The possibility of an acute conflict between the health of the individual and that of his society is a problem that has received scandalously little attention. Now the tables have been turning, and birth control has become fashionable and respectable, almost to the point of being advocated as a panacea for all developmental difficulties. Quantitative population control, however, is only a part of the general problem of what might be called societal health, which is not the same thing, incidentally, as public health. Public health concerns itself primarily with the environmental factors affecting the health of the individual. Societal health deals with the factors that determine the health of the whole society, and societies can be sick even when the individuals in them are medically well.

The problem of qualitative population control is beginning to rise seriously onto the human agenda. The eugenics movements of the nineteenth century were premature, and based on wholly inadequate genetic concepts. With the enormous advance in genetics in this century, however, the problems of the genetic composition of future populations are no longer as random as they used to be. Indeed, a recurrent nightmare is that all the medical advances will eventually prove ineffective simply because the improved techniques of individual survival will enable more and more adverse genetic strains to penetrate the population. In his argument against that position, Medawar says that if a genetic adaptation to medical knowledge produces more people who have to be kept alive by "artificial" means, nothing is particularly wrong with that, because genetics always adapts itself to the environment and medical knowledge is part of the environment of man.[2] The argument, however, is not wholly

satisfactory, simply because of the cost of medical care for those whose genetic constitution requires it. If the existence of medical care produces a population of the genetic composition which requires it, the whole system seems to be self-defeating. Whatever level of medical care is established, no matter how high and how elaborate, one can argue that in the long run the genetic composition of the population will deteriorate to the point where the established level of medical care becomes necessary. In this case the level of medical care creates its own need. No objective need exists which determines the level of medical care.

Looking to the rather long run, therefore, one would expect to find large payoffs in research devoted to altering the genetic composition of the population in directions which would minimize the cost of medical care. Conceivably, genetic control might eliminate medical care almost entirely, except for accidents; for some genetic constitutions are extraordinarily resistant to disease, and if these could be propagated in the population, the need for medical care would correspondingly decline.

In the next few decades, the possibility of changing genetic constitutions even after birth is not wholly off the agenda, although it certainly seems to be difficult. Even without that, however, the possibility of genetic control at the moment of conception opens up an enormous and rather frightening horizon to the human race, even though this would also open up enormous possibilities for good. Certainly the elimination of the more obvious genetic-related diseases or conditions would be a great gain. The ethical problems involved at this end of the scale, however, are just as severe as those at the other end relating to death. At what point, for instance, in the life history of a person does he have any rights? Opinion seems to have shifted in this regard toward the moment of birth as the point at which human rights are acquired. The increasingly favorable public opinion in regard to abortion would seem to imply that the embryo has no rights, whereas the infant does, as infanticide is still severely censored. If, however, the process of conception can be controlled and, for instance, selective gene structures implanted in the egg, the question of the human rights even of the fertilized egg becomes acute. That again is a problem because the ethical standards and ideas of the human race have been adapted to processes of birth and death which in the past have been essentially random, and substituting nonrandom for random processes always produces an acute moral crisis. Perhaps some consensus might be salvaged with elimination of certain obviously maladaptive genetic traits, for instance mongolism and obvious feeblemindedness. Even considering the elimination of hemophilia, enough distinguished people have had this disability to suggest that something might be lost by eliminating it. The ethical problems become even more acute with the proposal to alter genetic structures positively. The production of a race of supermen who would supersede the present generation might not be regarded favorably by ordinary mortals.

Underlying all this discussion is a seldom-discussed specter regarding the idea of health itself. Even assuming the very simple position that need involves merely the maintenance of homeostasis, the question as to what state of the organism is to be maintained still has to be answered. That is like the problem of at what temperature the thermostat should be set. Every homeostatic mechanism implies an ideal, and the question of the critique of the ideal itself, therefore, cannot be brushed aside. In particular, the conclusion cannot be avoided that within limits which may be quite broad, health is a matter of social definition. Societies and cultures do exist in which what is now defined here as ill health is somewhat admired. One recalls W. S. Gilbert's pale young curate, whose tubercular charms in the eyes of the village maidens even outweighed those of gilded dukes and belted earls. In some societies, epilepsy is regarded as a sign of divine favor. The limits of what is socially defined as physical health are so narrow that not much of a problem arises.

With mental health and human behavior in society, however, the limits seem to be broader, and the matter of social definition more important. For instance, should the problem of homosexuality be considered a problem in mental health, to be "cured," even if no cure seems to be currently available, or should it be regarded as a legitimate variation of human behavior, to be accepted and regulated by custom and law? A rather similar problem involving the acceptance of deviant subcultures has descended upon society with the development of the psychedelic drugs such as mescaline and LSD. Some claim that these are legitimate avenues to the expansion of human consciousness and others claim that these are dangerous drugs the use of which should be prohibited by law, except under medical supervision, and that unauthorized users should be punished as criminals. A similar conflict of voices is raised on behalf of marijuana, some people claiming that it affords a legitimate expansion of human consciousness and is no more dangerous than alcohol. The prevailing sentiment, however, is to lash out at the use of these drugs with all the ferocity of criminal law.

The failure to deal with alcohol, which has been with the human race for a long time and is certainly the earliest of the psychedelic drugs, is not an optimistic indication that society will be able to deal with a succession of new chemical and perhaps electrical devices, such as the "pleasure wire," which produce various types of euphoria. One remembers with a slight shudder the use of soma as a social tranquilizer in *Brave New World*. Even in the medical field, not very much is known about the impact on society of the enormous use of the tranquilizing drugs both in medical practice and in private life in the past few years. The frightening possibility of a society steeped in agreeable chemical illusions to the point where it becomes quite incapable either of recognizing or solving its real problems is by no means a matter only for science fiction.

Different societies have given very different answers to these questions, and they constitute merely one aspect of a much larger question as to the boundary between health, morality and law. In many fields the problem is defining the point at which behavior which is in some sense disapproved or regarded as below normal is defined as sickness or is defined as turpitude. In this society a long-term movement has attempted to push this boundary to define fewer things as turpitude and more things as sickness. Nevertheless, no golden rule dictates where this line should be drawn. In Samuel Butler's *Erewhon,* crime was treated by doctors and illness by policemen, and one has an uneasy suspicion that this might work too. The problem of the overall effects upon society of its system of punishment is very little understood, and the line between the need for medical care and the need for criminal prosecution is really quite hard to draw.

A question which is even more fundamental and still more difficult to answer, but which should not remain unasked, is whether the concept of ill health can be applied to moral and political ideas themselves. For instance, do diseases of the moral judgment exist, and if so, are they subject to epidemics? How are these epidemics spread? The rise of National Socialism in Germany and McCarthyism in the United States, of witch-hunting, war moods and irrational hatreds in innumerable societies, indicates that the concept of disease in the moral and political judgment is worth taking seriously, even though it is very hard to define. One may be able to define something like mass infections of unrealistic images of the world, if only one could be sure what is realistic. Whether these phenomena fall under the purview of the medical profession is, of course, a debatable point. The medical profession has long been

required in forensic medicine to advise on the medical status of a possible criminal act. Perhaps, one day it may be called in to determine the medical status of a political act or even of a moral exhortation. The difficulty here, and it is a real one, is that, up to now at any rate, a clear physical correlate of mental, moral and political ill health does not exist. The idea is not wholly far-fetched, however, to suppose such physical correlates do exist and that the discovery will be made one day of a drug against malevolence or another that increases good will. Even if the physical correlates are hard to find, the status of psychoanalysis as a medical speciality suggests possible extensions into therapeutic communication in moral, political and social systems.

Society is so accustomed to thinking of the problem of the interrelations of government, science and medicine in terms of the impact of government on science and medicine that people are at a loss when asked to consider the impact of science and medicine on government. Nevertheless, that may well become one of the major questions in advanced societies in the next generation or two. Political decisions are still made largely in the light of what might be called folk knowledge or at best literary knowledge. The scientist is supposedly to serve the values and interests of the folk but he is not to insert any values and interests of his own. He is supposedly an instrument of the state or at least of the people and not an autonomous creator of values and needs. That is the point of view of the famous aphorism that the scientist in government should be on tap but not on top, and that he would be a humble servant of folk and national values. That, however, is a most unrealistic estimate of the present situation. Science is not a passive servant of existing values. It has its own culture, it creates its own values, and because of its enormous impact on the world, it compels a re-examination of values everywhere.

The role of the social sciences in this respect is even more striking than that of the physical and biological sciences. The physical or biological scientist operates in a different field from that of the politician. The special skills of the scientist in, say, physics or physiology give him very little comparative advantage in attempting to answer a question in social systems. In respect to the economic system or the international system, the physicist or biologist has as much right to be heard as any intelligent citizen, but no more. The social scientist, however, occupies the same field as the politician and is in direct competition with him. The possibility of severe conflict between the folk culture and the scientific culture is thus present at this level. Up to now the conflict has been muted only because it has hardly begun; because the social sciences are only barely at the point where they can begin to challenge the folk wisdom of the politician. Economics already has a kind of establishment of "Lords Spiritual" in the Council of Economic Advisors and in the Joint Committee in Congress. The impact of this establishment is already noticeable in economic policy, and the United States is by no means the most advanced country in this regard. The other social sciences, and least of all what might be called the sociomedical sciences of clinical psychology and psychiatry, still seem to be a long way from any such status. The possibility, however, that one of the needs for medical care may be defined in the future as political mental health, though it may sound absurd at the moment, should not be taken lightly. Society is already beginning to see that the automobile is a problem in public health; to regard the Department of Defense as a similar problem is a simple logical extension of this position, for the present international system is almost certainly more dangerous to health than the automobile and far more dangerous than most communicable diseases.

Even at this point, the ambiguity can be maintained between demand as defined by the consumer and need as defined by the professional. All fields of life seem to feel the necessity for working out an uneasy compromise between these two concepts. Undiluted consumer sovereignty, whether in economics or politics, where it takes the form of the absolute sovereignty of the voter and the sovereignty of the nation, is ultimately intolerable and leads to corruption and disaster. On the other hand, total professionalization, in the case of the doctor, the economist, the sociologist or the political scientist, is likewise intolerable, if only for the reason that having that much father-image is intolerable; and the revolt against paternalism, no matter how benign, is an essential aspect of the human identity. Somewhere between the proposition that the customer is always right and the proposition that the public be damned must be an uneasy Aristotelian mean, and toward this the concept of professional need for medical care or for anything else uneasily steers itself.

The word need has a number of meanings, and the idea of homeostatic need or professional need which we have been discussing does not exhaust it. Another very important connotation of the word is that implied in the word "needy." One's need in this sense is not merely what some wise professional person thinks one ought to have, but what one cannot afford because he is poor. In this sense also, need is thought of as something which stands in contrast with demand, and the need for a concept of need arises because of certain deficiencies in demand as a principle of allocation. The concept of need as a criticism of demand here refers to the fact that effective demand is closely related to income and to the distribution of income. Need is an equalitarian concept. It recalls the famous communist slogan, "From each according to his ability, to each according to his need."

Demand, perhaps because of its very stress on autonomy and freedom, is libertarian rather than equalitarian, and liberty is seldom equally divided. If medical care is distributed according to demand, the rich will get most of it and the poor very little. One of the main concerns of society for the need for medical care, therefore, is the fact that a sizeable proportion of the population is "medically indigent" in the sense that its income is not large enough to provide a demand for the minimum medical care which a society, or a profession, identifies as need. That may be a part of the general problem of the social minimum. At present nearly all societies have a deliberate policy to establish a minimum standard life below which citizens are not supposed to fall. Whether the policy is in fact successful is another matter, for in almost all cases some people do fall below the minimum, and all the machinery of society is now powerful enough to elevate them. Nevertheless, the principle of a social minimum has been established for a long time and today is almost universally accepted.

Even the acceptance of a social minimum, however, does not necessarily resolve the conflict between need and demand. Some argue that insofar as the problem is one of poverty, the only solution to this is to make the poor richer, either by giving them money, by improving their skills or by integrating them more fully into the culture around them. Once the poor have been made richer, the problem of the need for medical care resolves itself essentially into the problem discussed earlier of a consumer's demand versus professional need, between which poles some uneasy compromise must be reached.

In the case of medical indigency, however, the temptation is to deny consumers sovereignty as the price of the relief of indigency, and to say that the poor must have what the professionals think is good for them whether they want it or not. This is part of a very old and still unresolved question as to whether the grants economy should content itself with grants of money, leaving the recipient to spend it as he will, or should consist essentially of grants in kind supplying needs as defined by the professionals. Those who are somewhat liberal are inclined to emphasize demand even in the case of the indigent, and to give them

at least some freedom to reject medical care if they prefer a short life and a merry one, though the liberty to preach against such behavior should also be preserved.

One of the great problems of the grants economy—which appears in the relief of medical indigency just as it does elsewhere—is that it can easily result in quite unintended administrative distortions of the price structure which in turn can cause social loss and quite unnecessary individual misery. If, for instance, a grant system bases a grant on a cost of service which is wrongly estimated, it can severely discourage the services which are undervalued and unnecessary and encourage the services which are overvalued. For example, certain casual administrative regulations in the social security system have stimulated a profitable practice of keeping indigent patients in nursing homes in bed, simply because the nursing homes are paid an extra amount for keeping people in bed. Hence nursing homes make more money on bed patients than on ambulatory ones. As a result of the strong financial pressure patients are kept in bed, in spite of the fact that this may be quite unwarranted medically and may contribute to the already bad enough miseries of old age and incompetence.

Generally any system which sets out to administer a price structure will get it wrong so that some things will be underpriced and some overpriced. The same problem may be seen in the universities, where teaching is underpriced relative to research, or where good administration is underpriced and bad administration overpriced. Under these circumstances a kind of universal Gresham's Law operates: the overpriced bad always drives out the underpriced good. No proposition as far as is known says that this problem is insoluble. Unless it is solved, however, socialized and administrative medicine will operate under some handicaps. The uneasy compromise between need and demand takes the form that if needs are to be well satisfied, demand, if it is not to be free, must at least be simulated. If administrative terms of trade are established in the system, it must also have an apparatus that can get feedback from their consequences and review them and adjust them rapidly in the way that the market does.

The last question of this discussion relates to the problem of the effectiveness of medical activity and research. Probably only in the last 100 years has the medical profession done more good than harm in promoting health. Now, although the direction of the effect is not in doubt, a certain amount of doubt remains about its magnitude. Certainly the most spectacular productivity of human activity in the production of health is only indirectly related to the medical profession as such. That is the kind of activity involved, for instance, in antimalaria campaigns, in cleaning up water supplies, in improving nutrition and even in teaching more desirable habits of child-rearing. This fact should not be surprising, nor does it redound to any discredit to the medical profession. Nothing is wrong with the assumption that the business of the doctor is sickness rather than health, just as the business of the garage mechanic is the repair of automobiles, not their production, or the provision of roads on which they may safely be driven. The medical profession is only a single input in the enormous network of social inputs which together determine the general level of health of the population. No one wishes the medical profession to lose its interest in sickness, for that is when a doctor is most needed. On the other hand, one also likes to see a strong interest in preventive medicine and in public health and in what might be called the larger environment of the health sciences. The need is also strong for the development of a social science of health, not only in economics but also in sociology and psychology. Considerable strides have been made toward this, but not in many centers in the world—to bring even one to mind is difficult—is the social science of health studied and taught as a whole.

One would like to see a research operation of at least the magnitude of the Rand Corporation, the object of which would be to study health in all its aspects, social, biological and physical, in a manner permitting a good deal of interchange among specialists. Such a study would clearly reveal that the need for medical services will depend on a very large number of other variables, economic, sociological, biological, and on the whole system of this planet. That answer may not satisfy those who are seeking quick results to solve administrative dilemmas, and the importance of administrative short-cuts cannot be denied. Nevertheless, in the long run, a very substantial intellectual endeavor still awaits mankind in the study of this problem, and at the moment its solution is not near.[3]

The Rand Corporation is used merely as a symbol of the magnitude of the research effort in the social science of health which would probably be profitable. Whether the effort should be concentrated in a single institution or scattered around the academic community is a matter of research strategy on which may rest very valid differences of opinion. Something is to be said for the theory of the "critical mass," especially in interdisciplinary research; and the extraordinary fruitfulness of the Center for Advanced Study in the Behavioral Sciences at Stanford, indicates that a critical mass of this kind may actually be quite small under some circumstances. On the other hand, a research strategy should certainly not be confined to any particular institution, and should envisage the whole intellectual community as its field. Research strategies which are too specific can easily do more harm than good, and even the concept of the need for research needs to be looked at with a slightly quizzical eye. The growth of knowledge is much more like an evolutionary than it is like a mechanical process, and this means that it is fundamentally unpredictable. This can be seen very clearly by asking the question, can anyone predict what will be known 25 years from now? The answer is obviously no, or it would be known now. If the results of a research program are known in advance, the point in doing it has been lost. Hence the growth of knowledge must always contain what is called fundamental surprise, and any research strategy must be built around the capacity to expect and react creatively to surprise.

If any research strategy emerges out of these considerations, it is that one should be extremely suspicious of research devoted specifically to finding out the need for medical care. Too much of such research has already been done, all of which has outlined "needs" which are absurdly inflated, and which, if allowed to be fulfilled, would justify themselves with the greatest of ease. A research program which concentrated solely on quantitative estimates of need would inevitably neglect the problem of demand and the problem of the price structure. A great deal in research depends on how questions are framed. If the question is asked, how does one use a combination of the grants economy and the price structure in producing a system of medical care that compromises between needs and demands, a much richer and more satisfactory answer will likely result than if one simply asks, what is the need for medical care? Almost everyone who has raised children has heard the anguished cry, "But I need—" and soon learns to interpret this as meaning, "I want something badly but I am not prepared to pay the price for it." This cautionary note seems a suitable place to end what is mainly an appeal to move gingerly into an inevitably uncertain future, without forgetting that the movement must be made.

DISCUSSION

If the concept of need for health services is to be made useful for research, it might better be restated or placed in a wider context, that of need in the health "system." Then the proper starting point becomes those factors that serve as the basis for a health system. The health services are only one of the several influences on health and a minor one at that, the others including environment, inheritance and behavior.

The goal of the system must be health, even if only understood as the absence of disease. The point is we do have a choice of goals. In effect, disagreement was being expressed with discussants of previous papers who had observed that meeting health service need is also a way of life for those who so serve and therefore must be counted among the goals of the system. However, by clinging to health as the goal of the system one can most clearly decide to what these services are to be directed. In fact, should they be directed to the kinds of economic incentives that have been allowed, even encouraged, to come into the health service system?

In respect to health services, if the goal is the ever-expanding potential for favorably influencing health through medical advance, problems currently deemed hopeless can be investigated, among them the plight of the aged sick. Evidence of progress is even here. In Oxford, under imaginative leadership, medical and social care of the elderly is at a standard well above that found in the nursing home situation of the United States.

As noted by the author, the concept of need cannot be considered without examining the rival concept of demand. The weaknesses in both concepts led to audience critique of the meaning and use of these terms. The author's denial of a single concept of need, especially in the case of need for health services, was not disputed. This being the case, objections could be raised against those who fault the concept of need as seeming to imply the single notion of want without limit.

The concept of medical need, as defined by Lee and Jones in their study, *The Fundamentals of Medical Care,* abstracting from ability to pay and representing professional judgment alone, since it was independent of personal awareness, was introduced for the purpose of discussion. One difficulty in applying this type of concept, aside from the author's contention that problems of demand and the price structure should not be ignored, arises in the doctor-patient relationship. What the professional perceives as need in his client may be in part a function of whether professional or client is in control of the relationship between them. The solo practitioner, being more dependent for his livelihood on the patient, is more apt to be responsive to the patient's wishes than is the physician in an institutional setting. The latter is more apt to appraise need by criteria within his span of initiative since he is in a position to be less sensitive to his patients' wishes. The concepts of need and demand must also be seen respectively as having social and political dimensions as well as individual and economic ones. The relativity of needs over time was also noted, with needs seen as constantly advancing in front of demand. In many situations the continuing compromise required between a capacity to cite needs and the capacity to satisfy them was seen in the view of one observer as having the nature of a hoax when compared with the reality situation. Although granting abuse in use of the concept, defense was noted, especially by physicians, for the validity for a concept of need aside from the separate question of how it was perceived or how it was expressed in terms of economic demand. In the view of the author, a certain tension exists between need and demand and this must also be represented in any research consideration of the need for health services.

On the question of whether the author's paper was likely to serve as a stimulus to research in the area under discussion, one commentator replied in the negative. He had expected that new vistas on need for health services would be explored, among them such matters as what effect do the economic arrangements under which the health services are available have on the need for health service? A second line of development that could have been employed concerns the social policies that might emanate from or be affected by research utilizing the

concept of need for health services. Another area of interest would be to hear in what ways systematic reorganization of presently available data might lead to further research. Something on the questions and methods that require investigation was seen as another alternative approach. Although the paper does contain imaginative and thoughtful ideas, even these had not been transformed into researchable areas by the development of a research strategy.

In defense of his paper, the author responded that his purpose was to ask questions and to urge everyone to think intelligently about research and this was stimulus enough. His questions involved issues, matters that are and will continue to be of common concern to investigators for many years ahead. Some of these are ethical questions, and a major problem is the evaluation of value systems. The greater the power acquired in science and medicine, or in any other walk of life, the more imposing these ethical problems become. When one has power, he has to start worrying about wanting the wrong things. Ethics is the study of why people want the wrong things.

In effect the author's paper, beyond serving as a critique of the concept of need for health services, must also be seen as a plea for study of certain related social phenomena and their dynamics, for example, study of the perception of need as more promising than the concept of need itself. Basic to such study would be examination of those matters which create saliency for perception within a social system. Perception depends on that, and behavior depends on perception. Even the behavior of organizations, among them those ranked as the most rational, are much influenced by salient events.

Such points as these only underscore the need to think about the information process as a totality in the social system, and research is only one part of this. The trend for research to separate increasingly from other information processes does not appear desirable and is leading to the development of a research subculture, a quasi-religion, an area thoroughly isolated from the rest of society. In other words, we need take a hard look at the problem, not of research, but of knowledge. How does one really come to know anything?

REFERENCES

1. Boulding, K. E., The Menace of Methuselah, *Journal of the Washington Academy of Sciences*, 55, 171–179, October, 1965.

2. Medaware, P. B., THE FUTURE OF MAN, New York, Basic Books, Inc., Publishers, 1960.

3. *See* Ginzberg, Eli, The Political Economy of Health, *Bulletin of the New York Academy of Medicine*, 41, 1015–1036, October, 1965.

6. Economic Aspects of Consumer Use

MARK V. PAULY *

Reprinted with permission from *Consumer Incentives for Health Care*. Copyright © 1974, PRODIST, 219-250.

The task of explaining the economic factors affecting the use of medical care would, in principle, be equivalent to the task of explaining all the economic influences in the medical-care market. To explain or predict use, one must know everything that determines what people will demand and everything that determines what providers will supply. Only satisfied demand and utilized supply result in actual use.

This paper does not take on the prodigious task of explaining everything but attempts instead the possibly more manageable task of summarizing and commenting on what we know and do not know about economic influences on the demand for medical care. In theory, whatever the difficulty in practice, the separation of knowns and unknowns is feasible for most consumer purchases. When we ask about demand we want to know what other factors affect the quantity the consumer would demand at a particular price. We also want to know how he changes the quantity he demands when prices change but the other factors do not. Then his use is that quantity at which, given a particular price, he demands exactly the same quantity that suppliers are willing to supply.

But with medical care the separate specification of demand influences is much more difficult, for two reasons. First, the price that is relevant to determining an individual's use, the marginal user price, is not taken by him as given, as it would be in a competitive market, nor is it even a datum to be manipulated unconstrainedly, as in a monopsony. Instead, the consumer can vary the user price he pays by purchasing customary forms of insurance. But, one way or another, he pays for price cuts in his insurance premium. Thus

* The author benefited in writing this paper from the helpful comments of David Salkever, Jon Joyce, and Joseph Newhouse.

the user price is not parametric, nor is it necessarily equal to the price producers receive. To explain demand for care, then, one must also explain demand for insurance, for it is the latter that determines the user price.

The second difficulty arises because there is reason to suspect that the supplier can manipulate demand relationship. In the more typical economic model of an undifferentiated good, the only way a provider of a good can increase the amount that people are willing to buy from him is by lowering the price. When goods are differentiated, it may be worthwhile for a provider to advertise, though advertising is costly and not always effective. It is also an influence not well incorporated into economic theory.

But it is alleged that availability of medical care—unfilled hospital beds, physicians seeing fewer patients than they would like—affects the quantity of care a person is willing to pay for. It has that effect not because price falls, but because the physician, in his role as advisor to the patient on the usefulness of care, can almost costlessly shift the patient's willingness to pay for care, perhaps within rather wide limits. For purposes of explaining demand, we must therefore know something about the extent of persuasion or advocacy by physicians. That means that, in a very critical sense, consumers' demand for care may not be independent of physicians' willingness to provide care. So in what follows insurance and supply must be discussed to explain demand.

Taxonomy of Economic Influences

To classify economic influences on the use of medical care, it will be helpful to begin with the paradigm of consumer choice that the economist employs in analyzing the demand for other goods and services. The paradigm does more than indicate which are important independent variables; it also indicates, for some of them, the direction of their effect. One purpose of this paper will be to examine the extent to which studies of empirical reality seem to fit the "economic man" paradigm.

In a sentence, the economist's model is one of an individual who maximizes his utility subject to a budget constraint. That constraint equates his money income to his expenditures on all goods, and those expenditures in turn are the products of multiplying quantity by price. The model implies that there are four main influences on demand for any good:

(1) things that determine the "shape of the utility function," called "tastes," and are assumed to be given,

(2) money income,

(3) the price of the good, and

(4) the prices of closely related goods, either substitutes or complements.

More sophisticated versions of the model differ in several ways. First, they recognize that income is more than just money income; in addition to a money-budget constraint, a person may face a time-budget constraint. Second, and similarly, not all prices are money prices—some services have time prices and inconvenience prices, which affect demand. Third, it is sometimes useful to view the household itself not as a final consumer but as a producer whose inputs are purchased goods, services, and time of household members and whose outputs are useful characteristics. In the case of medical care, for example, one useful characteristic may be "health," and medical care may be but one input into its production. Fourth, if a good adds to an individual's ability over time to earn income, in a human capital sense, the utility of the good is the present value of the extra income it permits a person to earn.

But these extensions are fully consistent with, though they are improvements upon, the simpler model described earlier. Consequently, in what follows, influences will be characterized as having predicted effects on use that are "price-like," "income-like," "taste-like," and so on.

Are there any peculiar characteristics of medical care that do not fit in this framework? One characteristic is uncertainty—uncertainty about the incidence of illness. In the case of medical care as in other contexts, the response of the risk-averse consumer is to purchase insurance. In its purest form, insurance affects only the money-income constraint, in effect transferring income from one possible state of the world to another. The insurance premium reduces income in no-loss states, but insurance benefit payments raise income in states that are insured against. Unfortunately for simplicity of analysis, typical medical insurance does more than transfer income. It also reduces the user price of some kinds of care. The implication of these remarks is that neither money income nor the price of the good is parametric when the consumer can choose his insurance coverage.

A second problem is that "tastes" for medical care may not be fixed. The most striking illustration is in the incidence of illness. One's "taste" for an appendectomy will vary, depending on whether or not he has abdominal pain. The problem could be handled with an ad hoc rule relating "tastes" to illness, or by defining health as the output and illness as a random reduction in the stock or flow of health. A second serious analytical problem is that consumers may be persuaded by physicians or by others to like or dislike various kinds of medical care. Unless such changes can be predicted, the explanatory power of the economic theory of demand is much reduced. To the extent that physicians are economically motivated, it may be possible to predict the effect of their advice on tastes.

Finally, the market for medical care may be such that demands are not fully satisfied. Then the pattern of use may be affected little, if at all, by demand elements and may simply reflect the curious behavior of suppliers.

In the following pages each of the influences on demand—income, prices, and tastes—will be examined, with comment on the normative implications of the findings for "appropriate" incentives to seek. An area of considerable importance, and one that is as yet relatively sparsely investigated, is that of interaction effects (the point has recently been made most strongly by David Salkever, of Johns Hopkins University). At question here is not the influence of prices when income, tastes, and illness incidence are held constant, but rather how responses to price changes vary with different incomes or tastes or illness states.

We might also wish to ask whether income affects use differently at high user prices than it does at low ones. So after indicating what we know and need to know about the direct effects on use, we shall consider interaction effects as well. Perhaps the omission of interaction effects, in most empiricial work, is the result of the multivariate regression analysis customarily used by economists; that analysis typically picks up the independent effect of one variable with the others held constant, but in doing so gives no information on interaction effects.

Effect of Income on Demand

A proper definition of income would distinguish between transitory and permanent income, with the latter being a measure of the true wealth constraint implied by theory.

Even if it were possible to measure permanent income, there are additional reasons why the "pure" effect of income on demand for medical care is difficult to estimate. The incidence of illness itself may be related to income (positively or negatively), and the existence of illness surely affects income. To get a pure income effect, we would have to determine the effect of income on use for given states of health, and that effect should be separated from any effect of income on health status. In principle, some of those separations can be made by using the concept of time. Income presumably affects health not instantaneously, but with a lag (as yet not too well known). Thus, two individuals with the same present income but with unequal income in the past should differ in their use of care. Illness may, of course, have the effect of reducing permanent income more or less immediately.

Pure Effect of Income

Why should we expect income to have an effect on use for a given condition? There are two reasons, but they point in opposite directions. First, there may be a time cost whose value varies directly with income, since the opportunity cost of time would be roughly proportional to income. Opportunity cost would, however, be even more appropriately measured by the wage rate, but no study has looked at the effect severity of illness has on the response of use for persons with different wage rates. Second, as income increases, persons have more to spend. One of the goods on which they spend more could be medical care. The only goods for which use actually declines with income are those goods for which higher priced substitutes exist, e.g., steak and hamburger. There does not seem to be a higher priced substitute for medical care in general, although the use of some kinds of care—clinics, physician—substitutes—may decline with income.

Relatively few studies have used data on state of health or illness as well as income. In one study, Richardson (1970) showed that income did indeed affect use, and in the expected way; the poor tended to use less care for a given state of health. A second study by him gave less conclusive results but looked at the effect of income with only seriousness of illness held constant, and did not control for other variables (Richardson, 1971). A study by Andersen, Anderson, and Smedby (1968) also indicated that income did affect use, and more strongly in the United States, where user prices are mostly positive, than in Sweden. Unfortunately, the only indicator of health used in the study was whether a person had a symptom; the seriousness of the symptom was not considered.

Surprisingly, there seems to be no large-scale, definitive data on the use of hospitals by individuals with given symptoms that would shed light on the effects of income. While there have been some studies of the variation of use with income by diagnosis, the severity of illness for a given diagnosis has not been considered, perhaps because of the difficulty of getting an independent measure of severity. An unpublished study in Rhode Island indicates that, for some kinds of illness, low income is likely to lead to more frequent hospitalization (e.g., for pneumonia and bronchitis) because desirable home-care alternatives are less readily available (see Scott, 1973). Moreover, the effect of income on care is obscured in simple cross-tabular analysis by the positive relationship between income and insurance coverage.

When medical condition is not included as a control variable, the effect of income on use becomes twofold. It affects both health and use.

Effect of Income on Health

There are at least four separate ways in which income might affect health, where health is defined as a stock that accumulates or depreciates over time. First, and most obviously, if income positively affects the use of medical care in each time period, and if additional medical care adds to the stock of health, rich people will be healthier. Second, other goods whose consumption increases with income—good housing, good food—may improve health. Third, still other goods may not affect health directly but may improve the efficiency by which health is produced; education is the prime example, although in theory it could also be considered as an input, like entrepreneurial capacity in the theory of the firm. Finally, other goods whose consumption increases with income may reduce the health stock at any point in time—goods such as rich food or liquor or even habits, such as reduced physical exercise.

Michael Grossman's recent work (1972) and that of his colleagues at the National Bureau of Economic Research, has shed light on the relationship between income and health (see, also, Auster et al., 1972; Silver, 1972). Surprisingly, Grossman's work indicates that income in itself does not affect the stock of health and that it affects the flow of health services negatively. What does affect both measures in the appropriate way is not total income but the wage rate, which is positively and significantly related to health.

Grossman interprets that finding in the context of an investment model. Since the wage is the "cost" of workdays lost, the higher the wage the fewer workdays a person will want to lose. Consequently, he will choose a larger stock of health and the flow of healthy days from that stock. Of course, wage income and total income are likely to be correlated, since the bulk of most peoples' income is from wages. But Grossman says that in his data "these variables are not so highly correlated that the results are dominated by multicollinearity." When wages are left out of the equation, income is positively related to health.

What do these results suggest about behavior patterns? Grossman's answer is that the negative relationship between income and health may be due to the fact that higher income induces people to buy more "bads" as well as "goods" and that the former dominate.

He interprets the results as indicating that health is not mainly wanted as a consumption good but as an investment good.

Taken literally, Grossman's results indicate that transfers of income (e.g., family assistance to the poor) that do not depend on work effort or that reduce the net wage rate will worsen health. Extra income allows people to buy things that are bad for them, at least those who are in the labor force, are white, and who have a record of not using sick time.

Grossman's results have two alternative explanations. The first is that those persons who have large nonwage components of income —the self-employed, moonlighters, etc.—may be in situations tending to affect their health adversely. The second is that a work-loss day provides leisure time. If leisure is a normal good, an individual will buy more of it as his income rises. Hence work-loss days will rise as income rises for a given "price" of a lost day of work. The rise occurs even if a work-loss day does not represent perfect leisure, in the sense that some illness is needed as a psychological excuse for staying home from work.

Grossman did not estimate the effect of income on the demand for medical care with health status held constant. Instead, he estimated an equation in which use of medical care was regressed on income, wage rates, age, sex, and family size. Note that no price variable was included. Here the wage rate is not significant, nor is education. Income has a significant positive effect, as it does in the "health demand" equations if the wage rate is left out. Insignificance of the wage rate probably stems from its two conflicting effects: A higher wage rate makes health more valuable and so induces a person to buy more care, but it raises the time cost of care, which tends to reduce use.

When Grossman estimates a "production function" for health, medical care has the right sign, it does contribute to health. But its significance is sensitive to the measure of health and to the particular set of variables excluded or included.

Measuring "Total Effect" of Income on Use

The permanent income elasticity of demand was the subject of an estimation attempt by Andersen and Benham (1970). Theory suggests that permanent income elasticity should be greater than transitory income elasticity, and their results confirm the theory. When a measure of quality is included, income elasticity of demand for physicians' services is 0.17 (i.e., a 10-percent increase in income increases use by 1.7 percent, but it is not significantly different from zero). When quality is excluded, the measure for income elasticity is 0.24.

In a study by Morris Silver (1972), the medical expenses of only currently employed persons are studied. The limitation should reduce some of the income-health relationship, since persons in very ill health (because of previously low income, for example) would not be included. Paradoxically, Silver found a high income easticity of demand in the range 1.2 to 2.0 for care as a whole, with lowest values for hospital and physician expenditures and highest values for dental expenditures. When Silver includes the earnings rate as well as income (though in his data the two valuables are highly correlated), income elasticity drops to the lower portion of the range. But because of data limitations, Silver was unable to separate out the effect of insurance, and insurance tends to be positively related to income.

Richard Rosett and L. F. Huang (1973) also estimated income elasticities that differ by income classes. They obtained measures for insured households ranging from 0.25 for those with incomes of four thousand dollars a year to 0.45 for those with ten thousand dollars a year. Feldstein (1971a) has estimated an income elasticity of demand for hospital bed-days of 0.54, using cross-section, state-aggregated data.

The results of the studies suggest that a good guess, if we had to pick a single number, would be an income elasticity of 0.5 or a little less. Note, however, that this is a "combined" or "total" income elasticity. If income does affect health status adversely (either in itself or as a proxy for wages), these measures overstate the pure or instantaneous effect of income on demand for care.

What we do not know is how the interactions occur. Theory would predict, for example, that the effect of income on use would decline as the user price declined. At the zero price extreme, people with the same utility functions would be likely to use about the same amount of care. Only Rosett estimated a "cross effect" term, which was positive and significant, suggesting the opposite. On the other hand, a study by K. Roghman and his associates (1971) indicated that differences in use remained even after people received Medicaid, indicating that full-coverage insurance did not remove all differences in use. Likewise, Andersen, Anderson, and Smedby (1968) found that income was more important in the United States, where the population is not fully insured, than in Sweden, where it is close to being fully insured. Another interaction effect is that of income and seriousness of illness. Richardson (1971) found, as we might expect, that the less serious the illness, the stronger the effects of income (and other economic influences).

Future Research

We are still ignorant about the relationship between income and the use of medical care. It appears that, as Paul Feldstein (1966) conjectured in 1965, the use of medical care does increase with income. Yet we are woefully ignorant of the pure effect of income on health, and Grossman's work is one of the few studies indicating that it may be wages, not income, that governs the relationship. There must be a more serious look at the effect of income on health, of medical care on health, and of income on use, given health status. What is clear, however, is that income transfers would affect the incentives people have to use health services.

The most important policy implications of findings about the disincentive effect of low income on use of care relates to some national health insurance proposals. One possible rationale for government interference in the financing of care is that some subsidization of care for the poor is necessary to make sure that the poor get what people in general regard as appropriate or needed care. To deal with presumably less use by the poor, several plans (Pauly, 1971b; Feldstein, 1971b) suggest arrangements in which reductions in user price via increased insurance coverage are used to offset the inability of the poor to afford care. The plans are appropriate only if lower income in fact leads to less use, and the subsidy depends in part on the extent to which use varies with income. The subsidy also depends on the responsiveness of use to price cuts. If there is no relationship between income and use, or if it is only a weak relationship, there would by that argument be no or almost no rationale for subsidization.

Tastes as a Determinant of Use of Care

The interest here is in those determinants of taste that are capable of direct economic interpretation. In this sense, they are taste-like variables, rather than the pure residual influences that the economist usually calls "tastes."

Education

Why should education affect the use of medical care? First, it may make consumers more aware of the utility and limitations of health care. The direction its effect will have on use is therefore unpredictable, since ignorance can lead to either too little or too much care. Second, education may enhance the value to the consumer of health. If he believes that care affects health, it may increase his use of care. If adjustment is made for wages, the only effect would be on consumption. Finally, as Grossman has suggested, education may enhance the "efficiency" with which the family produces health. Here its effect could be negative; education could make the family so efficient in producing health that it would use less medical care.

In most empirical studies, education and income are highly correlated, and education is perhaps better correlated with permanent income than with present income. When the wage rate was included, Grossman found that education had little effect on use. It is safe to say that we still do not know much about the pure effect of education on use.

Family Size and Composition

An individual's use of care will be affected by the kind of family of which he is a member. Although that influence is included here as a demographic determinant of "tastes," recent research suggests that in its economic influence it resembles both income and prices. If the family is viewed as a production unit that produces useful attributes employing goods as inputs, it does so constrained by the total amount of resources it has available. Those resources are obviously total family money income (and indeed family income rather than individual income or even family income per capita has customarily been employed in use or demand studies), but they also include the total amount of time available to the family and the total amount of human capital (e.g., education) available to the family as a whole. Similarly, the "price" of a unit of a family member's time in producing care for himself or others will vary with the alternative uses of his time.

The critical empirical question is whether alternative family configurations involve budget and price effects, and demand effects too, that will influence an individual's use, as suggested by a considerable amount of casual and less casual empirical evidence. Individuals who live alone, for example, use more care than others. That is doubtless because, in two-person families, one individual can produce care for the other that would otherwise have to be sought from the formal medical-care system. Other family characteristics, involving which person in the family is ill, whether the wife works and at what wages, and so on, are also relevant.

Recent economic research has begun to emphasize the "economics of the family," but relatively little has been done in health care. (The only research of which the author is aware is some yet unpublished work by Jon Joyce of Wesleyan University.) Even descriptive empirical work in the area might be very useful and have important policy implications. To give one example: There is a fair amount of evidence that hospital stays can often be shortened without adverse medical consequences and that many procedures can be done on an outpatient basis. Since such steps reduce costs incurred within the system, it is natural that many people consider desirable those arrangements that appear to produce these results, such as health maintenance organizations (HMO's). Yet in reckoning the true social cost of care, it is clear that the extra implicit costs imposed on the household must be considered. What does the household lose by virtue of the fact that it must produce care? Home care is desirable only if it "costs" less than institutional care. In the empirical studies of the advantages and disadvantages of reimbursement arrangements that reduce use, the offsetting cost imposed on the household is rarely considered.

Price and Price-Like Incentives

The economist naturally thinks of price as an incentive to encourage or discourage use. In a normative sense, the "wrong" price may provide an incentive to use too much or too little of a good. Conversely, given a definition of what constitutes appropriate use and given enough information, it is possible, at least theoretically, to design a price system that will induce individuals to choose that level of use.

While the role of price as an incentive has sometimes been recognized by noneconomist specialists in health care, there appears to be a curious sort of schizophrenic conventional wisdom in much of the policy-oriented work. Thus it is sometimes maintained that positive prices are likely to be bad because they discourage needed care, and at the same time there is an unwillingness to believe price has much effect on decisions to seek care. Recent research by economists and others has, however, increased our knowledge of the potential magnitude of price effects and has also provided some analysis of the appropriate use of prices. In both cases, research has served mainly to suggest that there are many more unanswered questions.

Why Price Might Affect Use

Price can affect use in two ways: First and most obvious is in the individual consumer's decision whether to seek care. If additional care has a positive cost to him, he will seek care only as long as he values the care he receives more than the other goods and services he might have purchased. The second way is in the effect the price paid by the consumer may have on the physician's decision about how much and what kind of care to render. The physician, acting properly in his role as proxy decisionmaker for the consumer, may decide that some kinds of beneficial care are not worth their cost to the consumer. Or a physician's orders for care may meet resistance from consumers who must pay the user price and acquiescence from those whose insurance pays the price. Even if the physician does not know the net or user price paid by a particular patient, he may adjust his behavior to an average level of the price that prevails among all his patients.

All this discussion is frankly speculative, since we know little about the precise way in which price affects the physician-patient decision nexus. In large part, our lack of knowledge is the result of a more basic ignorance about the way in which physician prices are set and the extent to which nonphysician charges affect the price the physician can get. We do not know, for example, whether a scheme in which physicians, rather than patients, were billed for hospital services would affect use and total cost to the consumer.

Concepts of Price

The true concept of the price that affects demand is broader than that of simple transfers of money. Obviously, what is relevant to a consumer's use of care is not the price charged for the services but the price he has to pay for them, the "user price." The higher the price charged or the greater his insurance coverage, the higher will be his premiums, but the effect of higher premiums in reducing spendable income will be spread over all his purchases and affect his purchases of medical care only slightly.

Prices can be paid in ways other than money. For many types of medical care price is the sacrifice of time, either in getting care or in traveling to a source of care, and psychological and physical pain and discomfort may be more important than money price. (Since medical insurance does not usually provide pain and suffering benefits, use is likely to be less than infinite even at a zero money price.) The cost of time is the value that time would have had in its next best use. Here again, we know relatively little about the effect of time on use, although Grossman's result of a zero wage elasticity of demand for care is suggestive, and there is currently some research being done on the effect of time costs on use.

Finally, a change in the price of a good affects more than just the demand for that good; it affects the demand for closely related goods. In the most extreme case, competition can be defined as an infinitely great cross-elasticity of demand between the price charged

by one seller for a given good and the quantity demanded from another seller for the same good. Thus, the price charged by one physician or hospital might affect the demand for other physician or
hospital services, and the user price in the outpatient department
might affect the use of care in physicians' offices.

Effect of User Charges on Use

Common sense suggests that the more "discretionary" the type
of care, the greater the effect of user charges. It is probably lack of
data that accounts for the fact that most documentation of the effect of user charges is on inpatient hospital care, probably the most
non-discretionary sort of care. In addition, many studies have
looked at the effects that represent combinations of incentives to
consumer (user charges), incentives to physicians and hospital administrators (reimbursement mechanisms), and organizational form
(solo practice, multi-specialty group). As a result, it is hard to isolate the effect of charges on demand.

The difficulty is particularly marked in a series of studies begun
in the mid-1950s and continued up to the present. The earlier studies have been summarized by Klarman (1965) and Donabedian
(1969). Their main message was (with some exceptions) that prepaid group practices had lower levels of hospital utilization and
lower inplan costs than did insurance plans that provided mainly
fee-for-service coverage for inhospital procedures.

But only rarely was it possible to tell whether observed differences in utilization were the result of the way physicians were paid,
the price incentives facing consumers, the mode of organization, or
the characteristics of plan members. In some of the studies, plan
members were matched to reduce the last problem, that of self-
selection.

A more recent study of the same sort done at the University of
California at Los Angeles has not been published, but some of the
results were the subject of a statement by the study director before
a congressional committee (Roemer, 1972). Extensive data on use
and demographic characteristics were obtained on three types of
plan (two examples of each): commercial indemnity, Blue Cross
service benefit, and prepaid group practice. Group practices had the
lowest hospital admissions, but the indemnity plan was a close second. The Blue Cross plans had the greatest use. The smallness of
the gap between indemnity plans and prepaid group practice was
attributed to the fact that indemnity plans covered better risks.
Length of stay is, however, much lower in the group-practice plans,
so that total hospital bed-days are much lower there. Ambulatory-
care use is least for the commercial plans and greatest for the Blue

Cross plans. Unfortunately, these gross findings have not yet been subject to multivariate analysis, so that their main cause is not known. And since only four noncomprehensive plans were studied, there will be at most only four possible values for user price.

Whatever the studies may tell us about the advantages of one particular plan over another, they do not provide answers to the general question of incentives. In addition to failing to separate effects, they are plagued by "small number" problems of two sorts. First, at best they compare half a dozen plans, surely a small sample. Second, they provide relatively few differential observations on alternative user prices. Consequently, some recent economic analyses have departed from the case-study approach in order to use larger or more diverse bodies of data.

Earlier work had indicated that higher levels of insurance coverage tended to be associated with greater expenditures in, and presumably greater use of, medical care. A recent, more sophisticated study by Martin Feldstein (1971a) used state-aggregated hospital admissions and mean stay as measures of use. Constructing a measure of user price by multiplying the gross price by an "average" measure of coverage for that state, he found that use was indeed responsive to coverage. An instrumental variable technique, not too clearly described, was used to avoid simultaneity problems.

Feldstein estimated that price elasticity of demand for hospital bed-days was about 0.67, with elasticity being somewhat greater for mean stay and less for admissions. All three are substantial elasticities and suggest that reduction from the present twenty percent to ten percent in the fraction of care costs would increase hospital expenditures by one-third. A somewhat similar estimate by Davis and Russell (1972), using similar data but a slightly different measure of insurance coverage and ordinary-least-squares regression analysis, estimated own-elasticity of demand to be 0.32 to 0.46.

A recent study by Richard Rosett and L. F. Huang (1973) used observations on coverage and total medical expenditures for individual spending units. Some ingenious methods of estimation were necessary to get around deficiencies in the data. Nevertheless, their estimates of elasticity range from 0.35 at a twenty percent copayment to 1.50 at an eighty percent copayment. Their figures suggest that, for example, going to zero copayment under a national health insurance plan from the present one-third level could as much as double expenditures.

Some other recent work, of a case-study nature, provides estimates of elasticity of demand for physicians' services (Scitovsky and Snyder, 1972; Phelps and Newhouse, 1972b). The work studied the effect of introducing a twenty-five percent copayment for physicians' services in one prepaid comprehensive group practice for employees of Stanford University. Imposition of the copayment reduced usage about twenty-five percent. The arc elasticity, using average price as a base, is calculated to be 0.14. A similar study of the introduction of a forty-one percent copayment in Saskatchewan indicated an arc elasticity of 0.13, although it is unclear whether this "use" elasticity is uncontaminated by supply as well as demand responses (Phelps and Newhouse, 1972a).

For the Stanford study, it is clear that results need not be comparable to what they would be in a more typical setting. Presumably there would already have been an incentive in that plan for physicians to keep physician use low (especially since hospital services were not obtained within the plan). Consequently, the possibilities for further reduction in use would have been limited. For the other studies, the low elasticities are a little more difficult to explain, although fixed prices might contribute to the Saskatchewan results. The results may also indicate rationing behavior by physicians, as Feldstein (1970) has suggested.

Finally, although one might have expected physician visits to be more price sensitive, the published results are certainly possible. Moreover, if the demand curve is linear rather than constant-elasticity, low levels of elasticity at low absolute prices are to be expected.

Can anything be said about the direction of bias in the Feldstein-Rosett-Huang-Davis-Russell estimates? The most serious aggregation problem arises because researchers have used an average rather than a marginal measure of insurance coverage. Since a typical policy will contain a deductible, the average fraction covered will ordinarily fall short of the marginal fraction covered. Thus, when a person with no insurance is compared with a person who has positive but relatively low average coverage but high marginal coverage, any increase in use will be attributed to the relatively slight increase in average coverage rather than to the large increase in marginal coverage. Consequently, estimates of the effect of coverage on use will be biased upwards.

The argument is correct as far as it goes, but it does not go far enough. An offsetting bias arises if it is true that marginal coverage is likely to remain high over a wide range of expenses. The change in marginal user price over such a range will be low or zero, while the change in average user price will be relatively greater. The change in expense associated with that change in average coinsurance will in fact reflect the zero or slight change in marginal coinsurance, and so a measure of the effect of coinsurance on use will be biased downward. The direction of bias in the estimate of the overall effect of coverage on use will depend on the strengths of the two effects, and there is no reason to suppose that the resulting bias will be necessarily upward.

A similar criticism is made in a paper by Newhouse and Phelps (1973); the results of Rosett-Huang's study are also properly criticized in it for omitting (because of data deficiencies) employer-financed coverage, leading to a large group of low-estimated coverage, low-estimated expenditure observations.

Insurance Effects

Another kind of omitted criticism is related to a problem endemic in all the studies of use so far completed. Results may be biased because the adjustment to user price caused by insurance is not exogenous. If individuals can choose their level of insurance coverage, potential expenditures and potential effects of coverage on use would affect the amount of coverage they buy. Even when obvious demographic characteristics are used to match populations, the fact that one individual chooses one form of coverage and another chooses a different form is evidence that they are not identical individuals. As long as insurance may affect use, the differences in individuals may likewise affect use.

There are no published studies that directly consider the simultaneity problem. Feldstein uses an instrumental variables approach rather than ordinary least squares, but it is not possible to tell whether the set of exogenous variables used to determine the instruments is the appropriate set. Attempts are presently being made, both at the RAND Corporation and elsewhere, to tackle the problem. It may be useful to consider the issues involved.

The endogenous nature of insurance can induce two sorts of bias into estimates of the effect of coverage on use. The biases arise from the problems of adverse selection and moral hazard.

Adverse selection occurs when premiums are not tailored to the expected losses of individuals. If, for example, all pay the same premium but have different expected losses (and hence different actuarially fair premiums), those for whom the premium charged is low in relation to what would be actuarially fair (the bad risks) will tend to choose high coverage, and those for whom the premium is high (good risks) will tend to choose low coverage. Coverage will then be related to losses, but the causal relationship runs from losses to coverage, not the other way around.

Adverse selection is less likely to raise estimation problems when geographically aggregated data are used. It arises when individuals have expected losses that differ from the average expected loss on which premiums are based. If a Blue Cross plan in a state is to break even, it must charge premiums that, on the average, cover its costs. If higher incomes increase medical-care expenses but premiums do not vary with income, and if other things (including risk aversion) are equal, higher income families would demand more insurance. But those are families with incomes higher than that of the average family on whose experience premiums are based, not necessarily families with higher absolute income. Families with high relative incomes may buy more insurance, but families with low relative incomes will buy less. The effect of income on insurance depends on the strength of the effects of each group's changes. This statement implies that one of Feldstein's reasons for attributing a possible positive effect to income in an insurance-demand equation was misleading (see Feldstein, 1973). So long as premiums are "experience rated" for a group, that group's average expenditure need not be affected by adverse selection. But unaggregated data, such as those used by Rosett and Huang, may give estimates that are biased upward.

Moral hazard will also affect the quantity of insurance bought. Families may differ in their responsiveness to user price changes. If so, families most responsive to price incentives will tend to purchase little insurance, because the "welfare cost" to them of such insurance will be relatively great. And families who do restrain use will purchase more extensive coverage (see Cummins, 1973). The differences would be accentuated if the marginal price of insurance reflected differential moral hazard, something that is plausible for experience-rated groups. If differential moral hazard does affect insurance choice, empirical estimates of the effect of additional coverage on overall use that ignore differential moral hazard will be biased downward. Families with little insurance are only those who, if given more coverage, would have much greater use than those who now have relatively extensive coverage.

In summary, it is fairly easy to come up with a number of reasons why existing estimates of the effect of insurance on use may be biased. Unfortunately, since even a guess at the direction of bias appears to be impossible, it seems appropriate to conclude only that prices do affect use.

Prices and Substitutes

Though a number of attempts have been made to relate the change in user price of a type of medical care to its use, there have been few empirical attempts to see whether changes in price can produce substitution between different types of care. It has always been an article of faith (or perhaps logic) that comprehensive coverage would reduce inpatient hospital use by reducing the user price of outpatient care to at least the level of inpatient care. (Indeed, the own-elasticity effects on outpatient care of such coverage changes have generally been ignored in policy-oriented discussion.)

That faith is confirmed in the study by Davis and Russell. Use of outpatient services is indeed affected by the price of inpatient care, with a cross-elasticity of 0.85 to 1.45. Outpatient care is also sensitive (elasticity = 1) to its own price. Since outpatient services are often very similar to the services a physician provides in his office, the numbers are also suggestive about own and cross-elasticities of demand for physician care.

There have been almost no estimates of the effect on use of prices charged for close substitutes, such as hospitals or physicians providing the same care. Although ostensibly similar hospitals may have very different charges, they do not necessarily have different user prices. A study by Newhouse (1970) in which he claimed that there was little competition between physicians was shown to be seriously flawed (Frech and Ginsburg, 1972). Lack of data on individual physician charges has prevented a direct approach to the problem. Yet if we are to determine if schemes that propose making the patient aware of differential hospital or physician charges are to be useful, we need to know more about the individual hospital or physician-level response of use to price.

Price as a Rationing Device

As noted above, there is now strong empirical evidence that user price is a feasible device for affecting use. The critical policy question is whether the device is desirable. It is commonplace to remark that, while price may discourage excess use, it may also inhibit needed care. But to make any sense out of the remark, we need a definition of "excess" and "needed."

There are at least three alternative notions of desirable levels of care: (1) medical necessity; (2) personal preferences; and (3) private and social benefits.

The notion of medical necessity as a method of specifying appropriate use is probably what most people have in mind. But it may not even be a feasible norm. It is clearly impossible to set up standards for appropriate treatment that apply to every individual case. Physical illnesses, patient personalities, and physician attitudes are too diverse. The most that could be expected is to set up standards for samples of identifiable diagnoses. While the appropriate length of stay for an appendectomy may vary, depending on the situation, the average length of stay (among a physician's patients, in a hospital) could be examined for conformance with a norm. Probably that is what the emerging professional standards review organizations will try to do, though it is not clear that sufficient agreement on proper care will be obtained.

Even if a consistent definition of medical necessity is possible, there still remains the question of whether it is a proper definition of appropriate levels of care. There are reasons to believe that it may not be. Within the scope of health per se, it is unlikely that what medical men are able to agree upon will correspond to that allocation which maximizes health. With limited resources, maximization of health implies care should be used only up to the point at which the health benefit (expected benefit, in an uncertain situation) from that care equals the benefit the same resources would produce if used for health elsewhere. In other words, care that may do an individual some good ought in some circumstances not to be given.

It is doubtful that the judgment of medical men will reflect that kind of thinking about trade-offs and cost, for their training is not usually in such terms. And if it is recognized that people have goals other than health, the appropriate question becomes the even more difficult one of whether extra medical care in a given situation provides as much benefit to the individual as would the same resources used for housing, for education, or even for entertainment. In summary, whether or not medical necessity in fact gets elevated to the status of a policy norm, there are important reasons to believe that it is not an appropriate norm.

A second kind of norm assumes that individual choices should determine the level of care. A rational individual will, of course, consult physicians and other experts to determine the possible benefits from care, but ultimately he will make a choice on whether to take care (or take a physician's advice about taking care) by considering both the costs and benefits to himself. Given such a norm, any reduction in user price caused by insurance is positively pernicious. It is likely to push price below cost and hence will induce the individual to use care which, as far as he is concerned, is worth less to him than its cost. Of course, he will have to pay the cost in the premium, so he is worse off with a reduction in user price than he would have been if his decision on use had reflected the full cost— that is, the full value of the alternative uses of his resources.

The dead-weight welfare cost of health insurance may, of course, be a necessary evil, in the sense that the individual may be willing to pay it in order to get coverage of risky expenditures, but the individual would still be better off if some way could be found to provide the same protection without reducing the user price. Indemnities of various sorts would be preferable to service benefits, and service benefits with some copayments would often be preferable to full coverage.

If an individual bought insurance at prices reflecting its cost, he would buy coverage up to the point at which additional risk-reduction benefits exactly offset additional welfare cost. In fact, various tax incentives are likely to induce the individual to buy too much insurance (Feldstein and Allison, 1972).

The thought here is that, by reducing insurance coverage, individuals are faced with a positive user charge, and the reduction in overuse may more than compensate for increased exposure to risk. The latter point should not be overemphasized, since much of present "first dollar" coverage does not cover ˙ ry risky situations. But there is some additional risk of expense associated with reductions in coverage. Is there no way "to have the cake and eat it too," to retain both appropriate price incentives and coverage of risk?

There is another form of insurance, used extensively outside the medical-care area, that does preserve incentives. It is indemnity insurance, insurance that as far as possible makes the insurance benefit depend not on expense, which is manipulable by the insured, but on the occurrence of a loss-producing event. To take a concrete example, a pure indemnity insurance would pay a fixed amount if tonsillitis occurred, regardless of the amount of care sought. The user price would be unaffected by such an insurance payment. Indemnities have, of course, sometimes been used in medical expenses cases, mostly for physicians' fees, but their importance is diminishing. Pure indemnities may not be feasible because of the practical impossibility of determining "medical condition" with sufficient accuracy. But some forms of indemnity modified to preserve both price incentives and risk coverage may still represent improvement over customary forms of insurance. The author has discussed such forms of indemnity coverage elsewhere (Pauly, 1971a); on a priori grounds it appears that, for many medical-care situations, indemnity coverage would be both feasible and desirable.

One legitimate objection to the analysis of user charges, and to calculations that make them benefit measures, is that they assume that individuals' choices are in fact made with "appropriate" information (which is not necessarily complete information if information is costly). One rather cavalier though correct answer is that, if information is deficient because of monopoly restrictions on supply or competition, then the appropriate remedy is more information on the benefits of care. A more useful response for the purposes of this discussion is that, even if individuals had appropriate information, (a) there is no reason to suppose they would buy the quantities of care they are induced to buy by existing or proposed insurances and (b) in an ideal situation, user prices should still be as close to true factor opportunity cost as possible. In other words, prices might still be appropriate incentives. Indeed, if it were possible to determine what individuals would buy if fully informed of benefits and costs, it might be better to structure insurance so that user prices induce persons who are less than fully informed to buy the same quantities. Such user prices might be above as well as below market prices. In summary, given this view of appropriate norms, prices are not only desirable as incentives, they are probably essential.

The third norm recognizes that society, in the sense of other people, may be concerned about the level of care an individual receives. Medical care may well be one of those goods whose consumption generates a kind of "external benefit" and not only in cases of contagious disease. Altruistic or humanitarian motivation may make individuals willing to pay something for care for others when that care would relieve perceived suffering (Pauly, 1971b).

Not all care would generate such benefits, since there may certainly be cases in which an individual buys enough care on his own so that others would perceive no benefit from additional care. But for those individuals who, if faced with the full user price, would buy what others regard as too little care, some device to increase use would be desirable. One device would be to reduce user charges by providing or subsidizing an "insurance" that gives more coverage (lower user prices) than any amount of insurance the individual buys on his own. Since empirical studies of the effect of income on demand indicate that the poor will use less care, the rationale given above suggests that relatively extensive coverage should be provided to the very poor, and then the extent of coverage should decline with income.

Individuals' willingness to pay for the care of others is reflected via the political process. While the expert adviser cannot tell the politician-representative what portion of his constituents' incomes should be spent on subsidizing health care, possible "reasonable" norms and their costs could be suggested. It would be useful to know, for instance, the cost of a scheme of price cuts needed to bring the poor up to the median level of use for various illnesses. Information would also be useful on the consequences of price cuts on use for different kinds of individuals, different kinds of care, and different types of illnesses. Or it might be worthwhile to consider a kind of "original position" approach, in which individuals are thought of as asking themselves what kind of public medical care subsidy, if any, they would wish to see if they were completely ignorant of what was to be their status, income, or position in life.

For different kinds of care, we have already seen that in general the measured response to price changes differs. What is perhaps more important to know is how the use of various kinds of care responds to price incentives for different kinds of illnesses. Almost all the studies by economists, and many of those by others, have failed to look at the relationship of price response to price incentives for different kinds of illness.

The only exception in the former group is in the study of the Stanford group practice by Scitovsky and Snyder (1972). They find some suggestion that a greater share of use reduction occurred in "minor complaints." They also find a decline in physical examinations (by 18.7 percent), which fell short of the overall decline in use (25 percent), but for some groups was in excess of the average decline. For male nonprofessionals the increase in user price cut physical examinations in half (from an already low base). Though one need not agree with their judgment that this was probably a reduction in "needed" care (since they have no standard of need), such information is clearly useful for those who must make policy decisions. Of course, Scitovsky and Snyder were only looking at a price change over one range, for one type of care, and for the grossest illness categories. More detailed study, and a method of summarizing results, would clearly be desirable.

Whatever the level of information obtained, it will never be possible to design a system of prices that guarantees that every person will use the right amount of care. Ostensibly identical people may respond in different ways to the same price, and some of the factors that affect use (level of education, family size) might themselves be distorted if user price varied with them. At any price, therefore, there will be some underuse and some overuse. As user price is reduced from any level, overuse will decrease as underuse increases. A balance will have to be sought, and it is surely possible that underuse might be regarded as worse than overuse. But it is unlikely that balance will be achieved in a system in which everyone is faced with a zero user price for every type of care. And even if the money price of care were zero, the time, distance, and inconvenience costs would still be positive.

One final comment should be made on the relationship between changes in user prices and severity of illness. It has sometimes been suggested that severity of illness and response to changes in user price might be related in a nontautological way. Zola (1964) suggested, for example, that the extent to which illness interferes with activities might be a better measure of that severity which is related to use than type of symptom.

The relevant point here is that an economic approach may also be useful in generating hypotheses about interrelationships between illness characteristics, user, charges, and use or demand. To take the simplest case, consider the "investment" approach suggested by Grossman, in which care is desirable only as it influences the stock of health and health is desirable only as it affects the ability to earn income. At any user price, care will be used for any illness up to the point at which the increment in earnings expected from the use of that care equals its user price. The expected increment in earnings can, crudely, be considered as the product of the effect that care has on illness and the effect that an illness change has on the ability to earn income. Only the latter second effect, the effect of illness on function, seems to correspond to Zola's measure of severity.

Now let the user price rise. By how much will care be reduced? It will be reduced relatively less for those kinds of illnesses for which an increase in illness severely limits activities and for which a small reduction in care use greatly increases the likelihood or severity of illness. Conversely, care will be reduced relatively more for those kinds of illness in which the marginal illness effect on income and the marginal care productivity of illness are low. Note that absolute severity of illness alone does not predict response; the marginal effect of illness on functioning and the marginal effect of care on illness must also be known. In principle, both concepts can be defined and measured empirically. A useful classification of illness might be based on this sort of analysis.

Supply Effects on Demand

Up to this point the author has tried to avoid discussing the effects on use of supply responses. But even though it was intended to discuss only demand effects on use, such a separation is not possible in any discussion of medical care. The reason is that there are strong theoretical and empirical grounds for believing that supply response affects demand directly, in addition to whatever other effects it may have on price or rationing or other determinants of use. The quantity of care people are willing to take at various prices may be affected by the incentives facing suppliers of care.

The theoretical reason is that people are sometimes unsure about the effects of medical care and tend to buy advice about how much care to use from the same persons or firms who supply that care. Especially if competition is not strong, it is possible that suppliers may be able to "shift" demand. One piece of empirical evidence to that effect is the substantial difference in use sometimes detected between prepaid group practice, where the incentive is to supply little care, and fee-for-service medicine, where the incentive is to supply as much care as yields the provider additional real income. Although some of the difference is undoubtedly due to self-selection in that the people who choose to belong to a prepaid group would have demanded a bundle similar to the bundle supplied, probably not all of it can be explained away. A second kind of empirical evidence, a little less substantial, is Feldstein's (1971a) finding that hospital beds, numbers of general patients, and numbers of specialists affect hospital use. The results are less substantial because the relationship could also reflect supply response to omitted demand parameters.

At the present time we know little about the extent to which suppliers can affect demand. It seems reasonable to conjecture that there are upper and lower bounds. Few people could be persuaded to have surgery for a cold or to take aspirin as a cure for a lacerated finger. It seems reasonable to suppose that the limits vary for the different kinds of illness or symptoms that individuals experience. It also seems reasonable to suppose that, within this range, incentives faced by providers will determine how much they shift or try to shift demand. Finally, one suspects that the effect of physician persuasion or other supply influences on an individual's demand should differ depending on the information he has; if more education really leads to more efficient production, for instance, it is likely that the demand of better educated people should be less influenced by supply influences. But other than these speculations and the gross empirical evidence mentioned above, there is little that we know.

Conclusion

In this essay I have discussed a number of economic or economically interpretable influences on use, but I have given the most stress to and spent the most space on the influence of user price. This emphasis is proper, since economics is, in a sense, about the influences price exerts on individuals' behavior. The general message is that, in medical care especially, price is not likely to be a "pure" incentive. Its interaction with other determinants of use, almost all of which are subject to economic interpretation, is an area in which both public policy and intellectual curiosity suggest that we should try to find out much more than we now know.

References

Andersen, R. J., O. W. Anderson, *and* B. Smedby
   1968   "Perception of and response to symptons of illness in Sweden and the United States." Medical Care 6: 18–30.
Andersen, R. J. *and* L. K. Benham
   1970   "Factors affecting the relationship between family income and medical care consumption." Pp. 73–95 in Klarman, H. M. (ed.), Empirical Studies in Health Economics. Baltimore: Johns Hopkins University Press.
Auster, Richard A., I. J. Leveson *and* D. K. Sarachek
   1972   "The production of health, and exploratory study." Pp. 135–160 in Fuchs, V. R. (ed.), Essays in the Economics of Health and Medical Care. New York: Columbia University Press.
Cummins, J. M.
   1973   Cost Overruns in Defense Contracting. Ph.D. dissertation, Northwestern University, Evanston, Illinois.
Davis, Karen A. *and* Lucille B. Russell
   1972   "Substitution of hospital outpatient for inpatient care." Review of Economics and Statistics 54 (May): 108–120.
Donabedian, Avedis B.
   1969   "An evaluation of prepaid group practice." Inquiry 6 (September): 3–27.
Feldstein, M. S.
   1970   "The rising price of physicians' services." Review of Economics and Statistics 52 (May): 121–133.
   1971a "Hospital cost inflation: A study in nonprofit price dynamics." American Economic Review 61 (December): 853–872.
   1971b "A new approach to national health insurance." Public Interest 23 (Spring): 93–105.
   1973   "The welfare loss of excess health insurance." Journal of Political Economy 81 (March/April): 251–280.
Feldstein, M. S. *and* E. E. Allison
   1972   "Tax subsidies of private health insurance: Distribution, revenue loss, and effects." Boston: Harvard Institute of Economic Research, Discussion Paper No. 237.
Feldstein, P. J.
   1966   "Research on the demand for health services." Milbank Memorial Fund Quarterly 44 (July): 128–165.
Frech, H. E. *and* P. B. Ginsburg
   1972   "Comment." Southern Economic Journal 38 (April): 573–577.
Grossman, M. J.
   1972   The Demand for Health: A Theoretical and Empirical Analysis. New York: Columbia University Press.

Klarman, Herbert E.
    1965   "Effects of prepaid group practice on hospital use:" Public
            Health Reports 78 (November): 955–965.
Newhouse, J. P.
    1970   "A model of physician pricing." Southern Economic Jour-
            nal 37 (October): 174–183.
Newhouse, J. P. *and* C. E. Phelps
    1973   "On having your cake and eating it too: A review of esti-
            mated effects of insurance on the demand for medical
            care." Preliminary draft. Santa Monica: The RAND Cor-
            poration, October.
Pauly, Mark V.
    1971a   "Indemnity insurance for health service efficiency." Journal
            of Economics and Business 32 (Fall): 53–59.
    1971b   Medical Care of Public Expense. New York: Praeger Pub-
            lisers, Inc.
    1972   An Analysis of Alternative National Health Insurance Pro-
            posals. Washington, D.C.: American Enterprise Institute.
Phelps, C. E. *and* J. P. Newhouse
    1972a   Coinsurance and the Demand for Medical Care. Santa Moni-
            ca: The RAND Corporation, R-964-OEO/NCHSRD.
    1972b   "Effects of coinsurance: Amultivariateanalysis."SocialSe-
            curity Bulletin 35 (June): 20–28.
Richardson, William C.
    1970   "Measuring the urban poor's use of physicians' services in
            response to illness episodes." Medical Care 8: 132–142.
    1971   Ambulatory Use of Physicians' Services in Response to Ill-
            ness Episodes in a Low-Income Neighborhood. Chicago:
            University of Chicago, Center for Health Administration
            Studies.
Roemer, Milton I.
    1972   Testimony before the House Committee on Ways and
            Means, June.
Roghman, K. J. et al.
    1971   "Anticipated and actual effects of Medicaid on the care pat-
            tern of children." Unpublished paper.
Rosett, R. M. *and* L. Huang
    1973   "The effect of health insurance on the demand for medical
            care." Journal of Political Economy 81 (March/April):
            281–305.
Scitovsky, Anne A. *and* Nelda M. Snyder
    1972   "Effect of coinsurance on the use of physician services."
            Social Security Bulletin 35 (June): 3–19.
Scott, H. D.
    1973   "Uses of hospital discharge data for community planning
            and quality assessment." Providence Evening Bulletin
            (April 5).

Silver, Morris

    1972   "An economic analysis of variations in medical expenses and work-loss rates." Pp. 97–118 in Fuchs, V. R. (ed.), Essays in the Economics of Health and Medical Care. New York: Columbia University.

Zola, I.

    1964   "Illness behavior and the working class: Implications and recommendations." Pp. 76–94 in Shostak, A. *and* W. Gomberg (eds.), Blue Collar World. Englewood Cliffs: Prentice-Hall.

7. Poverty and Health: A Re-examination

MYRON J. LEFCOWITZ

Reprinted with permission of the Blue Cross Association, from *Inquiry* Vol. X, No. 1 (March 1973), 3-13. Copyright © 1973 by the Blue Cross Association. All rights reserved.

Current discussions of health policies for the poor typically assume that poverty is a cause of medical deprivation. In these discussions there is much controversy over whether financial or structural barriers are more important in restricting availability and utilization of adequate health services by low-income populations. Whichever side of the argument is taken, two "facts" are accepted as true: 1) Poverty leads to less medical care; and 2) poverty results in diminished health.

In this paper available information that casts doubt on these two statements has been brought together. In addition to making the relationship of income to health problematic, the evidence at times suggests that level of education is a causal factor in individual health status and medical care utilization. When education is taken into account in analyzing the income-health relationship, the correlation is considerably diminished, usually to the point of disappearance. Education, within income levels, however, remains as a factor in health status and behavior. Hence, the observed correlation between income and medical deprivation appears to

be a consequence of education's relationship with both variables. Unfortunately, the published data provide only a few instances—although they are strategic—having to do with medical care for children and infant mortality.

Some possible implications of this evidence for the current health policy debate are suggested. The major objective of the paper, however, is to clear away some of the myths which have heretofore befogged that debate. Before beginning, two points need to be made. Although some of the material to be presented are recomputations of the available data, the following is primarily a discussion of information as it has been published in various reports of the U.S. National Center for Health Statistics.[1] We do not pretend, therefore, any originality in data analysis. Since the line being pursued is different from the prevailing—or, at least, published—consensus, the use of data well-known to professionals in the field would appear to be particularly appropriate.

Second, we do not want to debate the definition of poverty. Whatever it is, there is agreement that in general economic terms it is at least some minimum access to a bundle of goods and services.[2] One indicator of poverty in that sense is family income. Thus, we shall be using poverty, low income, plus equivalent adjectives synonymously.

Myron J. Lefcowitz, Ph.D. is on the staff of the Institute for Research on Poverty and is Associate Professor, School of Social Work, University of Wisconsin (1180 Observatory Drive, Madison, Wisconsin 53706).

The research reported here was supported by funds granted to the Institute by the Office of Economic Opportunity pursuant to the provisions of the Economic Opportunity Act of 1964. The author wishes to thank Burton Weisbrod, David Elesh, Robinson Hollister, Robert Lampman and Ray Munts for their comments on earlier drafts of this paper. However, the conclusions drawn in this paper are solely the responsibility of the author.

Medical Care

There has been almost universal agreement that the poor receive less than the non-poor in the way of actual medical care —both in quantity and quality. The Neighborhood Health Center programs sponsored by OEO and then HEW were designed, at least in part, to redress the imbalance. This inequity in medical care, moreover, is apparently observable.[3]

Quantity of Care

The most recent data, however, suggest that there is little correlation between average number of physician visits per person per year and family income. Based on information gathered from household interviews in 1969, the average number of physician visits was 4.8 for persons in families with less than $3,000 income, and 4.3 for persons whose income was over $10,000.[4] But, these averages mask a strong relationship for children under 15 years of age. When family income is under $3,000, the average number of physician visits from July, 1966 to June, 1967 was 4.4 for children under five, and 1.5 for those five to 14 years of age. When income is over $10,000, the averages for the corresponding ages were 7.2 and 3.5.[5] Taking education of the head of the family into account, however, the correlation between family income and average annual number of physician visits among children disappears (Table 1). This finding suggests that education of the family head is an important factor in medical care utilization for the young.

However, averages may not reflect the spread of utilization. Perhaps low-income persons visit the physician both less and more often than high-income persons; hence, the similarity in averages. There is little evidence, however, to support that suggestion. Although low-income persons are somewhat more likely than the high-income population *not* to have seen a physician, income is not related to a high frequency (five or more) of visits.[6]

Quality of Care

But what about the quality of that care? Unfortunately, the problem of medical care quality in general has barely been touched. It is an obviously complicated question both in definition and in measure-

Table 1. Number of physician visits per person per year by education of head of family and family income for persons under 15 years of age, July 1966-June 1967

| Family income | Education of head of family | | | |
	Under 5 years	5-8 years	9-12 years	13+ years
Under $5,000	2.1	2.2	3.2	5.4
$5,000 and over	1.4	2.6	4.1	5.0

Source: National Center for Health Statistics. *Volume of Physician Visits, 1966-1967*, Series 10-49 (1968) p. 23.

ment.[7] Hence, we ought to be wary of categorical statements on the relative inferiority of health care received by the poor.

One indicator of quality, however, is use of medical specialists. Specialists relative to other physicians deal more frequently with the diseases which come to their attention and are best-equipped to bring to bear the practices appropriate to management of the disease.[8] The three special services most frequently used, and for which information is available, are pediatrics, obstetrics-gynecology and eye care. In Table 2, the percent of the relevant population using those specialists from July, 1963 to June, 1964 is presented by family income and education of family head. In general, higher income persons had used these services more frequently than the population with incomes less than $4,000. Education also has an impact—one which appears to be sharper than income given the gross categories in Table 2. In almost all instances persons in families where the head had some college education were at least twice as likely to have used the service than when the head had less than nine years of education, regardless of income. These data, then, are consistent with the data reported on physician visits in general; which is, that education seems more strongly related to medical care utilization than income.

Another indicator of quality medical care is the use of private practitioners relative to public clinics. The poor are depicted as relying largely on public clinics and therefore are considered deprived in the quality of their health care compared

Table 2. Percent of population using selected types of medical specialists and practitioners by family income and education of head of family, July 1963-June 1964

Type of visit Income	Education of head of family		
	Under 9 years	9-12 years	13+ years
Pediatric			
Under $4,000	4	15	30
$4,000 and over	10	20	38
Obstetrics-gynecology			
Under $4,000	2	7	11
$4,000 and over	4	10	16
Ophthalmologic			
Under $4,000	4	5	10
$4,000 and over	5	6	11
Optometric			
Under $4,000	7	7	13
$4,000 and over	9	10	9

Source: National Center for Health Statistics. *Characteristics of Patients of Selected Types of Medical Specialists and Practitioners, July 1963-June 1964*, Series 10-28 (1966).

to the non-poor.[9] In fact, low-income persons are more likely to go to a hospital clinic or an emergency room than higher income persons—14 percent of physician visits from July, 1966-June, 1967 when family income is under $3,000 compared with 6 percent when income is over $10,-000. More important, however, 75 percent of the physician visits of low-income persons involved either a home or office visit with a private physician. This proportion, moreover, is the same for persons with higher income.[10] Thus, the image that the poor are at the mercy of public clinics for their medical care is a bit overdrawn.

This is not to argue that quality medicine is indeed distributed equitably across income classes. But, the little evidence available does suggest that an open mind on the issue is in order. Moreover, the data do suggest that when medical care varies by socioeconomic status, it is more across education levels than by family income.

Health of the Poor

But what about the health of the poor? If they are not as healthy as the non-poor, then similarity in medical care utilization would indicate that the poor are relatively deprived given their greater need. Assuming a corresponding demand, equal utilization may be a consequence of a relatively scarce supply of medical care in low-income areas.

Morbidity 病态

Taking age into account, however, there appears to be very little relationship between income and the presence of chronic diseases.[11] This information is based on interviews—and fewer people report ailments than are detected by clinical examination. For example, 6.2 million persons had heart conditions in 1963-1965 according to household interviews.[12] Based on the Health Examination Survey from 1960-1962, however, 14.6 million adults had definite heart disease.[13] This discrepancy might be proportionately larger at lower income levels where people may be less informed about the presence of less obvious chronic conditions. Consequently in an actual clinical examination many more unsuspected ailments could be discovered among low-income persons than among high-income ones. Thus, the correlation between morbidity and income would be increased.

With this possibility in mind, information from the National Health Examination Survey on heart and arthritic conditions, the two leading causes of activity limitation,[14] has been summarized in Table 3. The data presented are the differences between the actual rate per 100 adults, as diagnosed through the Health Examination, and the rate that would have been expected given the age composition of the subgroup. (See the appendixes of the various Health Examination Survey reports for a technical description of the derivation of the expected value.) Thus, a *negative* value indicates *less* actual disease than might be expected for that population and a positive value denotes more. The closer the value is to zero, the closer together are the actual and expected rates.

Looking first at hypertensive heart disease, we can see that there is no apparent

Table 3. Differences between actual and expected* prevalence rates per 100 adults of selected disease conditions by family income, sex and race, 1960-1962

Disease conditions	Family income				
	Under $2,000	$2,000-3,999	$4,000-6,999	$7,000-9,999	$10,000 and over
Definite hypertensive heart disease					
White men	−0.5	−0.8	0.7	−1.8	1.4
White women	3.8	−0.3	−0.7	−2.1	0.1
Black men	8.2	−6.6	−2.2	−6.9	11.9
Black women	2.7	−1.2	0.8	−6.4	−2.9
Definite hypertension					
White men	−1.6	0.4	1.0	−0.5	−1.6
White women	4.9	−0.7	−1.2	−0.7	−1.6
Black men	7.3	−5.4	−3.4	−13.8	6.5
Black women	4.3	1.9	−6.0	−0.4	−5.6
Definite coronary heart disease					
Men	−0.8	0.2	0.9	0.2	−1.7
Women	0.6	0.3	0.2	0.2	−1.2
Osteoarthritis					
Men	−2.8	0.3	−0.4	1.5	0.5
Women	0.5	0.0	−0.2	−1.0	2.0
Rheumatoid arthritis					
Men	3.0	−0.5	−0.6	−0.2	−0.1
Women	0.0	−0.5	0.7	−0.5	−0.5

*Standardized for age.

Sources: NCHS. *Hypertension and Hypertensive Heart Disease in Adults, 1960-1962*, Series 11-13 (1966) p. 24.
NCHS. *Coronary Heart Disease in Adults, 1960-1962*, Series 11-10 (1965) p. 23.
NCHS. *Osteoarthritis in Adults by Selected Demographic Characteristics, 1960-1962*, Series 11-20 (1966) p. 11.
NCHS. *Rheumatoid Arthritis in Adults, 1960-1962*, Series 11-17 (1966) p. 22.

relationship between family income and the difference between the actual and expected rates per 100 adults. For example, white men with under $4,000 family income have less definite hypertensive heart disease than expected; the next highest income category has more; the next less; those adults with incomes over $10,000 have more. For white women the pattern is quite different—the difference between the actual and expected rates decreases with income from 3.8 to −2.1 in the $7,000-$10,000 category and then increases to 0.1

for the highest income category. Black men exhibit a similar curvilinear pattern as white women—positive in the extreme income categories and negative in the middle categories. Among black women, however, there is no apparent relationship.

For hypertension, the curvilinear pattern appears for both white and black men, but in opposite directions. For women, however, the difference between actual and expected prevalence of hypertension does decrease as income increases (Table 3).

The general relationship is not clear, therefore, between income and hypertension, or income and hypertensive heart disease. Hypertension and hypertensive heart disease can stand for all the disease conditions reported in Table 3—that is, the negative relationship between income and these diseases is problematic. Given the relative importance of heart and arthritic conditions in limiting the activities of people, this conclusion would seem to be significant.

What about other impairments or conditions? The clinical data on diabetes,[15] anemia,[16] vision[17] and hearing[18] are generally consistent with the above conclusion. The available evidence from the Health Examination Survey, then, is consistent with data obtained from household interviews. The only conclusion is that the relationship between health and poverty—as indicated by morbidity—is not proven.

Mortality Rates

Some persons have argued, however, that mortality rates, particularly infant mortality, are a better indicator than morbidity rates of the health status of a population.[19] In general, past research has supported the generalization that these rates decrease with increased socioeconomic status. Nevertheless, the findings have not been unambiguous.[20] Data, however, are now available which permit us to obtain a fix on the variation in infant mortality rates by family income and parents' education. The necessary information was obtained by a follow-back survey of national samples of births and infant deaths for 1964-1966. The data presented suggest that for white births, family income has no consistent relationship with infant mortality when parents' education is taken into account. At all income levels, however, education, whether mother's or father's, is negatively related. For blacks, the patterns are not as clear although both income and education appear to have an impact on infant mortality rates.[21]

This evidence again forces us to be more skeptical about the presumed relationship between poverty and health even when the index of the latter is infant mortality. Rather, as our thesis contends, education appears to be the socioeconomic variable most closely related.

Education and Medical Deprivation

The policy implications of the apparent effect of education on medical deprivation and the concomitant diminution of the income-health correlation when education is taken into account are not readily apparent. In this section a general interpretation of the relationship of education to health will be presented; on the basis of that framework some policy directives are suggested.

Weber[22] pointed out that people are distributed in society along three dimensions —class, status and power. Class refers to economic positions, status to life styles (prestige), and power to control of others. Since persons are distributed with reference to each, policies can be directed to redistributing the values which locate people on each dimension; or, at least by producing enough of the values, we can attempt to move all members of society above some minimum level. Hence, poverty is reduced by increasing family income —and hopefully, the poor's relative share of total income is increased.

In this context, our hypothesis is that health-related and health-oriented behaviors are primarily a function of valued life styles and that education is a primary agent in the development of such tastes. Put some-

what differently, every family—within reasonable limits—has access to any part of the market bundle of goods and services available. How it selects, given its income, from that bundle is the family's life style. Education is a primary determinant in the ordering of those priorities.

What are the dynamics which link education and health? We start with the assumption that reduction of illness and prolongation of life are desired states. Education, in the first instance, is a process that increases the level of information about factors related to those desirable states. It does so directly through what is taught, at least up through the secondary level, but more probably through the acquisition of skills which enable the person to be both more sensitive and more alert to relevant information. Thus, for example, we expect that the more educated a person is, the more likely he is to be aware of the relationship between health and diet or physical exercise, topics much discussed in the mass media. Therefore, we would hypothesize that: The more educated a person is the more likely he is to have the opportunity to be exposed to, to expose himself to, and to be influenced by health information. His opportunities are greater because the mass media to which he is exposed is more likely to provide that information. He is more likely to expose himself because he is more alert to such information. Moreover, he is more influenced because he is more accepting of the claims of science in matters affecting day-to-day life.

Also, through education, the individual develops a life style which may have a greater impact on health status than what he or she may do directly. Diet, for example, may be more a consequence of food preferences or of physical aesthetics than concern about its apparent relationship to health.

This function of education is not explicit in that preferred choices are taught at each level, but rather that the level of education provides the basis for entry into social statuses; and during the distributional process different life styles are acquired—consciously or unconsciously.

More concretely, our educational system is directed toward fitting people into urban society. In that society, for instance, small families are apparently preferred— possibly because the costs for children are larger in cities. Therefore, we should expect that birth rates are related to residential background and education. And, that is indeed the case. Low rates are found for women of nonfarm origin and nonfarm residence. On the other hand, women with a farm background rapidly approach the birth rate for women who have a nonfarm background as farm women's educational level increases.[23] Moreover, family income is unrelated to birth rates in urbanized areas.[24] Whatever the primary social or economic function of small family size, it probably has the additional consequence of affecting the health status of the offspring. Evidence indicates that, in general, infant mortality increases with parity;[25] and moreover, this relationship remains even when socioeconomic status as measured by occupational categories is taken into account.[26] Thus, we can infer that the decreasing number of children per family which flows from increased education has the secondary consequence of reducing infant mortality and, hence, improving the health status of the population concomitantly, albeit indirectly.

One more example of the possible indirect effects of education on health status relates to accidents. The accident rate for a population is in some degree a consequence of the potentiality for injury inherent in that population's physical location and movement within a social environment. Presumably, this location and movement is a function of life style. Therefore, it is interesting to note that although income, controlling for age, is only slightly related to the current injury rate, education, again taking age into account, is strongly and negatively related in general. Thus, for persons 25-44 years of age, the current injury rate per 100 persons per

year drops from 35.2 for persons with only some high school to 20.5 for persons with a college degree.[27]

One explanation is that education is also negatively related to the accident potential in occupations. Some evidence for this hypothesis is that men have higher injury rates than women at all age levels up to 65. This difference is largely attributable to the much greater incidence of work injuries among men. Following the same reasoning, we would also expect that nonwhites would have a higher accident rate than whites; that is, they are more likely to be in accident-risking situations—particularly at work. On the contrary, the nonwhite accident rate is two-thirds the white one for persons under 45 and about the same for persons over 45. These data at least bring into question occupation as an explanation for the relationship between education and injury rate. We would suggest that differential life styles may be the explanation.

Consumption Patterns and Permanent Income

An alternative explanation for the analytic importance of education relative to income for health status and health care is that consumption patterns are more directly tied to permanent income, for which level of education is a proxy. There is no way using available data, however, to test directly the permanent income hypothesis. Presumably, the relationship of education to family consumption of medical care and to infant mortality rates might be explained in part by the permanent income hypothesis. However, since most physician visits are a direct response to an illness and injury—only about 20 percent of the visits by children under 15 are for a general check-up or immunization and vaccination[28]—permanent income might be less important in the consumption of medical care than in expenditures for durable consumer goods.

Unfortunately, the above is only supposition. Efforts to find published data which could provide a more direct test was, with one exception, largely unavailing. The exception relates to cigarette smoking. We would expect in that case that average number of cigarettes smoked per day by men would increase with income—and indeed it does among present smokers. What we also find is that income is positively related to the age-adjusted percentage of men who have *never* smoked and who are former smokers. The same relationship holds for education.[29] It would be difficult to predict the fact that higher income is positively associated with not smoking cigarettes from a permanent income hypothesis. Actually, we would be more likely to predict the opposite in keeping with the generally positive relationship between income and the consumption of other goods and services.

Given the current state of our knowledge, however, the permanent income hypothesis is not so easily disproven. The above data do bring it into question, while leaving the life-style hypothesis untouched. Probably both mechanisms are in operation so that the main issue is their relative importance.

If our contention is correct that preferences (life styles) are of more moment in health behavior than access to a market basket of goods and services, what does this hypothesis have to say about whether to emphasize a financial or structural approach in our health policy? If the hypothesized lower preferences for health care among the less educated is correct, the price elasticity with respect to health care is small. Moreover, our data suggest that the income elasticity is also small (see Table 1). Although reduction in cost would clearly increase utilization (we assume, of course, that supply increases correspondingly or is already sufficient to handle the increased demand), the change would be small if the elasticities are as predicted. Whether the magnitude of that effect is optimum from society's viewpoint —that is, whether the consumption of medical services by the lower educated will move up to some level of adequacy—is problematic given the hypothesis.

The problem, then, is to increase the preference for health care and other health-inducing behaviors among the lower educated. This guideline suggests that alterations in the structure of the delivery system, as it relates to the less well-educated, be considered the appropriate policy direction. Most discussions of structural reform focus on increased supply and/or proximity of services, none of which addresses the heart of the problem as here stated. What is needed are changes that will decrease the psychic distance and that will enhance the significance of modern health practices for the medically deprived. Such programs as outreach workers sensitive to the life styles of the low-educated, medical translators to facilitate communication between the practitioner and client, reinforcement of preferred behaviors which are causally linked to health (e.g., making available at low cost preferred food which provides an adequate diet) appear to be mechanisms which in the short-range policy horizon would be more conducive to improving the health and medical care of the population concerned. An examination of the social-anthropological literature on the introduction of modern health technology among underdeveloped groups might be most instructive for our own society. If programs of this type were directed toward the low-income population, they would, by their nature, scoop in a large part of that subset which is deprived as a result of their life patterns.

Health and Poverty Restated

But what about the consequences of illness? It is our contention that illness and medical care have more serious consequences for lower income populations than for the affluent. In economic terms, the costs of illness are inequitably distributed among the income categories and hence may cause or increase impoverishment. We claim no originality for this idea for which the supportive data are generally known. What we do assert is that incorrect policy implications have been drawn.

First, even though the prevalence of persons with one or more chronic ailments

Table 4. Percent of adults with family incomes under $3,000 by their chronic condition and activity limitation status, 1965-1966

| | Percent under $3,000 income | | | | |
| | | Persons with 1+ chronic conditions | | | |
Age	Persons with no chronic conditions	No limitation of activity	Limitation, but not in major activity	Limitation in amount or kind of major activity*	Unable to carry on major activity
17-44	12	11	16	24	41
45-64	12	13	21	36	51
65+	43	47	54	55	57

*Major activity refers to ability to work, keep house, or engage in school or preschool activities.
Source: NCHS. *Limitation of Activity and Mobility Due to Chronic Conditions, 1965-1966*, Series 10-45 (1968) p. 26.

is unrelated to income, persons whose chronic conditions limit their major activity are much more likely to have incomes under $3,000 than where the ailment is less restrictive (Table 4). This relationship is particularly true for non-aged adults. In the 17-44 age group, among those who have no chronic conditions, one out of every eight or nine has a family income under $3,000; in the same group among those unable to carry on their major activity two out of every five have family incomes under $3,000 (Table 4). The pattern is similar for 45-64 year olds. Among the aged, where advanced years restrict activity in any case, low income is much less related to the limitations imposed by chronic conditions.

This finding is not surprising. Income and the physical demands of occupational activity are, in general, negatively related. Among persons with similar ailments, moreover, we would expect those engaged in physical labor to be more restricted in their work activity than persons in non-manual occupations.

Some evidence for this hypothesis is presented in Table 5. Among currently employed persons over 44 years of age who report one or more chronic conditions, those in farm and nonfarm labor occupations are most likely to say that their condition limited their major activity. Alternatively, professional, technical, and clerical workers are least likely to report such restrictions (see Table 5).

Haber[30] presents corroborating data from the Social Security Disability Survey. The occupations in which the workers are most limited are also somewhat more likely to include workers having one or more chronic conditions (Table 5). Thus, it is possible that the chronic condition may be a consequence of work, particularly farm work, itself. That possibility aside, however, the data are consistent with, but do not confirm our thesis that the economic consequences of poor health are more serious for persons in more physically demanding occupations.

Income and Work Days Lost

Unfortunately, these data are not available by employment status and income. However, we do have, by income, the average number of days lost from work during 1968-1969 for currently employed persons. What is instructive to note is that income is correlated with work days lost for men between 25 and 64 years of age. Moreover, the relationship is quite strong. Men 25-44 years old lose twice as much time from work if their income is less than $3,000 than if it is over $10,000. Among men 45-64 years old, those with less than $3,000 income lose more than twice as many days as men with more than $10,000 family income. Thus, precisely among primary wage earners, the differential cost of illness is greatest.[31]

Lower income families, then, lose a greater proportion of their income as a result of illness than do more affluent per-

Table 5. Chronic conditions and limitation of major activity by occupation of currently employed persons over 44 years of age, 1965-1966

Occupation	Of all in occupation, percent with chronic conditions	Of all with 1+ chronic conditions, percent with limitation of major activity
Professional, technical	68	7
Managers, officials proprietors (nonfarm)	69	15
Clerical	68	9
Sales	72	15
Craftsmen and foremen	67	14
Operative	66	13
Service, except private household	69	15
Private household	77	24
Laborers, except farm and mine	69	24
Farm laborers and foremen	72	33
Farmers and farm managers	77	33

Source: NCHS. *Limitation of Activity and Mobility Due to Chronic Conditions, 1965-1966*, Series 10-45 (1968) pp. 48-49.

sons. This conclusion assumes that days lost from work means wages lost for everyone. But, it is plausible that persons in higher paying jobs are more likely to have sick leave benefits, formal or informal, and therefore, are less likely to lose any income as a result of illness. In fact, that is the case. The higher the family income, the more likely are currently employed persons to report that they are reimbursed for work time lost through illness.[32] Thus, the impact on income for wage earners in the lower income categories is even greater relative to high-income persons than just missing more days at work.

Costs of illness, obviously, can also mean direct out-of-pocket expenses for the necessary treatment and care. Such out-of-pocket costs are proportionately greater for lower income families.[33] In 1961, families with less than $4,000 money income after taxes spent between 7.5 and 10 percent of it on medical care compared to 6 to 7 percent for higher income families.[34] Family income was negatively and sharply related to coverage by hospital and surgical insurance.[35] Since the proportion of persons hospitalized in a given year does not vary by income,[36] we can assume that lower income persons are more likely to be confronted with a large medical bill than are persons with higher incomes. For example, of those persons hospitalized for surgical treatment, where family income was under $2,000, about one-third of the discharges had some part of the surgeon's bill paid for by insurance compared with four-fifths when the income was over $7,000.[37] The threat of a catastrophic medical bill is underlined by the fact that hospitalized lower income persons tend to be in the hospital somewhat longer than their higher income counterparts.[38]

The conclusion that illness has a greater financial impact on the poor than the more affluent is hardly surprising. After all, Medicare and Medicaid are attempts to correct this inequity—at least insofar as direct out-of-pocket costs are concerned—as are the various health bills currently in the Congressional hopper. What the data point to, however, is that vocational rehabilitation and cash transfer programs may be more productive in ameliorating the consequences of poor health than are health programs.

Conclusion

This paper has attempted to focus the available, mostly published data about income and health on the public debate over whether financial barriers or structural barriers are more important in restricting availability and utilization of adequate health services to lower income populations. This debate has assumed in part that medical deprivation is caused by poverty. Through reviewing the data, however, that assumption has been questioned. Hence, insofar as the policy controversy has been based on poverty as a causal factor in poor health and inadequate medical care, the demarcation of alternative approaches to improving health standards and increasing medical care utilization has rested on an unstable assumption. Instead, the evidence presented indicates that education is negatively related to health and health care.

Policy Directions

The policy directions for intervention between education and health status and care are not immediately apparent. We have suggested that education functions to distribute the population by valued life styles (preferences, in economic terms) and that these styles include elements which directly or indirectly affect health and utilization of health services. Presumably, as the educational level increases, the health status of the population will improve in response to the hypothesized change in life styles. At the same time, effective demand for health care will also increase. It is very difficult, of course, to demonstrate both trends as well as their causal relationship to education. If the general hypothesis is correct, however, it does suggest that policies designed to reduce medical deprivation on the basis of poverty as a cause are misguided. In this framework the current policy issue may be reformulated: What changes in health policy—financial and/or structural—will increase utilization among the less educated given their relatively lower preference for health care?

A policy explicitly for the less educated does not appear reasonable. We would hardly want to add a taste test as an analog to the means test. Since education and income are highly correlated, a health policy directed toward the poor would cover a large portion of the low-educated population. But, which type of remedy—financial or structural—should be emphasized?

The argument is presented that the ef-fect of a financial policy would lead to only a small increase in health care utilization and/or health-improving behavior among the low-educated. The basis for that hypothesis is that both income elasticity and price elasticity with respect to such behavior are small. Thus, if we are interested in the medically deprived, policies directed to changing the preferences and/or to reinforcing existing health-inducing preference patterns are required. This conclusion suggests, then, that structural changes be given central consideration over financial changes in the health arena.

But, can we then ignore the poor as such in our development of policy? The evidence presented in the paper does support the notion that a loss of health and the use of medical care are more costly to the poor than non-poor. This cost is twofold. First, the share of income required for medical care is greater for the poor. Any policy which picks up the tab for services can to that extent redress the inequity. Clearly, however, this objective is more income-distributional than health-improving. Second, poor health can drastically affect earnings, making poor out of previously non-poor and creating a barrier to movement out of poverty for those persons already there. Policies designed to reduce the income consequences of ill health would focus on transfer payments during an illness or disability period (e.g., broader disability insurance both in coverage of working population and to other than work-related disabilities) and/or an expansion of our vocational rehabilitation programs.

To a large extent, then, a serious attempt to deal with the health and poverty issue would involve only in part what is typically considered a health program and would address itself to the relative cost inequities between poor and non-poor.

References and Notes

1 See the following National Center for Health Statistics (NCHS) publications for a more detailed description of their surveys: *Origin, Program, and Operation of the U.S. National Health Survey,* Series 1-1 (1963); *Cycle I of the Health Examination Survey: Sample and Response,* Series 11-1 (1963); and *Plan and Initial Program of the Health Examination Survey,* Series 1-4 (Washington, D.C.: GPO, 1964).
   Since the Government Printing Office is the publisher for all NCHS publications, that information will not be repeated.
2 Watts, Harold. "An Economic Definition of Poverty." In: Moynihan, D.P. (ed.) *On Understanding Poverty* (New York: Basic Books, 1969) pp. 316-329.
3 White, Elijah L. "A Graphic Presentation on Age and Income Differentials in Selected Aspects of Morbidity, Disability and Utilization of Health Services," *Inquiry* 5:18-30 (March 1968).
4 NCHS. *Age Patterns in Medical Care, Illness, and Disability, 1968-1969,* Series 10-70 (1972) p. 10.
5 NCHS. *Volume of Physician Visits, 1966-1967,* Series 10-49 (1968) p. 19.
6 *Ibid.*, p. 39.
7 Roth, Julius. "The Treatment of the Sick." In: Kosa, John, *et al.* (eds.) *Poverty and Health* (Cambridge: Harvard University Press, 1969) pp. 222-226.
8 Mechanic, David. *Medical Sociology* (New York: The Free Press, 1968) p. 354.
9 Roth, *op. cit.,* pp. 217-218.
10 NCHS. Series 10-49, *op. cit.,* p. 30.
11 NCHS. *Limitation of Activity and Mobility Due to Chronic Conditions, 1965-1966,* Series 10-45 (1968).
12 NCHS. *Age Patterns in Medical Care, Illness, and Disability, 1963-1965,* Series 10-32 (1966) p. 55.
13 NCHS. *Heart Disease in Adults, 1960-1962,* Series 11-6 (1964) p. 7.
14 NCHS. Series 10-45, *op. cit.,* p. 6.
15 NCHS. *Blood Glucose Levels in Adults, 1960-1962,* Series 11-18 (1966).
16 NCHS. *Mean Blood Hematocrit of Adults, 1960-1962,* Series 11-24 (1967).
17 NCHS. *Binocular Visual Acuity of Adults, by Region and Selected Demographic Characteristics, 1960-1962,* Series 11-25 (1967).
18 NCHS. *Hearing Level of Adults by Education, Income, and Occupation, 1960-1962,* Series 11-31 (1968).
19 Lerner, Monroe. "Social Differences in Physical Health." In: Kosa, *et al.* (eds.) *Poverty and Health, op. cit.* p. 91.
20 Mechanic, *op. cit.,* pp. 244-257.
21 NCHS. *Infant Mortality Rates: Socioeconomic Factors,* Series 22-14 (1972) pp. 13-14.
22 Weber, Max. "Class, Status, Party." In: Gerth, H. H., and Mills, C. Wright. (trs.) *From Max Weber: Essays in Sociology* (New York: Oxford University Press, 1946) pp. 180-195.
23 Duncan, Otis Dudley. "Farm Background and Differential Fertility," *Demography* 2:240-249 (1965).
24 Sweet, James. "Some Demographic Aspects of Income Maintenance Policy." In: Orr, Larry L.; Hollister, Robinson G.; and Lefcowitz, Myron J. (eds.) *Income Maintenance: Interdisciplinary Approaches to Research* (Chicago: Markham Press, 1971).
25 Illsley, Raymond. "The Sociological Study of Reproduction and Its Outcome." In: Richardson, Stephen A., and Guttmacher, Alan F. (eds.) *Childbearing: Its Social and Psychological Aspects* (Baltimore: Williams and Wilkins, 1967) pp. 96-98.
26 Chase, Helen C. "Infant Mortality and Weight at Birth: 1960 United States Birth Cohort," *American Journal of Public Health* 59:1618-1628 (September 1969).
27 NCHS. *Types of Injuries: Incidence and Associated Disability, 1965-1967,* Series 10-57 (1969) p. 7.
28 NCHS. *Volume of Physician Visits by Place of Visit and Type of Service, 1963-1964,* Series 10-18 (1965) p. 26.
29 Hedrick, James L. *Facts on Smoking, Tobacco, and Health* (National Clearinghouse for Smoking and Health, 1968) pp. 10-11.
30 Haber, Lawrence D. "Disability and Social Planning: Implications of The Social Security Disability Survey." Paper presented at the annual meeting of the National Conference on Social Welfare, June 3, 1970, Chicago, Illinois.
31 NCHS. *Time Lost From Work Among the Currently Employed Population, 1968,* Series 10-71 (1972) p. 15.
32 *Ibid.*, p. 23.
33 Tucker, Murray A. "Effect of Heavy Medical Expenditures on Low Income Families," *Public Health Reports* 85:419-425 (May 1970).
34 U.S. Bureau of Labor Statistics. *Consumer Expenditure Survey Report, 1960-61,* Report 237-93 (Washington, D.C.: GPO, 1965) p. 16.
35 NCHS. *Family Hospital and Surgical Insurance Coverage, 1962-1963.* Series 10-42 (1967) pp. 13-17.
36 NCHS. *Persons Hospitalized by Numbers of Hospital Episodes and Days in a Year, 1965-1966.* Series 10-50 (1969).
37 NCHS. *Proportion of Surgical Bill Paid by Insurance, 1963-1964.* Series 10-31 (1966) p. 8.
38 NCHS. Series 10-50, *op. cit.,* p. 14.

8. Insurance, Copayment, and Health Services Utilization: A Critical Review

PAUL B. GINSBURG AND LARRY M. MANHEIM

Reprinted with permission from *Journal of Economics and Business* 25. Copyright © 1973, Temple University, 142-153.

Discussions of the issues involved in National Health Insurance have often raised the question of the efficacy and desirability of having consumers share in the costs of purchasing medical care. If consumers do pay a portion of the cost, such as through coinsurance and deductible provisions, federal and possibly total expenditures on health services covered by National Health Insurance would be reduced.[1] If the consumers must contribute too large a share, important benefits of the program would be lost.[2]

Coinsurance and deductible provisions have long been used by commercial insurance companies in their health insurance plans. One purpose has been to achieve a reduction of what the companies call "moral hazard." When consumers have a degree of control over the events which are insured (in this case utilization of medical care), they tend to cause those events to occur more frequently than in the absence of insurance (use more medical care). The companies have felt that if consumers agree to pay part of the cost of insured health care, they will not increase their consumption so much, and will moderate insurance rates.

Cost-sharing takes four major forms. Under a deductible scheme, the consumer pays all expenses up to a certain point, where the insurance begins. With a coinsurance scheme, the consumer pays a specified percentage of the insured

expenses. Under a copayment arrangement (a term used for cost-sharing schemes) a fixed charge per unit of insured service is paid by the consumer. Finally, indemnity payments provide a fixed payment to the consumer per unit of service used regardless of actual charges, which in most cases results in cost-sharing.

Deductibles and coinsurance are the forms of cost-sharing most commonly in use. Over time, deductibles have tended to be included in a larger proportion of health insurance policies. In 1956, 22 percent of group comprehensive major medical insurance policies had a deductible of at least $50 [14]. In 1970, 48 percent of new group policies in this category had a deductible provision exceeding this level [15]. It is not possible to document a trend in the use of coinsurance provisions, but when coinsurance is used, 20 percent and 25 percent are the most common rates among commercial insurers (the rate for the Medicare program is 20 percent).

Formulation of an optimal cost-sharing arrangement for National Health Insurance plans is dependent upon the answers to two key research questions. First, one needs to know whether coinsurance and deductible provisions have a substantial effect on utilization. If the impact should be small or negligible, then the benefits of cost sharing are a reduction in the excess burden of the taxes required to finance the program, while its costs are a diminution of the risk-reducing benefits of insurance and the costs of administering a collection system. In addition, imposition of cost-sharing requirements affects the distribution of income, with the provision weighing most heavily on the poor and the sick. The policy decision with regard to cost-sharing is not a simple one in this case, but it is conceptually clearer than that for the case in which utilization is affected. When cost-sharing reduces the use of health services, an evaluation of the effects of the reduction on social welfare must be coupled with the above considerations. In the abstract, economists might regard this reduction as a benefit, as it would result from bringing the costs of medical care faced by consumers closer to

Dr. Ginsburg is assistant professor of economics at Michigan State University, and Mr. Manheim is an economist at the National Center for Health Services Research and Development, where the work reported here was conducted. They wish to thank John Rafferty, Ted Frech, Dan Walden, William Lohr, and Jere Wysong for helpful comments on this study. The authors assume sole responsibility for the views expressed.

1. This paper does not get involved with the details of the various plans proposed for universal entitlement. An abstraction with features common to most of the proposals is envisioned when National Health Insurance is mentioned. Most plans provide a subsidy to the major part of the population to consume health services and accomplish this subsidization through financing rather than government production of health care.

2. In a limiting case, a program with a 100-percent coinsurance rate would be a nonprogram and achieve nothing.

the costs incurred by society. Others may place their own valuations upon the change in utilization.

The evaluation of a reduction in utilization should not be carried out on too aggregated a basis. A given coinsurance charge places a larger burden on the poor than the wealthy. Likewise, medical care for the sick is weighted differently than that for the relatively healthy and perhaps for the young as opposed to the old. Value judgments about the distribution of health care are the basis for these decisions. If research should show that coinsurance and deductible provisions do affect the use of medical care, defining optimal copayment arrangements will require knowledge of the magnitudes of the reductions for various age, income, and health-status groups.

It should be noted that the presence of insurance or of copayment provisions is not the only factor that impinges on utilization of medical services. The organization of the health-care system is also of substantial importance to utilization, and National Health Insurance undoubtedly will foster changes in its structure. The influence of cost-sharing can be examined to a large degree independently of organizational factors. Imposition of a coinsurance provision need not change the structure of the medical-care industry. While the organizational framework in which an insurance change takes place may affect the magnitude of the change in utilization, the problem is handled by studying it in different organizational contexts.

A fairly large number of studies have already been completed on the issue of the effect of copayment on utilization of health services. While the studies have not provided sufficient information as yet, they comprise a useful base on which researchers can build. Pointing out the serious deficiencies which plague a large number of the studies should assist future researchers in avoiding these pitfalls. Discussing previous research within the context of the design of National Health Insurance Plans should assist those contemplating studies on the subject to focus most directly on the relevant issues.

Effects of cost-sharing on utilization

The theory of consumer choice demonstrates how a consumer's demand for a good is a function of its price, the prices of other goods, income, and other factors such as tastes. The demand for medical care can be viewed in this way. A health insurance benefit granted by the government is usually in the form of a price subsidy to the consumer of medical care.[3] When insurance pays all of the bill, the effective price to consumers is zero, and they can be expected to demand the quantity that they would have demanded at a zero price. This demand will be finite because of the discomfort of medical care, the time input necessary to consume it, and other reasons.[4] Coinsurance and deductibles are seen as altering the degree of subsidization by insurance. The net price is raised from zero to (in the case of coinsurance) a proportion of the market price. Since the quantity demanded is an inverse function of price, imposition of copayments reduces the quantity demanded.

The theory is somewhat more complex when individuals purchase health insurance. They may desire copayment provisions to reduce the insurance premium. Choice of a coinsurance rate involves a tradeoff between the value of the risk-reducing effects of insurance, and the additional premium costs due to the higher utilization that results from the subsidy effect of insurance. It follows that those with the poorest expected health status and strongest tastes for medical care will choose insurance policies with the smallest copayment provisions.[5] Thus, in private health insurance the copayment rate and the extent of health services utilization are determined simultaneously.

Additional complexity is added to the theoretical framework when the supply of medical services is considered. The price of a given health service and the quantity of it that is exchanged depends upon both supply and demand factors. Isolating the influence of demand thus provides only part of any model of market adjustment. Ignoring supply considerations causes further difficulties when the market for medical services is organized as a monopoly. Frech and Ginsburg have demonstrated that the impact of governmental insurance benefits on medical care utilization depends upon market structure [11]. In addition, health insurance benefits often affect market structure, further altering the effect on utilization.

The discussions thus far are based on market clearing. This may not always occur in the short run (which might be quite long), causing problems of "access" to medical services by consumers, and causing the demand model to overestimate the impact of copayment on utilization. In this case nonprice rationing may occur, causing a short-run diagnostic mix to vary with total utilization as has been measured for hospitals by Rafferty [19].

A topic of continuing debate involves whether consumers have very much choice at all in medical care utilization decisions. If physicians play an important role in these decisions, then a supply factor directly enters the demand relation. This factor does not alter the direction of the

---

3. An "ideal" health insurance benefit would compensate for illness rather than consumption of medical care, but practical considerations prevent this arrangement from being used extensively.

4. The cost of time is likely to be especially important for blue collar workers who cannot leave their jobs without loss of pay.

5. This statement is based on the assumption that those who would demand more care do not pay high enough premiums because they pay community rates. Akerlof notes that under a private insurance system, adverse selection may prevent community-rated insurance sales from taking place at any market price since the average medical condition of insurance applicants deteriorates as the premium rises [2].

relationship between copayment and utilization, but, like the other supply considerations, it does affect magnitudes.

Research methods

In order to determine the effects of coinsurance and deductibles on the utilization of medical services, it is important to know the price elasticity of demand (or the responsiveness to price changes) for medical services. Among individuals, demand will be dependent upon tastes for medical care (often reflected by age, sex, race, education, and socio-economic status), health status, income, and the presence of medical care providers. In order to measure responsiveness to price accurately, these other factors must be held constant. Concern with holding factors other than pr ce constant is the dominant theme in research design.

A further problem is that the responsiveness to price changes is different among various groups in the population identified by age, income, sex, and other characteristics. As each group has a different price elasticity, an estimate of the overall elasticity for the entire population loses a lot of information for policymakers. It is essential to identify the persons whose use of medical care will be reduced most and least by coinsurance so that the overall reduction in utilization can be evaluated. The notion of different price elasticities for different groups of people also poses problems for the estimation of overall elasticities. For example, one cannot estimate the price response of the entire population by studying a sample composed entirely of the elderly. These considerations suggest disaggregation whenever practicable. Both simulations of controlled experiments and regression analysis have been used to estimate the response of utilization to price. The method used is largely dictated by the available data.

The ideal controlled experiment is one in which a randomly selected experimental group is subjected to a change in price while the control group continues to face the original prices. While such controlled experiments rarely occur naturally and tend to be prohibitively expensive to undertake strictly for research, close approximations are available by studying situations where changes have been made in the benefits of group health insurance policies. While the control group is not present, the insurance change can often be identified as exogenous. Adjustment for trends and exceptional circumstances must be made on an ad hoc basis—a potential source of error.

Earlier studies of this type often committed the error of allowing the control group and the experimental group to be self-selected. The result was that those planning to consume more medical care chose the group with the lower coinsurance deductibles, causing the effect of price on utilization to be overestimated. Hall quotes an insurance executive: "Our company indicates an uncanny ability on the part of laymen to choose, when offered an option in coverages, that which later events will prove benefical of them" [12, p. 256].

Response to a change often differs according to the time period under consideration. In some studies, the initial response was found to be larger than the long-term change. Several factors may be responsible for such behavior. For example, if the price is increased with advanced warning, price expectations would shift the timing of short-run utilization, increasing demand for care shortly before the price change and decreasing it shortly thereafter. If one views medical expenditure as an investment in human capital, it is noted that when the quantity of medical care an individual demands is decreased his expected health status will decline in future periods, increasing his expected demand curve for health services in those periods. If price increases, the immediate quantity demanded decreases more sharply than in the long run when a new steady-state equilibrium is reached, and vice versa with a price increase.

Working in the opposite direction is the usual economic argument that price response will be larger in the long run than in the short run due to such factors as habit and increased ability to substitute between medical care and other health-improving activities in the long run. Results confirming this type of behavior are also available, for studies over a short period must be interpreted cautiously. One further problem occurs when the prices for only some medical services are changed. The estimates are relevant only to the particular services under study, and in addition the price response may be overestimated because of substitution between the services under study and other services.

Major difficulties inherent in group comparisons are that natural experiments are uncommon, that the time period for observation is necessarily limited, and that the sample may not be sufficiently varied in composition to generalize the results to the entire population. An advantage is that the insurance provisions faced by the group before and after the change are easy to compare.

Regression analysis methods use survey or claims data on utilization, prices faced, and characteristics such as income and age.[6] While these characteristics are held constant, the variation in utilization caused by different prices is measured. However, when individuals can choose their insurance plan, they can be expected to do so on the basis of planned consumption. This adverse selection will bias the estimates of price response upward. This problem may be overcome by limiting the sample to individuals who had no choice of policy, by using state observations adjusted for demographic factors instead of those on individuals, or by estimating a simultaneous equation regression model which includes an equation for the demand for insurance. An argument can be made for separate regression equations on various age groups and income groups to estimate the differential elasticities across these characteristics.

Thus far the discussion has been conducted on the assumption that the supply of the relevant medical services is completely elastic, that the producers will produce any quantity of care that is desired of them at the going price. This assump-

---

6. State populations may be used as units of observations in place of individuals.

tion is clearly not realistic, especially in the short run. If an insurance plan alters demand for a substantial number of people in an area, price will be higher and the quantity demanded lower than in the case of elastic supply. It will not be possible to allocate the overall quantity change to supply and demand factors respectively unless additional information is available. As the elasticity of supply varies by area, it is impossible to generalize from the results without knowledge of the separate effects of supply and demand.

Most studies overcome this problem. A number consider an insurance change which affects a small enough proportion of consumers in an area that the change in the quantity demanded by the community is negligible. While this methodology finesses the problem of supply factors to some extent, the relevance to the national health insurance issue is open to question. A National Health Insurance benefit would affect the demand of a large proportion of the population in an area. As all areas would be affected, the results of the long-run equilibrium cross-sectional analysis would not apply either. What is most desirable is a model which explicitly takes supply into account.

A diversity of opinion exists on the issue of the effectiveness of coinsurance and deductibles on health services utilization. This diversity is reflected in two surveys of providers of insurance, which arrived at assorted conclusions. Diokno's survey of Michigan insurers obtained a view of effectiveness of cost-sharing in reducing utilization [6]. Fifty-two percent of the respondents felt that coinsurance was effective, while 14 percent felt that it was ineffective, and 34 percent claimed that they did not know. A recent survey of Blue Cross and Blue Shield Plans found an evenly split opinion on whether cost-sharing affected utilization [4]. There was a consensus, however, that reductions are often in "needed care." Furthermore, they felt that serious financial hardship resulted from high copayment provisions. It should be noted that views about cost-sharing correlate well with the long-standing policies of commercial insurers and Blue Cross-Blue Shield Plans toward this issue. While these opinions reflect judgment of people active in the field, almost none were based on studies of the issue.

A large number of studies have been completed to date. However, most run into one or more of the methodological problems already discussed. Recently, some of the work has shown promise of the sophistication necessary to provide the quantitative information policymakers require. It is these latter studies that will consume most attention here.

Experimental simulations

Diokno used data from 1956 to 1958 to construct two-year comparisons of the experience of companies with indemnity insurance plans covering less than full medical expenses as opposed to data of those with Blue Cross-Blue Shield full-benefit hospital service type plans [6]. The companies compared were in the same line of business and were located in the same metropolitan

area. The data collected allowed for adjustment for age and sex, although some failure to report age caused problems. The fact that company policies were examined should have severely limited the bias that arises from individual selection of policies. In general, Diokno found significantly lower utilization under indemnity programs even when age and sex were accounted for, but the results were more impressive for females.[*] Quantifying the effect of an indemnity as opposed to full coverage is very difficult because of different benefit structures for different services and, more importantly, because it is difficult to obtain actual prices of services in relation to indemnity payments. What should be noted is a large variability in results among age and sex brackets. While this is no doubt partially due to uncontrolled differences in the groups, it apparently also reflects two recurrent themes in all these studies—that aggregate elasticities will obscure many differences among age, location, and sex brackets and that the price effect, while it is often important, is usually dominated by changes in other variables when they cannot be held constant. Dividing hospital admissions into surgical and nonsurgical cases does not appear to provide any additional insights, but the study does provide strong evidence as to the qualitative significance of copayment.

In the Diokno study, as in those that follow, the question of evaluating the decrease in utilization with regard to whether it represents the elimination of "unneeded" or "needed" care (disregarding all the ambiguity inherent in these terms) is left unanswered. Wirick used two methods to approach this problem [28]. First he found that data for admissions for eighteen common diagnoses in twenty-two Michigan hospitals showed the percentage of "inappropriate" admissions to be higher in cases covered by third-party insurance than in those of self-paying patients, but the result was not statistically significant. In a second study, he assessed the effect of insurance on length of stay. Comparing lengths of stay to a norm determined with reference to standard medical practice by a panel of physicians, Wirick observed that 11.2 percent of patients paying the entire bill had understays as compared to 5.6 percent of patients with some insurance. For overstays, the percentages were 6.7 and 11.8 percent, respectively. These results underestimate the differences in understays and overstays because of case-mix differentials.

In one of the first studies on the effect of different insurance schemes on utilization, the Columbia University School of Public Health and Administrative Science found in 1958 no major differences between three representative types of hospital health coverage—insurance with deductibles, full coverage insurance, and Kaiser hospital plans (see Jesmer and Scharfenberg [17]). On the other hand, Perrott found that those covered by the Federal Employees Health Benefit

---

7. "Significantly" will be used in terms of rejection of the null hypothesis of no difference between two populations at the 5-percent level. While it is much more helpful to have numbers associated with statements on significance, in many cases this was not possible here due to a lack of details on any meaningful numbers.

(FEHB) program, non-maternity hospital days per thousand covered were Blue Cross, 729; Indemnity Plans, 708; Prepaid Group Practice, 454 [18]. Since, the comparison between the Blue Cross and Indemnity Plans is not very meaningful without a detailed comparison of the different benefit structures, there may be no important differences in the effective coinsurance rate between the two plans. More interesting is the different utilization experience for the high and low option policies for each insurer. The utilization rates for the Blue Cross-Blue Shield Plans are 882 and 520 days per thousand and for the Indemnity Plans are 760 and 481, respectively. These numbers demonstrate the magnitude of the combined effects of adverse selection and the price elasticity of demand. In both studies the data on prepaid group practice must be considered in a different context due to the financial incentives to reduce costs by lowering utilization and substituting ambulatory for inpatient care.[8]

Ackart found that after the Blue Cross Plan of Virginia attached a $50 deductible provision for hospital payments and an additional copayment if hospital room charges exceeded $12 per day, admission rates for individuals decreased by 6.7 percent [1]. Ackart thought this might have been larger except that supplementary insurance could be purchased. Jesmer and Sharfenberg note that Ackart's figures did not include many one-day stays under the deductible plan since these, under $50, were not reported [17]. Their calculations on the effect of this bias used a different plan and found this nonreporting would cause an illusory 2.9 percent difference in admission rates. Thus, Ackart's figures must be adjusted downward by something of this order.

Williams used a large population and compared deductibles and copayment with full benefit hospital insurance within geographically homogeneous Blue Cross Plans [27]. The data from a survey of Blue Cross plans made in 1964 include information on plan enrollment and utilization by age and sex. Individuals within each of three groups were given a choice between full benefit and deductible plans ($10-$25 deductible per admission), and those individuals with the deductible coverage had 12.3 percent less, 8.2 percent less, and 18.1 percent more admissions per 1,000 (adjusted for age and sex) than individuals in the same groups with full insurance coverage. The latter increase is explained by greater benefits under the deductible plan for this specific group. Length of stay was somewhat longer for the deductible plan, but again some one-day stays may not have been reported under the deductible plan which would reduce the differences reported. Even had one-day stays been

reported, such a difference would be explained by the fact that a deductible will discourage short visits more than longer visits. (This is more plausible than Ackart's rationalization that patients try to "make up" for the deductible.) For two other group plans, a choice between a copayment scheme (insured pays $4 per day for the hospital room) and full-benefit insurance was available, and individuals under copayment had admission rates of 136 and 135 per 1,000, as compared with 156 and 144, respectively, for the full-benefit scheme. The lengths of stay were about the same. Given the ability to select on the part of the insured, the effects of cost-sharing are overestimated, but the numbers are useful in establishing an upper bound for price elasticity.

A recent study of two Pennsylvania Blue Cross Plans by Hardwick et al. compared a group having a full-service benefit contract with a group having a copayment clause (insured pays $5 per day for the first 15 days of inpatient hospitalization). Adjusting for age and sex, they found that utilization of hospital services was not significantly different for the two groups. Specifically, they reported: "The overall conclusion of this study is that five-dollar per day copayment has had no significant effect on hospital use as measured by five indices: 1) average length of stay, 2) average benefits per admission, 3) average benefits per day, 4) admissions per 1,000 members, and 5) patient days per 1,000 members" [13, p. 9]. Unfortunately, these conclusions are based on what can only be described as a less than careful analysis of data implications. The data collected are biased because the fully-covered population almost exclusively used Pittsburgh metropolitan area hospitals while those with copayment plans were dispersed throughout Western Pennsylvania. This difference in residence will reflect differences in supply (availability of beds), urban-rural patterns of medical care demand, income, and education. All these factors suggest that even if both groups paid the same price for their medical care, the rural group would have less patient days per 1,000 members. Since the rural group is the one with copayment, one would expect the rural group to have lower statistics for patient days per 1,000 as long as there was not a large positive price elasticity. In most age-sex categories the Pittsburgh group had much lower utilization rates suggesting not a perverse positive price effect, but rather large structural differences of unknown origin between the two groups. Patient days per 1,000 for females are presented as a dramatic indication of these results;[9] the figures for males were much less decisive. As the article itself takes no cognizance of these strange happenings, the results probably should be ignored.

---

8. The Columbia Study's results regarding Kaiser are contrary to all other data and may represent poor experimental design. In another set of studies comparing full coverage of union health insurance policies to full coverage of H.I.P. of New York, Densen finds that active union control of their full coverage plan can help to eliminate utilization differentials [5]. As racial composition was not taken into account in this study, and as it is probably a significant factor in the union plans studied, the results are subject to some questions. They do suggest another variable which may dominate any price effects.

9.

	Patient Days per Thousand	
Females	Rural Copay Group	Urban Fully-insured Group
Age 60-64	2,353.7	1,000.0
50-59	1,277.3	813.8
40-49	1,054.3	495.5
30-39	837.5	741.9
20-29	499.0	423.9

Source: Hardwick [13]

In 1965, a contract study of the Michigan Blue Cross Plan by Vaughn compared comprehensive and deductible plans obtained both by groups and by individuals; only 10 percent chose the deductible [25]. Utilization under the deductible plan had been running 50 to 75 percent of that under full insurance. It was found that while child dependents were fully covered under both schemes, those whose parents or the group to which they belonged chose the deductible plan showed significantly lower utilization rates, tending to confirm the existence of bias when individuals or even groups are allowed to select their own schemes. Since the utilization figures do not take into account observed age and geographical differences—differences which we have already found to exert large effects upon utilization—specific quantitative estimates from the data on selectivity bias are not feasible.[10]

One important hypothesis is that a change in prices to the insured may not change utilization except when price goes to zero. If this hypothesis is true, then small copayments might be effective. This is the tentative conclusion reached by Weisbrod and Fiesler who looked at the hospitalization experience of two large groups of persons under Blue Cross hospital plans before and after one group chose to obtain more comprehensive Blue Cross coverage [26].[11] Differences between the standard and the preferred coverages pertained to ancillary services (many more of them were covered) and private room accommodations (went from $10 to $12 per day room allowance). A significant increase in hospital use by those in the preferred plan occurred, but it was concentrated among females over 55. Ancillary services were increased significantly for those under the preferred plan relative to the lower coverage plan, but among those who entered the hospital, use of private rooms did not significantly increase. Since the price drop to zero for ancillary services increased utilization substantially, while room price changes had no such effect, Weisbrod and Fiesler arrived at the tentative hypothesis that price response may only be substantial as price to the consumer goes to zero.[12] It may be more likely that ancillary prices dropped to zero from quite substantial heights, and it was the magnitude of the drop in prices that was responsible for their results.

Hall surveyed a number of companies which changed from full-benefit payment to some co-payment scheme, usually to attempt to cut spiraling costs. The results were conflicting, but three studies do indicate a substantial decrease in hospital utilization due to deductibles of $25 and $50. Lack of reporting of individual claims may account for some of this, as may the fact that those most affected may cancel. Hall concludes that, while the effect of coinsurance and deductible provisions in health services and facilities is difficult to quantify, "there is considerable evidence which supports the intuitive conclusion that these provisions do act as a brake on utilization, yet there are sufficient examples of no or negative correlation to cast a lingering doubt as to the exact role which they play" [12, p. 262].

Only one study has attempted to measure the effect of imposing a change in price on one group, while using another distinct but similar group to control for time-trend factors. But data limitations that researchers faced at the time make the control meaningless. Heany and Riedel surveyed a sample of data covering 1966-68 gathered by Connecticut Blue Cross, which had changed half of its group plans from indemnity coverage (up to $15 per day maximum benefit) to full coverage of hospital room and board charges (semi-private room option for new plan) [16]. They arranged the groups by size and found that in five of seven instances the rate of admission increased following the increase in benefits, but in no case was the increase statistically significant. Overall, the admission rates went from 4.56 to 6.09 per 100, which (though quite substantial) also was not significant.[13] The average length of stay increased slightly less than one day (7.26 to 8.17 days) for those fully covered, and there was a markedly significant increase in the day rate under the new benefits (33.17 to 41.66 days per 100). It must be noted that the study covers only six months after the increase in benefits, not long enough to infer any strong conclusions. While roughly half the groups were used as controls, the authors were not able to study the control groups over the same twelve-month period. Thus, extraneous factors affecting utilization which changed during the year could not be eliminated. Indeed, Heany and Reidel did not even correct for seasonal variations. And the substantial changes that, in fact, occurred within the control group when the first six months are compared with the last six months of the year studied, illustrate the importance of taking into account other factors which change over time.

The Saskatchewan Medical Insurance Plan (SMIP), established in 1962, provides universal and comprehensive insurance coverage to Saskatchewan residents for almost all physician services. It is supported by annual premiums with Provincial and Federal contributions from general revenues, and physicians are paid on a fee-for-service basis. In 1968, a copayment of $1.50 for an office visit and $2.00 for a home emergency or outpatient visit was instituted. R. G. Beck analyzed the effect of these utilization fees in 1968 and found, after adjusting for age-sex distribution and

---

10. The differentials among children were roughly about 50 percent of that found for parents when group policies were surveyed and about the same as for parents when coverage was by conversion policies.

11. Actually, individuals in this group had the chance to choose whether they wanted the additional coverage with 75 percent taking this coverage. This adverse selection bias is noted by the authors.

12. Some support for this view comes from a study of a program of insured prescription drugs in Saskatchewan which looked at the effect of raising the coinsurance charge from 20 percent (which had been imposed in 1948) to 50 percent in 1959. The effect varied with age, sex, and degree of urbanization. Utilization actually increased for males, age 25-44. According to the Royal Commission on Health Services, "it is worth recording that these cocharges have not had the deterrent effect originally hoped for, even though they were followed by an overall reduction in drug utilization."

13. It is not clear how significance is obtained—their enumerated method suggests they assumed some known variance.

Table 1			
Annual Percent Change in Adjusted per Capita Utilization of Services			
Year	Percent Change	Year	Percent Change
1964	5.75	1968	− 3.07
1965	2.43	1969	0.39
1966	4.52	1970	8.91
1967	3.69	Average Annual Rate of Change 1963-70	3.23

Source: Saskatchewan Insurance Commission [22].

Table 2			
Annual Rate of Physicians' Calls per 1,000 Beneficiaries			
Year	Office	Home	Hospital
1952	2,187	398	1,239
1953*	2,136	158	1,259
1954	1,812	175	1,416
1955	1,904	181	1,451
1956	1,789	187	1,359
1957	1,942	236	1,440
1958	1,991	222	1,393
1959	2,056	231	1,370

* Copayment charges adopted in 1953 (home charge of $2 during the day or $3 at night instituted in January and office charges of $1 instituted in August).
Source: Straight [24, p. 77].

a time trend, that the introduction of the copayment caused an overall reduction in the utilization of services of about 6 to 7 percent [3]. Larger families and families headed by the aged, probably low-income families, exhibited a proportionately greater reduction in utilization of services. As can be seen from Table 1, 1970 utilization rates jumped sharply, possibly implying that the introduction of copayments often has a transitory shock effect which disappears several years later. Supporting this notion is research on the Swift Current Health Region Program established in 1946 for part of the southwest corner of Saskatchewan [24]. The insurance covered physician and hospital services (see Table 2). The institution of a coinsurance charge appeared to reduce utilization of home visits dramatically. The coinsurance charges, however, were limited to home and office visits, and thus coincident with this reduction was an increase in the fully-covered hospitalization and minor surgery. Relevant to the transitory shock hypothesis, the lower utilization rates were somewhat less clear in later years. The investigator, Straight, noted that beneficiaries found that the coinsurance was less likely to be actually collected in later years. Similarly, an increase in the number of medical specialists from 1969-70 might have some significant role in explaining the greatly increased utilization under SMIP in 1970. These varied hypotheses indicate the value of a control group in isolating utilization factors. A time trend appears to be a poor substitute.

While the 1970 jump in utilization plus the time trend problem in general cast some doubt on Beck's results, his study is one of the most careful and successful attempts to examine the problem thus far and will be discussed in more considerable detail.

Beck has data for 1963-68 physician visits for families in Saskatchewan, as well as data on income, the age of family head, number of children, location, and welfare status. He uses only age and number of children as independent variables when estimating the differential effect of the copayment. Implicitly he assumes that no significant change in the other variables had taken place in 1968 relative to the 1963-67 trend.[11] From 1963 to 1967 there were no patient fees for physician visits. By regressing the number of visits upon age and the number of children, coefficient estimates are obtained. Then, for each coefficient, a regression on the five coefficient

observations from 1963-67 is obtained and used to predict what the coefficient would be in 1968 if the relationship remained unchanged. This method provides estimates of age-sex variable coefficients for families in the absence of the utilization fee. Using these coefficients, one could predict the physician utilization for the average family in a given age-sex bracket if no utilization fee had been in existence. Beck then compares this prediction to actual utilization to compute the effect of the utilization fee. As a check of his time-trend predictions of the coefficients, Beck compares the predicted coefficients to actual ones from January to April 15, 1968 (the date when copayments were instituted), and finds the predictions reasonable.

Clearly, one problem is that some structural change might have occurred in 1968 which may equally explain what happened in 1970. Supply factors are not considered and will be an important consideration when an entire region is being considered. From Beck's analysis there is a tentative feeling that large changes in supply factors did not take place. The one exception to this supposition is that in the middle of 1968 physician fees went up from 85 to 95 percent of a published fee schedule. But the resulting increase in the quantity of service physicians would be willing to supply at the established fee schedule would tend to increase utilization so that the estimates of the effect of the copayment will be underestimates. Examples of the change in the quantity of service for a family as a result of the introduction of utilization fees are presented in Table 3. Another reason why these figures should underestimate the decrease is that not all visits were covered by the utilization fee.

Research by Scitovsky and Snyder estimated the effect of coinsurance on utilization by a group of about 2,500 Stanford University employees covered by a comprehensive prepaid medical care plan [23]. In 1967, members began to be charged 25 percent of the scheduled fee for all physician (including inpatient) and outpatient ancillary services. The utilization under the plan was compared in 1966 and 1968, the two full calendar years before and after the change. Per capita physician services declined by 24 percent for the group as a whole and by varying degrees for every age-sex-occupation subgroup. Home visits decreased most (51.6 percent), office visits about average (24.9 percent), and hospital surgery least (4.8 percent). These results are consistent

---

14. The effect of income had previously been found to be quite small under the insurance plan.

Table 3

Percent Change in Quantity of Services for Couples
with Head of the Household 45-54 Years Old[15]

Size of Family	Total Quantity of Services	Home and Emergency Visits	Hospital Visits	Major Surgery
0 children	− 5.06	− 10.00	− 10.28	− 1.45
1 child	− 14.21	− 22.22	− 11.28	− 7.59
2 children	− 12.58	− 17.76	+ 2.98	− 7.06
3 children	− 17.39	− 19.70	− 20.13	− 11.00
4 children	− 18.03	− 24.84	− 7.86	− 18.87
5 children	− 14.19	− 26.37	− 7.89	− 8.77

Source: Beck [3] Tables 6.11-6.18.

with economic expectations. The problem of no control to allow for a time trend is unfortunate, but unlike the Beck study, since these employees constitute only 16 percent of the clinic's population, supply can be considered elastic.

Regression studies

A number of economists have used regression analysis to explain health services demand. Paul Feldstein's survey of medical-care-demand studies confirms that price effects had received little attention, probably because the price paid by the consumer was so difficult to isolate [9]. Since Feldstein's survey, some results have appeared.

Paul Feldstein and Ruth Severson estimated price elasticity from 1958 cross-sectional data obtained by the National Opinion Research Center at the University of Chicago. From this data, sixty-six primary groups were formed—how this was done was not explained—and by using these groups as observation points, price elasticities for various medical care utilization measures were computed. In addition to the price variable, income, age, family size, location, education, free-care situations, and the percent of bill paid for by insurance were used as explanatory variables. The price variables used in each regression were generated by dividing net expenditures for the relevant care component by the quantity of services consumed. The estimated price effects reported are reproduced in Table 4. How much confidence can be put in these estimates? As the authors note, since net expenditures (which were used in generating a price variable) may represent differences in quality as well as prices, the price effect may be underestimated. Including both an insurance variable and a price variable in the same equation provides, in effect, two price variables in the equation. If the percent of the bill paid by insurance is highly correlated with the price

variable, which is what one would expect, the full effect of prices upon utilization may not be accounted for by looking at the coefficient on the price variable. This fact may explain the insignificance and perverse estimates in some regressions. As the method of primary grouping is left unexplained, adverse selection bias among groups may again be an important factor.

Rosenthal used 1962 data for New England short-term general and special hospitals to estimate the effect of price upon length of stay [20]. The estimated equations adjusted for age and sex and run for a number of diagnostic categories were

$$Y = a_1 X_1^{b_1}$$

$$Y = a_2 X_2^{b_2}$$

where Y is length of stay, X_1 is cash outlay as a percent of the total bill, X_2 is average daily room charge, and b_1 and b_2 are price elasticities of demand. Neither variable actually represented price paid by the patient, and Rosenthal inexplicably did not give us the results of running the more reasonable equation $Y = a(X_1 X_2)^b$ where $X_1 X_2$ would be a true price variable (although a biased one due to the different services X_1 and X_2 measure). At any rate, average daily room charge was by far the more successful variable with a greater elasticity and more explanatory power. Tonsillectomies and adenoidectomies tended to have the highest price elasticities while more serious diagnoses had lower elasticities. The price elasticities for length of stay varied from some perversely positive estimates to price elasticities of −0.7. The variation in elasticities among diagnoses conformed to theoretical expectations and showed the value of diagnostic disaggregation. While the specific quantitative results are questionable because of the price variables used, it is true that if the percent of bill paid by insurance was not correlated with the average charge, the average charge coefficient would provide a price elasticity. One major bias was the lack of quality control—higher priced patient days may result from more intensive care which would shorten stays even with zero price elasticity.

A tour-de-force of econometric manipulation by Rosett and Huang provides price elasticity estimates for physician and hospital expenditures from the 1960 Bureau of Labor Statistics *Consumer Expenditure Survey*. This data includes insurance premium payments, and direct medical payments, but none on benefits paid by insurance companies. Assuming equal premiums represent

---

15. An amount equal to $1.50 for office visits and $2.00 for home, emergency, or hospital outpatient visits is deducted from the payment to physicians for these services, but the physician is permitted to recover this deduction in the form of a direct charge to the patient. This charge was not always made. While there was no copayment for physician hospital visits for major surgery, a per diem hospital copayment of $2.50 was assessed on the patient as of April 1968. The per diem charge probably acts similarly to copayment for a physician's hospital visit. Surgery, which also decreased considerably, may be related to this per diem charge and to ambulatory charges. The latter case would imply that either many people who decreased their visits to a physician did so in spite of a need for major surgery or that doctors do a lot of discretionary surgery.

Table 4

Effect of a 10-Percent Increase in Price on the Consumption of the Various Components of Medical Care

Type of Medical Care Expenditures	Percent Change	Significant at 5% Level?
Physician visits (total):	− 1.9	Yes
Physician visits (home, office):	− 1.4	No
Physician expenditures:	+0.2	No
Hospital admissions:	+ 1.1	No
Hospital patient days:	+ 0.2	No
Hospital expenditures:	+ 4.3	Yes

identical policies, the authors arrive at the percent of total bill paid for by insurance. Price responses by consumers in different health categories are computed on the assumption that all insurance can be represented as a single coinsurance variable, where the percent of the total bill paid by the consumer is the coinsurance payment. Sex, education, age, family size, location, race, saving-income ratio, and attitude toward pain as reflected by dental expenditures are used as control variables.

Rosett and Huang's estimates of price elasticities are a function of the coinsurance rate. For an average family, the price elasticity is −0.35 for a coinsurance rate of 20 percent and increases in absolute value with higher coinsurance rates. The elasticity at an 80 percent rate is −1.5. The large variation in price elasticity estimates for different prices explains some of the variance in results among the other studies. While the study is quite ingenious, the data used is poor for the purpose at hand. Adverse selection bias is probably important here. It should be noted that, given their estimated elasticities, Rosett and Huang find that those insured at risk, especially lower-income families, would be better off buying insurance for the most expensive and least likely events, but to self-insure the more usual minor expenses. Martin Feldstein, using state data, has come to a similar conclusion—if insurance coverage were reduced, the utility loss from increased risk would be more than outweighed by the gain due to lower prices and the reduced purchase of excess care [7]. Of course, these conclusions depend crucially upon the price elasticity estimates.

Recently, Martin Feldstein has estimated elasticities for hospital demand in terms of a full supply and demand model [8]. He used aggregate state data for 1958 to 1967, necessitating an assumption that average and marginal coinsurance rates are equal, to estimate price elasticities. As he did adjust utilization data for age, sex, and color, and as one would not expect the distribution of preferences for health care, given these adjustments, to vary markedly among states, adverse selection should not be a problem here. The regression equations control for the usual demand and supply factors aside from price which influence utilization. Feldstein arrives at demand price elasticity estimates of −0.435 (standard error 0.061) for hospital admissions and −0.236 (standard error 0.041) for mean stay (i.e., −0.671 total demand price elasticity for hospital days). In such cross-sectional analyses, there is no reason to believe the estimates are transitory rather than equilibrium estimates.

In order to test whether there is a lag in adjustment to the new prices, Feldstein adds a lagged utilization variable. He finds that the short-run (one year) price elasticity is only about one-half of that found in the long-run (the above estimates). This may be due to slowly changing habits on the part of consumers or physicians or the slow emergence of new, higher medical norms as the community increases its ability to pay. One further interesting result of this research is that the number of beds and number of general practitioners and surgeons enters the demand equation directly (as well as influencing utilization through the supply equation), suggesting the importance of physicians in determining consumer demand for hospital services.[16] As all these regression estimates are based on the assumption that price elasticity is constant over different socio-economic groups, an assumption at odds with the results discussed in the last section, these estimates should be applied to particular groups (e.g., the aged) with great care.

Newhouse and his associates at the Rand Corporation are engaged in a project to determine, among other things, the impact of the price to the consumer on the demand for various medical services. Using household survey data, he plans to estimate a model with three sets of simultaneous questions. Sets of equations estimate the demand for medical insurance, provider choice, and the response of utilization to price and other variables. The last set of equations will be more disaggregated than similar studies in the past. A similar model will be tested with claims data from insurance company files; however, an assumption will be made that there is no consumer choice in purchase of group insurance so that the first set of equations will be eliminated for analysis of claims data. The simultaneous equation model employed by the Rand project should eliminate the adverse selection bias that plagues the Rosett and Huang study. Preliminary analyses point to price elasticities substantially lower than those of Rosett and Huang and also less than estimates by Martin Feldstein.[17]

Conclusions

While many of the studies reviewed suffer problems in research methods, the evidence is strong enough to conclude that consumer cost sharing does affect medical care utilization. The greater the proportion of cost that the consumer bears, the lower will be utilization.

Clear evidence is also present that the responsiveness to cost-sharing (or price elasticity of demand) varies by demographic group, by price and by medical service. One finding showed that females over age 55 were particularly sensitive to changes in coinsurance rates. This is not to be confused with high utilization—the statement implies only that this group experienced the largest change in the percentage of utilization in response to a common change in the proportion of cost sharing. It has also been shown that the price elasticity of demand (responsiveness of utilization to changes in price) varies with price or the coinsurance rate. Rosett and Huang found that responsiveness to price was greater when consumers paid a higher proportion of the cost [21]. Further, Rosenthal gave evidence of differences in price elasticity by diagnosis [20].

---

16. Demand for hospital admissions increases as the number of surgeons and hospital beds increases and as the number of general practitioners decreases.
17. The estimates, while lower than those of Martin Feldstein, may be explained by the fact that Rand is working with data on individuals while Feldstein used data by state. Aggregate data may present a greater price response if community norms play a large part in determining utilization and if consumer norms, in turn, are determined by community average net price of care to consumers.

Variations in price elasticity of demand for medical care explain some of the major differences in results encountered among the experimental simulation studies. For instance, demographic variations among the groups under study are probably not negligible. Changes in price occur also from different levels in the various experimental situations and/or will affect different mixes of medical services. Regression studies are usually not subject to these problems as the data base often encompasses the entire population or a random sample of it.

Presently, there is a need for further studies of the problem. Only a few of those studies completed or in progress are free from serious error in methods and reflect the entire population. Confirmation of their results with studies using other data sources is desirable. As there are many important price elasticities instead of just one, a particularly important need is for disaggregated studies. These studies can be accomplished within the framework of either experimental simulation studies or regression analysis. For instance, if the population in the simulation is sufficiently broad, results for subgroups can be found. With regression analysis, separate equations can be estimated for each population group and for each medical service group. Alternatively, interaction terms may be incorporated into a single regression equation.

Studies of this sort should be useful in estimating the impact of alternative National Health Insurance proposals on medical care utilization and on the budget of the federal government. However, a number of related research topics must also be addressed. One is the issue of supply response. Many of the studies reviewed tended to avoid the need to estimate supply response to major changes in the demand for medical care. Martin Feldstein is an exception [8]. This omission cannot be avoided in predicting the effects of National Health Insurance. In addition, research on the dynamics of price response to utilization changes is useful in evaluating universal entitlement. Finally, studies on the effect of alternative methods of physician and hospital reimbursement would complement the results of these demand studies as a basis for policy analysis.

The results of disaggregated coinsurance studies should be useful in designing optimal cost-sharing arrangements for National Health Insurance Plans. In addition to yielding quantitative estimates of the overall effect of coinsurance and deductibles, the studies should be able to identify which groups and which types of medical services will be affected most drastically. This should make the evaluation of utilization changes easier and more meaningful.

REFERENCES

[1] Richard Ackart, "Pre-Paid Medical Care," Virginia Medical Monthly, 88: 276-77 (May 1961).

[2] G. A. Akerlof, "The Market for 'Lemons': Quality Uncertainty and the Market Mechanism," Quarterly Journal of Economics, 84: 488-501 (August 1970).

[3] R. G. Beck, An Analysis of the Demand for Physicians' Services in Saskatchewan, unpublished doctoral dissertation, University of Alberta, 1971.

[4] Blue Cross and Blue Shield, "The Effect of Deductibles, Coinsurance and Copayment on Utilization of Health Care Services—Opinions and Impressions from Blue Cross and Blue Shield Plans," September 1971.

[5] Paul Densen et al., "Comparison of a Group Practice and a Self-Insurance Situation," Hospitals, November 16, 1962.

[6] A. W. Diokno, "Relationship Between Benefit Levels and Hospital Utilization," in Hospital and Medical Economics, vol. 2, ed. W. J. McNerney et al., Chicago, Hospital Research and Education Trust, 1962, pp. 1087-1116.

[7] Martin Feldstein, "The Welfare Loss of Excess Health Insurance," Journal of Political Economy, 81: 251-80 (March-April 1973).

[8] ———, "Hospital Cost Inflation: A Study of Nonprofit Price Dynamics," American Economic Review, 56: 853-872 (December 1971).

[9] Paul Feldstein, "Research on the Demand for Health Services," Milbank Memorial Fund Quarterly, 44: 128-165 (July 1966).

[10] ——— and Ruth Severson, "The Demand for Medical Care," Report of the Commission on the Cost of Medical Care, vol. 1, Chicago, American Medical Association, 1964, pp. 56-76.

[11] H. E. Frech and P. B. Ginsburg, "Imposed Health Insurance in Monopolistic Markets," discussion paper No. 3, Economic Analysis Branch, National Center for Health Services Research and Development, 1971.

[12] Charles Hall, Jr., "Deductibles in Health Insurance: An Evaluation," The Journal of Risk and Insurance, 33: 253-63 (June 1966).

[13] C. P. Hardwick, S. B. Myers, Shlomo Barnoon, and Larry Shuman, "The Effect of a Copay Agreement on Hospital Utilization," Research Series No. 9, Blue Cross of Western Pennsylvania, July 1971.

[14] Health Insurance Association of America, A Profile of Group Health Insurance in Force in the United States, December 1956, Washington, D.C., 1957.

[15] Health Insurance Institute, New Group Health Insurance Policies Issued in 1970, New York, 1970.

[16] Charles Heany and Donald Riedel, "From Indemnity to Full Coverage: Changes in Hospital Utilization," Blue Cross Reports, Research Series 5, October 1970.

[17] Shirley Jesmer and R. J. Scharfenberg, "Problems in Measuring the Effect of Deductibles upon Hospital Utilization," Blue Cross Reports, vol. 6, October 1968.

[18] G. S. Perrott, "Utilization of Hospital Services," American Journal of Public Health, 56: 56-64 (January 1966).

[19] J. A. Rafferty, "Patterns of Hospital Use: An Analysis of Short-Run Variations," Journal of Political Economy, 79: 154-65 (January 1971).

[20] Gerald Rosenthal, "Price Elasticity of Demand for Short-Term General Hospital Services," Empirical Studies in Health Economics, vol. 2, ed. H. E. Klarman, Baltimore, The Johns Hopkins University Press, 1970.

[21] Richard Rosett and Lien-fu Huang, "The Effect of Health Insurance on the Demand for Medical Care," Journal of Political Economy, 81: 281-305 (March-April 1973).

[22] Saskatchewan Insurance Commission, Annual Report, 1970, table 3.

[23] Ann Scitovsky and Nelda M. Snyder, "Effects of Coinsurance on Physician Services," Social Security Bulletin, 35: 3-19 (June 1972).

[24] B. W. Straight, "Reducing the Incidence of Office and Home Visits in a Medical Service Plan by Use of Coinsurance Charges," Proceedings of the Conference of Actuaries in Private Practices, vol. 11, 1961-62, pp. 73-79.

[25] H. F. Vaughn, Jr., "Deductibles Contract Study," Michigan Hospital Service, August 1965.

[26] Burton Weisbrod and Robert Fisler, "Hospital Insurance and Hospital Utilization," American Economic Review, 51: 126-32 (March 1961).

[27] Robert Williams, "A Comparison of Hospital Utilization and Costs by Types of Coverage," Inquiry, 3: 28-42 (September 1966).

[28] G. C. Wirick, "Appropriateness of Admission and Length of Stay," in Hospital and Medical Economics, vol. 1, ed. W. J. McNerney et al., Chicago, Hospital Research and Education Trust, 1962, pp. 473-77.

9. Non-Monetary Factors in the Demand for Medical Services: Some Empirical Evidence

JAN PAUL ACTON

Reprinted from "Non-Monetary Factors in the Demand for Medical Services: Some Empirical Evidence," from *Journal of Political Economy* 83, by Jan Paul Acton by permission of The University of Chicago Press.

Nonmonetary factors are expected to assume an increasingly important role in determining the demand for medical care as the out-of-pocket money price falls (due to spreading health insurance coverage or the enactment of the federal health insurance legislation). A utility maximization model is used to develop predictions for the demand for "free" and nonfree care. A simultaneous-equation system is estimated on a survey of users of New York City's "free" outpatient departments and municipal hospitals. The empirical results support the major predictions that nonmonetary factors such as travel distance will function as prices in discouraging demand and that earned and non-earned income have different impacts. A number of implications for public policy are suggested, including the possibility of substituting income maintenance for the direct provision or insurance of medical care.

I. Introduction

The demand for health care would deserve close scrutiny by researchers if only because of the size of the health sector. In addition to its size, the health sector has been one of the most inflationary in recent years, causing increasing interest by the public and policymakers alike. Finally, the growing numbers of proposals for significant changes in the health care system, especially proposals for federal health insurance legislation, make imperative a better understanding of the determinants of demand. This research is part of a growing literature that studies the demand for medical

This paper is a revised version of a RAND report, "Demand for Health Care When Time Prices Vary More than Money Prices," which was delivered to the winter meetings of the Econometric Society, 1972. The report was prepared for the Office of Economic Opportunity and the Health Services Administration of New York City. Raymond Lerner, of the State University of New York at Stony Brook, provided survey data for analysis. William Butz, David Chu, Michael Grossman, John Koehler, Joseph Newhouse, Charles Phelps, Norman Shapiro, Finis Welch, and a careful reviewer made comments on an earlier draft. Without trying to implicate them, I am grateful for their assistance.

services using disaggregated data.[1] It differs from previous literature in concentrating on alternative mechanisms that may arise to determine demand for medical care as money prices to the patient fall through insurance.

The out-of-pocket money price of medical care has been decreasing as a proportion of total price in recent years, primarily because of the spread of health insurance and the rising opportunity cost of time (and perhaps increased time needed to receive care). There is every reason to believe that money prices will continue to fall in relative importance because of the secular trend in insurance coverage and opportunity cost of time and, perhaps even more important, the prospect of national health insurance. With the decreasing relative importance of money prices, it is reasonable to expect an alternative mechanism to control demand. A mechanism involving time is quite likely to assume this role since medical care usually requires a payment in both travel time and waiting time.[2] Indeed a substantial increase in queues and waiting lists was one of the widely noted results of the enactment of the National Health Service legislation in Britain (see Harris [1951] and citations therein).

This paper considers the effects of travel distance in determining the demand for medical services in New York City, an especially good "laboratory" in which to try to examine the effects of nonmonetary prices because of the long-standing availability of free care in the city's municipal hospitals and clinics.[3] After developing a formal model of the demand for medical services that includes a payment in money and in time for private care, the predictions are tested on a cross-sectional survey of about 2,600 users of city hospital outpatient departments (OPDs).

Although limitations of the data base indicate cautious interpretation, the empirical results lend support to the model's major predictions. Empirical verification of the conjecture that time is important in determining the demand for care raises a number of important policy issues. These not only include the effect on the distribution of services to recipients of care; they also indicate powerful policy instruments for increasing the medical access of target populations. Some of these policy options—which include the location of clinics and the substitution of income maintenance for subsidized care—are discussed at the end of this paper.

[1] See, among others, Grossman 1972b; Phelps and Newhouse 1972; Acton 1973a; and Rosett-Huang 1973.

[2] The importance of time as a determinant of demand was suggested by Becker (1965), its application to the demand for medical care by, among others, Leveson (1970) and Holtman (1972).

[3] In a related study, Acton (1973a) examined the role of travel time and waiting time in the demand for medical services using two surveys of poverty neighborhoods in New York. This study differs from the previous report in a number of ways. First, it is based on a survey of the users of outpatient departments (OPDs) rather than a survey of the general population in a neighborhood. Consequently, we know that everyone had nonzero utilization of the health sector. This allows the specification of a simultaneous set of equations to describe the demand at several different sources of care. Second, the chief measure of price paid for "free" public care is travel distance to the clinic. Further, travel distance is specified as endogenous in this system. In the previous study, the large proportion of observations on the limit value of zero health sector utilization forces the estimation of reduced-form equations using Tobit estimation technique.

II. Model of Demand for Medical Services

The underlying theoretical model for this study is developed in detail in Acton (1973a, 1973b).[4] The model concentrates on the role of money prices, time prices, and earned and nonearned income. For simplicity, the model is developed in terms of only one provider of services, but the implications for several providers can easily be drawn. In the theoretical and empirical sections to follow, I will be studying the demand for care at alternative providers—free city clinics, private physicians, and hospitals.

Assume two goods enter the individual's utility function: medical services, m, and a composite, X, for all other goods and services. Using an assumption of fixed proportions of money and time to consume m and X and the full income assumption, the model can be represented as follows:

Maximize

$$U = U(m, X) \tag{1a}$$

subject to

$$(p + wt)m + (q + ws)X \le Y = y + wT, \tag{1b}$$

where

U = utility,
m = medical services,
X = all other goods and services,
p = out-of-pocket money price per unit of medical services,
t = own-time input per unit of medical services,
q = money price per unit of X,
s = own-time input per unit of X,
w = earnings per hour,
Y = total (full) income,
y = nonearned income, and
T = total amount of time available for market and own production of goods and services.

A more complicated specification of the model was not used because this simpler formulation yields most of the same predictions and because the data do not permit estimation of the unique implications of the richer specification.[5]

---

[4] Similar models can be found in Becker (1965), Grossman (1972a), and Holtman (1972).

[5] Grossman (1972a) allows the amount of medical services, m, to influence the total amount of time, T, available for production. Phelps (1973) makes the selection of insurance parameters, and therefore p, endogenous to the system. Some researchers (notably Grossman [1972a, 1972b] and his followers) have taken the Lancaster (1966) formulation of letting the argument "health" enter the utility function and then deriving a demand for medical services. The present data do not allow us to estimate the relation transforming medical services into health.

Effects of a Change in Price

It can be shown that the assumptions sufficient to make money function as a price in determining the demand for medical services are also sufficient to make time function as a price, producing negative own-time–price elasticities of demand and positive cross-time–price elasticities. One of the chief interests in this study is the relative importance of money prices and time prices in determining the demand for medical services. If we let Π equal the total price per unit of medical services (i.e., $\Pi = p + wt$), then the elasticity of demand for medical services with respect to money price is

$$\eta_{mp} = \frac{p}{\Pi} \eta_{m\Pi}, \tag{2a}$$

and the elasticity with respect to time (which equals the elasticity with respect to wt) is[6]

$$\eta_{mt} = \frac{wt}{\Pi} \eta_{m\Pi}. \tag{2b}$$

Comparing these two elasticities yields the second prediction from the formal model, namely, that $\eta_{mt} \gtreqless \eta_{mp}$ as $wt \gtreqless p$. Clearly, as p goes to zero and wt does not, the time-price elasticity will exceed the money-price elasticity. In other words, as the out-of-pocket payment for a unit of medical services falls, because of either increasing insurance coverage or the availability of subsidized care, demand becomes relatively more sensitive to changes in time prices. Further, this implies that the demand for free medical services should be more sensitive to changes in time prices than demand for nonfree services, because time is a greater proportion of the total price at free than at nonfree providers.

Effects of a Change in Income

Exogenous changes in income can arise either from a change in earnings per hour or from a change in nonearned income. The two effects are not, in general, equal. The assumptions that are sufficient to make money function as a price are also sufficient to mean that an increase in nonearned income will produce an increase in the demand for medical services.

The effects of a change in the wage rate cannot be determined a priori because of offsetting influences. An increase in earnings per hour produces an income effect, which acts to increase demand. It also raises the opportunity cost of time, which reduces demand for time-intensive activities. The net effect on the demand for medical services depends on the time intensity of the price of medical services relative to the time intensity of the price of all other goods and services. It can easily be established (see Acton 1973a or 1973b) that the substitution effect of a

---

[6] These elasticities are only approximate in the long run if insurance premiums are adjusted to reflect the changes in utilization.

change in the wage rate on the demand for medical services is positive if and only if

$$\frac{ws}{(q + ws)} > \frac{wt}{(p + wt)}, \tag{3}$$

that is, if the time price is a larger proportion of the total price for the composite good, X, than it is for medical services, m. The substitution effect is necessarily negative for free sources of medical care since the condition in equation (3) will not be met as long as there is a nonzero monetary price for X. Of course, the net effect of a change in wages may still be to increase the demand for medical services if the income effect exceeds the substitution effect. Intuitively, however, the effect of a wage change on the demand for medical services is more like a price effect for free sources of care (and therefore more likely to be negative) and more like an income effect for nonfree sources of care (and therefore more likely to be positive).

Predictions from Other Formal Models

As noted above, the model developed here is deliberately simplified because it is adequate to produce testable hypotheses for the variables of primary interest. There are some additional hypotheses regarding the effects of education and age from the Grossman (1972a) investment model that can be tested with these data. Grossman argues that medical services are combined with other inputs the individual supplies to produce health and that it is health that enters the utility function. Now, if education raises health productivity (e.g., more highly educated people are more skillful in combining inputs to produce health) and if the price elasticity of health is less than one, then education will have a negative effect on the demand for medical care.[7] The second implication of Grossman's work involves the effect of age on consumption of health services. If the price elasticity of demand for health is less than one, then the demand for medical services will be positively correlated with the depreciation rate on health. In general, empirical evidence suggests that the depreciation rate increases over the life cycle, causing a positive effect of age on consumption of medical care.

III. The Empirical Base

The data used for this study come from a 1965 survey of users of the out-patient departments of New York City municipal hospitals. Respondents were selected from a random sample of persons at the clinic; hence, the probability of being interviewed is proportional to the frequency of use

---

[7] In the consumption model, given a "neutral" effect of education on all household activities, the elasticity with respect to wealth must also be less than one to produce a negative relationship between medical care and education (Grossman 1972b, pp. 36–37).

of the clinics. The Appendix defines and presents the mean values of the variables used in this analysis. In addition, the means are reported when observations are weighted by the inverse of the number of clinic visits. These weighted means indicate the mean characteristics of people who ever use the clinics, rather than the mean characteristics of the patient loads at the clinics.

The respondents were questioned about their previous year's medical use and a number of sociodemographic characteristics from the previous year. The interviews at each of the OPDs were conducted in four waves spread throughout the year to cancel seasonality in usage.[8] There are advantages and disadvantages to using survey data. One of the advantages is that disaggregated data provide a more precise description of individual behavior because individual rather than aggregate values can be used for explanatory variables. This overcomes the bias away from zero that is frequently encountered in using average values in aggregate data.[9] Other advantages include the much larger sample size typically available in surveys so that variance of coefficients can be reduced. The chief disadvantage of survey data in general is that it relies on recall by the individual. This frequently leads to an underreporting of some variables, particularly medical utilization and income.[10]

Some responses to the surveys were checked independently, increasing the validity of the data, while others were coded poorly for present analysis. The number of outpatient department visits (OPD) and hospitalizations (HOSP) in the preceding year were verified with providers. The distance (DIST) to the hospital of interview was calculated from the person's home address. The number of private physician visits was coded in intervals and had to be calculated. This calculation and all important variables are discussed in detail in Acton (1973b).

---

[8] Details of the study and selected analysis (chiefly analysis of variance) can be found in Lerner and Kirchner (1967) and Lerner, Kirchner, and Dieckmann (1967, 1968).

[9] See Newhouse and Phelps (1974) for an elaboration of this point.

[10] Recall for ambulatory care seems to be extremely accurate for physician use in the last 2 weeks and for hospital use in the last year, according to Regina Loewenstein (personal communication, 1971). Underreporting will generally bias the coefficients of explanatory variables toward zero. The estimated elasticities, however, need not be biased. If all people recall k proportion of their utilization in the previous year, then the estimated elasticity of demand for care with respect to, say, price is

$$\eta_{mp} = \frac{\partial km}{\partial p} \cdot \frac{p}{km} = \frac{\partial m}{\partial p} \cdot \frac{p}{m},$$

which is the same as the elasticity that would have been estimated with full recall. By the same argument, the cross-price elasticities and the elasticity of substitution of one type of provider for another should be unbiased. There is further potential bias in this particular study because of the fee structure at the municipal hospitals. In order to receive free care, the individual was supposed to be unable to pay for private care (although I am told that it was well known at the time that anyone who asserted he was entitled to free care would receive it without challenge). This institution, however, might have caused some persons to underreport income or utilization of private facilities. There is no evidence that such an error was introduced and the interview opened with a statement of confidentiality, but in the absense of verified income data the possibility exists.

IV. Estimation Results

The demand for health care by type of provider is estimated from a simultaneous-equation system using two-stage least squares. Four structural equations are specified and 28 exogenous variables are used for estimation. All the equations are overidentified by several variables.[11] After a brief overview of the model, this section describes first the structural equations and then the reduced-form equations.

Overview of the Model

The four structural equations describe the volume of ambulatory and inpatient services demanded and the distance traveled to the free ambulatory care.[12] The last year's volume of OPD visits and the number of visits to a private physician (PRIVE) are the two alternative sources of ambulatory care. They are technical substitutes for one another. The volume of private-physician visits and the number of hospitalizations are entered as right-hand endogenous variables in order to measure substitution and complementarity effects among different types of providers. We would prefer to enter the money price of private-physician visits and the cost of a hospitalization and examine the cross-price effects, but this information is not available in the survey. Since substitution or complementarity is important both theoretically and empirically in medical care, we wish to measure the effects as best possible and limit the bias in the remaining coefficients. One consequence of entering quantities on the right-hand side is to make price elasticities different from the usual elasticities, as discussed next.

The distance (DIST) to the outpatient department where the interview was conducted is specified as an endogenous variable in this system. It is the chief measure of the price of an OPD visit and functions as a cross-price term for PRIVE and HOSP.[13] Distance actually measures several things. It includes the physical distance one has to travel and the money and time costs of travel, and it is associated with higher informational costs. The informational costs represent the fact that patients generally have less difficulty in finding out about the quality and suitability of a close-by clinic (for instance, by asking neighbors or by having experienced the care themselves) than in finding out about a distant clinic. The money costs and informational costs will tend to be positively correlated with the

---

[11] Since a number of the variables are dummy variables for health status or mode of transportation, they really contain less information than their number indicates. Therefore, in checking the number of excluded exogenous variables for purpose of identification, I counted a set of mutually dependent dummy variables as one variable.

[12] Some of the "exogenous" variables in this cross-sectional survey are really endogenous in a larger system that includes life-cycle behavior (such as labor-force participation and family size) and a broader set of economic decisions. Since we are specifying only a subset of these relations, it is possible that some of these exogenous variables are really proxies for common underlying theoretical variables. I tried to limit the possibility of such undesirable interference by specifying such variables as family health status only in the equations where their principal effects could be anticipated.

[13] An imprecise measure of waiting time is included. If the person says he waits longer at an OPD than at a private physician's office WAIT take the value one.

distance traveled. However, those who previously lived near one clinic and now live farther away (perhaps nearer another) have a lower information cost with the former, more distant, clinic. Therefore, the coefficient on HABIT should be positive in the structural equation for distance, but it will capture only part of the differences in information costs in this and other equations. DIST is endogenous in this system because the distance a person travels to the OPD is influenced by a number of the same underlying variables influencing demand for medical care, including the opportunity cost of time, the health status of the user, and his sociodemographic characteristics. Consequently, the only way to see the total effect of these variables is through the reduced-form coefficients. The result of this specification is that the elasticities with respect to DIST are not identical with the usual price elasticity of demand because they show the effect of distance holding constant the level of all other things, including other forms of medical care. With three or more goods, it is not possible to sign bias without stronger assumptions about the utility function.[14]

The important exogenous economic variables in this system are earned and nonearned income (GRWAGE and NWAGE), assets (LIQUID and EQUITY), and health insurance (INSF). The insurance variable is very imprecise and indicates only that at least one member of the family had some coverage (this was before Medicare and Medicaid). Additional important variables in this system include the mode of transportation used for the named sources of care (the suffix letter P indicates mode of private care), health status, and a number of sociodemographic variables.[15]

The Structural Equations

The specifications of the structural equations and their estimated coefficients are given in table 1.[16] In the absence of an explicit utility function, there is no unique set of structural equations. A linear specification is employed. The principal value of the structural equations is to show the effects of endogenous variables on one another. The net effect of exogenous variables is clear only from the reduced-form coefficients in table 2.

[14] With only two goods, the own-cross-price elasticities estimated holding constant the quantity of the other good are lower bounds (in absolute value) for the normal elasticities. With three or more goods, we need stronger assumptions (such as, hospitalizations are complementary to one form of ambulatory care and substitutes to the other form) because of offsetting effects to determine the sign of the bias unambiguously.

[15] It can be argued that the method of transportation is an endogenous variable just as is the distance traveled to OPD care. For both conceptual and practical reasons, it is considered exogenous in this model. First, it can be viewed as exogenous if before the period of observation the person has already made a decision about the methods of transportation he will use for various types of trips. We can argue that he is unlikely to alter this choice significantly during the course of the year. A more practical reason is that making the method of transportation endogenous means that the normal assumptions about the distribution of the error term would not be satisfied, and either a Tobit or probit model would be more appropriate. Estimating a simultaneous Tobit system with 12 or so endogenous variables is probably unwarranted with this data base.

[16] The t-values reported are the asymptotically normal values. By multiplying these by the t-adjustment factor, the Dhrymes (1969) t-statistics for 2SLS result.

TABLE 1

Coefficients of Structural Equations from 2SLS Estimation*

Variables	OPD (Eq. [1]) Coef.	t	η	PRIVE (Eq. [2]) Coef.	t	η	HOSP (Eq. [3]) Coef.	t	η	DIST (Eq. [4]) Coef.	t	η
Endogenous:												
OPD				−0.052	3.45	−.27	0.006	1.58	.14	0.021	0.36	.08
PRIVE	−0.577	3.20	−.11				0.023	2.80	.10	⋯	⋯	⋯
HOSP	11.144	5.22	.47	1.312	2.69	.29				⋯	⋯	⋯
DIST	−0.552	2.51	−.14	0.050	0.99	.07	0.029	2.40	.18			
Exogenous:												
GRWAGE × 10^{-4}	1.010	1.02	.04	0.452	2.02	.09	−0.098	1.80	−.09	0.117	0.76	.017
NWAGE × 10^{-3}	0.329	1.47	.04	0.171	3.40	.10	−0.035	2.94	−.10	0.052	1.47	.02
LIQUID × 10^{-4}	−0.161	0.14	−.00	0.419	1.65	.01	0.037	0.58	.00	⋯	⋯	⋯
EQUITY × 10^{-3}	−7.047	0.52	−.02	0.047	1.56	.01	0.014	1.91	.01	⋯	⋯	⋯
INSF	−0.347	0.75	−.02	0.285	2.76	.07	0.054	2.17	.06	−0.049	0.61	−.01
WAIT	0.401	0.78	.01	1.174	12.16	.23	⋯	⋯	⋯	⋯	⋯	⋯
FAMH	0.972	2.30	.04				−0.101	2.08	−.03	0.263	1.45	.01
EX	−1.726	1.90	−.02	−1.406	7.14	−.09	−0.075	2.15	−.11	0.285	2.29	.07
GOOD	−1.083	1.65	−.07	−1.152	8.23	−.36	−0.015	0.44	−.01	0.014	0.14	.00
FAIR	−0.788	1.30	−.03	−0.880	6.63	−.18	−0.019	3.05	−.21	0.025	0.70	.04
AGE × 10^{-1}	0.811	7.59	.38	0.046	1.74	.11	0.055	1.87	.07	−0.240	2.20	−.05
BLACK	−2.312	4.51	−.12	−0.382	3.19	−.10	0.016	0.51	.02	−0.261	2.53	−.05
PR	−1.643	2.95	−.07	−0.446	3.51	−.10	0.005	1.80	.09	⋯	⋯	⋯
EDUC	−0.131	2.77	−.11	0.007	0.64	.03	0.094	4.26	.11	0.158	2.24	.03
MALE	−1.863	4.35	−.09	−0.340	3.47	−.09	0.064	2.14	.05	⋯	⋯	⋯
WELF	−0.827	1.50	−.03	−0.411	3.36	−.07	−0.059	1.92	−.03	0.095	0.69	.01
WORK				0.251	1.99	−.03	⋯	⋯	⋯	0.505	3.10	.01
NMAIN	−2.372	2.48	−.01	⋯	⋯	⋯	⋯	⋯	⋯	−0.004	0.54	−.01
HABIT	0.137	4.72	.09	⋯	⋯	⋯	⋯	⋯	⋯	1.067	12.35	.23
BUS1	⋯	⋯	⋯	⋯	⋯	⋯	⋯	⋯	⋯	2.444	25.01	.28
BUS2	⋯	⋯	⋯	⋯	⋯	⋯	⋯	⋯	⋯	2.524	14.72	.06
CAR	⋯	⋯	⋯	⋯	⋯	⋯	⋯	⋯	⋯	1.393	10.85	.06
TAXI	⋯	⋯	⋯	2.986	17.49	.13	⋯	⋯	⋯	⋯	⋯	⋯
BUS1P	⋯	⋯	⋯	3.193	13.75	.74	⋯	⋯	⋯	⋯	⋯	⋯
BUS2P	⋯	⋯	⋯	2.125	7.70	.47	⋯	⋯	⋯	⋯	⋯	⋯
CARP	⋯	⋯	⋯	2.958	9.95	.43	⋯	⋯	⋯	⋯	⋯	⋯
TAXIP	⋯	⋯	⋯	⋯	⋯	⋯	⋯	⋯	⋯	−0.099	0.71	−.09
CLINS	⋯	⋯	⋯	⋯	⋯	⋯	0.240	3.50	⋯	0.515	1.80	⋯
CONSTANT	5.636	4.30	⋯	1.363	4.47	⋯	0.347	⋯	⋯	0.763	⋯	⋯
t-adjustment factor	0.19			0.55			⋯			⋯		

* Scaling factors adjust only coefficients, not elasticities. Elasticities calculated at the means of unweighted data.

TABLE 2

COEFFICIENTS OF REDUCED-FORM EQUATIONS*

VARIABLE	OPD (Eq. [5]) Coef.	η	PRIVE (Eq. [6]) Coef.	η	HOSP (Eq. [7]) Coef.	η	DIST (Eq. [8]) Coef.	η
GRWAGE × 10⁻⁴	−0.245	−.01	0.353	.07	−0.089	−.08	0.111	.02
NWAGE × 10⁻³	−0.129	−.01	0.139	.08	−0.031	−.09	0.049	.02
LIQUID × 10⁻⁴	0.100	.00	0.477	.01	0.048	.00	0.002	.00
EQUITY × 10⁻³	0.070	.00	0.064	.01	0.016	.01	0.001	.00
INSF	0.150	.01	0.360	.09	0.063	.07	0.003	.00
WAIT	0.025	.00	1.205	.23	0.026	.02	−0.048	−.01
FAMH	1.050	.05	−0.046	−.01	0.006	.01	0.022	.00
EX	−2.600	−.03	−1.450	−.09	−0.143	−.04	0.208	.01
GOOD	−1.709	−.10	−1.190	−.37	−0.106	−.15	0.249	.06
FAIR	−0.713	−.03	−0.895	−.18	−0.040	−.04	−0.0003	−.00
AGE × 10⁻¹	0.631	.30	−0.0003	−.01	−0.014	−.16	0.037	.06
BLACK	−1.661	−.08	−0.269	−.07	0.031	.04	−0.275	.05
PR	−1.354	−.06	−0.402	−.09	−0.009	−.01	−0.290	−.01
EDUC	−0.089	−.07	0.018	.08	0.005	.09	−0.002	−.05
MALE	−0.854	−.04	−0.171	−.04	0.090	.10	0.140	.03
WELF	−0.0004	.00	−0.337	−.05	0.057	.04	−0.000	−.00
WORK	−0.805	−.02	0.222	.02	−0.057	−.03	0.078	.01
NMAIN	−2.705	−.02	0.167	.01	0.001	.00	0.449	.01
HABIT	0.149	.10	−0.007	−.02	0.001	.01	−0.0004	−.01
BUS1	−0.299	−.02	0.110	.03	0.031	.04	1.063	.23
BUS2	−0.683	−.02	0.251	.04	0.072	.05	2.429	.28
CAR	−0.706	−.00	0.259	.01	0.074	.01	2.509	.06
TAXI	−0.390	−.00	0.143	.01	0.041	.01	1.385	.06
BUS1P	−1.079	−.01	3.125	.14	0.065	.01	−0.023	−.01
BUS2P	−1.148	−.01	3.342	.08	0.070	.01	−0.024	−.00
CARP	−0.763	−.00	2.224	.05	0.046	.01	−0.016	−.00
TAXIP	−1.063	−.00	3.095	.05	0.064	.00	−0.022	−.00
CLINS	0.027	.01	−0.010	−.01	−0.002	−.01	−0.099	−.08
CONSTANT	8.237	...	1.412	...	0.340	...	0.687	...

* Scaling factors adjust only coefficients, not elasticities. Elasticities calculated at the means of unweighted data.

The OPD Equation

The structural equation for OPD visits (1) includes the other three endogenous variables. Private-physician visits are technical substitutes for OPD visits, producing an elasticity of −.11. Hospitalizations appear to be significant technical complements to OPD care with an elasticity of .47. This complementarity is reasonable, first, because inpatient care frequently requires ambulatory follow-up. Second, hospitalizations produce a budget effect that may increase the demand for less expensive forms of ambulatory care. Third, the municipal OPD clinics act as ports of entry to municipal hospitals.

One of the important predictions of the formal model developed above is that distance to the OPD would function as a price in determining demand. Equation (1) supports this prediction, producing an elasticity of −.14. It is likely that the elasticity with respect to travel time is greater (in absolute value) than −.14 because people traveling farther will tend to take more rapid forms of transportation.[17] The mode of transportation to OPD care has its major influence on the distance traveled and is included in the DIST structural equation.

The PRIVE Equation

The structural equation for private physician care complements the estimates from the OPD equation. Again, PRIVE and OPD are substitutes and PRIVE and HOSP are complements. DIST functions as a cross price to PRIVE, producing an elasticity of about .07. The estimate of .07 is considerably smaller than the cross-time elasticities of about .6 estimated for private care in Acton (1973a). Again, it is likely that the elasticity with respect to travel time is greater. An additional downward bias in the coefficient may be caused by the omission of a measure of travel distance from the structural equation for PRIVE. All we have to measure travel distance are the dummy variables for method of transportation. In this structural equation, the partial effects indicate that walkers demand the least care, while taking the bus, subway, or taxi all have about the same effect. The statistically significant coefficients on mode of transportation suggest that distance is playing an important role in demand (this conclusion is supported by the reduced-form coefficients reported in table 2).

The Hospitalization Equation

The structural equations for hospitalization reveal effects for the endogenous variables consistent with the other equations. Clinic and private-

---

[17] For instance, it may not be worth taking a bus a few blocks, but it is worthwhile when crossing town; similarly, it may be worthwhile to switch to an express train for part of a longer journey by subway and then return to a local. The own-price elasticity of demand for public ambulatory care with respect to self-reported travel time is estimated between −.6 and −1.0 in Acton (1973a).

physician visits are complements to hospitalization, with elasticities around .14 and .10. The coefficient on distance to an OPD has a positive sign (elasticity = .18)

The Distance Equation

The only included endogenous variable in explaining distance to the OPD is volume of OPD services, arguing that those who go more frequently will want to reduce the travel price they have to pay. The results of equation (4) show a coefficient not statistically significantly different from zero. The distance equation is specified as a function of a number of the exogenous variables that are common to the medical care equations— including earned and nonearned income, mode of transportation, health status, and sociodemographic characteristics. The most important theoretical prediction for this equation is that those with a higher opportunity cost of time should travel shorter distances for OPD care. The coefficient on GRWAGE in equation (4) does not support this prediction, although its t-ratio is only 0.76. The general effects of the opportunity cost of time follow the predictions as indicated by the coefficient on GRWAGE in the reduced-form equations for medical care.

The Reduced-Form Equations

The chief value of the reduced-form equations is to indicate the net influence of the exogenous variables on the dependent variables. Consequently, the effects of a few key variables will be examined across equations, and the estimated coefficients will be compared with the predictions of Section II.

The Role of Travel Distance and the Value of Time

There were several predictions about the role of time on the demand for various types of care. The first prediction, that time (and travel distance) would function as a price, was supported by the structural equations. They reveal a negative (own-price) coefficient on the variable DIST in the OPD equation and a positive (cross-price) coefficient in the PRIVE and HOSP equations. Second, we expect those with a higher opportunity cost of time to demand less time-intensive care. Both working people and people with a higher opportunity cost of time demand less time-intensive OPD and hospital care and more private-physician care. A further hypothesis, that the higher wage rate would shorten travel distance, was not supported by equation (4).

Income and Assets

Unless service from a provider is an inferior good, the nonearned income elasticity should be positive. Equations (5), (6), and (7) show a positive elasticity of demand for private-physician services and a negative elasticity for OPD and hospital care, suggesting that private outpatient care is a normal good and municipal health care is an inferior good (in an economic sense). The effects of earned income depend on the time intensity of medical goods relative to other goods and services. The model predicted that earned income would function more like a price effect in the demand for free care and more like an income effect in the demand for nonfree care. The reduced-form coefficients show a positive elasticity of demand for private outpatient care with respect to GRWAGE and a negative elasticity of demand for public care. This supports the popular impression that OPD and hospital care are time intensive relative to private physicians' care and relative to all other goods and services.

Education and Age

Two other predictions from the formal models involve the effects of education and age. Grossman suggested that, if those with more education were more efficient producers of health, education would have a negative coefficient (as long as the price elasticity of demand for health is less than one). Equations (5) and (6) show a negative effect of education on OPD visits and a positive effect on private-physician visits. However, the decrease in the number of OPD visits is only partly made up by increases in the number of private visits so that the net change in ambulatory visits produced by an increase in education is negative. This finding is compatable with the predictions of Grossman's (1972b) model discussed above. The investment model also predicted a positive correlation of age and the depreciation rate on health. The present data on ambulatory utilization show a negative (but very small) elasticity for PRIVE and a positive net effect of age for OPD care. The OPD finding supports the hypothesis that depreciation in the health stock increases with age. The negative coefficient on age in the hospitalization equation may indicate older persons going to nursing homes.

The remainder of the coefficients describing health status, insurance, and sociodemographic characteristics of the population generally conform to the expectations based on other studies. As found by most researchers, those in poorer health demand more inpatient and outpatient care. They also travel shorter distances to receive their OPD care. The effect of at least one family member's having fair or poor health (FAMH) reinforces the health status effects. In general, the positive correlation of health status in the family and the budget effect of a very sick member should either increase utilization at each source of care or cause a shift to public care; FAMH is positive in the OPD equation (5). Although it is an imprecise variable, if anyone in the family has health insurance, the person will seek more medical services, both public and private. Blacks and Puerto Ricans generally receive less care of all types than do their white counterparts, and they travel shorter distances to receive it. Finally, men seek less ambulatory care and more inpatient care than women. This finding provides further support for the suggestion of Acton (1973a) that males may let their health deteriorate further than females do before seeking medical care, so that when they go they require more intensive care.

V. Conclusion

This study supports the prediction that travel time (as measured by distance) functions as a price in determining the demand for medical services when free care is available. This survey of users of the municipal OPDs indicates negative own-price elasticities with respect to travel distance at free providers and positive cross-price elasticities for nonfree providers of care. Further, the estimated distance elasticity approaches or equals the money-price elasticities that have been estimated by a number of researchers.[18] The predicted negative effect of earned income on distance was not found, but persons with higher earned income are more likely to use the private sector, which is relatively less time intensive, than the public sector.

There are a number of policy implications of this study. Two of the most important involve (1) the redistribution in services that will be caused by a change in money and time prices and (2) the possibility of using income subsidies rather than direct provision of goods to meet public objectives. As money prices out of pocket are reduced, because of either the continued spread of private insurance or the enactment of a federal health insurance scheme, demand will become more responsive to time prices. In turn, this will permit persons with a lower opportunity cost of time to bid services away from those with a higher opportunity cost of time because they will face a price that is relatively less costly. This conclusion holds even if there is not differential coverage by income class and even if there is no supply side response increasing the time prices. It is likely that a shift in demand will be accompanied by an increase in the time needed to receive a unit of medical services.[19] This will further increase the relative shift in favor of those with a lower opportunity cost of time. The significant effect of travel distance on the demand for medical services suggests a policy instrument for delivering more services to target groups. By moving clients closer—either by improving transportation, locating clinics closer, or by establishing satellite clinics around central facilities—the consumption of selected populations can be increased.

A second important policy implication is for alternative means of meeting the objective of increasing medical services consumed by target

[18] Feldstein (1971), Davis and Russell (1972), and Rosett and Huang (1973) have all reported money-price elasticities in the range $-.5$ to -1.0, although there is reason to believe these estimates are biased upward (see Newhouse and Phelps 1974). Other more conservative measures of the money-price elasticity (using several data sources) place it around -0.15 or less (see Phelps and Newhouse 1974).

[19] This supply response is likely for a number of reasons. First, it may be optimal from the point of view of the provider to have a queue to even out the variation in demand that he experiences without having to invest in significant excess capacity. A shift in demand will generally cause the optimal queue length to change (for instance, the opportunity cost of an idle moment of the supplier's facility is higher). Second, the suppliers may not be profit maximizers, so that they do not respond to a shift in demand by charging the highest possible monetary prices but instead allow time prices to increase. In particular, physicians may be income satisfiers rather than maximizers. See Newhouse (1970), Frech and Ginsburg (1972), and Newhouse and Sloan (1972) for a discussion of physician pricing behavior. Third, there may be a conscious attempt to redistribute services by discriminating in favor of those with a lower opportunity cost of time. See Nichols, Smolensky, and Tideman (1971) for a discussion of the first and third points.

populations. In one form or another most proposals reduce to a sub-sidized provision of services, whether through social insurance schemes such as Medicaid or various federal health insurance proposals, or through direct provision of care as in neighborhood health centers or the requirement that Hill-Burton hospitals provide charity care. But as Davis (1972) has correctly noted, there is seldom a consideration of the extent to which changing the income distribution will alleviate the desire to subsidize the medical purchase. Even in the administration's proposals for income maintenance (FAP) and subsidized medical care for the poor (FHIP) there was little discussion of the degree to which one can be substituted for the other. The proposed comprehensive health insurance plan (CHIP) now before Congress provides an opportunity to illustrate the tradeoffs.

Income subsidy will not, in general, meet the objective of risk spreading for medical expenses (unless it induces a significant demand for health insurance), but it will raise the average demand for medical services in the subsidized population. The equations reported in tables 1 and 2 put us in a position to address this question of substituting income maintenance for subsidized medical care to achieve a given increase in medical services consumption. Since income maintenance is a nonearned source of income, the elasticity of demand for medical care with respect to changes in nonearned income is used. A hypothetical example, not based exactly on FAP and CHIP provisions, will serve to illustrate. The estimation results in table 2 indicate that a $1,100 increase in nonearned income for a family with a current nonearned income of about $400 and earned income of about $2,900 (in 1965) will produce an increase of about 11 percent in the demand for private practitioners' care per person. If the money-price elasticity of demand for ambulatory medical services is around $-.15$ over the range under consideration,[20] and the out-of-pocket expenditure is reduced from 25 percent of money price to 15 percent (the upper limit on CHIP's coinsurance rate and the rate for an insuree with income of $3,000), then the demand for private care will increase by 7.5 percent. Clearly, one means of increasing private medical consumption by the poor is income supplementation, and the magnitude of the change may be comparable over the range of subsidy and income guarantee under consideration.

Appendix

Definition of Variables Used and Their Mean Values[21]

AGE = Age in years. Means = 35.6, 31.1.
BLACK = Dummy variable equaling one if Negro or indeterminable, or other than Puerto Rican, Mexican-American, American Indian, or other white. Means = 0.38, 0.41.

---

[20] The actual money-price elasticity may be even lower than this. See Phelps and Newhouse (1974) for a discussion of the price elasticities in several published reports.

[21] The first mean value is for the unweighted data and the second is for the data weighted by 1/OPD to adjust for the probability of being sampled.

BUS1 = Dummy variable equaling one if patient's usual means of transportation to the clinic requires one bus or train. Means = 0.42, 0.42.

BUS2 = Dummy variable equaling one if patient's usual means of transportation to the clinic requires two or more buses or trains. Means = 0.23, 0.21.

BUS1P = Dummy variable equaling one if patient's usual means of transportation to private doctor requires one bus or train. Means = 0.07, 0.08.

BUS2P = Same as above except two or more buses or trains. Means = 0.03, 0.03.

CAR = Dummy variable equaling one if patient's usual means of transportation to the clinic was by car driven either by individual or a friend. Means = 0.05, 0.06.

CARP = Same as above except to private doctor. Means = 0.03, 0.03.

CLINS = Total number of clinics used last year. Means = 1.71, 1.29.

DIST = Distance in miles to the hospital of interview. Means = 2.14, 2.13.

EDUC = Highest grade completed, in years. Means = 6.25, 6.23.

EQUITY = Equity in home. Means = $207, $198.

ERNRS = Number of earners in the family. Means = 0.83, 0.91.

EX = Dummy variable equaling one if health status of patient is excellent. Means = 0.095, 0.13.

FAIR = Dummy variable equaling one if health status of patient is fair. Means = 0.30, 0.27.

FAMH = Dummy variable equaling one if all family members reported health as good. Means = 0.34, 0.33.

GOOD = Dummy variable equaling one if health status of patient is good. Means = 0.46, 0.48.

GRWAGE = Gross annual earnings from all wage earners in the family. Means = $2,929, $3,215.

HABIT = Number of years patient has been coming to current clinic. Means = 5.03, 4.10.

HOSP = Number of hospitalizations last year. Means = 0.32, 0.30.

HSSIZE = Number of persons in individual's household. Means = 3.67, 3.92.

INSF = Dummy variable equaling one if any family member has medical insurance. Means = 0.35, 0.36.

LIQUID = Liquid assets. Means = $177, $207.

LNGWT = Dummy variable equaling one if patient had to wait a long time before being taken care of at the hospital where he was interviewed. Means = 0.59, —.

MALE = One if male, zero if female. Means = 0.38, 0.39.

NMAIN = Dummy variable equaling one if main source of medical care is other than the same clinic as at time of interview. Means = 0.047, 0.064.

NWAGE = Nonearned family income in last year. Means = $878, $802.

OPD = Number of visits in last year to a physician in a clinic. Means = 7.65, 2.97.

PR = One if Puerto Rican; zero otherwise. Means = 0.34, 0.35.

PRIVE = Number of visits in last year to a physician in his private office. Means = 1.46, 1.63.

TAXI = Dummy variable equaling one if patient's usual means of transportation to the clinic was by taxi. Means = 0.091, 0.095.

TAXIP = Same as above except to his private doctor. Means = 0.021, 0.020.

WAIT = Dummy variable equaling one if patient had to wait longer in the hospital where he was interviewed than in private doctor's office. Means = 0.28, —.

WELF   = Dummy variable equaling one if individual had some type of welfare assistance. Means = 0.24, 0.22.
WORK   = One if indivudal worked either full or part time. Means = 0.16, 0.20.

References

Acton, Jan Paul. "Demand for Health Care among the Urban Poor with Special Emphasis on the Role of Time." Memorandum R-1151-OEO/NYC, RAND Corp., April 1973.(*a*)

——. "Demand for Health Care When Time Prices Vary More than Money Prices." Memorandum R-1189-OEO/NYC, RAND Corp., May 1973.(*b*)

Becker, Gary. "A Theory of the Allocation of Time." *Econ. J.* 75 (September 1965): 493–517.

Davis, Karen. "Health Insurance." In *Setting National Priorities: The 1973 Budget*, edited by Charles Schultze et al. Washington, D.C.: Brookings Institution, 1972.

Davis, Karen, and Russell, Louise. "The Substitution of Hospital Care for Inpatient Care." *Rev. Econ. Statis.* 54 (May 1972): 109–20.

Dhrymes, Phoebus. "Alternative Asymptotic Tests of Significance and Related Aspects of 2SLS and 3SLS Estimated Parameters." *Rev. Econ. Studies* 36 (April 196ɔ): 213–26.

Feldstein, Martin S. "An Economic Model of the Medicare System." *Q.J.E.* 85 (February 1971): 1–20.

Frech, H. E., and Ginsburg, Paul B. "Physician Pricing: Monopolistic or Competitive: Comment." *Southern Econ. J.* 38 (April 1972): 573–77.

Grossman, Michael. "On the Concept of Health Capital and the Demand for Health." *J.P.E.* 80, no. 2 (March/April 1972): 223–55.(*a*)

——. *The Demand for Health: A Theoretical and Empirical Investigation.* New York: Columbia Univ. Press (for Nat. Bur. Econ. Res.), 1972.(*b*)

Harris, Seymour E. "The British Health Experiment: The First Two Years of the National Health Service." *A.E.R.* 41 (May 1951): 652–66.

Holtman, A. G. "Price, Time, and Technology in the Medical Care Market." *J. Human Resources* 7 (Spring 1972): 179–90.

Lancaster, Kevin. "A New Approach to Consumer Theory." *J.P.E.* 74, no. 2 (April 1966): 132–57.

Lerner, Raymond C., and Kirchner, Corinne. *Municipal General Hospital Outpatient Population Study: Social and Economic Characteristics of Patients in New York City Outpatient Departments, 1965: Financial Eligibility under Medicaid and Potential Reimbursement to the City.* Report no. 1. New York: School Public Health and Admin. Medicine, Columbia Univ., 1967.

Lerner, Raymond C.; Kirchner, Corinne; and Dieckmann, Emil. *Municipal General Hospital Outpatient Population Study: Social and Economic Characteristics of Patients in New York City Outpatient Departments, 1965: Methodology.* Report no. 2. New York: School Public Health and Admin. Medicine, Columbia Univ., 1967.

——. *New York Municipal General Hospital Outpatient Population Study, 1965: Data on Background, Medical Care Utilization and Attitudes of Outpatients, by Hospital.* Report no. 3. New York: School Public Health and Admin. Medicine, Columbia Univ., 1968.

Leveson, Irving. "Demand for Neighborhood Medical Care." *Inquiry* 7 (December 1970): 17–24.

Newhouse, Joseph P. "A Model of Physician Pricing." *Southern Econ. J.* 37 (October 1970): 174–83.

Newhouse, Joseph P., and Phelps, Charles E. "On Having Your Cake and Eating It Too: A Review of Estimated Effects of Insurance on Demand for Health Services." Memorandum R-1149-NC, RAND Corp., April 1974.

Newhouse, Joseph P., and Sloan, Frank A. "Physican Pricing, Monopolistic or Competitive: Reply." *Southern Econ. J.* 38 (April 1972): 577–80.

Nichols, D.; Smolensky, E.; and Tideman, T. N. "Discrimination by Waiting Time in Merit Goods." *A.E.R.* 61, no. 3, pt. 1 (June 1971): 312–23.

Phelps, Charles E. "Demand for Health Insurance: A Theoretical and Empirical Investigation." Memorandum R-1054-OEO, RAND Corp., July 1973.

Phelps, Charles E., and Newhouse, Joseph. "The Effects of Coinsurance on Demand for Physician Services." Memorandum R-976-OEO, RAND Corp., June 1972.

———. "Coinsurance, the Price of Time, and the Demand for Medical Services." *Rev. Econ. and Statis.* 56, no. 3 (August 1974): 334–42.

Rosett, Richard N., and Huang, Lien-fu. "The Effects of Health Insurance on the Demand for Medical Care." *J.P.E.* 81, no. 2 (March/April 1973): 281–305.

SECTION III

PRODUCTION

10. The Internal Organization of Hospitals: Some Economic Implications

JEFFREY E. HARRIS

Reprinted with permission from *Bell Journal of Economics* 8. Copyright © 1977, American Telephone & Telegraph Company, 467-482.

This paper investigates the economic implications of the hospital's internal organizational structure. It concludes: (1) The hospital is actually two separate firms—a medical staff (or demand division) and an administration (or supply division). Each half of the organization has its own managers, objectives, pricing strategies and constraints. (2) Within this dual organization, the medical staff and administration have devised a complicated system of nonprice allocative rules. (3) This internal allocative scheme is subject to repeated breakdowns, especially when the medical staff's internal demands exceed the short-run capacity supplied by the administration. (4) Our current regulatory policy toward hospitals is almost exclusively directed at the supply side of the organization. Unless we revise our definition of "hospital" to include the doctor part of the firm, this policy is doomed to failure. (5) Ultimately, a rational public policy toward hospitals requires a change in the internal organization of the hospital itself.

1. Introduction

■ Economists frequently point out our lack of an adequate economic theory of the hospital. Those simple models which have been proposed do not seem to capture the essential institutional details or have great predictive power. The hospital has so many complicated features—the absence of equity capital, an abundance of regulatory controls, near complete insurance subsidization, to name a few—that no single overriding principle fits all the facts. Certainly, many of these characteristics also apply to ordinary business firms, and the conventional theory has been criticized for similar reasons. But the hospital appears to be an extraordinary case.

The hospital is special, this paper suggests, because it is actually two firms in one. There is one part run by doctors and another run by hospital administrators. This split in authority has been emphasized repeatedly in the organizational literature.[1] But it remains the source

---

The author is also a Clinical Fellow, Medical Services, Massachusetts General Hospital. Important criticisms by P. Diamond, P. Samuelson, R. Solow, P. Temin, M. Weitzman, T. Willemain, and the Editorial Board are greatly appreciated.

[1] For some earlier references, see Smith (1955), Henry (1960), and Perrow (1963). More recently, see the contributions in Georgopoulos (1972).

of considerable confusion in existing economic models. In some versions, doctors are regarded as independent entrepreneurs separate from the hospital. In others, they are assumed to be subordinate to the administration and trustees. In others, doctors have *de facto* control over the administration. Sometimes, the entire question of the identity of the firm's decisionmaker is avoided.[2]

My task in this paper is to begin to make some sense out of this confusion. I shall ask some basic questions about internal resource allocation and internal conflict resolution which, hopefully, will be reflected in future models of the hospital. It turns out that this organizational schizophrenia has considerable importance for our current public policy approaches to the hospital sector.

My main conclusions are as follows:

> (1) There is an important ambiguity in the relation between doctor and hospital in this country. On the one hand, the physician is a specialized member of a complicated, decentralized "fire-fighting" organization. On the other hand, the doctor-patient relation renders the physician's medical practice contractually separate from the rest of the hospital. The net result is one organization split into two disjoint pieces, each with its own objectives, managers, pricing strategy and constraints.
>
> (2) Within this organization, the medical staff and administration are locked in a noncooperative oligopoly-type game. This internal foray is resolved not by strategic bargaining at a joint conference committee, but through the short-run internal allocation process itself. Frequently, the only way to resolve conflicts over the control of hospital capacity is for the firm to get bigger and more complicated.
>
> (3) Our current regulatory policy toward hospitals is too one-sided. Attempts to control expenditures or restrict the supply of investment funds to hospital administrators without accompanying incentives at the level of the physician-patient relation will lead to queues, bitterness, and bad medical care.
>
> (4) As an alternative, we must devise policy measures directed jointly at both halves of the organization. Ultimately, this means a change in the internal organization of the hospital itself.

After this introduction, Section 2 discusses the complexity of the internal allocation problem in hospitals. Section 3 considers the reasons for the institutional separation of doctors and hospital in this country. Section 4 discusses the interplay between medical staff and administration in determining short-run capacity levels. Section 5 considers some policy implications.

Any discussion of this type must confront the fact that a very special ethical tone pervades the hospital. Business as usual in hospitals is, after all, a continuous sequence of potential crises. I do not want to exploit or dissect the "myth of uniqueness" surrounding medical care. But it should be understood that the organization is set up to protect the doctor from behaving as economic man. Some might

---

[2] For critical analyses of existing models, see Feldstein (1974) and Jacobs (1974). See also Newhouse (1970), Feldstein (1971), Lee (1971), Clarkson (1972), Davis (1972), Manning (1973), Pauly and Redisch (1973).

regard this as a mere artifact of the insurance system. Others would elevate it to the level of ideology. Whatever, it cannot be ignored in the analysis.

■ The hospital is a firm specifically designed to solve a complicated decision problem—the diagnosis and treatment of illness. Because of the uncertainty inherent in human disease processes, this task requires an organization which can adapt rapidly to changing circumstances and new information. In this section, I emphasize: (1) hospitals have developed a specialized system of very short-run internal resource allocation to handle this coordination problem; and (2) this allocative scheme forms the basis for the split organizational structure characteristic of hospitals in this country.

2. The internal coordination problem

☐ **The diagnosis and treatment of illness.** For heuristic purposes, consider the following hypothetical case history:

Mr. X comes to Dr. A with a fever and a cough. A chest X ray reveals a density. He is hospitalized. Penicillin is administered. Although the fever subsides with this treatment, a repeat X ray shows that the density has not disappeared. A sputum cytological examination is performed and lung cancer is diagnosed. Further studies suggest that the cancer can be removed surgically. An operation is performed. Unfortunately, massive postoperative bleeding occurs. Matched whole blood is administered. Despite this treatment, a cardiac arrest ensues and an emergency resuscitation (code call) is announced. Mr. X is transferred to Intensive Care with chest tubes and a respirator. A special contrast study (angiogram) reveals the site of bleeding. A repeat operation is performed.

In this story, Mr. X's doctor did not just figure out the correct diagnosis and then apply the appropriate treatment. Instead, Mr. X's hospital care involved a complicated sequence of adaptive responses in the face of uncertainty.

All necessary actions taken by Dr. A were obviously not spelled out before Mr. X's hospitalization. Dr. A could have suggested to Mr. X that the X ray density might be cancer, but the number of necessary units of blood required for his postoperative hemorrhage was not predictable in advance. What Mr. X bought was not an operation or blood, but a more general guarantee to be given appropriate medical care whatever his fever and cough turned out to be. In this situation, neither Dr. A nor Mr. X can know at the start the price of the package Mr. X is buying. And once the promise is entered into, it becomes very difficult to stop when the cumulative price reaches some fixed amount. This implicit promise is as much a part of the doctor-patient "contract" as any specific therapeutic measure.

This is not to deny that each of Mr. X's problems had a textbook treatment. For many routine hospital cases, in fact, the actual course of action does not vary much from that planned initially. But the point is that any medical problem can have numerous idiosyncrasies. Not every case of lung cancer presents with pneumonia. Mr. X could have been penicillin-allergic. He might have had diabetes as well. In principle, the complete set of actions required to care for Mr. X was potentially different from that of any other patient.

Moreover, failure to take the necessary actions at precise times and in an exact order could have disastrous consequences. Matched whole blood was required for Mr. X only in the minutes and hours after bleeding. Mr. X's code call (emergency resuscitation) was necessary only at the time of his postoperative cardiac arrest. This does not apply just to emergencies. Even the penicillin had to be given at certain time intervals and dosages.

This "fire fighting" aspect of hospital care is critical to the firm's organization. In contrast to the standardized assembly line production process, each patient receives customized attention. Such a regime of special cases requires a considerable degree of decentralization of decision making.

Any organization designed to care for Mr. X must obviously have a certain amount of standby capacity. But in the hospital, this is not merely a matter of stocking the appropriate physical inventories. Mr. X's emergency resuscitation involved highly specialized human inputs. As a component of his medical care, the code call had to be organized just at the time it was required. Even the task of providing a chest X ray on demand required that a technician and radiologist be available to take, develop, and interpret the picture. And since many services are specially adapted to the particular patient (for example, whole blood thawed and cross-matched for Mr. X), they are not always substitutable from one patient to another.

I do not want to give the impression that every aspect of hospital care involves fixed coefficients. There is a putative set of scientific standards which serve to define the minimum acceptable level of each medical input. But exceeding that minimum is not the same as failing to satisfy it. How far it is exceeded has something to do with the "quality" of medical care the patient receives. If Mr. X bleeds, then his blood pressure and blood count must be checked frequently, but he gets better care if they are watched even more frequently. Although Mr. X stabilized after his repeat operation, he might be better off staying in the intensive care unit another day. The real problem is that in a decentralized regime of special cases, it may be operationally impossible for anyone but the patient's doctor to determine where these minimum cutoff points lie. As a result, production must be organized *as if* every input received by the patient is potentially an absolute necessity. I shall return to this point below.

☐ **The split organization:** To solve these coordination problems, the hospital has developed a characteristic division of labor. This division of labor does not in general depend on the type of hospital ownership (nonprofit, proprietary, government, etc.). The idea is basically this. The firm is made up of an array of specialized suppliers and demanders. On the supply side, certain functionally-oriented departments, such as the pharmacy, operating rooms, and blood bank, stand ready to assemble and deliver a particular input. These inputs are called "ancillary services" and the suppliers are called "ancillary departments." On the demand side, various doctors such as Dr. A decide which patients need which ancillary services and when. Thus, Dr. A recognized the need for sputum cytology and ordered it, and in response the pathology department supplied it. Then Dr. A ordered an operation, and the operating room department made a surgical suite and technicians available. Then postoperatively, an angiogram was ordered and the radiology department performed the service, and so on. The patient care process becomes, in effect, a sequence of spot demands and deliveries.

This separation of internal supply and demand functions is really what distinguishes the hospital from other forms of physician enterprise. In a solo or group office practice, for example, the doctor serves to a great extent as both the patient's medical decision maker and as the manager of the firm's inputs. But in the hospital, the supply function has become too specialized for doctors to handle by themselves. Hence, when Dr. A ordered an X ray, he did not also purchase and stock the film. Nor did he hire the radiological technician, finance the equipment, or plan for the availability of these inputs on demand. Dr. A's decision that Mr. X needed a particular test created an internal demand for that ancillary service, which someone else in the firm then supplied—namely, the hospital's administrator.[3]

This separation of functions is reflected in the formal "organization chart" of the hospital (see Figure 1).[4] The typical voluntary

FIGURE 1
HOSPITAL ORGANIZATION CHART

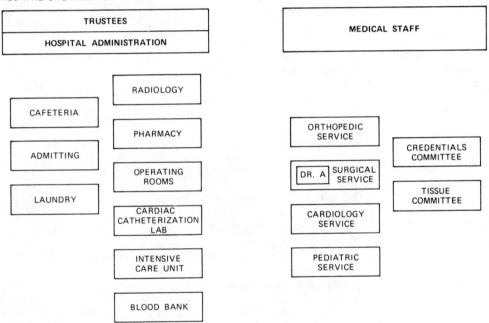

hospital, for example, is a nonprofit corporation with a board of trustees as its ultimate authority. Although the trustees delegate operating responsibility to the hospital's administration, there is also a second separate line of authority emanating from the medical staff, which constitutes the hospital's affiliated physicians. The exact de-

---

[3] For certain medical inputs, doctors are also suppliers. Dr. A (or possibly a surgical consultant) both ordered and performed Mr. X's operation. But the operation could not have taken place unless an operating room, sterile equipment, and scrub nurses were also supplied. It is the physician's decision making role, not his technical skill, which is the critical factor here.

[4] The voluntary hospital, the most prevalent type in this country, will be discussed here. Figure 1 is a stylized version of the organization chart required by the Joint Commission on Accreditation of Hospitals. To adapt the Figure to proprietary or government hospitals, it would be necessary to replace the Trustees (sometimes called the Governing Board) with some alternative form of ownership arrangement. However, in all but the smallest hospitals, this basic organizational split prevails. For an example of a more complete hospital organization chart, see American Hospital Association (1969, p. 7).

partmental divisioning of the administration and the accompanying hierarchy varies among hospitals.[5] The important point is that the administration does not make patient care decisions. The information it uses to plan capacity for ancillary and support services is derived basically from the set of internal demands of individual doctors.[6]

The organization of the medical staff also varies considerably among hospitals. It is usually divided into "clinical services" according to the specialty branches of the member physicians, e.g., Dr. A belonged to the surgical service. There is often no clear hierarchy of physicians. There may be a full-time chief of the medical staff and various department heads and executive committees, but their authority is quite variable. Sometimes a medical staff member is appointed to the trustees. Sometimes there is a "joint policy committee" of medical staff and trustees, which is designed to bring the two lines of authority together on matters of long-run strategy.[7]

3. The doctor-hospital problem

■ In this section, I emphasize that the two-part organization of Figure 1 is actually an extreme and unusual case. For all intents and purposes, the typical hospital is two firms loosely connected by a complex set of nonmarket relations. The basis for this extreme organizational split is the special relation between the doctor and the hospital.

The mere fact that an organization has two parts is not by itself very unusual. Many service organizations have similar division of labor. A large-scale auto repair shop, for example, may have separate service and parts divisions. In the service division, an auto mechanic fixes up cars much like Dr. A "fixed up" Mr. X. And when the mechanic needs a particular gadget, he orders it from inventory just as Dr. A ordered penicillin from the pharmacy. What then is the difference?

If we consider only uncertainty and technological complexity, then our image of the doctor is that of a specialized decision maker in a very decentralized organization. In fact, there would be every reason to think of the doctor as an employee-specialist tied to the hospital in some sort of continuous supply arrangement.[8] To fulfill his contract to take care of Mr. X, Dr. A needed assured access to the hospital's ancillary services. It would be difficult to imagine how Dr. A could

---

[5] In addition to the ancillary departments, the administration has operating responsibility for an array of support services such as admitting, housekeeping, cafeteria, etc. These are not formally considered ancillary services, as they are generally supplied to all hospital patients and not specifically ordered by doctors. Also, some nursing functions are considered to be part of the basic service package rather than as ancillary services, even though doctors' orders routinely include instructions for specific nursing activities.

[6] Some ancillary departments are headed by physicians. This is especially the case for radiology, anesthesiology, and pathology, where, as a rule, these doctors do not admit their own patients. There are also some interesting cases where practicing physicians are ancillary department administrators. The role of these physicians in the organization will be discussed in Section 4 below.

[7] In much of the organizational literature, the trustees are thought of as a third line of command separate from the administration. Frequently, the nursing staff is considered a fourth dominant group. Sometimes the chief executive in the administration is an M.D. I am abstracting away from these complicated institutional considerations to focus on the critical separation of the medical staff and the rest of the hospital.

[8] The parallel with university faculty is obvious.

treat Mr. X if he had to enter into a market sales arrangement for every angiogram or code call.

Anyone who has ever been seriously ill, however, knows that something else is going on. Whatever this ''something else'' is, it is an ethical factor quite apart from the doctor's legal status as a professional. The doctor-patient relation creates a much stronger expectation of fidelity than is present in other agent-client arrangements.[9] The doctor is saddled with a moral burden of ultimate responsibility for the outcome of the case.

In a sense, Mr. X regarded his doctor as his own professional ''gun for hire.''[10] As an implicit part of his contract, Dr. A was supposed to take a single-minded devotion to his assignment. He was expected to do everything which was *scientifically indicated* for his patient without reference to price. By contrast, negotiations between a car owner and mechanic usually go to some length to specify an exact price—or at least a maximum price—for the job. The mechanic is much more a member of the auto repair business than a professional agent for his client. Dr. A, however, was supposed to be on Mr. X's side.

I am not saying that doctors ignore the magnitudes of their own fees or their patients' abilities to pay them. On the contrary, one function of the fee-for-service system is to seal the ethical bond between the doctor and patient. I am also not saying that doctors are prevented from ever making informal inquiries about the costs of nondoctor inputs. My point is that no patient such as Mr. X would want his doctor to be compelled to make repeated marginal decisions about the costs and benefits of an angiogram or unit of blood. People who are seriously ill do not want doctors who are cost-effective agents of the organization or of society. That would dilute the doctor's role as a paladin.

Many readers, I suppose, would argue that this is purely an artifact of the insurance system. Admittedly, if consumers were totally ignorant about cars and had full insurance for car repairs, then they might let mechanics do what doctors do. I must emphasize, however, that there is an unusual feature to this agency relationship. Even if Mr. X had full knowledge and no insurance, there would still be some social requirement for an agent who could make noneconomic decisions on his behalf. There is a special negative externality in an arrangement in which one makes repeated marginal decisions about life and death. This externality is so important that the physician's participation in the ''market'' for angiograms and code calls is explicitly foreclosed. Whether or not it is justified, this notion has an important influence on the way the hospital is organized.[11]

The net effect of all this is a sort of contracting dilemma. The patient buys a promise from the doctor to be fixed up. The hospital in turn (that is, the administration part) supplies the necessary inputs to the doctor. The technology of hospital care is such that the doctor and the hospital must be closely linked. On the other hand, there is a **strong ethical presumption that the doctor be left alone to do what-**

---

[9] For an earlier reference to this point, see Arrow (1963).

[10] The analogy is from Halberstam (1971).

[11] One might ask whether this special ideology prevails in other countries. It seems to me that the closer relationship between doctors and hospitals found in many parts of Europe is traceable to a weakening of this ideology.

ever is necessary for the patient's well being. Somehow, the doctor must be isolated from the rest of hospital, even though he is really a part of it.

This problem is solved by setting up a separate contract between the patient and the hospital-supplier. Rather than buying the doctor's and the administration's services together in one package, the patient buys the two separately. This is not just a matter of Mr. X's getting a breakdown of "labor" and "parts" costs. Dr. A is not even supposed to get involved in the sale to Mr. X of the hospital-supplied operating room, penicillin, and X rays. It is, literally, not his business.

To go along with this contractual scheme, there must be a system of operating rules and property rights. In fact, the whole hospital seems to be "split down the middle" just so this three-way arrangement will work. Thus, there is a set of sanctions which permit the doctor to conduct his practice without interference from the administration or trustees. Only the doctor decides what patients shall be admitted, how long they will be hospitalized, and what inputs they shall receive.

Moreover, the doctor does not pay a user toll for the right of access to the hospital's inputs.[12] Instead, "staff privileges" are rationed by a system which is basically controlled by the medical staff. Although there is a variety of open and closed staffing policies, restricted admitting privileges, salaried faculty, professional corporations, fellowships, house officers, and so forth,[13] all of these are in effect dictated and policed by the medical staff. With few exceptions, the medical staff can dismiss or discipline one of its members.[14] It alone has rules of professional conduct, ethics, extra-hospital activities, and type of patients admitted.

Although there is a varied, complex and ever-changing system of hospital charges and cost-reporting schemes, their common feature is the separate pricing of the doctor's product and the hospital's product. Most physicians' fees are not even included in such cost reports. Those physician-originated costs which do end up in the hospital's accounts are separated into a "professional component," which is then reported separately. It is this definition of total cost (net of doctor inputs) which is the base for hospital rate regulation.

There are admittedly many other reasons why the hospital is set up this way. One could argue that the separation of an autonomous medical staff and the phenomenon of closed staffing are basically designed to perpetuate an organized medical monopoly. One could focus on the issue of the profession's self-policing of physician qual-

---

[12] Physicians may pay in nonpecuniary ways such as administrative duties or teaching. In some nonprofit hospitals, there is a significant amount of physician philanthropy. There has also been a recent increase in the number of medical office buildings incorporated into hospital facilities. These methods of "buying in" are, however, far from universal.

[13] See Roemer and Friedman (1971).

[14] As Ludlam (1970) indicates, the courts have become increasingly involved in the protection of the doctor's right to due process in these disciplinary procedures. Their basic rationale for intervention is that private hospitals, when acting upon staff membership applications, are exercising a fiduciary power for the public good. This seems to me to be further evidence that our society does not want a market-oriented "hire or fire" relationship between doctors and hospitals.

ity.[15] My interpretation here is that the doctor-hospital separation is intended to eliminate the necessity for repeated cost calculations in the clinical care of patients like Mr. X. Hence, doctors get assured access to hospital inputs by becoming "members" of the firm. Yet, unlike employees, they do not get told what to do.

The doctor and hospital are, therefore, really part of the same firm. But there is a whole system of institutional constraints designed to make doctors look like individual entrepreneurs who happen to conduct their business on the hospital's premises.[16] Certainly, there is a market between doctor and hospital-supplier in the sense that doctors can admit patients in many hospitals. And, as I have suggested, there may be some good reasons why rights of access to hospitals should be rationed by the staff privilege system rather than by the price mechanism. But, as I shall suggest below, the failure to recognize that doctors and hospitals are linked by a strong bond of joint production is at the basis of many of the hospital's inefficiencies.

■ Except for some preliminary suggestions about the hospital's pricing behavior and methods of third-party reimbursement, I have said nothing so far about the external market and regulatory environment in which this firm operates. Clearly, any theory of the hospital must take these things into account. But before we construct such a theory, it must be recognized that the medical staff and administration each has its own objectives, decision variables, and constraints. Furthermore, there must be an important set of rules specifying how the two sides get along.

There are many possible ways of analyzing this problem. One might consider some kind of bargaining model in which group decision rules are derived from many utility functions. Admittedly, it is interesting to see how joint committees of trustees, doctors, and administrators decide whether to buy a new computer software package or to discontinue open heart surgery. But it seems to me that the institutional barrier between doctors and hospitals creates a more basic team problem. That is, in the absence of explicit prices, what kinds of decision rules or signals are passed between the two sides of Figure 1 to accomplish the short-run allocative task of individual patient care? What I am really asking is how the hospital manages to work at all. Why is there not a continuous mad scramble for beds, operations, and blood?

I want to tell the story here of a complicated system of rationing

4. The capacity problem

---

[15] One could take the historical approach. Hospital care was not always so complicated as Section 2 suggests, nor was doctor-oriented medical care always the function of hospitals. With increasingly complex technology, the administrative role became more distinct, and the loose association of doctors and hospitals became more formalized as the medical staff.

[16] In the well-known Darling case (*Darling* v. *Charleston Community Memorial Hospital*, 33 Ill 2d 326 (1965); cert. denied, 383 U.S. 946 (1966)), the court moved toward the interpretation of joint production when it ruled that the hospital trustees as well as the physician were liable for malpractice. On the other hand, in a more recent case (*St. John's Hospital Medical Staff* v. *St. John's Regional Medical Center, Inc.*, Docket No. 11746, Supreme Court of South Dakota, Sept. 3, 1976), the court held that the medical staff was a separate legal entity with its own bylaws. See also Curran (1977).

devices, uncodified rules, and subtle maneuvering, conducted in a sanctified atmosphere of "life and death." Most of the time, this system seems to allocate resources fairly well. But as the degree of capacity utilization increases, previously stable risk-sharing arrangements break down. Doctors, fearing that they will not have access to necessary inputs, grab up their own exclusive shares to keep themselves protected. The hospital becomes a sort of noncollusive oligopoly in which each of the main actors is vying for his own separate empire.

Let me pose the problem this way. In the short run, the hospital administration must set capacity levels for each of its inputs. Although bed size is probably more rigid than the total capacity for, say, angiograms or respirators, I am concerned with the very short-run frame of reference in which all these parameters are essentially fixed. In principle, these capacity decisions should not be much different from the standard inventory problem. One has to know the joint probability distribution of demands for the firm's inputs as well as the right- and left-hand side loss functions associated with holding excess or insufficient capacity. Once the optimal magnitudes of these "defensive positions" are determined, it is then a question of doctors' figuring out which of these inputs their patients need and the administrations' making sure that each patient gets the right inputs in the right combinations at the right time.

Although this problem may seem straightforward, anyone who has been in a big, metropolitan hospital will recognize that things do not always work so well. There are queues in front of radiology. The supply of a certain type of blood is exhausted. The floor stock of chest tubes is found to be out just when Dr. A declares Mr. X's life-saving need for one. This is not just because hospital administrators failed to take courses in operations research. And it is not (as far as I can tell) because the observed level of mistakes is acceptable. In fact, there is considerable conflict within the hospital over the appropriate magnitudes of these defensive positions. It is really because the capacity problem itself is extremely complicated. And the actual solution observed is very much determined by the basic institutional split between doctor and hospital.

One complication is that the joint probability distribution of demands for hospital inputs is not exogenously given, but is under the control of doctors. If all illnesses were truly textbook cases with a known set of optimal input combinations and fixed coefficients, then the firm might do quite well estimating this probability distribution from exogenous epidemiologic data. To a certain extent, this is what hospital administrators are supposed to do. But the difficulty is that the demand for intensive care beds is as much a matter of doctors' discretionary judgments as it is a question of heart attack statistics.

As I emphasized above, hospital medical care is very unstandardized, with every case requiring the doctor's unique and individual attention. Even in those peaceful cases where nothing goes wrong, there must be a doctor standing ready to put out fires. In this decentralized regime of special attention, it is very costly to monitor what demands of doctors are really "necessary" as opposed to discretionary.[17] Furthermore, there is a strong moral sanction against interfer-

---

[17] It is not my purpose to pass judgment on schemes of concurrent review which attempt to monitor unnecessary utilization. The point is that special cases like Mr. X's

ing in the doctor-patient relationship. The net result is a very sanctified atmosphere in which "doctor knows best."

I cannot overemphasize the influence of this ideological tone on the allocation process. Doctors are in a position to deem all sorts of demands as necessary for their patients. This is not the same thing as saying doctors order useless tests to satisfy some ulterior motive. Additional demands for inputs above the hypothetical scientific minimum are going to be regarded by doctors as improvements in quality. And the fact is that doctors have an almost inexhaustible repertoire of things that will make their patients better off. Hence, doctors will demand some minimum very inelastically, but given the opportunity, they can slide down their demand curve with ease.

An additional complication is that the hospital administration and the members of the medical staff will attach different weights to the right- and left-hand side loss functions in this inventory problem. The administration—whether it is trying to maximize profit or break even—must consider the expected costs of holding extra capacity and the expected revenues obtained from utilizing that capacity. Although hospitals are by no means pure price takers, it is nevertheless true that if charges are based on ancillary services and patient days, then revenue will be related to the degree of utilization of capacity. Hence, it generally pays administrators to keep the hospital full. This does not mean that administrators are completely oblivious to circumstances of excess demand. No administrator wants a front-page newspaper headline about the little old lady who died after being turned away from his hospital. But the point is that the cost side of the loss function is weighted heavily. On the other hand, the institution is set up so that doctors do not have to worry about the costs of holding a certain capacity. Doctors weigh only the possible losses incurred from excess demand. Dr. A cares little about an empty bed. But he will not be very happy if he cannot get one for Mr. X.

This means that there is going to be internal conflict over the size of the hospital's short-run defensive position. And the special institutional constraints embedded in the problem make it difficult to see how this conflict is resolved. If, for example, administrators find the hospital to be underutilized and losing potential revenues, then they would want doctors to admit more patients and increase their established margins over the scientific minimum. But such an improvement in "quality" may create pressure on capacity which the medical staff would find uncomfortable. Somehow, everyone has to get his signals straight.

Before examining what actually goes on, let me suggest that an internal price system could not by itself perform the necessary job.[18] This is not merely because doctors have no incentive to pay attention to decision rules in which, say, costs per case are minimized. Rather, it would be inappropriate to require a price system to regulate the capacity of, say, a code call. Like many of the hospital's inputs, a code call must be produced and delivered on demand; it is poorly

---

are really the rule rather than the exception. Although Mr. X may have used resources in excess of some established guidelines for cases of lung cancer, it is not clear how such standards can be enforced.

[18] I do not want to get into the more general problem of why internal price systems are not used in certain organizations. The argument I make here is similar to that put forward by Weitzman (1974).

substitutable among patients; and it cannot be stockpiled as physical inventory. In these situations, both the administrator's supply curve and the doctor's demand curve will be highly inelastic. There is just no way to ration the excess demand without going below the minimum standard. Moreover, all sorts of small numbers problems of the type usually associated with failure of the price system would develop. It would be intolerable to have Dr. A and Dr. B haggle over the market clearing price of, say, one available intensive care bed which was immediately needed by both of their patients.

To be sure, there are many situations in which the transfer price for, say, an additional discretionary day in the intensive care unit would be a valuable allocative instrument. Although it is not entirely clear to me why this allocative instrument has not been tried, perhaps it is a question of making difficult distinctions with insufficient information. Even the most routine test could turn out to provide life-saving information for Mr. X. And even if it were not so crucial, Dr. A could say it was. It is not clear, therefore, where the price system would be formally applied and where exceptions would be made. In any case, it is a known fact that doctors in this country do not know the costs of blood, angiograms, or intravenous penicillin.[18]

Like many other organizations, therefore, the hospital must solve this capacity problem with a rather wide variety of nonprice-related decision rules. There are loosely enforced standards, rules of thumb, side bargains, cajoling, negotiations, special contingency plans, and in some cases literally shouting and screaming.[19] As the hospital approaches short-run full capacity utilization, these allocative devices become increasingly important. Various rules which are usually loosely enforced are suddenly invoked to curtail doctors' powers of fiat. The nurse refuses to administer certain treatments which are not in her job description. The floor secretary wants a written requisition for a procedure usually ordered by telephone. The hospital admitting office manipulates the elective waiting list. The radiology dispatcher decides who goes next. Doctors' orders, which are classified into "routine" and "stat" priorities, all become "stat." Special clearance must be obtained for angiograms and other ancillary services. Doctors hedge against the possible short supply of a particular test by ordering it far in advance. If the patient later does not need the test, it is cancelled. Doctors bargain over which patient will receive the last available intensive care unit bed. Rules for sharing operating room availability are invoked. Interns and residents become masters at the art of bed juggling.

Certainly, the kind of wild maneuvering described above does not occur in all hospitals all the time. In many small hospitals, there seems to be a tacit understanding among medical staff and administration that this allocative scramble must be avoided. Complicated patients like Mr. X are transferred to other hospitals. Only routine or "rest home" type cases are admitted. Inputs such as beds and operating rooms are pooled and available for any doctor's use. In this

---

[18] For a recent review, see Skipper *et al.* (1976).

[19] In an interesting case study of a psychiatric hospital, Strauss *et al.* (1963) characterized this type of allocational process as "negotiated order." In another context, see Powell's 1977 discussion of the variety of pressure tactics, complaints, and maneuvering found in the execution of Soviet economic plans. See also Ward's discussion of the interwar U.S. Navy (1967, pp. 190ff).

"quiet life" model, physicians think of their shares of this internal market as stable.

At the other extreme, these risk-sharing arrangements have broken down. Instead, each clinical service of the medical staff is constantly striving to maintain and expand the magnitude of its own defensive position. Rules are established to differentiate orthopedic beds from general surgical beds. Operating rooms are held exclusively for special uses. Each service gets its own intensive care unit. Each intensive care unit gets its own laboratory. The idea behind all of these arrangements is to ensure the exclusive availability of a set of inputs to a small group of demanders. In that way, no one is going to get bumped.

One interesting instance of this hoarding phenomenon is the practice of joint appointments. A particular medical staff physician is designated to be a "manager" of a supplying ancillary department. One frequently observes such staffing titles as "Associate Cardiologist and Clinical Director of the Cardiac Catheterization Laboratory." The same rules governing the organizational separation of cardiologists and cardiac catheterization apply. The staff physicians do not pay for the department's inputs. But now the cardiologists can control the rationing of cardiac procedures in times of tight capacity.

It could be argued that this is all just the specialization which accompanies technologically complicated medical care in bigger hospitals. But it seems to me that the causality is actually reversed. It is the constant noncooperative scramble to expand one's own defensive position which drives the hospital to bigness and betterment. I have in mind here a disequilibrium model in which everyone behaves as if the hospital is not big enough. The administration, on the one hand, wants the hospital filled. But the doctors want bigger defensive margins. The administration will expand capacity only if doctors can fill up the beds. Since there is internal conflict over the control of these defensive margins, doctors will expand utilization and increase quality to obtain their share. As a result, the administration will tolerate the creation and perpetuation of these separate empires even though it negates the advantages of risk pooling.

To a certain extent, this is not much different from the kind of quantity-quality maximizing model which has been used to explain hospital cost inflation in the post-Medicare period (see Feldstein, 1971). There is a built-in drive to expand size and complexity. When external constraints are relaxed (e.g., increased insurance coverage, increased availability of investment), then the hospital grabs up the slack. The story I have told, however, seems to have a number of other important implications.

5. Implications and future directions

■ In this section, I consider a few of the policy implications of the above discussion. Rather than providing a series of complete analyses, I merely want to be suggestive. Some of these ideas I hope to explore in future papers.

□ **Technological change.** In general, it strikes me that the right way to look at the extensive spread of increasingly expensive technology in hospitals is to ask how it affects the game which administrations and physicians play. The above discussion suggests that pressure for new innovations is really built into the hospital's internal organization. In the same way that doctors use "quality" improvement to expand capacity, they will also use new innovations as weapons in the conflict. Instead of new diagnostic and treatment schemes which increase hospital efficiency—in the sense of permitting fewer resources per case—one would expect innovations which allow doctors to do more things for their patients. In other words, one would expect innovations which complement rather than substitute for existing capacity.

I am not saying that coronary care units, left ventricular assist devices, and bypass surgery had nothing to do with the desire to improve the survival and life style of heart patients. And there is no denying that physicians have been trained to favor sophisticated gadgetry. But in a regime of constant technical change, it is important to understand why certain innovations are selected and others are not. Certainly, these innovations have done little to decrease the intensity of resource use per case of cardiac disease. On the contrary, the current research thrust is to include a much wider class of patients as potential users of our new coronary technology.

☐ **Hospital regulation.** Current regulatory policy toward the hospital sector does not give careful consideration to its effects on the internal organization of the hospital, the behavior of the medical staff and administration, and the internal allocational process itself. Without such careful examination, we are bound to produce maladaptations which run counter to our intended goals.

This is particularly obvious in the case of hospital rate regulation schemes. What the hospital actually sells to patients is the diagnosis and treatment of illness (the promise to be "fixed up"), not a collection of ancillary and support services. The product to be priced is actually the joint output of both doctors and hospital-suppliers. A pricing scheme which separates out the administration's part and the doctor's part of the product will not work as long as the doctor has control over both his own and the hospital's inputs. It has never been clear to me how a rate regulatory commission can seriously require hospital administrators to limit hospital costs attributable to say, radiology, when the doctors, not the administrators, order the X rays. Even if the administrator eliminates 25 percent of technical inefficiency in the radiology department, what keeps the doctor from raising "quality" and ordering 50 percent more X rays?

One might respond that a budget constraint on the administrator will eventually end up as a constraint on doctors' decisions. If for no other reason, these rate setting and cost control regulations, along with P.S.R.O.'s, Certificate of Need rules, and complicated accounting schemes, are all going to strengthen the hand of the administration. When this happens, doctors, seeing these constraints, will start sending the patients home earlier and ordering fewer tests. But this ignores the short-run possibilities. If doctors want to spend more than administrators have available, the hospital may be converted into the type of mad scramble I outline above. In the short run, such a constraint may lead to an increase in resources used per case as doctors grab up what they can before capacity becomes too tight. Hospitals with apparent capacity excesses or cost overruns may actually be in a deceptively stable equilibrium. Any threat to choke off defensive positions may only lead to queues and more madness.

The more rational approach, it seems to me, is to concentrate on the relation between doctor and patient and on the relation between doctor and hospital. Under the current institutional arrangement, the critical price is the physician's fee for hospital care and not the administration's reimbursement. This conclusion does not depend on the relative magnitude of the doctor part and the nondoctor part of total hospital expenditures. If the doctor makes the short-run allocative decisions, then it is the doctor's yield from those decisions that matters.[20]

□ **Organizational changes.** With all of the recent enthusiasm over prospective reimbursement, expenditure caps, and cost-reporting according to case mix, there will be nothing but the ravages of excess demand unless the cost-minimizing incentive is transferred directly to the doctor part of the organization. As long as we continue to define "hospital" as the left-hand side of Figure 1, this is going to be no easy task. One might be able to devise some very complicated internal operating and enforcement rules. But, ultimately, there must be a change in the current institutional and legal structure of doctor-hospital relations.

One possible clue to this change is a particularly interesting property of the patient care technology—namely, its tendency toward decomposability (Harris, 1975b). It turns out that the resource transfers between medical staff and ancillary departments go predominantly only in certain directions. The cardiac catheterization laboratory is used primarily by cardiologists. The operating rooms are used primarily by surgeons. Special orthopedic appliances are ordered primarily by orthopedic surgeons. Brain scans and brain angiograms are ordered primarily by neurologists. To be sure, a number of ancillary services are supplied to all demanders in the organization. Nevertheless, these partial decomposability properties suggest a method of reorganizing the hospital along separate "product lines" rather than across functions (Harris, 1975a). Cardiologists would run the cardiac catheterization unit. Neurologists would run the neuroradiology unit. Surgeons would run the operating rooms, etc. This type of system is in effect a generalization of the "separate empire" phenomenon described above, but with the important additional feature that a much simpler set of operating rules can be imposed. In particular, it may be possible to introduce cost-minimizing incentives at the clinical decision making level. But these ideas must await another paper.

References

AMERICAN HOSPITAL ASSOCIATION. *Internal Control and Internal Auditing for Hospitals.* Chicago: American Hospital Association, 1969.

ARROW, K. "Uncertainty and the Welfare Economics of Medical Care." *The American Economic Review,* Vol. 53, No. 5 (December 1963), pp. 941–973.

CLARKSON, K. W. "Some Implications of Property Rights in Hospital Management." *Journal of Law and Economics,* Vol. 15, No. 2 (October 1972), pp. 363–376.

---

[20] Many studies have suggested a substantial elasticity of hospital length of stay with respect to the rate of coinsurance. As far as I can tell, in all of these experiments the rates of coinsurance on both the hospital's charges and the doctor's attending fees are varying simultaneously. For a recent review, see Newhouse and Phelps (1974).

11. A Conspicuous Production Theory of Hospital Behavior

MAW LIN LEE

Reprinted with permission from *Southern Economic Journal* 38. Copyright © 1971, University of North Carolina, 48-58.

Amidst the growing concern over rapidly rising prices and costs of hospital services, both time series studies of hospital cost increases and cross-section studies of hospital cost and production relationships have been undertaken [for example: 4; 8; 10]. However, such studies have been handicapped by the absence of a generally accepted theory concerning the economic behavior of the hospital.[1] The reason for this handicap is rather obvious. In the classic, competitive model of the firm, the concept of profit maximization provides an effective assumption about the behavior of business firms. Most hospitals, however, are not profit-oriented enterprises and therefore the assumption of profit maximization does not shed much light on hospital behavior.

In recent years, there have been several attempts to develop a theory of hospital behavior. In his recent paper R. G. Rice [17] proposed a sales maximization model of the hospital.[2] J. Newhouse [12], on the other hand, suggests that hospital decision-makers have both quantity of output and prestige in their maximand. In contrast to these two theories, K. Davis [5] assumes that hospitals maximize short-run net reve-

nue in her study of the demand, cost, and production of hospital care. Also, M. Pauly [14] has recently proposed that hospitals attempt to maximize profit.

In this paper, an alternative theory of hospital behavior is proposed. The theory is based on the propositions that the preferences of hospitals are interdependent[3] and certain inputs are acquired for purposes other than to meet the requirement of ordinary production.[4] It is because of the similarity of the latter proposition to Veblen's concept that our theory is called conspicuous production theory.

I. SOME RELEVANT CHARACTERISTICS

In this paper, it is assumed that hospital administrators attempt to maximize utility. Such an approach was suggested initially in connection with business firms where ownership and management do not coincide. Under these circumstances, it was argued that management might consistently make some decisions that were inconsistent with profit maximization, but which would improve management's welfare in other ways—rugs on the floor, pretty secretaries, business trips to Hawaii, etc. [1, 157–183]. While the usefulness of this assumption has been challenged in the case of business firms, such an approach appears reasonable for non-profit institutions [7]. For this reason, the utility function is assumed to be the objective function of hospital operations.

The utility function, as used here, is a

---

* The author wishes to thank Edward Greenberg, Teh-Wei Hu, Paul Junk, David Kamerschen, Paul Smith, and Ernst Stromsdorfer for their comments on this paper. He is especially grateful to Richard Wallace for his contribution to this study. This project was supported in part by the Missouri Regional Medical program under a Public Health Service grant (USPHS, RM 00009-3 PEC). The author assumes responsibility for the views expressed in the paper and for any errors.

[1] For simplicity sake, the motivation or behavior of "decision-makers within a hospital" is simply referred to as that of "the hospital" throughout this paper.

[2] This model is similar to the sales-maximization hypothesis of Baumol [3, 295–310].

[3] The concept of interdependent preferences of consumers has been examined by Duesenberry [6, 17–46] and Leibenstein [9] in terms of demonstration, bandwagon, and snob effect.

[4] "Ordinary production" is used here to represent the type of production function that will be adopted by a firm motivated by profit maximization.

199

broad concept meant to include all those variables which affect the well-being of the administrator. Such variables include salary, prestige, security, power, professional satisfaction among others. This definition of utility function is based on that of organizational theorists. In addition, organizational theorists have argued that the salary, prestige, security, power and professional satisfaction of decision makers are dependent on the prestige and status of the organizations with which the decision makers are associated [2; 18; 20]. This implies that the utility of hospital administrators is a function of the status of the hospitals in which they serve. Thus, it is assumed that the drive for status has become a socially recognized goal among hospital administrators and that this drive plays a dominant role as hospital administrators strive to maximize utility.

As a result of such behavior, there are forces of competition at work in the hospital industry—not for profits but for status.[5] This nonprice competition results from the drive for self-esteem on the part of hospital administrators. As will be argued below, it is reinforced by the nature of the relationship of the medical staff to the hospital. In contrast to price competition among profit-oriented firms where the result is protection of the consumer's interest, the competition for status among hospitals lies at the root of some of the fundamental economic problems facing the hospital industry today.

The status of a hospital is an abstract, nonmeasurable concept. It is a relative concept which exists in the mind of people who pass a judgment on a hospital. Since a judgment of this nature is concerned with the status of a hospital as a producer of hospital care, it is usually based on visible objects or symbols. For this reason, attention of hospital administrators has been focused on the variety, quantity, and complexity of the inputs available in the hospital. Thus, the status of a hospital is assumed to vary directly with the range of services available and the extent to which expensive and highly specialized equipment and personnel (including M.D.'s) are available.

The attention of hospital administrators to inputs is reinforced by the particular importance of the physician to the hospital. Not only will judgments concerning the status of the hospital depend on the reputations of the M.D.'s practicing therein, but the hospital also is dependent on the medical staff for its patients. As the size and quality of the hospital's medical staff increases, it can expect its patient load to increase.

The result is another important aspect of the competition among hospitals. In order to attract and maintain physicians, hospitals are responsive to the demand of their medical staffs.[6] In producing health care, a hospital acquires inputs for the care of the patients, and these inputs are utilized by physicians in their practice of medicine—the inputs are provided for physicians' use without charge. To physicians, hospitals are "free" workshops or factories: the better and more fully a hospital is equipped, the greater the reward to physicians is implied. Thus, competition among hospitals for physicians also results in expanding and improving the investory of inputs. In this respect, a part of the expense incurred for expansion of inputs may be regarded as an implicit payment to physicians—a price paid to attract physicians.

---

[5] The assumption that hospitals are competitive is not consistent with the widely held belief that competition does not prevail in the health sector. In addition to the absence of a profit motive, it is believed that a hospital is in a monopolistic position because, where there is a choice, physicians select hospitals for consumers. However, this is merely a short run phenomenon. In the long run, not only do consumers change physicians, but physicians also change their hospital affiliations.

[6] In some hospitals the medical staff has the power to make all vital decisions. In other hospitals, the administrators are profoundly influenced by physicians.

The particular role of inputs described above implies that equipment, facilities and personnel are used as status symbols and represent the price paid to physicians. Because of this, hospitals strive to acquire certain inputs without adequate regard for the extent to which such inputs will be used for actual production.[7] Such a result is facilitated by at least three factors. First, the public has had great confidence in the hospital sector. This trust or confidence is based in part on the fact that most hospitals are non-profit enterprises. The general public may interpret this to mean lower costs and a sincere effort to meet medical needs. The trust is based in part on the public's ignorance about the nature of a hospital—anything that has to do with "life and death" must be entrusted to the experts.

Second, the acquisition of inputs without adequate regard for their actual utilization is facilitated by the impersonalization of payment procedures. A substantial portion of a hospital's total revenue is provided by third party payers—government and private health insurance. For this reason, consumers do not feel the full impact of the magnitude of hospital charges at least in the short-run. Hospitals feel that third parties, instead of consumers, are paying the bills. Thus, it has been a relatively easy matter for hospitals to pass increased expenditures along in the form of higher prices. To the extent these increases have been scrutinized by third party purchasers, it has amounted to an examination of the extent to which the hospital's actual expenditures for inputs has increased. There has been little scrutiny of the necessity for adding new inputs or of the efficiency with which inputs are combined.

Third, the acquisition of inputs without adequate regard for the value of output is facilitated by the practice of average cost pricing of individual hospital services. Hospital administrators readily acknowledge that there are certain "losers" among the services that hospitals produce and that the losses on these services must be covered, at least in part, by the charges for other hospital services. In addition to the question concerning the equity of such a procedure where the result is subsidization of one group of patients by another group of patients, an important question concerning efficiency also arises. This practice facilitates the provision of new services, equipment, and personnel so long as a general increase in hospital rates will cover the additional expenditure. There is no necessity for the increase in expenditure associated with new input to be matched by an equivalent increase in revenue realized from the sale of the output produced by that input. The new input may add little to the hospital's actual output of services, but it may be acquired so long as its cost can be spread over hospital prices in general.

The acquisition of inputs without adequate regard to actual production implies that hospitals use more resources than required to produce a given output stream. This may result from relatively expensive pieces of equipment standing idle much of the time, the actual use of greater quantities of factors than necessary to produce a given output, or the use of higher quality inputs than necessary to do a given task.

II. THE MODEL

This study assumes that, as a producer of health care, each hospital has a desired status (S^*) and an actual status (S). The community delegates to the hospital a mission to produce health care, and the nature of this delegated mission defines the desired status of a hospital.[8] However, the actual status will differ from the desired

---

[7] Such behavior might have been both a cause and an effect of the way in which government grants are awarded and philanthropic contributions are made. Both government grants and philanthropic contributions favor physical plant, equipment and facilities.

[8] Hospitals, as agents of the community, are trying to do a job expected of them by the community and justify their actions on the grounds that they must do what other hospitals do in order to maintain the status quo.

status if there is a discrepancy between the behavior and activity which are expected of a hospital and the actual behavior and activity of the hospital. The basic hypothesis of the conspicuous production theory is that a hospital attempts to minimize the gap between its desired status (S^*) and its prevailing status (S). That is,

minimize $(S^* - S)$, where $S^* \geq S$.

Three aspects of the hypothesis should be noted. First, minimization of the status gap implies maximization of utility on the part of hospital administrators. Second, the assumption that hospitals strive to minimize the status gap rather than maximize status implies that the efforts of hospitals are defensive in nature. The fundamental reason for proposing such a defensive postulate is that hospitals justify their activities on the ground that other hospitals are undertaking similar activities—they must emulate other hospitals in order to maintain their relative status. Third, the defensive nature of the postulate in no way implies that the forces due to defensively motivated behavior under interdependent conditions are weaker than those due to offensively motivated behavior when behavior is independent. In fact, the former may well be stronger than the latter.

As previously indicated, inputs are used as status symbols, or, in other words, the pattern of input utilization defines the status group to which a hospital belongs. One practical implication of the use of inputs to define status is that for each status group at a particular time, there is a set of desired inputs (I^*). The actual inputs (I^a), however, determine the actual status of the hospital. Thus, the assumption that a hospital attempts to minimize the gap between its desired and actual status may be restated as:[9]

Minimize $(I^* - I^a)$ where $I^* \geq I^a$ (1)

subject to the budget constraint

$$Y = R'I \qquad (2)$$

where R and I are respectively $(n \times 1)$ vectors of prices and quantities of inputs acquired or utilized.

To complete the behavioral model of the hospital, it is necessary to specify a desired input function (I^*), and this function is determined by the sociological structure of the hospital sector. The hospital sector consists of hospitals in various status groups, and it is a well known sociological phenomenon that a member of a particular status group is expected to meet the behavioral standard of other members in the group. This implies that a hospital desires to use the same inputs as other hospitals in the same status group.[10] The desired inputs of, say, the ith hospital is assumed to be a function of the inputs utilized by other hospitals.[11] Thus:

$$I^* = f(I_1{}^a, I_2{}^a, \cdots). \qquad (3)$$

The assumption underlying the desired input function also may be justified by the relationship between medical staff and a hospital. As pointed out in the previous section, a part of the expenditures incurred for hospital expansion and improvement in

---

[9] This implies that our attention is directed away from status to input which is the means by which the status gap is minimized. The argument underlying this procedure is similar to the argument underlying the managerial discretion model developed by Oliver E. Williamson [21]. Although

Williamson is concerned with behavior of profit-oriented business firms, he considers that the expansion of staff and the expansion of physical plant and equipment provides general opportunities for managerial satisfaction.

[10] The relevance of sociological factors to human behavior was pointed out by Duesenberry in his discussion of interdependent preferences of consumers [6, 28–32].

[11] Conceptually, the pattern of inputs utilized by a hospital may be influenced by all conceivable hospitals in existence. But, in fact, the pattern of inputs utilized is likely to be influenced by only a few hospitals, most of which are in the same geographical area. The determination of the desired level of inputs in hospitals given by relation (3) differs significantly from that of business firms. In the theory of investment behavior, the desired level of capital is assumed to be proportional to output or to profit. For stock types of inputs, the determination of the rate of replacement must also be specified.

fact represents an implicit payment to physicians. It is a price paid to attract physicians, and the "price" that one hospital has to pay depends on the price that other hospitals are paying.

There is an important aspect of the desired input function that must be noted. If one hospital increases its stock or flow of inputs, other hospitals can be expected to follow suit. But if one hospital reduces the inputs, other hospitals are not likely to follow.[12] This characteristic of behavioral interdependence in the hospital system is similar to that in the oligopolistic or oligopsonistic market structure. Hospitals compete primarily in terms of the methods of treatment and the pattern of equipment and personnel utilization. Any unfavorable comparison in terms of input utilization gives rise to the motivation for acquiring the inputs utilized by other hospitals. The utility derived from a unit of an input depends not only on its contribution to output, but also, on its contribution to demonstrating the capacity of the hospital to produce a certain mix of health care. Thus, hospitals can acquire certain inputs without adequate regard for the output of services that can be produced with such inputs.[13] This second component of utility is based on what members of the community and the health profession think of the hospitals as a producer of health care. This aspect of the demand for inputs in hospitals is similar to that underlying the conspicuous consumption aspect of consumer demand.

III. EFFECTS OF TECHNOLOGICAL CHANGES

It is important to note that, even though the desired status of a hospital may not change over time, the factors which affect its status and the behavior and activities

which are expected of it change rapidly. Such changes are closely related to advances in medical science and technology. For this reason it will be useful to consider the process through which technological change is diffused through the hospital industry.

For the purpose of this analysis, the research-teaching hospitals, which are in the forefront in developing new medical technology, constitute the "highest" status group.[14] In general, new methods of treatment and new types of equipment are developed and utilized on an experimental basis in a few of the research-teaching hospitals. As the effectiveness of the new technology is demonstrated, it will be acquired by other hospitals in this same status group. The utilization of the new technology then will spread to one or more hospitals in lower and lower status groups. In this way, desired inputs, I^*, of all hospitals are changing as a result of developments in medical technology, and hospitals have to make constant efforts to adjust their actual pattern of input utilization because the desired pattern of input utilization for a given status group is changing.

The pattern of technological diffusion in the hospital sector differs from that in the business sector in two ways. First, the business and hospital sectors differ greatly in the constraints that are imposed on the adoption of innovation. In the business sector, the adoption of an innovation is a function of the demand, profitability, and size of investment involved [11]. A hospital is not concerned about the profitability of investing in the new technique but simply

---

[12] If a hospital reduces the inventory of inputs, it implies a reduction in "price" paid to physicians. Other hospitals therefore would not follow.

[13] The acquisition of equipment and facilities without appropriate regard for actual output is an important characteristic which distinguishes hospital investment behavior from business investment behavior.

[14] Although hospitals in the highest status group include both teaching and research hospitals, the theory developed here pertains to the production aspect of hospital operations only. A low status hospital might have aspirations to acquire a teaching-research staff and become a teaching-research hospital. But legal, institutional and financial constraints make it impossible for such aspirations to materialize. However, a non-research hospital may adopt teaching-research procedures of higher status hospitals which result in the use of teaching and research methods for routine treatment.

in whether its budget can be increased by enough to cover the cost, and as pointed out previously, the increase in cost may be spread over hospital rates in general. Second, in the business sector, the originators of technological change are not confined to a special group of firms, and it is not possible to predict with a high degree of certainty who will be the originator and what will be the direction of technological diffusion. In the hospital sector, innovation and invention come from a particular group of hospitals, and it is possible to predict with reasonable accuracy the direction of technological diffusion. In other words, the leaders and followers in the process of technological diffusion are determined by the status group to which hospitals belong.

IV. RELATION OF BUDGET CONSTRAINT TO CONSPICUOUS PRODUCTION

In the formulation of the conspicuous production theory it was assumed that a hospital attempts to minimize the gap between its desired and actual inputs subject to a budget constraint. In this section, the relationship between the budget constraint, hospital pricing, hospital costs, and hospital expenditures will be discussed.

For purposes of this paper, we differentiate between costs and expenditures. The cost of producing a particular level of output is the expenditure that would be incurred for producing that level of output in the most efficient manner. Expenditures, on the other hand, are the outlays made for all inputs regardless of their appropriateness for the production process. In the case of hospitals, what are called "costs" indeed are expenditures.

The hospital's budget, which is the sum of income received for services rendered plus contributions (both government and otherwise), sets an upper limit on its expenditures. Even if it is assumed that contributions are fixed and output is beyond control of the hospital itself, it is still possible for the hospital to increase

its budget and hence its expenditures by increasing its prices.

In order to illustrate the relationship between pricing and a hospital's internal adjustment, the budget constraint (Y) is rewritten as:

$$Y = PQ + B \qquad (4)$$

where P and Q are respectively price and quantity of output, and B is philanthropic contribution.[15] Rearranging,

$$P = (Y - B)/Q. \qquad (5)$$

By relation (2), we have

$$P = (R'I - B)/Q.$$

Since inputs acquired (I) are in general a proportion of the differences between the desired and actual inputs, we may write

$$I = k(I^* - I^a).$$

It follows that

$$P = [kR'(I^* - I^a) - B]/Q. \qquad (6)$$

Equation (6) depicts the pricing policy of hospitals. That is, the pricing procedure of hospitals is a special case of full cost (in fact, full expenditures) pricing policy.[16] On the surface, the price-setting procedure does not contain anything unusual. However, the desired inputs are a function of the pattern of inputs utilized by other hospitals and are not a function of production of output. As a consequence, the total expenditure of a hospital and its prices may increase without any change in output. In fact, there is a two-way relationship between prices and expenditures.

[15] For the purpose of analytical convenience, output may be measured in terms of patient days. This measurement is justified on the ground that each patient day contains a certain quantity or mix of services provided by hospitals.

[16] In hospitals, the rates of charge are not set on the basis of costs (average or marginal) of *specific* services. Instead, the rates are set in such a way so that the total revenues from all sources are sufficient to meet the total expenditures. The term "price" as used here refers to the rate of charge assessed on the use of hospital facilities regardless of the methods of payments.

In some cases, needs for increased expenditures associated with efforts to minimize the gap between the desired and actual inputs will be the motivating force for an increase in the price of services. In other cases, price increase will facilitate increased expenditures. This implies that we have to seek additional sources of explanation for the prices of hospital care. This explanation, however, can be found in that hospitals have traditionally charged what the traffic will bear. This practice had been possible because over the relevant range the price elasticity of demand for hospital care is zero or nearly so [5, 8].

Since the extent to which the traffic will bear increased prices of hospital care depends on consumer disposable income (M), health insurance (H), and government programs (G), the price of hospital services may be assumed to be a function of these variables. That is,

$$P = f(M, H, G). \qquad (7)$$

An increase in disposable personal income, expansion in health insurance, and efforts of governments to shift a larger proportion of GNP to health care indirectly facilitate an increase in prices paid to hospital inputs. This also facilitates the increase of inputs acquired or utilized. This is exactly what happened after medicare and medicaid programs went into effect in 1966.

V. IMPLICATIONS OF CONSPICUOUS PRODUCTION

In the previous discussion, it was implied that hospitals can be ranked in terms of the status groups to which they belong. The patterns of input utilization characteristic of higher status groups are regarded as superior and are preferred over those utilized by lower status hospitals. If one or more hospitals in a given status group adopts the patterns of input utilization of higher status hospitals, the desired inputs of other hospitals in the same status group will change.

A given hospital may adopt the patterns of inputs utilized by hospitals in higher status groups under a number of circumstances. First, the action may be initiated by members of the community (in which the hospital serves) who visualize the desirability of a particular new pattern of inputs and therefore initiate and facilitate the acquisition of such inputs. Second, the action to adopt new inputs may be initiated by hospital administrators.

Finally, but most important of all, a hospital may acquire or introduce new inputs as a basis for attracting physicians or in response to the demands of physicians already on the staff. The competition for physicians is probably the most powerful force behind the acquisition of inputs utilized by a higher status hospital.

In general the case mix of services (actual output) for hospitals in higher status groups is much more complex than in lower status groups, and for this reason, health services provided by hospitals in high status groups are characterized by the application of relatively large quantities of a wide variety of highly specialized inputs. Even though lower status hospitals may strive to simulate this input pattern, there is no reason to expect the case mixes in lower status hospitals to change accordingly.[17] Even if the adoption of the more complex pattern of input utilization alters the product mix in lower status hospitals, there is no assurance that these hospitals can treat more complex cases effectively.

The major consequences of conspicuous production may be summarized in qualitative and quantitative terms. Qualitatively, we would expect conspicuous production to result in the use of inputs

---

[17] The increase in variety and degree of specialization of inputs is accompanied by increased impersonalization of care. This is detrimental to the quality of care and therefore may offset any improvement that would have resulted. The case mixes will remain unchanged because the demand mixes remain unchanged.

superior to those warranted by production requirements. Highly trained personnel may be employed to perform tasks suitable for persons with less training, and equipment of advanced and complex design may be used for tasks not requiring such sophisticated equipment.

Quantitatively, we would expect conspicuous production to result in undue duplication, over-equipment, and over-hiring of staff.[18] Equipment, facilities, and staff will be underutilized, and what the hospital is equipped to produce may be quite different from its actual output.[19] The importance of this factor is enhanced by the relatively large initial investment and maintenance expenditures required for many types of hospital services. For these services, the fixed costs will be very high, and for low volumes of output, cost per unit of output will be very high. As previously indicated, the costs of these services will be spread over prices charged for other hospital services, and a part of the bills for many patients will be for services which they never received.[20]

As a result of the quantitative and qualitative factors, we would expect the average product curves under conspicuous pro-

duction to be lower than those existing under ordinary production. Similarly, the cost curves of hospitals subject to the influence of conspicuous production will be higher than under ordinary production.[21]

Finally, it may be useful to consider the compatibility of the conspicuous production theory with the evidence of input substitution reported in several recent studies of hospital costs and production relationships [4, 8]. In particular, these studies indicate: (1) a direct relationship between the wage rate and capital intensity; and (2) an inverse relationship between the wage rate and labor intensity. Both these relationships would be expected for privately owned firms where managers are striving to maximize profits. However, the relationships also are consistent with conspicuous production. Under a budget constraint, a hospital cannot afford the desired level of each input, and this means the hospital must choose among alternatives. In making decisions to purchase inputs, the hospital will be influenced by relative input prices, and we would expect the limited budget to be spent so that the marginal dollars being spent on each input add the same amount, in the opinion of the administrators, to the status of the hospital.[22] As the price of an input in-

[18] This implication of conspicuous production is consistent with the view expressed by Reder [16]. There are in fact three aspects to the quantitative consequences of conspicuous production. These are: the application of excessively large quantity of inputs; overstock of inputs; and overcapacity from the viewpoint of the society as a whole. In addition, the variety and the degree of specialization of inputs utilized are also not warranted by production requirements.

[19] Superficially, this problem appears to be similar to that of public utilities which build reserve capacity to meet peak period demand. But the problem of conspicuous production is quite different from the problem of building capacity to meet peak period demand.

[20] It may be argued that the costs of conspicuous production are not necessarily passed on to consumers if philanthropic contribution is large enough. But philanthropic contribution has become less and less an important source of hospital revenues in the past two decades. Also new inputs would enable hospitals to provide new types of care, but because of the absence of adequate demand, such inputs are unemployed or employed ineffectively.

[21] Such costs of conspicuous production are passed on to and are borne by the consumer (except for philanthropic contribution). One may, therefore, argue that consumers are deriving benefits from conspicuous production. This argument would have merit if the consumer were knowledgeable about the nature of hospital care. In fact, most or all consumers are ignorant about the nature of hospital services and a consumer's demand for such services is prescribed for him by physicians. Because of the ignorance and the absence of free choice, we cannot say that consumers are deriving benefits from conspicuous production even though they are paying for the costs of such behavior.

[22] The possibility of input substitution under conspicuous production may be illustrated with isoquants. That is, in the place of an isoquant, define an equal status curve as the locus of points representing different combinations of two inputs which yield a given level of status. In the context of such equal status curve analysis, and given a budget constraint, it can be demonstrated that a

creases, the contribution of the marginal dollar being spent on this input will fall. This calls for some substitution of other inputs for the input affected by the price increase. It should be noted that the basic motivation for the substitution is status gap minimization and not profit maximization. The end result, in terms of inputs utilized, may be quite different from that which would result from the profit maximization motivation.

VI. CONSISTENCY OF THE CONSPICUOUS PRODUCTION THEORY WITH AVAILABLE EVIDENCE

It was evident from previous discussion that the conspicuous production theory implies a number of testable hypotheses. Unfortunately, the necessary data for a systematic test of these hypotheses are not available. However, we can point to several factors concerning the hospital industry which are consistent with the implications of the theory. The purpose of this section is to describe briefly such evidence: (1) the rapid increase in the use of inputs per unit of output over the past two decades; (2) the rapid growth of corporate hospital chains; and (3) specific evidence of conspicuous production with respect to open heart surgery.

While the Consumer Price Index for all items increased from 67.7 (1957–59 = 100) in 1945 to 131.3 by the end of 1969, the hospital room rate component of the CPI increased by 32.5 to 267.9 over the same period. Although a number of factors contributed to this very rapid increase in hospital rates, a substantial increase in inputs used per patient day of care was an important contributing factor. For example, the number of hospital personnel per 100 patient census increased by approximately 80 per cent from 1948 to 1968. The value of plant assets per bed in con-

stant dollars more than doubled over the same period. No doubt, a very rapid rate of change in medical care has resulted in the availability of improved treatment methods both for some diseases that were treatable in 1946 and for diseases that were not treatable (or not recognized) in 1946. Yet it is unlikely that improvements in the quality of care can explain increases in factor use of the magnitudes observed over the past twenty five years. This is because the diseases for which the methods of treatment have improved constitute only a relatively small fraction of total incidence of diseases.

The analysis of the implications of conspicuous production suggests that the voluntary sector of the hospital industry is inefficient. If this is true, profit hospitals may be able to produce services at lower costs, and, if so, we would expect the relatively small, private sector of the industry to have gained in relative importance. Despite formidable legal, social, and tax obstacles, this segment of the industry has been showing signs of vigorous growth and indications are that private hospitals are able to produce services at lower costs [13].

The voluntary hospitals claim that privately-owned hospitals fail to supply the essential services required to meet the medical needs of a community. In particular, the money-losing services are omitted. While there may be some merit to this position, it is interesting to note that the argument is consistent with the most important implication of the conspicuous production theory. Specifically, the voluntary hospitals will tend to provide too many of the "money losing" services most of which represent needless duplication of facilities. In other words, aggregate demand is not adequate to justify the maintenance of such facilities in a large number of hospitals.

The increase in inputs per unit of output and the growth of for-profit hospitals de-

hospital can reach the highest equal status curve by combining inputs in such a way that the ratio of the marginal contributions of the inputs is equal to their price ratio.

TABLE I
OPEN AND CLOSED HEART SURGICAL FACILITY UTILIZATION IN 1961

Type of Procedure	No. of Hospitals Reporting Such Facilities	Percent of Hospitals with Specified Cases Per Year				
		None	1–9	10–49	50 or more	Unknown
Open Heart	327	11	30	36	17	6
Closed Heart	777	30	43	18	6	4

Source: [19]

scribed above are evidences consistent with the implications of the conspicuous production theory. A direct evidence of such behavior is found in a study of heart surgical facilities [19]. This study revealed that of the 327 hospitals equipped to perform open heart surgery in 1961, 11 per cent did not have a single case during the year and only 17 per cent had 50 or more cases. Also, of the 777 hospitals equipped to perform closed heart surgery in the same year, 30 per cent did not have a single case while only 6 per cent had 50 or more cases. These figures are summarized in Table I.

Even more startling, the President's Commission reported that "cardiopulmonary laboratories and cardiac surgical facilities with the highest frequency of complications are those with the least experience" [15, 10–11]. Apparently, practice was an important determinant of the skill with which open heart surgery could be performed. This is a particularly important finding with respect to the conspicuous production theory for it would indicate negative social value associated with the provision of heart surgery equipment in hospitals where the facilities are used infrequently. On balance, the patients treated in these hospitals would be better served if transferred to hospitals with more practice in this delicate procedure.

VII. CONCLUSION

In concluding this study, it will be useful to make a brief comparison of the conspicuous production theory with other theories of hospital behavior. The conspicuous production theory is based on the assumption of status gap minimization (in connection with utility maximization), while the other theories of hospital behavior are based on the assumptions of sales-maximization, output and prestige maximization, short-run net revenue maximization, and profit maximization. The conspicuous production theory also postulates defensive behavior under interdependent conditions while no such assumption is made in other theories.

In the past two decades, the stock of certain inputs has been increased without corresponding increase in output. The result is undue duplication, overequipment, and overcapacity. Because of the increase in inputs without corresponding increase in output, the assumptions of sales- and output maximization do not provide a satisfactory explanation of the actual behavior in the hospital industry. Nor do the assumptions of net-revenue maximization and profit maximization provide a satisfactory explanation because without an increase in output increased expenditures on the stock of inputs have not been accompanied by increased revenue.[23] Also, the assumption of prestige maximization is inconsistent with the nature of the mission delegated to most hospitals.

In contrast to these theories, the conspicuous production theory provides a logically consistent explanation of: (1) why hospitals acquire inputs without adequate regard for the extent to which such inputs are used in actual production and (2) why there is overspecialization, extensive duplication, overequipment, and

[23] A large part of the increase in hospital revenues comes from increased prices.

overcapacity. The theory also contains a dynamic property depicting the cumulative process of undue duplication, overequipment, and excessive capacity resulting in continuous inflation in the hospital sector.

The conspicuous production theory of hospital behavior presented in this paper should be regarded as tentative. Both the theory and its implications require further refinement and verification. In view of the importance of the quantitative and qualitative implications of the theory, investigation concerning the use of inputs in hospitals should shed some light on how to improve resource allocation and on how to contain costs in the hospital sector. Such research should be concerned with both the quality of the inputs being used for particular tasks and the extent to which inputs are being utilized.

REFERENCES

1. Alchian, A. A. and R. A. Kessel, "Competition, Monopoly, and the Pursuit of Pecuniary Gain," *Aspects of Labor Economics*, National Bureau of Economic Research Special Conference Series, Vol. 14. Princeton, N. J.: Princeton University Press, 1962.
2. Barnard, C. I., *The Functions of the Executive*. Cambridge, Massachusetts: Harvard University Press, 1968.
3. Baumol, W. J., *Economic Theory and Operations Analysis*. Englewood Cliffs, N. J.: Prentice-Hall, 1965.
4. Berry, R. E. Jr., *An Analysis of Costs in Short-Term General Hospitals*. Final Report to Social Security Administration. Cambridge, Massachusetts, October 1968.
5. Davis, K., "Production and Cost Function Estimation for Nonprofit Hospitals," unpublished manuscript.
6. Duesenberry, J., *Income, Savings, and Consumer Behavior*. Cambridge, Massachusetts: Harvard University Press, 1949.
7. Kamerschen, D. R., "The Influence of Ownership and Control on Profit Rates," *American Economic Review*, June 1968, 432–477.
8. Lee, M. L. and R. L. Wallace, "Prices and Costs of Hospital Services," paper presented at the Midwest Economic Association meetings. April 1970.
9. Liebenstein, H., "Bandwagon, Snob, and Veblen Effects in the Theory of Consumers' Demand," *Quarterly Journal of Economics*, May 1950, 183–207.
10. Mann, J. K. and D. E. Yett, "The Analysis of Hospital Costs: A Review Article," *Journal of Business*, April 1968, 191–202.
11. Mansfield, E., *Industrial Research and Technological Innovation*. New York: Norton, 1968.
12. Newhouse, J., "Toward a Theory of Nonprofit Institutions: An Economic Model of a Hospital," *American Economic Review*, March 1970, 64–74.
13. Owens, A., "Can the Profit Motive Save Our Hospitals," *Medical Economics*, March 1970, 76–101.
14. Pauly, M. V., "A New Model of Nonprofit Hospital Behavior and Investment," unpublished manuscript.
15. President's Commission on Heart Disease, Cancer, and Stroke, *A Report to the President: A National Program to Conquer Heart Diease, Cancer, and Stroke*, Volume II. Washington, D. C.: U.S.G.P.O., 1965.
16. Reder, M., "Some Problems in the Economics of Hospitals," *Proceedings of the American Economic Association*, May 1965, 472–480.
17. Rice, R. G., "Analysis of the Hospital as an Economic Organism," *Modern Hospital*, April 1966, 87–91.
18. Simon, H. A., *Administrative Behavior*. New York: Macmillan, 1965.
19. Spencer, F. C. and B. Eiseman, "The Occasional Open-Heart Surgeon," *Circulation*, February 1965, 161–162.
20. Thompson, V. A., *Modern Organization*. New York: Knopf, 1961.
21. Williamson, O. E., "Managerial Discretion and Business Behavior," *American Economic Review*, December 1963, 1032–1057.

12. The Not-for-Profit Hospital as a Physicians' Cooperative

MARK V. PAULY AND MICHAEL REDISCH

Reprinted with permission from *American Economic Review* 63. Copyright © 1973 American Economic Association, 87-99.

The private, nonprofit hospital has usually been regarded by economists as an organizational anomaly. In particular, it has been alleged that the predominance of the not-for-profit structure within the American hospital system is associated with a weakening of the usual market constraints of competition and profit orientation. As a result, this critical element in any analysis of the medical care system in the United States has usually been modeled with a mixture of anecdote and *ad hoc* assumption. It is typically assumed that "all objectives of nonprofit organizations can be described in terms of some type(s) of output (broadly defined) or capital stock."[1] William Baumol and Howard Bowen describe these goals as "bottomless receptables into which limitless funds can be poured" (p. 497).

Model variation occurs as investigators place combinations of key variables in either the objective function or the constraint set of the hospital. Joseph Newhouse (1970) and Martin Feldstein (1971) studied the implications of the maximization of quantity-quality subject to a budget constraint. Millard Long's model is one of quantity maximization subject to both a budget and a quality constraint. Paul Ginsburg assumed maximization of weighted output subject to a budget and an availability of capital constraint. Maw Lin Lee included types of physical capital in the hospital objective function. And Melvin Reder talked of hospitals trying to maximize "the weighted number of patients treated (per time period), the 'weights' being the professional prestige to the doctors attending them" (p. 480).

This last model is the only one to (even) hint at a nonpassive role for the physician in a model of hospital behavior.[2] In this paper we propose an alternative model in which the physician emerges as a traditional income maximizing economic agent who is "discovered" in a decision-making role within this not-for-profit enterprise. Our model is similar to the model of the firm customarily used by economists, in that it is based on the assumption of net income maximization. Only a somewhat unusual definition of net income is needed to enable us to apply in our short-run analysis many of the conclusions of the orthodox model of the firm. In the longer run, however, our model, while still based on net-income maximization, yields different predictions about the institution's response to changes in demand and supply parameters. Furthermore, it may be possible to generalize parts of our model to other private, nonprofit service firms such as universities and symphony or-

* Northwestern University and the Office of Health Policy Analysis and Research, Department of Health, Education, and Welfare, respectively. Research support was provided by the Health Services Research Center of Northwestern University and the American Hospital Association and the Health Economics Research Center of the University of Iowa. Portions of this paper were presented at the Health Economics Session of Allied Social Sciences Meetings, December 1969. Helpful comments were received from R. Tollison, C. M. Lindsay, and James Buchanan. Views expressed are those of the authors.

[1] See Paul Ginsburg, p. 42.

[2] Paul Feldstein and Carl Stevens have discussed the role of the physician in the hospital, but have not provided an explicit model.

chestras, which produce and sell services to individual consumers, many of whom are not poor.

Specifically, we assume that the group of attending physicians on the hospital's staff enjoys *de facto* control of the hospital at any point in time. Given this assumption, we develop a model in which the hospital operates in such a way as to maximize the net income per member of the physician staff. Results are obtained which are similar to those derived from models of producers' cooperatives in Yugoslavia and collective farms in the *USSR*. The physician plays a role analogous to that of the Yugoslav worker and the Russian peasant. Our results are also similar to those obtained from the "theory of clubs," developed by James Buchanan and others.

I. The Model

We simplify the problem initially by assuming that patients pay the full market price for care, and that the decision-making group in the hospital is able to impose its collective will on individual members. The implications of weakening these assumptions to allow for customary forms of health insurance and for imperfect cooperation among controlling individuals will be discussed in later sections.

The product produced in the hospital is hospitalization services. We shall assume that this output can be represented by a single variable Q.[3] To produce this output, physical capital (K), nonphysician labor (L), and physician or medical staff labor (M) are used. The production process can

be summarized by the production function

$$(1) \qquad Q = F(K, L, M)$$

In European countries in which physicians who treat patients in the hospital are employed by and paid by the hospital, this three-input production function is the obvious one.[4] But in the United States, the hospital patient is subject to two separate billings. The hospital charges him only for the use of capital and nonphysician labor. The physician presents a separate bill for the use of his "personal" physician's services. This dual billing system has led to a conceptually false dichotomy in much of the health economics literature. The physician and hospital are often viewed as independent economic entities selling services in functionally segmented health markets. This view appears to provide the rationale for the hospital-administrator-oriented, output-maximization theories of hospital behavior discussed earlier.

We propose an alternative view. It seems obvious that the patient's demand is primarily for the service produced by the physician and hospital acting in combination, not for the separate components, even though there probably is a separate demand for some attributes, such as amenities, or additional patient days for recuperating, that the hospital alone produces.

The critical assumption of our model is that the physician staff members enjoy *de facto* control of hospital operations and see to it that hospitalization services are produced in such a way as to maximize their net incomes. The appearance of physician control is not hard to establish. The staff physicians have direct control over the number and types of patients admitted and over the types of services

[3] Derivatives of two quite different surrogates for hospital output have been used most often by economists doing empirical research. One is based on the number of inpatient days and outpatient visits at the hospital while the other is concerned with the number of cases treated in the hospital. The "case treated" corresponds most closely with the measure of output implied by our model.

[4] This was the form used by M. Feldstein (1967) in in his study of hospitals in the United Kingdom.

they receive; they control output. The staff physicians can determine, within rather broad limits, what use of the hospital will be made in treating a patient; they control many of the production decisions. They have indirect control over many other aspects of the hospital's operation, such as capital investment and the level of nursing care, in the sense that no administrator can afford to incur the displeasure of the medical staff, interfere with medical staff prerogatives, or make decisions which will deter large numbers of physicians from remaining on the hospital's staff or using that hospital for their patients. The trustees, who have nominal control over the hospital's operation, usually look to the medical staff when making decisions on operations or capital investment.

We first assume that the physicians on the staff of a hospital at any point in time act in such a way as to maximize the sum of the money incomes of all staff members. Such an assumption implies a process of group decision making resulting in a kind of perfect cooperation not likely to be observed in practice. It also ignores nonmonetary components of a physician's income, such as leisure time and prestige, which are likely to be of some importance. Nevertheless, this model is useful as a bench mark from which to consider the effects of alternative assumptions.

We postulate an economic short-run period as one in which the number of physicians on the hospital staff, M, remains constant. Each physician is presumed to supply a constant, homogeneous amount of medical input.

The patient's demand is primarily for the service produced by the physician and hospital acting in combination, not for separate components. This can be formalized by postulating a demand function for "hospitalization services" faced by the physician staff that takes the form

$$(2) \qquad Q = Q(P_T), \qquad \frac{\partial Q}{\partial P_T} < 0$$

where P_T is the combined price paid by the patient for the physician and hospital components.[5,6]

We also assume that the hospital component of P_T is set so as to allow the hospital to just break even, with no gain or loss.[7] That is, we assume that the hospital price P_h is set to produce the equality:

$$(3) \qquad P_h Q = wL + cK$$

where P_h is the unit price the hospital charges for use of nonphysician labor and capital, w is the wage rate for nonphysician labor, and c is the user cost of capital.[8]

[5] Some empirical justification of this assumption may be found in Donald Yett et al, where it was estimated that the elasticity of demand for *hospital* output with respect to *surgeons'* fees is 0.7.

[6] If the market for output is perfectly competitive, $|\partial Q/\partial P_T|$ will be infinite; otherwise, the individual hospital demand curve for output will have a negative slope.

[7] If the hospital received contributions, it may set a target loss equal to the contributions, but this will not alter our analysis. Moreover, after the fact the hospital may have a profit or loss, but this is assumed to result wholly from stochastic factors.

[8] The interpretation of the user cost of capital c is worth comment. When capital is provided through borrowed funds, the interpretation is clear; c is equal to $(r+d)P_K$, where r is the interest rate at which the funds were borrowed, d is the depreciation rate, and P_K is the price of capital goods. When unrestricted donations are used to pay for the marginal unit of capital, the user cost is $(r'+d)P_K$, where r' is the opportunity cost of using contributed funds for hospital physical capital, i.e., the rate which could have been earned on those funds if they had been invested elsewhere (say, in government bonds). When donations are made with the restriction that they be used for physical capital investment, they will affect the marginal user cost of capital only if the hospital receives so much in donations that it does not have to turn to any other source for funds for capital investment (unless, of course, the conditions for contribution of restricted funds specify a certain amount of the hospital's own funds as matching payments). If restricted donations fall short of the amount which, given the interest rate r, the hospital wishes to invest so that the hospital borrows, the relevant *marginal* user cost of capital must involve the interest and depreciation rates. Except for the case in which restricted donations are so large that the amount

The hospital is to be run so as to maximize the net incomes of the physicians on the staff at any point in time. If the number of physicians in the short-run analysis is taken as given at $\overline{M}$, the problem is to maximize $P_T Q - P_h Q$ (which is equal to $P_T Q - wL - cK$) subject to the production function (1), with the level of M set at $\overline{M}$, and the demand curve (2). This problem is obviously identical to that facing an orthodox profit-making firm with one input held constant. The marginal conditions for optimal employment of labor and capital are the same, namely, that marginal factor costs equal their respective marginal revenue or value products.[9]

It may be useful at this stage to contrast the model of the nonprofit hospital just developed with the orthodox model of the profit-maximizing firm. In the latter case, all labor inputs and capital services financed by debt are paid their competitive costs. Nondebt capital then obtains the residual income, which is usually assumed to consist of payment of the opportunity cost of that capital (normal profits) and economic profit. The only difference between this model and the physician-profit maximization model of the hospital is that in the latter it is the physician input, rather than the nondebt capital input, which obtains economic profits, the residual income. If a profit-maximizing firm submitted two bills for its services—one just covering the cost of labor and debt-financed capital, produced in a "nonprofit" firm, and the other from a separate legal institution covering the services of equity capital, the analogy would be complete.

II. Long-Run Individual Hospital Equilibrium

The number of physicians on the staff of any hospital obviously is not fixed, but is variable over time. What determines the size of the hospital's staff? The answer to this question depends critically on the assumption made about the hospital's staffing policy. We shall outline the results of three alternative policies—closed staff, open staff, and a policy in which new physicians can be hired by the hospital.

Closed staff

Many hospitals in the United States restrict staffing privileges; they do not permit any physician to join the hospital's staff just because he wishes to do so, even if he is licensed to practice medicine and surgery. The decision on whether or not to admit a new member to the staff (or whether to replace a member who has left) is made by the existing members of the hospital's staff of physicians. If we

---

of capital that is bought with them exceeds the amount which would be indicated by the marginal conditions, donations, whether unrestricted or restricted, are really equivalent to lump sum subsidies. Only if the hospital's price and output policies affect contributions (and within wide margins, they do not seem to) should contributions be treated as other than lump sum grants. In a world of uncertainty, however, the total of donations past and present may affect a lender's willingness to lend, since they provide collateral. Even in this case, current donations are likely to be important only if they are large relative to total nonborrowed capital.

[9] The model implies cost minimization in the sense that, given the physician input, quantities of labor and capital are chosen which, given their marginal supply prices, minimize costs. Cost minimization is also a characteristics of output-maximization models. However, normative conclusions that have been derived from empirical cost function studies regarding socially optimal scale of hospital facilities are considerably weakened when it is realized that there is no reason to suppose that, in comparisons across hospitals or over time, the physician input actually is constant, or even variable in a random way. The physician input has been left out of cost and production function studies of U.S. hospitals. Unless the physician input is specified or is known to be a constant ratio to K and L, there is no way of knowing the true social costs of all the inputs associated with any scale of output, and hence no way of determining the cost-minimizing scale. Observed decreasing hospital costs, for instance, may only represent a systematic increase in physician input with size. Furthermore, when we allow imperfect cooperation of the physician staff in our model in a later section, we will find that minimization of even nonphysician costs in the technical sense by the hospital is a very unlikely conclusion.

ssume that once a physician is admitted) the staff, he has privileges identical to nose of the existing members, the appropriate maximand for the hospital appears to be the maximization of net income per physician, Y_M. Physicians will e willing to add members to the staff as)ng as it causes each member's net income to rise.

This implies that the objective function) be maximized is

$$4) \qquad Y_M = (P_T Q - cK - wL)/M$$

ubject to the production function (1) and he demand curve (2). The necessary first-rder conditions for an extremum become

$$5a) \qquad w = P_T \frac{\partial Q}{\partial L} + \frac{\partial P_T}{\partial Q} \frac{\partial Q}{\partial L} Q$$

$$5b) \qquad c = P_T \frac{\partial Q}{\partial K} + \frac{\partial P_T}{\partial Q} \frac{\partial Q}{\partial K} Q$$

$$5c) \qquad Y_M = P_T \frac{\partial Q}{\partial M} + \frac{\partial P_T}{\partial Q} \frac{\partial Q}{\partial M} Q$$

In long- or short-run equilibrium, the physician-hospital conglomerate firm that ve have postulated will equate the marginal supply price of all nonphysician inputs to their respective marginal revenue or value products. However, in our model, physicians all share equally in the residual income of this health enterprise, the shares depending on their assumed equal shares of a total output. Condition (5c) states that physician staff size is determined in ong-run equilibrium by equating the marginal revenue product of physicians to the net average revenue product of the physician staff. This makes intuitive sense. The hospital "pays" for new physicians by allowing them a proportionate share of total output and, hence, of net revenues. Staff physicians will want to welcome warmly a new member as long as his contribution to total revenues of all staff physicians is greater than the average

current income per physician which he receives.

Of course, condition (5c) cannot be satisfied unless there are physicians willing to work at the hospital for the earnings available. That is, the equilibrium value of Y_M must be at least as large as the income stream available to a physician in his next best opportunity. There will be a supply curve of physicians to any hospital. The shape of this curve will depend in part on the income a physician could get in other hospitals, and his valuation of other uses of his time, both as leisure and as office practice.

Figure 1 depicts the long-run equilibrium position of a hospital operating in an urban, physician-intensive environment. The physician supply curve, SS, may therefore be assumed to be approximately infinitely elastic, and we also assume that it is at a low level relative to income possibilities in this particular hospital. Within the hospital, capital and nonphysician labor take on short-run optimal values as physician staff size, M, varies along the horizontal axis. ABC thus represents the maximum attainable income per physician for each specific value of M. Returns to scale and elastic demand lead initially to the upward sloping segment of ABC, but eventually decreasing returns and diminishing marginal revenue cause the curve to turn down. The maximum maximorum, Y_M^*, of this set of short-run maximums is reached at the intersection of the marginal revenue product and net average revenue product curve, when physician staff size reaches its long-run equilibrium value of M^*.

This model is very similar to those developed by Benjamin Ward (1958, 1970), Evsey Domar, Walter Oi and Elizabeth Clayton, Jaroslav Vanek, and others who explain the economic behavior of the Soviet collective farm or the Yugoslav producers' cooperative. The physician

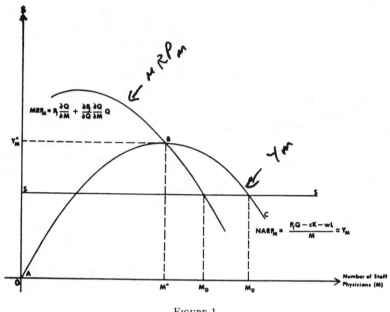

Figure 1

plays a role analogous to that of the Russian peasant and the Yugoslav worker. Institutionally, the arrangements differ because the physician receives his "share" of the enterprise's income directly from the sale of his output, whereas the worker on a collective receives it from a common pool. But this is because, in the case of the hospital, output can usually be directly assigned to particular staff members.

Our model of the hospital shares certain of the seemingly paradoxical conclusions of these cooperative-collective models. Supply response to changes in product and factor market conditions can be in perverse directions. An upward shift in the demand curve for hospital output could result[10] in a new equilibrium with higher price levels, *lower* output, and *fewer* physician staff members to share the greater total net revenues of the physician-hospital conglomerate enter-

prise. "Members have an incentive to con tract membership to hoard the spoils" o a demand increase (see Oi and Clayton p. 43). An increase in a factor price ma lead to an expansion of operations to help spread the misery around among a large group of individuals. On the other hand, lump sum subsidy, such as a philanthropic contribution, will decrease output and staff size. "Even when the co-op moves in the same direction as a capitalist firm its response is usually more sluggish. For market stability, the picture is not par ticularly reassuring" (see Domar, p. 739)

The reason for this result can be sketched out briefly:[11] Suppose a hospital faces a given price for output, and price increases by some amount. This will produce a proportionate increase in the marginal revenue product of physicians assuming that K and L are held constant but the income per physician (Y_M) will increase more than proportionately. The

[10] Unambiguous results concerning the direction of supply response cannot be determined unless specific restrictions are placed on the nature of the demand shift and the form of the production function.

[11] For a more extensive development, see the references cited in the preceding paragraph.

maximum average income would be attained at a smaller value of M.

The values of K and L will not, of course, remain constant. They will increase in response to increases in their marginal products. But M^* will still decline unless increases in K and L increase the marginal revenue product of physicians and do so by a large enough amount to offset the increase in average income. This need not happen; Q and M^* may decrease, or not increase much, whereas in a profit-seeking firm the use of an input and the amount of output would almost certainly increase with a rise in the price of output.

Discriminatory Sharing or Hiring Model

To consider the consequences of altering the "equal sharing" assumption, we suppose that the hospital depicted in Figure 1 is allowed to hire physicians at the supply price, OS. The hospital will then organize production in the same way as would a profit-maximizing firm. The physician input will be increased until the marginal revenue product and the marginal supply price of physicians' services are equal to each other. Staff physicians will be able to capture, in their own incomes, the excess of the marginal products of the inframarginal hired physicians over their supply price. Equilibrium will be at M_D. But note that there is explicit discrimination in returns to homogeneous labor in this situation; the ability to sustain a stable equilibrium under these circumstances is highly suspect. As Pauly has shown, a system of clubs in which some identical persons receive less than others is not likely to be stable. It may well be that the internship-residency programs so prevalent in the United States may be an institutionalized method of getting around the inherent instability in the discriminatory hiring model by creating artificial, functionally viable distinctions among homogeneous

physicians.[12] Determination of the ratio of "partner" physicians to "hired" physicians is likely to be arbitrary. The economic well-being of those physicians left with full staff privileges varies inversely with this ratio.

Open Staff Model

Alternatively, we can retain the "equal shares" assumption, and examine the economic behavior of hospitals that do not restrict entry to their physician staff. Any licensed physician who chooses to do so may become a "full partner" in the firm. Equilibrium at M_o in Figure 1 is characterized by equality of average income per member of the physician staff and the marginal supply price of physicians services.

Of course, for a hospital in a rural area with few physicians, or in an area where many physicians have attractive alternatives to membership on that hospital's staff, the situation might be somewhat different. Faced with a sharply rising supply curve for physicians' services, $S'S'$ in Figure 2, the physician staff will be in equilibrium at M_{oo}. The hospital might as well call its policy "open staffing," since it would be willing to add new members in order to move up the rising part of the net average product curve and increase income per staff member. Such a "frustrated closed staff" hospital only needs to adopt a closed staff policy when the number of staff members reaches M^*.

Note that the discriminatory-hiring and open-staff hospitals, either the "true"

---

[12] Interns and residents serving in *U.S.* hospitals currently comprise about 15 percent of all MD's and, of course, provide a considerably higher percentage of hospital based physicians' services. In several of the cost function studies, there have been attempts to estimate the effect these physician trainees have on hospital costs and revenues. Our model would suggest that it might prove more fruitful to analyze the ways in which trainees can increase the incomes of those physicians with regular staff privileges.

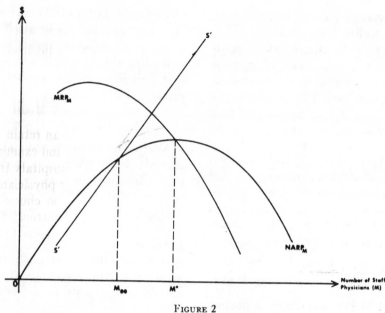

Figure 2

open-staff hospital or the frustrated closed-staff one, do not exhibit the potentially perverse supply responses that were uncovered in the closed staff model. Increases in demand will lead to increases in physician staff and output.

III. Long-Run Industry Equilibrium

The closed-staff hospital in the long run tries to adjust its physician staff size to achieve maximum income per physician. But if physicians in a hospital achieve incomes below those of other identical physicians on the staffs of other hospitals in that area or in other areas, the low-income physicians may wish to join the staffs of high physician-income hospitals. If they are prevented from joining the staffs of existing hospitals, as would occur if those hospitals were large enough so that average income was maximized, it will be worthwhile for M^* of those rejected physicians to join a new hospital, a duplicate in size of the old one. Indeed, the formation of new hospitals will continue as long as higher incomes can be earned, bidding up the supply price of physicians and bidding

down the price of final output (and hence the curve of average income) until a position of long-run equilibrium is attained at which average income, marginal income, and marginal supply price are equal to each other and equal across hospitals. In the open-staff model, long-run equilibrium is also reached by the formation of new hospitals, but here the new hospitals draw off excess members from existing hospitals, raising average incomes since average size shrinks. This process will continue until formation of a new hospital does not raise average income. Finally, in the discriminatory-hiring model, physicians who are paid less than staff physicians (i.e., hired) will find it advantageous to try to join a hospital of their own in which they are all staff members and receive incomes equal to those of physicians in existing hospitals.

Thus these models have identical long-run industry equilibria (when the number of firms is variable), but the closed-staff model has a radically different long-run firm equilibrium, and may move in a perverse direction from that of the discriminatory-hiring firm. The open-staff model, on he other hand, responds in the same way s would the discriminatory-hiring (or rofit maximizing) hospital, but is likely o have a quantitatively different response. Although the final industry outcomes nder these institutional arrangements are he same, the adjustment process by which hat outcome is reached is very different in ach case.

IV. Imperfect Cooperation on the Hospital Staff

In this section we wish to relax the ssumption of perfect cooperation by the hospital's staff of physicians. The *individual* physician may in fact have direct control over the process of producing output. He is able to order use of nursing and other nputs for his patients, in his character of professional expert. At best, "the hospital" can determine only a stock of inputs; the physician controls the flow of services from them. This is in contrast to a producers' cooperative (or even a nonprofit university) in which, presumably, a central management is somewhat more able to prevent individualistic behavior. Moreover, each physician's income from the hospital-connected services depends entirely on his own output, in contrast to the producers' cooperative model in which an individual worker's income partly depends on his own output but also depends on his share of total profits or surplus income. The physician shares group income insofar as he shares group output.

We assume, as before, that the hospital price is set at a level which permits the hospital to break even. It is now easier to see why this assumption is itself a consequence of the physician profit-maximization hypothesis. Other things being equal, hospital profits mean higher hospital prices, which reduce physician incomes. To be sure, hospital profits could be used for capital investment which may enhance future physician incomes, but 1) physi-cians may not want to invest in the hospital—and 2), as Eirik Furubotn and Svetozar Pejovich have noted, the fact that property rights are not vested in investment from profits makes it even less desirable than owned investment.

Since prices for services are not (yet) set at marginal cost,[13] and since the physician does have the power to direct the application of labor and capital services in producing his output, noncooperative behavior can occur. Suppose the hospital follows the policy of charging an all-inclusive daily rate. Suppose ordering the use of more labor in the production of some output will permit the physician to charge more for that unit of output, because the "quality" of the output is enhanced. If the application of more nonphysician labor raises the price P_T^i that can be charged by the ith physician but if the same price P_H is charged for all units of hospital output, regardless of whether or not extra labor is ordered, the physician will want to use labor for his Q_i patients up to the point at which the following equality is satisfied:

$$(6) \qquad \frac{\partial P_T^i}{\partial L} Q_i = \frac{Q_i}{Q} w$$

That is, the individual physician only considers a fraction Q_i/Q of the cost of the labor he orders to be employed, whereas group profit maximization would require him to take account of the costs his action imposes on other physicians' patients. Consequently, imperfect cooperation leads

[13] In fact, it does not appear that hospitals do price at marginal cost. They have moved away from the use of an all-inclusive daily rate, the same for all patients, toward itemized bills, but they are still far from charging marginal cost as a price. And in theory, it is unlikely that prices could be set equal to marginal cost. Unless marginal cost just equals average cost, marginal cost pricing by the hospital of its services would violate the no-profit, no-loss constraint assumed above. Moreover, the use of different prices for different qualities of outputs involves transactions and information costs, which may be substantial.

to the use of too much labor relative to the amount that would be used if group incomes were maximized with perfect co-operation.

How great these departures from perfectly cooperative usage will be depends upon how well the staff as a group can control the actions of its individual members. It seems reasonable to suppose that the magnitude of the departure from cooperative behavior should get larger as the size of the staff gets larger.[14] There are at least three reasons for making this assumption. 1) When the staff size is small, each physician bears a larger share of the cost of his own actions. 2) When the staff size is small, departures from cooperative behavior on the parts of others are more noticeable to any single member. 3) When the staff size is small, mutually agreeable group decisions are more likely to be arrived at, since the cost of decision making is less.

In terms of the geometric analysis, introduction of imperfect cooperation in this way shifts the curve of net revenue per member down and to the left. The conclusion is obvious; lack of perfect co-operation makes the (second best) optimal size of the staff and hospital smaller than it would otherwise be.

V. The Effect of Insurance

To this point we have assumed that patients confronted the full market price for care. Insurance coverage of medical costs may weaken the applicability of this assumption. The hospital is typically paid on the basis of costs incurred. If there are no copayments or deductibles at all, this arrangement effectively eliminates market control over the hospital component of the

price of hospitalization, since higher hospital costs and prices have no effect on the cost actually paid by the patient (except through the premium, which only matters if the premium rises so high that the person drops coverage). Moreover, the allocation of costs within the hospital to insured patients, especially Blue Cross members, is often done on average cost basis. The only restraint on the physician's prescribing the use of hospital capital and labor for his fully insured patient is the upward pressure his behavior would exert on the prices paid by his noninsured patients. Conversely, under average cost allocation some of the market discipline is lost for the noninsured by the transfer of some costs to the insured.

If every patient had full coverage cost-based hospital insurance, there would be no constraint on the amount of capital and labor that physicians combine with their services. Capital and labor would therefore be employed up to the point at which the marginal contribution of each to the physician's revenue was zero. This produces "Cadillac-quality" medicine. The only constraint on the use of these inputs would be offered by the upper limit on the number of things a hospital can do for a patient which might have some justification. Over time, technological change might be expected to relax even this constraint.

When insurance covers part of each patients' hospital bill, the factor prices of hospital inputs K and L are effectively reduced as far as the group of physicians is concerned. One would expect an increase in the usage of hospital inputs relative to physician inputs for producing a given output. Hospital unit costs would rise. Thus our model provides an explanation of the positive relationship between hospital insurance coverage and hospital unit prices and costs found by M. Feldstein (1971). In addition, our model yields the important result that, ceteris paribus, increased

[14] A similar analysis of the effect of size is provided by Mancur Olson. Other applications to medical care can be found in the work of Newhouse (1972) and Mather Lindsay.

ospitalization insurance should increase physician prices and physician incomes.

VI. Toward a Theory of the Not-For-Profit Enterprise

To this point we have taken the not-for-profit nature of the typical American hospital as given. In this section we offer an explanation of why this organizational form has arisen.

There are two ways in which the hospital might operate if it were on a profit-maximizing basis. It might combine the services of nonphysician labor and physical capital, and sell them to or through the physician, who combines them with his own input to produce the output of hospitalization services. Alternatively, the hospital might perform the job of combination itself, hiring the physician input and selling the final output. In either case the direct control over the use of nonphysician labor and capital would not be held by the physician. In the first case, he would have to use the market for control, which is not always efficient in the sense of minimizing all costs, including transactions costs, as direct control. In the second case, he himself would be under the direction of the supplier of equity capital. It is surely possible that there are some products which are not produced efficiently when a representative of the owners of equity capital directs their production, or when the market is used to organize the production process instead of the use of direct controls within a single organization. The most efficient method might be for the supplier of an important component of the labor input to direct the production process.

This would tend to happen when human capital is important in the production of some output and when the flow of services of that human capital cannot well be directed from outside, but is controlled by the person in whom the capital is embodied. As Armen Alchian and Harold Demsetz have noted, the wage system tends to break down when marginal products cannot be monitored closely. This may be a reasonable conjecture in the case of the production of hospital services. Many of the decisions the physician has to make are decisions which cannot be supervised directly, and which have contingent outcomes. There probably needs to be some incentives for the physician. Financial interest in the outcome of his actions is one such incentive, and that incentive is at its greatest when the physician bears the full residual income, when the consequences of his actions are not spread over suppliers of physical capital.[15]

The production process requires some physical capital. In a labor-managed firm in which most of the assets of labor are embodied in nontransferable human capital, not all of the physical capital can be borrowed, since collateral cannot be provided. Another necessary condition therefore for the emergence of the not-for-profit form would seem to be the willingness of individuals to contribute for its equity capital. In principle, contributions could either be voluntary or provided through government. Where voluntary contributions are sufficient, government contributions would not be expected to emerge. On the other hand, voluntary contributions may arise in precisely those cases in which the government fails to act. They may also arise in cases in which the government through tax deductibility

[15] To see this, think of each physician as a "firm." The socially most efficient institutional arrangement is the one which maximizes the net present value of this firm. The present value is a contingency, depending on the state of nature (for example, what's really wrong with his patients, whether an epidemic occurs, etc.) and the amount of effort that the physician makes. The amount of effort, in turn, depends upon the share of profits the physician receives. The appropriate share for the physician, even given the greater risk he bears, may be approximately equal to one.

subsidizes private contributions. The source of contributions, whether unsubsidized voluntary, subsidized voluntary, or governmental, is not critical to the argument, except to the extent that one form (for example, government) implies more external control over physicians' actions than another.

These contributions could be motivated by a desire on the part of contributors to make output available to themselves or to those whom they would like to see consume it. That is, the motivation could either be based on the potential receipt of private benefits or of external benefits. Contributions are a logical way for potential purchasers of the outputs of labor-managed firms to make possible production of the output, which they or those about whom they are concerned will use. If there are barriers to entry by profit-seeking firms (as there are in higher education and, to some extent, in the hospital industry as well), potential consumers may be willing to contribute if that is the only way that output, which yields them consumers' surplus, can be made available. It is not surprising that private not-for-profit firms which sell output—hospitals, universities, symphony orchestras—tend to provide output which is used *not* by the poor, but partly by the contributors themselves.[16]

VII. Conclusion

The main thrust of the model we have suggested here, and the one which differentiates it from models of the not-for-profit hospital that have been suggested

[16] This last point is an important consideration. It is sometimes alleged that these firms have attained a nonprofit status so that they may better provide services to the poor. However, the recent experience in this country is for the poor to receive health services from government operated hospitals, to receive education in government operated institutions, and not to partake at all of the output of symphony orchestras, theatre groups, or private universities.

by others, is the use of the maximization of physicians' income as the characteristic function. The potential absence of perfect cooperation distinguishes it from similar models of producers' cooperatives. In a methodological sense, our model seems to be more attractive than those which simply assume that the not-for-profit organization maximizes a variable such as "quantity of output," because it explains what the organization does in terms of the economic motivation of those who control it.

More importantly, it appears to provide an appealing explanation of some peculiar characteristics of not-for-profit hospitals. The supposed quality consciousness of such hospitals, for example, is easily explained; "quality" is a synonym for application of nonphysician labor and capital in physician-income-enhancing ways, and noncooperative behavior could easily lead to "too high" quality. "Duplication of facilities" probably owes its existence to closed staffing and lack of perfect cooperation. Other aspects of hospital behavior could also be explained by considering their effect on physicians' income; the pattern of investment, for example, might be best explained by changes in the ability of capital to enhance physicians' incomes. The inelastic supply response of hospitals to Medicare and Medicaid is also consistent with our model.

Even the average size of hospitals, which seems, by most accounts, to be below the optimal or cost-minimizing level, can easily be explained. In the first place, empirically observed cost curves may be misleading, if we add the physician input. But more importantly, in a period of rising prices our model shows that hospitals will tend to be small, and for two reasons. First, smallness tends to permit maximization of net income per physician. Second, smallness is necessary to permit coordination of the medical staff.

A narrower range of possible observations is consistent with our model than with the general utility-maximization model. Appropriate choice of the variables to enter the utility function can make almost any observed behavior consistent with utility maximization. In particular, the definition of quality is not clear. Our model specifies the variable in the objective function. In principle it will also predict quantitative as well as qualitative responses, in the sense that physician income can be measured while utility cannot. Unfortunately, at present hospital-specific data on physicians' incomes or prices do not exist which would permit us to provide a conclusive test of the model. Nevertheless, we hope that more data can be made available to test this model.

REFERENCES

A. Alchian and H. Demsetz, "Production, Information Costs, and Economic Organization," *Amer. Econ. Rev.*, Dec. 1972, *62*, 777–95.

W. J. Baumol and H. G. Bowen, "On the Performing Arts," *Amer. Econ. Rev. Proc.*, May 1965, *55*, 495–502.

J. Buchanan, "An Economic Theory of Clubs," *Economica*, Jan. 1966, *32*, 1–14.

E. Domar, "The Soviet Collective Farm as a Producer Cooperative," *Amer. Econ. Rev.*, Sept. 1966, *56*, 734–57.

M. Feldstein, *Economic Analysis for Health Service Efficiency*, Amsterdam 1967.

———, "Hospital Cost Inflation: A Study of Nonprofit Price Dynamics," *Amer. Econ. Rev.*, Dec. 1971, *61*, 853–72.

P. Feldstein, "Research on the Demand for Health Care," *Millbank Memorial Fund Quart.*, Part II, July 1966, 128–65.

E. Furubotn and S. Pejovich, "Tax Policy and Investment Decisions of the Yugoslav Firm," *Nat. Tax. J.*, Sept. 1970, *23*, 335–57.

P. Ginsburg, "Capital in Non-profit Hospitals," unpublished doctoral dissertation, Harvard Univ. 1970.

M. L. Lee, "A Conspicuous Production Theory of Hospital Behavior," *Southern Econ. J.*, July 1971, *38*, 48–59.

C. M. Lindsay, "Supply Response in the Financing of Medical Care," unpublished doctoral dissertation, Univ. Virginia 1968.

M. F. Long, "Efficient Use of Hospital," in *The Economics of Health and Medical Care*, Ann Arbor 1964, 211–26.

J. Newhouse, "Toward a Theory of Nonprofit Institutions: An Economic Model of a Hospital," *Amer. Econ. Rev.*, Mar. 1970, *60*, 64–73.

———, "The Economics of Group Practice," *J. Hum. Resources*, forthcoming 1972.

W. Oi and E. Clayton, "A Peasant's View of a Soviet Collective Farm," *Amer. Econ. Rev.*, Mar. 1968, *58*, 37–59.

M. Olson, *The Logic of Collective Action*, Cambridge 1962.

M. Pauly, "Clubs and Cores," *Publ. Choice*, fall 1970, *9*, 53–65.

M. Reder, "Some Problems in the Economics of Hospitals," *Amer. Econ. Rev. Proc.*, May 1965, *55*, 472–80.

C. Stevens, "Hospital Market Efficiency: The Anatomy of the Supply Response," in H. Klarman, ed., *Empirical Studies in Health Economics*, Baltimore 1970.

J. Vanek, *The General Theory of Labor-Managed Market Economies*, Ithaca 1970.

B. Ward, "The Firm in Illyria: Market Syndicalism," *Amer. Econ. Rev.*, Sept. 1958, *48*, 566–89.

———, *The Social Economy*, New York 1970.

D. Yett, L. Drabek, M. Intriligator, and M. Kimball, "A Macroeconomic Model for Regional Health Planning, *Econ. and Bus. Bull.*, fall 1971, *24*, 1–21.

13. The Relationship of Cost to Hospital Size

W. JOHN CARR AND PAUL J. FELDSTEIN

Reprinted with permission of the Blue Cross Association, from *Inquiry*, Vol. IV, No. 2 (June 1967), pp. 45-65. Copyright © 1967 by the Blue Cross Association. All rights reserved.

The primary purpose of this study is to estimate the net, or independent, effect of hospital size upon the cost of providing care. In the process, estimates of the approximate effects of a number of other factors upon cost are also derived. The results indicate that, other things being held approximately equal, average cost per patient day falls initially as size is increased because of the economies associated with the use of specialized personnel and equipment and then probably rises at very large size levels due to increased managerial problems of communication and control. Apparently, the greater the capability of a hospital to provide a wide range of diversified services, the more rapidly average cost initially falls with increased size.

The study was undertaken by applying multiple regression analysis to data from 3,147 U.S. voluntary short-term general hospitals collected by the American Hospital Association. The variables utilized in the study were: total cost, hospital size, number of services provided, number of outpatient visits, whether or not the hospital had a nursing school, number of

student nurses, number of different types of internship and residency programs, number of interns and residents, whether or not the hospital was affiliated with a medical school, and average wage rate. An initial analysis was undertaken by using data from all of the hospitals in the study. Separate analyses were then conducted for five groups of hospitals in order to determine the effect of differences in the capability of hospitals to provide a wide range of service upon the cost-size relationship.

An enormous amount of work has already been dedicated to the achievement of an efficient distribution of hospital facilities. But this is a task that can never be completed. Shifts in the size and distribution of the population, variations in the prevalence of disease, disability, and pregnancy, and changes in medical technology continuously alter the optimum number, size, and geographic distribution of hospitals.

At first glance, it may appear that each case for areawide planning demands a unique approach since conditions in individual communities, and even in the same community over time, are of such a varied nature. Although it has been recognized that hospital planning is best undertaken on a local level, enough common ground has been found, however, to make the development of general guidelines and principles worthwhile.[1]

W. John Carr is Research Associate, John Fitzgerald Kennedy School of Government, Harvard University, and Paul J. Feldstein is Associate Professor, Program in Hospital Administration, the University of Michigan.

The work on which this article is based was performed by the American Hospital Association under a contract with the U.S. Public Health Service, Division of Hospital and Medical Facilities. Funds were also provided by Community Health Project Grant #CH-00236-01. The authors would like to thank Ann Morton for her editorial assistance.

[1] For this reason, the American Hospital Association and the U.S. Public Health Service have issued reports embodying principles ap-

The major purpose of this study is to describe and estimate one of the fundamental relationships which underlies the apparent diversity of individual planning situations—namely, the effect of hospital size upon the cost of providing care. Because our results can be most meaningfully understood and applied within the more comprehensive theoretical structure of areawide planning, we shall devote some attention to determining their position within this broader framework.[2] In this brief discussion, emphasis will be placed upon planning as it relates to the inpatient care functions of hospitals while matters of outpatient care, teaching, and research will be largely ignored.

THE RELATIONSHIP OF HOSPITAL COST TO AREAWIDE PLANNING

When viewed from a comprehensive standpoint, the areawide planning prob-

lem can be divided into two major parts. First, what is the need or demand for hospital services in a given area, and, second, what distribution of facilities and personnel will most efficiently provide the care to be utilized.[3]

It has been increasingly recognized that certain socio-demographic and economic characteristics of the population have an important effect upon both the need and demand for hospital care and ought to be taken into account in planning. Quantitative estimates of the independent effects of these factors may be applied to projected population measures in order to forecast levels of need or demand for an entire planning area.[4]

Given the level of demand or need, one is faced with the problem of determining the optimal distribution of hospital resources. This problem may be divided into three interrelated parts: (1) what is the best distribution of various types of personnel and facilities among hospitals, (2) what are the optimal sizes (and number) of these institutions, and (3) what is the optimal locational pattern for hospitals. Finding the answer to any one of these questions involves the simultaneous determination of the answers to each of the others and, in addition, the simultaneous de-

plicable to the organization and operation of areawide planning agencies. See, particularly, Joint Committee of the American Hospital Association and Public Health Service, *Areawide Planning for Hospitals and Related Health Facilities* (Public Health Service Publication No. 855 [Washington, D.C.: U.S. Government Printing Office, 1961]), and U.S. Public Health Service, *Procedures for Areawide Health Facility Planning, A Guide for Planning Agencies* (Public Health Service Publication No. 930-B-3 [Washington, D.C.: U.S. Government Printing Office, 1963]).

[2] Economic characteristics of the medical care field which suggest the need for planning (or some other form of market intervention), as opposed to substantial reliance upon market mechanisms to allocate resources among hospitals, are pointed out in M. W. Reder, "Some Problems in the Economics of Hospitals," *American Economic Review*, Vol. 55, No. 2 (May, 1965), pp. 472-480, and Burton A. Weisbrod, "Some Problems of Pricing and Resource Allocation in a Nonprofit Industry—The Hospitals," *Journal of Business*, Vol. 38, No. 1 (January, 1965), pp. 18-28.

It should be noted that hospital care is only one of many components, or factors, used in the production of medical care and that to some extent these components are substitutable. This means that hospital planning should not be considered in isolation from the rest of the medical care system. See Paul J. Feldstein, "Research on the Demand for Health Services," *Milbank Memorial Fund Quarterly*, Vol. 44, No. 3, Part 2 [Health Services Research 1] (New York: The Milbank Memorial Fund, July, 1966), pp. 128-165.

[3] By demand, we mean the amount of care for which persons are willing and able to pay. Given the distribution of income, need may be defined as the amount of service (including prepayment or insurance) which fully informed, or knowledgeable, consumers would purchase plus any amount arising from external benefits to other members of society. The use of a need criterion of this sort within the context of hospital planning raises certain practical problems. In particular, although it may be possible to reduce demand which exceeds need by some means, such as the establishment of utilization review committees, building facilities to serve needs which are not reflected in demand may only result in underutilization.

[4] Empirical estimates of the net effects of various socio-demographic and economic characteristics upon hospital utilization may be found in Gerald D. Rosenthal, *The Demand for General Hospital Facilities* (Chicago: American Hospital Association, 1964), and Rosson L. Cardwell, Margaret G. Reid, and Max Shain, *Hospital Utilization in a Major Metropolitan Area* (Chicago: Hospital Planning Council for Metropolitan Chicago, 1964).

termination of the quantity demanded or needed.[5] Since no satisfactory method for the simultaneous solution of this problem is yet available, and because of their limited powers to initiate change, areawide planners have proceeded by seeking the optimal solutions to a series of partial alterations in the systems for which they are responsible. While there is no guarantee that this process will converge upon an optimum distribution of resources for the entire system, some inefficiencies should be avoided.

The Cost-Size Relationship

For the present, we shall ignore these difficulties and concentrate our attention upon the effect of hospital size and other factors on the cost of providing care and, in turn, upon the general relationship of these considerations to the optimal distribution of facilities and personnel among hospitals and the determination of optimal hospital sizes and locations. Let us first consider the independent effect of size upon cost, given the capability of a hospital to produce "products" (diagnoses and treatments) of various sorts and the mix and quality of products actually produced.

Economists have distinguished certain factors which make the production of products and services more economical as the size of an organization is increased and others which cause efficiency to decline with larger size. Two important factors which make large scale production of products and services more economical are the gains obtained from the use of more highly specialized personnel and the economies associated with the more extensive use of large or specialized equipment.[6] Off-

FIGURE I

Cost per Patient Day in Relation to Hospital Size

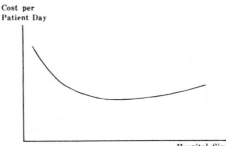

setting these advantages is the greater proportion of time and effort required to coordinate and control work in large organizations.

In general, for sufficiently small outputs, efficiency increases with size because the advantages that accrue from the use of specialized labor and equipment far outweigh the increased cost of management. As size increases, however, the reduction in per-unit cost afforded by greater and greater specialization begins to decline and is eventually outweighed by increased costs of coordination and control.[7] Other things being equal, hospital cost per patient day may thus be expected to decline initially and then rise as size is increased as shown by the U-shaped curve in Figure I.

---

[5] This is the case because, according to the above definitions, the quantity of care demanded or needed is dependent upon economic factors, including price (which, in turn, should reflect cost).

[6] In addition, dealing with large quantities of supplies may result in savings from low record handling costs, quantity discounts, re-

duced per-unit freight costs, and relatively low inventory requirements.

To some extent, small hospitals may circumvent the various diseconomies associated with their size by purchasing auxiliary services from outside firms. For example, 40 percent of voluntary short-term general and other special hospitals with less than 200 beds had their laundry service provided by cooperative ventures and outside firms whereas only 11 percent of similar hospitals with 200 or more beds entered into such arrangements. Source: *Hospitals*, Vol. 38, No. 15, Part 2 (August 1, 1964), p. 516.

[7] For an extensive discussion of factors affecting the cost-size relationship, see E. A. G. Robinson, *The Structure of Competitive Industry* (Chicago: University of Chicago Press, 1958).

FIGURE II

Cost of Basic Care and of a Specialized Service per Patient Day in Relation to Hospital Size

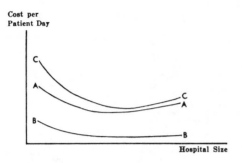

FIGURE III

Hospital and Travel Cost per Patient Day in Relation to Hospital Size

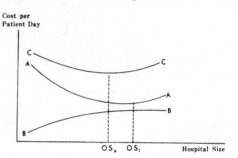

Service Capability and Cost

Let us now turn to the question of the effects of differences in the capability of hospitals to produce different types of care and in the mix of services they actually provide upon cost. For simplicity, we may conceive of a hospital as producing both a component of basic care (room, board, and routine nursing care) and a number of distinct, specialized services. In general, there may be economies associated with the large scale production of each individual service as well as with the provision of basic care. In Figure II, line AA indicates the cost of providing basic care in relation to hospital size and line BB the cost of providing a fixed average number of units of a given specialized service per patient day in relation to size. From line CC, which indicates the sum of these costs, we may infer that, other things being equal, the greater the number of specialized services provided: (1) the higher the level of average cost per patient day at any given size and (2) the more rapidly over-all average cost initially falls with increased size.[8]

A second factor affecting the relationship between the provision of individual

[8] The provision of additional services may also accentuate the rise in average cost due to managerial problems at large size levels because of the greater organizational complexity involved.

services, average cost, and the degree of economies of scale is the extent to which each service is utilized, on the average, by hospital patients. In general, more extensive utilization of a service per patient day will result in higher average costs at any given size level. However, it is not possible to determine the effect of the degree to which services are utilized upon the rapidity of the fall in average cost as size increases without knowledge of the shapes of the relevant cost curves.

Costs External to the Hospital

Determination of the optimum allocation of hospital resources involves consideration of both the costs incurred by hospitals themselves and the costs associated with hospitalization which are borne by patients, visitors, and the hospital staff. Perhaps the most obvious external cost is travel cost, measured in terms of both dollar outlay and the psychological cost of time consumed.

In any given community, average travel cost per patient day will depend upon a complex array of factors such as the geographic distribution of hospitals of various types, the distribution and characteristics of the population, and the configuration of travel routes. In general, however, it is safe to assume if the sizes of hospitals were increased (with constant utilization rates), their geographic service areas would expand and, consequently, average travel cost would rise.[9] In Figure III, line AA represents the relationship of average cost per patient day incurred by the hospital to the size of the institution, line BB represents average travel cost, and line CC indicates their sum. Note that the optimum size of a hospital is reduced (from OS_1 to OS_2) when travel cost is taken into account.

From the foregoing discussion, it is evident that both the scope of services offered and the cost of travel affect the optimum size (and, thus, number and location) of hospitals and ought to be taken into account in planning.[10] In this study, only the costs incurred by hospitals, and reflected in their accounts, will be analyzed.[11] Once the relationship between hospital costs and size is known, however, the effects of other factors can be readily brought into consideration.

---

[9] In addition to travel cost, account should be taken of possible increases in morbidity and mortality arising directly from the time it takes to get to hospitals.

[10] In addition, the relationship of costs to short-run variations in demand should be considered by those engaged in areawide planning. To some extent, the cost of maintaining "standby" facilities and personnel may be offset by delaying or discouraging admissions, releasing patients sooner than usual, shifting patients or "swing beds" among departments within a hospital, or by centrally allocating patients to hospitals. See Millard F. Long, "Efficient Use of Hospitals" in *The Economics of Health and Medical Care* (Ann Arbor, Mich.: The University of Michigan, 1964), pp. 211-226. Each of these methods will affect the cost-size relationship and thus the optimum hospital size as determined by the above analysis. A study in which consideration was given to the effect of both hospital size and short-run variations in demand on hospital and travel cost (for obstetric care in the Chicago area) may be found in Millard Long and Paul Feldstein, "The Economics of Hospital Systems: Peak Loads and Regional Coordination," *American Economic Review* (May, 1967).

[11] A number of other hospital cost studies, with varying objectives, data, and methodologies, have been conducted in the last few years. See Ralph E. Berry, "Returns to Scale in the Production of Hospital Services," to be published in *Health Services Research;* Harold A. Cohen, "Variations in Cost Among Hospitals of Different Sizes," *Southern Economic Journal,* Vol. 33, No. 3 (January, 1967), pp. 355-366; Robert E. Coughlin, *Hospital Complex Analysis: An Approach to Analysis for Planning a Metropolitan System of Service Facilities* (unpublished Doctoral Dissertation, University of Pennsylvania, 1965); Martin S. Feldstein,

METHODOLOGY

Factors Affecting Hospital Cost

In the previous section, we have outlined the basic theory of the cost-size relationship and have pointed out how variations in service capability affect it. A number of additional determinants of hospital cost must, however, be taken into account if statistical measures of the independent effect of size on cost are to be obtained. For the purposes of this study, we need only consider those factors that have a potentially important nonrandom effect. After selecting and classifying these, we shall be better able to adjust for their influence on hospital cost.

The primary long-run determinants of hospital costs, other than size, can be divided into three major groups:

(1) variation in the capability of a hospital to provide different types of care and in the mix of "products" actually produced;

(2) differences in the prices paid for the factors used in production (except to the extent that such prices are affected by size);

(3) variation in the efficiency with which hospitals operate (except to the extent that efficiency depends upon size).

"Hospital Cost Variation and Case-Mix Differences," *Medical Care,* Vol. 3, No. 2 (April-June, 1965), pp. 95-103; Paul J. Feldstein, *An Empirical Investigation of the Marginal Cost of Hospital Services* (Chicago: Graduate Program in Hospital Administration, University of Chicago, 1961); Thomas Fitzpatrick, Symond Gottlieb, and Grover Wirick, "The Nature of Hospital Costs," (Ann Arbor, Mich.: Bureau of Hospital Administration, The University of Michigan, 1964 [mimeo.]); Mary Lee Ingbar and Lester D. Taylor, *Hospital Costs: A Case Study of Massachusetts* (Cambridge, Mass.: Harvard University Press, 1967); and Kong Kyun Ro, *A Statistical Study of Factors Affecting the Unit Cost of Short-Term Hospital Care* (unpublished Doctoral Dissertation, Yale University, 1966); John F. Deeble, "An Economic Analysis of Hospital Cost," *Medical Care,* Vol. 3, No. 3 (July-Sept., 1965), pp. 138-146.

A critical discussion of most of these and some additional cost studies may be found in Judith R. Lave, "A Review of the Methods Used to Study Hospital Costs," *Inquiry,* Vol. 3, No. 2 (May, 1966), pp. 57-81.

1. Mix of Products—There are considerable differences in the type of patient care which hospitals are capable of producing and in the distribution of types of cases for which they normally provide care. This distribution reflects the aggregate demand for various kinds of care in an area and, more importantly, the way in which this demand is apportioned among different hospitals. Also, there are differences in the quality of care hospitals provide for the same medical conditions, both in terms of medical outcomes and in the degree of amenity provided to patients, and these variations affect the costs incurred.[12]

Hospitals operate a number of patient care programs in addition to inpatient service that may have a significant effect upon cost. The most pervasive of these is general outpatient services, but other programs, such as home care, may be of importance in a few cases. Research and educational activities, such as nursing education and internship and residency programs, may also have a fairly substantial effect upon costs, particularly in large institutions.

2. Prices Paid for Factors Used in Production—The prices paid for the factors of production used in providing hospital services can be divided into two major groups: labor inputs and materi-

al inputs. The wages paid to hospital employees vary considerably from one region to another and between urban and rural areas.[13] There would appear to be much less variation in the prices of material inputs, although differences in transportation cost may affect the prices of supplies and equipment.

3. Efficiency—Finally, the factors of production may be combined with varying degrees of efficiency to produce a given mix of products. The efficiency attained will depend, in large part, upon the managerial competence of a hospital's administrative staff, the techniques and methods passed down from previous generations of management, the activities of the medical staff, and the nature of the physical plant. In addition, the level of efficiency attained may be affected by the pattern of incentives associated with the form of organization under which the hospital operates (i.e., proprietary, voluntary, governmental).

These three factors — product mix, factor prices, and efficiency—constitute, together with size, the basic categories of long-run cost determinants. In the following statistical analysis, we have used eight measures of service capability and product mix variation because of their potential importance and because of the number of different types of data available. Because of lack of data, the number of factor-price measures used was limited to one—the average wage rate. In view of the relatively small variation expected in material price, however, a price variable covering these factors probably would not have contributed much to the accuracy of the estimates of the cost-size relationship. We were unable to find adequate measures of efficiency for use in the statistical analysis, but this should not be a serious shortcoming. All of the hospitals included in this study are of a single organization type (voluntary nonprof-

[12] In studies of a number of diagnostic conditions based upon data from England and Wales it was found that case-fatality rates are usually higher in non-teaching hospitals. See J. A. H. Lee, S. L. Morrison, and J. N. Morris, "Fatality from Three Common Surgical Conditions in Teaching and Non-teaching Hospitals," *Lancet*, 2 (London: Proprietors, The Lancet, Ltd., October 19, 1957), pp. 785-790, and J. A. H. Lee, S. L. Morrison, and J. N. Morris, "Case-fatality in Teaching and Non-teaching Hospitals," *Lancet*, 2 (London: Proprietors, The Lancet, Ltd., January 16, 1960), pp. 170-171; and L. Lipworth, J. A. H. Lee, and J. N. Morris, "Case-fatality in Teaching and Non-teaching Hospitals 1956-59," *Medical Care*, Vol. 1, No. 2 (April-June, 1963), pp. 71-76. These differences, no doubt, reflect both the distribution of medical resources among hospitals and advantages that arise directly from the educational process. It appears plausible that hospital size and a number of other factors may also affect the quality of care, but it would be very difficult to put weights (e.g. dollar values) on the resulting quality differences even if they were known.

[13] For empirical evidence on the extent of wage rate differences, see Harold A. Cohen, *op. cit.*

it). Thus, to the extent that variations in efficiency are not dependent upon size, they can be considered as largely random in nature.

The Measure of Size

In a study of this type, the variable used as a measure of size is of critical importance. If hospital sizes are overstated or understated, incorrect conclusions may be reached about the effect of size on cost.

The most obvious measure of hospital size that comes to mind is bed capacity. However, this is not an adequate standard, if size is defined as the average number of patients for whom care can be provided in an optimal manner. Since hospital admissions (and discharges) are to a large extent randomly distributed in time, a hospital administrator must operate his institution, on the average, at a level of occupancy somewhat lower than maximum capacity in order to provide enough space for unforeseen variations in demand. Because the relative degree of variation in census level is greater for small hospitals than it is for large institutions, small hospitals must operate at lower average occupancy than large hospitals to maintain the same probability of having available beds.[14] Thus, using number of beds to measure hospital size overstates the size of small hospitals.[15]

One solution to this problem is to use an adjusted bed size measure, which may be determined by subtracting the average number of unoccupied beds at each size level from reported bed capacity figures. Another solution is to use average daily census (i.e., actual output) as an estimate of size.

Each of these variables is subject to some degree of error as a measure of the capacity of a hospital to provide care for a given average number of patients in an optimal manner. The use of average daily census as a size measure involves the implicit assumption that all of the factors used in producing care, such as building space, equipment, and personnel, have been adjusted to a level appropriate to each hospital's average output. Since utilization cannot be predicted perfectly and because there is an inevitable time lag between changes in average output and the quantity of productive factors utilized, some hospitals will be operating at average output levels for which they were not designed and incurring costs which differ from long-run optimal values.[16] To this extent, average daily census will provide an imperfect measure of size.

Measures based upon the adjusted values of reported bed capacity are also subject to error, however, because of the well-known variations in the criteria which hospitals use in determining what shall be counted as bed capacity. Since yearly average data will be used in the

---

[14] The optimal average occupancy rate also depends upon other considerations such as the number of patient care units into which a hospital is divided and among which patients are not normally transferred. See Mark S. Blumberg, " 'DPF Concept' Helps Predict Bed Needs," *Modern Hospital*, Vol. 97, No. 6 (December, 1961), pp. 75-81.

[15] The standby cost associated with the relatively high proportion of normally unoccupied beds in small hospitals provides an additional reason to expect the existence of economies of scale.

[16] If an output measure which primarily reflects very short-run changes (such as daily census or average daily census computed on a monthly basis) is used, hospitals operating at abnormally high levels of output will have below normal per-unit costs and *vice versa* because of delays in the adjustment of factor inputs. This phenomenon, which is a variant of the so-called regression fallacy, was pointed out by Milton Friedman in "Discussion" in *Business Concentration and Price Policy* (Princeton, N. J.: Princeton University Press, 1955), pp. 230-238. It is discussed further in J. Johnston, *Statistical Cost Analysis* (New York: McGraw-Hill, 1960), pp. 188-192, and A. A. Walters, "Expectations and the Regression Fallacy in Estimating Cost Functions," *Review of Economics and Statistics*, Vol. 42, No. 2 (May, 1960), pp. 210-216.

On the other hand, if an output measure covering a relatively long time period is used, hospitals operating at higher than optimal levels of average output may incur average costs that are either above or below the amounts which obtain at optimal average output levels because in short-run equilibrium the factors of production utilized are combined in nonoptimal proportions.

empirical part of this study and because most hospital costs are incurred for factor inputs, supplies and personnel (rather than capital consumption), which can be adjusted over this time span, it appears that average daily census will provide a reasonably accurate measure of size. This variable will therefore be used in the empirical analysis to follow.[17]

Method of Analysis

We have used the statistical technique of multiple regression analysis to estimate the net, or independent, effect of hospital size upon cost per patient day. Estimates of the net effects on cost of each of the other factors included in the analysis were also obtained from application of the regression technique.[18]

In essence, multiple regression analysis consists of deriving estimates of the coefficients of an equation relating a dependent variable (in our case, total cost) to a number of independent variables (in our case, size and other factors believed to affect cost).[19]

---

[17] The wide range of values of size utilized relative to the expected amount of error in average daily census as a measure of size suggests that any biases in measures of the cost-size relationship arising from this source are likely to be relatively small.
Analyses were conducted using adjusted bed capacity as a measure of size, with a separate measure of output variation, but the results (available from the authors upon request) did not differ materially from those based upon the average daily census measure of size.
[18] An introduction to regression analysis can be found in Mordecai Ezekial and Karl A. Fox, *Methods of Correlation and Regression Analysis: Linear and Curvilinear* (3rd edition; New York: John Wiley & Sons, 1959). A more advanced treatment of regression methods, with particular attention to the problems encountered in applying them to economic data, is contained in J. Johnston, *Econometric Methods* (New York: McGraw-Hill, 1963).
[19] Total, rather than average, cost was used in the regression analyses of this study primarily in order to avoid spurious correlation that may arise when data are ratios. Under certain conditions, however, this may not be a very serious problem in cost studies based upon cross-section data. See John R. Meyer and Edwin Kuh, "Correlation and Regression Estimates when the Data Are Ratios," *Econometrica*, Vol. 23, No. 4 (October, 1955), pp. 400-416.

In the analyses to follow, we will utilize an equation of the form:

$$TC = a + b\,(ADC) + c\,(ADC)^2 + d\,(OPV) + \ldots,$$

where TC = total cost, ADC = average daily census, and OPV = number of outpatient visits. Given values of TC, ADC, OPV, and the other variables included in the equation for each of the hospitals included in the analysis, the regression technique, when properly applied, yields estimates of the coefficients (e.g., a, b, and c) which best represent the average net effects of each of the independent variables upon total cost. For example, if the d coefficient turned out to be $6.50, we could say that, on the average, each additional outpatient visit adds about $6.50 to total cost.

There are a number of considerations which should be kept in mind in order to increase the likelihood that application of the regression technique will provide accurate, unbiased measures of the relationships considered. One of these is that each of the factors having a potentially important effect upon the dependent variable (total cost) be included in an equation which correctly represents the relationships which are hypothesized to exist. For example, in the section on the cost-size relationship, we hypothesized that cost per patient day would initially fall and then rise as hospital size increases. In order to determine whether the above equation is capable of representing a relationship of this type, both sides may be divided by ($365 \times ADC$) in order to convert the dependent variable to total cost per patient day (i.e., average cost):

$$TC/PD = (a/365)\,(ADC)^{-1} + b/365 + (c/365)\,ADC + \ldots.$$

Now, if a, b, and c are each positive, the value of the $(a/365)\,(ADC)^{-1}$ term of the equation will fall at a decreasing rate as ADC increases, the value of the b/365 term will remain constant, and the value of the $(c/365)\,ADC$ term will

FIGURE IV

Relationship of Total Cost per Patient Day to Hospital Size Described by the Terms of a Hypothetical Regression Equation

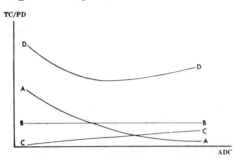

meaningful measures of the potential degree of error in the regression coefficients may be calculated. These measures will be introduced in the empirical-analysis section to follow, and conditions which may effect both their accuracy and the efficiency of the regression technique (in terms of minimizing potential random errors in the regression coefficients) will be pointed out.

THE EMPIRICAL RELATIONSHIP OF
COST TO HOSPITAL SIZE

Two sets of analyses relating cost to hospital size were conducted. In the first analysis, data from all of the hospitals in the study were used in calculating the coefficients of a regression equation. In the second stage of the study, hospitals with different numbers of facilities, services, and programs were grouped together according to service capability and each group was then analyzed separately in order to detect any substantial differences in the degree of economies of scale. Our expectation was that the greater the capability of a hospital to provide a wide range of diversified services, the more rapidly average cost would initially fall with increased size.

increase at a constant rate, as shown by the lines AA, BB, and CC, respectively, in Figure IV. The sum of the values of these terms of the equation is represented by the U-shaped DD curve in Figure IV, indicating that it is possible for the above total-cost equation to represent the hypothesized relationship between average cost and size.[20] The other variables utilized, and their relationship to total cost will be introduced in the section on empirical analysis.

Another important consideration affecting the accuracy of the regression coefficients is the possibility of errors in the independent variables. This matter has already been discussed with respect to the measure of size, but it should be kept in mind that similar considerations may affect the other variables included in the analysis.

Finally, the regression coefficients derived may differ randomly from their "true" values because they are affected by random errors in the cost data. If all of the important independent variables have been measured with little error and included in a correctly specified mathematical model, however,

Analysis Based on all Hospitals

The following cost-affecting factors were included in the regression analysis as independent variables.[21]

(1) Hospital size, as measured by average daily census (ADC). In addition, average daily census squared (ADC)^2 was included to

---

[20] We have implicitly assumed, here, that all of the costs associated with the *a* term of the total cost equation may be attributed to inpatient care and that none of the other variables included in the equation represent part of the cost-size relationship (i.e., that size is measured exclusively in terms of inpatient care).

[21] Our analyses use 1963 data on 3,147 United States short-term voluntary general hospitals registered by the American Hospital Association and taken from the A.H.A. annual survey of hospitals accepted for registration. Some additional information, relating to internship and residency programs, was derived from the American Medical Association's report on internships and residencies.

allow for the possibility that average cost first falls and then increases with hospital size.

(2) The number of facilities and services available (S).[22] In addition, the number of facilities and services available times average daily census (S × ADC) was included in the regression equation. These measures were intended to reflect a component of long-run cost associated with the provision of specialized services which is relatively constant regardless of size and a component which is relatively constant per patient day, respectively.[23]

(3) The number of outpatient visits (OPV).

Five additional variables were added in order to hold constant the costs associated with operating important research and educational programs:

(4) Existence of a hospital-controlled professional nursing school (NS).

(5) Number of student nurses (N).

(6) Number of types of internship and residency programs offered (IRP).[24]

(7) Number of interns and residents (IR).

(8) Affiliation with a medical school (MS).

In addition to the variables listed above, the level and structure of wage rates may have an important effect upon hospital cost. Because detailed information on geographic differences in the wage rates of hospital employees throughout the United States is not available, it was necessary to use the differences between the average wage rate of the employees of each hospital and the average wage rate of all hospital employees as a basis for adjustment. The adjustment was accomplished by multiplying the number of full-time-equivalent employees in each hospital by the average yearly wage rate paid by all hospitals in order to obtain an adjusted payroll cost figure. This amount was then added to nonpayroll cost to obtain the adjusted total cost (ATC) measure used as a dependent variable in this study.[25]

In addition to taking account of geographic wage-rate differences, this method will effect an adjustment for variations in the average skill level of employees among hospitals. Therefore,

---

[22] This variable consists of a count of the number of facilities and services present in a hospital out of the first 28 listed in *Hospitals*, Vol. 38, No. 15, Part 2 (August 1, 1964), p. 14.

[23] The following qualifications need to be made about variable 2:

(1) Using a count of the number of facilities and services available as a variable involves the assumption that the costs associated with them are approximately equal.

(2) In counting the number of services, we have also made the implicit assumption that the variety of services provided within each service classification and the degree of utilization of each service is constant among hospitals of different sizes. However, it appears plausible that the variety and perhaps the amount of service per patient day rendered within each classification increases with hospital size.

(3) Some of the services listed by the American Hospital Association are not inpatient care units. However, to the extent that their output is correlated with hospital size, the costs incurred in operating them should be adequately held constant by the services variable utilized.

[24] To form this variable, the existence of internship programs, regardless of the number of types, was counted as one and added to a count of the number of different types of residency programs in a hospital out of the 28 listed in *Directory of Approved Internships and Residencies* (Chicago: American Medical Association, 1964), p. 129. In addition, the existence of a cancer program approved by the American College of Surgeons was counted as one and added to the total.

[25] As noted above, we could not make an adjustment for price differences in the other important factors of production (e.g., supplies) because of lack of data. A more refined analysis would also take account of the possibility that differences in the relative prices of the factors of production may cause the proportion in which they are used to vary among hospitals. For an elegant mathematical treatment of this idea, see Marc Nerlove, "Returns to Scale in Electricity Supply," in Carl F. Christ, *et. al.*, *Measurement in Economics* (Stanford, Calif.: Stanford University Press, 1963), pp. 167-198.

there are a few qualifications associated with its use:

(1) The optimal average skill level of employees may be affected to some extent by hospital size. For example, a large hospital may require a greater proportion of supervisory personnel who are paid at above average wage rates. On the other hand, it is also probable that in a large institution there is a greater opportunity to save money by delegating tasks requiring lesser knowledge and skill, thus making more effective use of supervisory and professional manpower. Although these differences are probably small, and will tend to cancel, ideally no adjustment should be made for wage rate differences resulting directly from size.

(2) The optimal average skill level of employees will also be affected by the mix of products produced by a hospital. We would generally want to hold costs associated with variations of this type constant in estimating the cost-size relationship. However, this will result in biases in the coefficients of variables reflecting product-mix variation because, when adjusted, they will indicate only those cost differences resulting from nonpayroll factors and the number of full-time-equivalent personnel utilized.[26]

The results of the regression analysis based upon data from all hospitals are as follows (the size measure has been converted from average daily census to patient days, PD, for ease of comprehension) :[27]

$$\text{ATC} = \qquad\qquad -\$307{,}568$$

$$+ \ \$0.0000351 \ (\text{PD})^2$$
$$(\$0.0000029)$$
$$- \ \$0.31 \ (\text{S} \times \text{PD})$$
$$(\$0.07)$$
$$+ \$23{,}188 \ (\text{NS})$$
$$(\$31{,}593)$$
$$+ \ \$5{,}034 \ (\text{IR})$$
$$(\$617)$$
$$+ \ \$34.70 \ (\text{PD})$$
$$(\$1.19)$$
$$+ \ \$33{,}827 \ (\text{S})$$
$$(\$3{,}619)$$
$$+ \ \ \$4.81 \ (\text{OPV})$$
$$(\$0.34)$$
$$- \ \ \$1{,}805 \ (\text{N}) \qquad + \$55{,}347 \ (\text{IRP})$$
$$(\$295) \qquad\qquad (\$5{,}480)$$
$$+ \$174{,}796 \ (\text{MS})$$
$$(\$43{,}744)$$

The following interpretation may be made of the results obtained:

(1) An increase of one patient day raises predicted long-run cost by about $34.70 plus an amount associated with the $(\text{PD})^2$ measure. The coefficient of the $(\text{PD})^2$ measure was statistically significant, suggesting that the relationship between adjusted total cost and size may be curvilinear.

---

[26] In general, we would expect the coefficients of variables representing products which require a high level of skill to be biased downward and *vice versa*. This expectation was borne out in a comparison of regression analyses using total cost and adjusted total cost as dependent variables (available from the authors upon request), but the dependent variable utilized did not substantially affect the estimate of the cost-size relationship.

[27] The regression coefficients shown may differ randomly from their "true" values because of random errors in the cost data. An estimate of the degree of potential error in each regression coefficient arising from this source is indicated by the standard error measure shown in parentheses below it. Subject to the quali-

fications mentioned below, and in the methodology section, we may say, with a 95 percent chance of being correct, that the estimated effect of each variable upon total cost plus or minus about two standard errors describes a range encompassing the true effect.

In general, as hospital size rises, the degree of absolute error in the total cost measure will increase and this condition (a case of heteroscedasticity) will bias the standard errors of the size-related regression coefficients downward. (It will not bias the regression coefficients themselves.) More importantly, heteroscedasticity will result in a loss of efficiency in the estimation of the size-related regression coefficients as compared with estimation based upon average cost data (or, more properly, by means of weighted least squares). For regression analyses covering a rather wide range of sizes, however, the loss of efficiency in terms of the resulting increase in the true standard errors of the regression coefficients will not be inordinately great. See the examples given in J. Johnston, *Econometric Methods* (New York: McGraw-Hill, 1963), pp. 207-211.

The proportion of variation in the dependent variable, adjusted total cost, accounted for by the independent variables is indicated by the coefficient of determination (R^2). For this equation $R^2 = 0.947$.

(2) The average constant component of cost associated with each additional facility or service was estimated at $33,827. However, the coefficient of the (S × PD) measure, which was intended to represent the average increase in cost per patient day per additional service was apparently significantly negative. This unexpected result may have arisen from the high degree of correlation between the (S × PD), PD, and (PD)² measures accompanied by errors in these variables.[28] The average amount of service rendered per patient day no doubt increases with hospital size. Thus, to the extent that errors in the (S × PD) measure may be relatively greater than errors in the PD measure, we would expect the cost of providing a given number of services per patient day to be partly reflected in the coefficients of the PD and (PD)² variables, and, thus, to bias them upward. This phenomenon may also account for the fact that the constant term of this regression equation was, unexpectedly, negative.[29]

(3) On the average, each outpatient visit apparently added about $4.81 to total cost.

[28] The correlation coefficient of (S × PD) and PD was 0.986 and of (S × PD) and (PD)² was 0.898. This condition of high correlation between independent variables (known as multicollinearity) when accompanied by errors in the independent variables, may result in possible errors in the associated regression coefficients that are larger than those indicated by their respective standard errors. See the discussion of case III multicollinearity in J. Johnston, *Econometric Methods* (New York: McGraw-Hill, 1963), pp. 206-207.

[29] Suppose, for example, that three types of hospitals have total cost curves as described by the lines AA', BB', and CC' of Figure V. The height of each curve at any given size level depends upon the service capability and product mix produced by each type of hospital. Assume that hospitals of type CC' tend to be larger than those of type BB', which, in turn are generally larger than those of type AA' (hypothetical observations from each type of hospital are represented by the a's, b's, and c's, in Figure V). A simple regression equation based upon these data (indicated by the line RR') may have a negative constant term (OR) even though the constants of the "true" cost equations (OA, OB and OC) are positive. A similar phenomenon will occur in multiple regression analyses if the adjustment for service capability and product mix is not completely adequate.

FIGURE V

Hypothesized Actual and Measured Relationship Between Total Cost and Hospital Size

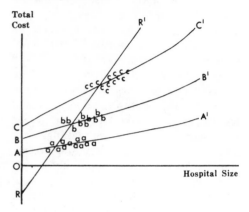

(4) The variable representing the existence of a hospital-controlled professional nursing school (NS) was intended to reflect the constant costs associated with nursing education. The coefficient of this variable turned out to be positive, but it was not statistically significant. The coefficient of the student nurse variable (N) was intended to account for the average incremental cost associated with each additional student-nurse year. This would normally include the cost of training and of food, housing, and other living expenses. These costs would of course, be offset somewhat by the value of the students' clinical experience to the hospital. Unexpectedly, the coefficient of N turned out to be very significantly negative, indicating that total costs were about $1,805 lower per additional student-nurse year. A discussion of the possible reasons for this result is deferred to the summary and conclusions section.

(5) The IRP variable was intended to take account of the educational, research, and increased patient care costs associated with the operation of internship and residency programs. The coefficient of this variable indicated an average increase in cost of about $55,347 per program. The number of interns and

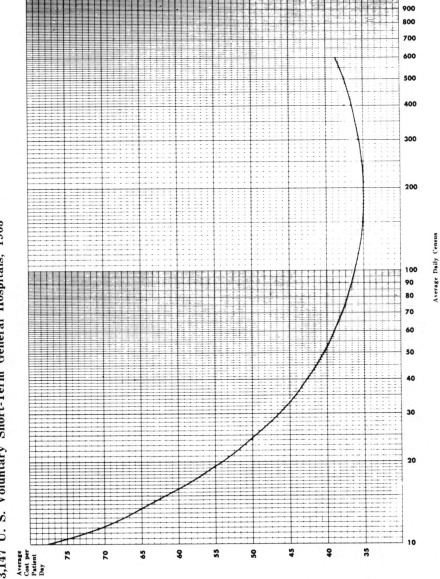

FIGURE VI

Estimated Average Cost Per Patient Day in Relation to Average Daily Census, 3,147 U. S. Voluntary Short-Term General Hospitals, 1963

Average
Cost per
Patient
Day

Average Daily Census

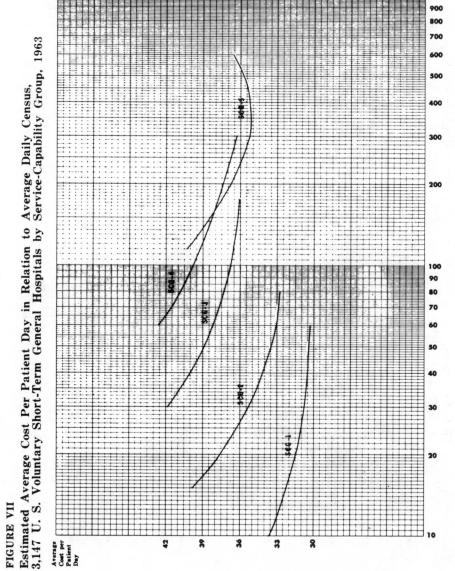

FIGURE VII

Estimated Average Cost Per Patient Day in Relation to Average Daily Census, 3,147 U. S. Voluntary Short-Term General Hospitals by Service-Capability Group, 1963

residents was included as a variable (IR) to hold approximately constant the additional cost associated with their presence. This amount turned out to be about $5,034 per person.

(6) An average incremental cost of $174,796 was shown by the coefficient of the variable representing affiliation with a medical school. It should be recognized that this estimate reflects only those cost differences which exist after the costs associated with internship and residency programs and other foregoing factors have been taken into account.

The main findings of the analysis based upon all hospitals were those related to the cost-size relationship itself. The regression results, stated in terms of adjusted total costs, were converted to adjusted average cost (AAC) by assuming the presence of the mean number of services (14.15) and the absence of all the other cost-affecting characteristics (e.g., nursing school, interns and residents). In order to obtain estimates of average cost at various size levels, the relevant terms of the regression equation were divided by patient days, to yield the following equation:

$$AAC = \$171,085 \ (PD)^{-1} + \$30.31 + \$0.0000351 \ (PD)$$

The relationship between adjusted average cost and size (measured in terms of ADC) described by this equation is portrayed graphically in Figure VI.

The results indicate that as hospital size increases, average cost declines until it reaches a minimum level at about 190 ADC and then begins to rise. However, to the extent that the constant term of the regression equation may be biased downward and the coefficient of the $(PD)^2$ term biased upward, as noted above, the degree of the initial decline in cost will be underestimated and the amount of the rise in cost at large size levels will be overestimated.[30] There-

fore, we decided to carry out a second series of analyses that would account more satisfactorily for the influence of the number of facilities and services upon the cost-size relationship.

Analyses by Service-Capability Group

For these analyses, the hospitals were divided into five service-capability groups (SCGs) according to the number of facilities, services and programs they provide as shown in Table 1. A separate regression equation was then fitted to the data from hospitals in each group.

As in the case of the all-hospital analysis, we decided to use adjusted rather than reported total cost as the dependent variable in order that geographic wage differences and wage variation associated with product mix could be held approximately constant. Of the independent variables used in the all-hospital analyses, only (S), the number of facilities and services, was not included. The differences in constant cost associated with facilities and services were largely accounted for by the division of the hospitals into service-capability groups. However, an (S × PD) variable was included to reduce the degree of possible bias in the PD and $(PD)^2$ regression coefficients and, thus, in the constant term.

The results of the regression analyses based upon the five service-capability groups are presented in Table 2. Positive constant terms that become greater as service capability increased were estimated, suggesting that the initial decline in costs is more rapid with greater service capability. The results were

---

[30] It should be noted that no measures of the degree of economies of scale or confidence limits

to be attached to them have been presented. Although such measures would be subject to the potential biases noted above, and it is not presently clear as to just what type of measures would be most useful for areawide planning purposes, it should be possible to calculate them from the means and joint confidence regions of the regression estimates. See, for example, H. Gregg Lewis, "On the Distribution of the Partial Elasticity Coefficient," *Journal of the American Statistical Association*, Vol. 36, No. 215 (September, 1941), pp. 413-416.

TABLE 1
Hospitals by Service-Capability Group

Service-Capability Group	Number of Facilities, Services and Programs (S)	Number of Hospitals	Mean Average Daily Census (ADC)
SCG 1	0 through 9	680	26
SCG 2	10 through 12	693	46
SCG 3	13 through 16	729	93
SCG 4	17 through 19	490	170
SCG 5	20 through 28	555	294

converted to average cost per patient day by a method similar to the one described in the all-hospital analysis. The estimated relationships between average cost and size, for the range of sizes encompassed by the regression analyses, are shown in Figure VII.

Economies of scale in the provision of care appear to exist over a wide range of sizes in each of the service-capability groups. As the number of services increases, the size level at which a relatively low level of average cost is attained apparently increases. Possible diseconomies of scale were indicated only for hospitals in the upper size range of the highest service capability group.

In the analyses of service-capability groups 1 through 4, the coefficients of the (S × PD) measure were positive. This suggests that product-mix variation was more adequately taken into account in the analyses by service-capability group than in the all-hospital analysis. The fact that the (S × PD) coefficient decreases with increased service capability suggests that the less commonly available services cost less per patient day on the average, no doubt because they are utilized less intensively on a patient-day basis.[31]

The following interpretations may be made with respect to the other variables

included in the service-capability-group analyses:

(1) The lower cost per outpatient visit in hospitals in the lower service-capability groups appears to be a result of the type of care typically provided in the outpatient clinics of those hospitals. Such care consists primarily of normal emergency and clinic services of lower cost per visit than the more specialized services available in the referral programs of hospitals in the higher service-capability groups.

(2) The effect of the nursing-school variable on hospital cost was generally insignificant, perhaps because the relatively constant cost of operating a nursing school is likely to be a small percentage of total hospital cost. The presence of student nurses generally appears to have a negative effect on total cost; that is, total cost decreases with increased numbers of student nurses. This result is particularly apparent for hospitals in the highest service-capability group, which are those with the largest number of student nurses.

(3) As expected, total cost increases with the operation of internship and residency programs and the presence of interns and residents. However, the increased cost of having interns and residents is smaller in hospitals of higher service capability. Since the average number of interns and residents in these hospitals is relatively high, a possible explanation for this is that there may

[31] The variation in the coefficients of the PD, $(PD)^2$, and (S × PD) measures may also be partially explained by the high degree of correlation among these measures.

TABLE 2
Regression Coefficients, Adjusted Total Cost in Relation to Patient Days and Other Characteristics, 3,147 Voluntary Short-Term General Hospitals, by Service-Capability Group, 1963

	Service-capability group				
	SCG 1	SCG 2	SCG 3	SCG 4	SCG 5
Number of hospitals	680	693	729	490	555
R²	0.844	0.861	0.875	0.850	0.896
Constant	13,422	55,003	83,756	134,677	570,398
Variable	Regression coefficients				
PD	21.36	9.58	27.76	36.19	27.25
	(3.06)	(4.50)	(4.49)	(6.85)	(5.25)
(PD)²	−0.0000182	0.0000667	0.0000146	−0.0000149	0.0000370
	(0.0000515)	(0.0000294)	(0.0000165)	(0.0000148)	(0.0000069)
S × PD	1.1151	1.8130	0.4301	0.0270	−0.0479
	(0.3260)	(0.3835)	(0.2849)	(0.3671)	(0.2152)
OPV	1.78	1.29	2.36	1.86	6.20
	(0.47)	(0.69)	(0.83)	(0.69)	(0.85)
NS	239,157	−129,390	−70,969	−83,077	5,404
	(71,728)	(63,977)	(41,698)	(59,329)	(104,622)
N	−1,456	3,260	234	−52	−2,621
	(918)	(891)	(585)	(591)	(760)
IRP	6,075	86,147	8,374	11,085	70,491
	(17,661)	(30,308)	(17,533)	(15,459)	(12,705)
IR	34,767	21,547	18,578	7,928	4,157
	(9,387)	(5,482)	(3,744)	(3,099)	(1,315)
MS	*	☆	−34,707	127,469	171,734
			(96,867)	(86,670)	(107,551)

* None of the hospitals in these groups were affiliated with medical schools.

be economies of scale in the operation of internship and residency programs.

(4) Although the results for costs of affiliation with a medical school are not statistically significant, they indicate that such costs are rather small. This may be because some medical school costs are reflected in the accounts of other organizational entities (e.g., a university), or because they are partly reflected in the internship and residency variable or in other variables.

SUMMARY AND CONCLUSIONS

The main purpose of this study has been to estimate the net relationship between patient-day cost and the size of hospitals. It was hypothesized that, according to economic theory, average cost would initially decline as size is increased—primarily because of the gains resulting from specialization—but that, after some point, average cost would begin to rise because of increased problems of internal control and communications. If the net relationship of cost to size could be determined, hospital construction plans could be appropriately adjusted and great savings could be made.

Two approaches were used to empirically estimate the independent effect of size on cost. In the first analysis, data from 3,147 U. S. voluntary short-term general hospitals were used to relate total hospital cost to hospital size and a number of other variables by means of multiple regression analysis. Although the primary reason for the inclusion of the other variables was to eliminate their effect on hospital cost, estimates of their independent effects on cost were also derived. The additional variables utilized were the number of services in the hospital, the number of outpatient visits, the presence or absence of a nursing school, the number of student nurses, the number and types of internship and residency programs, the number of interns and residents, and affiliation or non-affiliation with a medical school.

The major finding of the first analysis was consistent with our hypotheses. Average cost initially declined with increased hospital size but, after a point, began to increase with size. However, the results of the all-hospital analysis were not considered conclusive because the adjustments for variations in the services provided by hospitals of different sizes were apparently inadequate.

Therefore, in a second series of analyses, the effect of the amount of specialized service provided upon cost was partially held constant by dividing the hospitals into five categories according to the number of facilities and services provided. Regression coefficients were then calculated for each group of hospitals, using essentially the same variables as in the first analysis. The results confirmed the general relationship determined in the previous all-hospital analysis. For hospitals with a given number of services, economies are associated with increased size. As the number of services increases, a relatively low level of average cost is reached in hospitals of successively larger size. Only for the largest hospitals in the highest service-capability group were diseconomies of scale indicated within the size range covered by the regression analysis.

Additional studies of hospital cost could provide more refined knowledge of the cost-size relationship. For instance, in future studies, the extent of economies of scale could be determined for individual services and facilities; then the interrelationships of different services could be ascertained to determine what facilities and services should be provided together in the same hospital. In addition to making possible a more accurate estimate of the over-all cost-size relationship, such a study would make it possible to determine the number of hospitals that should provide certain facilities and services in any given area.

In any case, our findings on the net relationship of cost to size are useful as they stand. They provide estimates of the independent effect of size upon cost and, more broadly, they indicate the range of practicable hospital sizes.

Our findings suggest that small hospitals with high service capability should not generally be built because they are likely to be of uneconomic size. Large hospitals having low service capability are also likely to be uneconomic, since there are few or no additional economies associated with increased size to offset the greater transportation costs incurred.

The most interesting of our findings relating to variables other than size concerned nursing education. The coefficient of the student-nurse variable (N) was negative in both the analysis based on all hospitals and in the separate analysis of service-capability group 5. In each of these cases, the student-nurse coefficient was statistically significant in the sense that the associated standard error measure was relatively small.

These results are broadly consistent with the relationships found for 1951 and 1952 in the study of the Commission on Financing Hospital Care. At the time of that study, average expense per patient day was found to be 11 percent lower in small hospitals with nursing schools than it was in similar hospitals without such schools.[32]

These findings are surprising in view of the available evidence showing that the cost of maintaining and educating student nurses substantially exceeds the value of the services they provide during their clinical training. In a recent analysis of the costs associated with diploma programs in nursing, it was found that the average gross cost incurred by the parent institution was about $2,400 per student-year. The average value of the students' clinical experience to the parent institution was estimated at $600 per student-year.[33] This leaves an estimated net cost to the hospital of $1,800 per student-year.

One explanation for this apparent contradiction may be that the lower cost per patient day in hospitals with nursing students is a reflection of factors other than the direct value of students to hospitals. For example, the National League for Nursing study suggested that hospitals which operate nursing schools have an advantage in the recruitment of professional nursing personnel.

In conclusion, we should like to make a few comments about factors affecting optimal hospital size that may not be reflected in the results of our statistical analyses.

First, it should be pointed out that hospitals operating above the lowest levels indicated on the least-cost curves are not necessarily inefficient. For example, certain teaching and research programs may require a hospital large enough to furnish a certain number of medically specialized cases, even though this size level would be uneconomic if only the patient care operations of the hospital were considered.

Another factor—mentioned earlier in this paper—that may affect optimal size is travel cost, including both the monetary and non-monetary costs associated with distance. Now that an estimate has been made of the magnitude of internal economies of scale, we are in a better position to determine in later studies the "trade off" between the increased travel costs involved in having fewer, larger hospitals and the loss of economies of scale involved in having more but smaller hospitals closer to prospective patients.

Finally, it should be recognized that our analyses are based upon historical costs as they are reflected in hospital accounting records. The costs relevant for planning purposes, on the other hand, are often those associated with new facilities. And they are always those which will be incurred in future time periods. More generally, all planning activity is directed toward the future, and statistical studies based upon past data (as they must be) have value, in this context, only to the extent that they allow us to draw inferences about expected future relationships.

[32] See John H. Hayes, ed., "Factors Affecting the Costs of Hospital Care," *Financing Hospital Care in the United States,* Vol. 1 (New York: The Blakiston Company, 1954), pp. 119-120.

[33] See National League for Nursing, "Cost of Basic Diploma Programs," *Study on Cost of Nursing Education.* Part I (New York: National League for Nursing, 1964), particularly pp. 68-70.

14. The Effects of Patient Mix and Service Mix on Hospital Costs and Productivity

HENRY W. ZARETSKY

Reprinted with permission from *Topics in Health Care Financing* 4. Copyright © 1977, Aspen Systems Corporation, 63-82.

Topics in this chapter include:

EVALUATING HOSPITAL PER-
FORMANCE
THE COST FUNCTION
THE DATA
EMPIRICAL RESULTS
EFFECTS OF CONTROLLING FOR
SERVICE AND CASE MIX
ECONOMIES OF SCALE
COST FUNCTION AS A USEFUL
TOOL

IT IS WELL KNOWN that comparison of costs among hospitals is less than straightforward. This is because different hospitals produce different products in terms of the patients they treat and the services they provide; a patient day in one hospital may be a quite different product from a patient day in another hospital. Simple comparison of cost per day or per admission among hospitals will result in large variation.

EVALUATING HOSPITAL PERFORMANCE

In evaluating hospital performance, it is essential to know how much of the cost variation among hospitals is due to variation in product and how much is due to operating efficiency. Effective and equitable economic regulation requires a sound method of comparing hospitals.

The project on which this article is based was supported by National Center for Health Services Research, HEW Grant Number HS01104-02.

Hospital Classification

For example, hospital reimbursement restrictions under Medicare are determined through hospital classification based on hospital size and area per capita income. The Medicare-Medicaid Administrative Reform Act (S. 1470) currently before Congress seeks to establish an incentive payment structure based on hospital classifications and proposed additional developmental work in this area. In addition, various state rate-setting programs make use of hospital comparisons either as guidelines in reviewing budgets or as establishing reimbursement ceilings.

In the project on which this article is based, costs and productivity among diverse hospitals were compared and studied. The insight gained into the various factors determining hospital cost variation is a step toward selecting data items and appropriate comparison techniques to be used in a statewide financial reporting system.

Hospital costs were compared through

evaluation of a statistical cost function for hospitals. A cost function is a mathematical relationship between a firm's costs, in a given time period, and the firm's rate of output and other factors influencing costs, such as location and product mix. This technique enabled comparison of hospital costs, taking into account, simultaneously, a large number of cost-influencing factors and estimation of the effects of each of these factors on costs.

Service and Patient Mix
Affect Hospital Costs

The results of this method of comparison suggest that service mix and patient mix, particularly the latter, are highly important and statistically significant factors affecting hospital costs.

Failure to account for scope of service and patient mix leads to the erroneous conclusion that cost per admission is positively related to hospital size.

Failure to account for scope of service and patient mix leads to the erroneous conclusion that cost per admission is positively related to hospital size. The simple positive correlation between hospital size and costliness is due to the fact that larger hospitals, in general, treat more complex patients and provide more costly services than do smaller institutions; and does not point to inefficiencies in large-scale institutions. This has cru-

cial implications for planning and economic regulation.

THE COST FUNCTION

The cost function—a mathematical relationship between a firm's total costs per a given time period and the firm's rate of output—has its origin in economic theory and has certain theoretical properties based on assumptions about management objectives, characteristics of product and factor markets, and short-run versus long-run applicability. The cost model, for our purposes, is a convenient method of analyzing hospital costs as they relate to a variety of cost-influencing factors.

The cost function can be denoted as $C = C(y, z)$, where C is total costs of production, say per year, y is total output per year and z is a set of other variables influencing costs. The relationship between cost and output indicates the extent, if any, of economics or diseconomies of scale. That is, are higher or lower unit costs associated with larger volumes of output? The economies of scale issue has crucial implications for health facilities planning. Is efficient health care delivery prompted through relatively few large institutions or a greater number of small institutions in a hospital service area?

Failure to adequately account for variation in product mix leads to the erroneous conclusion that large hospitals are less efficient than small hospitals. Moreover, hospital productivity and efficiency cannot be appropriately

:valuated without holding constant
lifferences in product mix.

Application to Hospitals

The cost variations among hospitals in
California were examined to determine
:he extent of economies of scale and the
effects of differences in product mix
'case mix and service mix) on hospital
:osts. Work on this activity is explained
n detail in *Analysis of Hospital Costs
Controlling for Service Mix and Case.*[2] ed

The cost functions were estimated on
1971 data from 176 acute care California
hospitals, incorporating data on patient
nix broken down according to ICDA
:ategories, in addition to cost and utiliza-
:ion data.   " DA

Most cost (or production) function
studies of industries other than the hospital industry have not been specifically
:oncerned with product heterogeneity. A
disproportionate amount of cost and
production function studies have involved
public utilities and railways; the remainder have involved manufacturing
and agricultural industries. This mainly
reflects availability of data (in addition to
public policy implications regarding
economies of scale in the regulated industries). Product mix and quality variation are not central issues in these industries. The multiproduct nature of hospital production and the wide variability
of patient types across hospitals has
tended to make "product mix" adjustments the major consideration.

Early research on the hospital cost
function, most likely due to scarcity of
data, did not explicitly consider case mix.

More recent work demonstrates
imaginative approaches to dealing with
case mix variation.[3,4,5,6] In general, the
studies that did not explicitly consider
case mix of patients did account for
service capability (i.e., number and types
of services offered).

The Cost Model

The cost model discussed here is
illustrated, COST/ADM = f(ADM,
FLOW, SERVICE, CASEM, URBAN),
where **COST/ADM** represents cost per
admission; **ADM** represents number of
admissions; **FLOW** represents case flow
(admissions per bed); **SERVICE**
represents service capability; **CASEM**
represents diagnostic mix of patients;
and **URBAN** is a dummy variable indicating whether a hospital is located in an
urban area. (This variable is assigned the
value of unity if a particular hospital is
located in an urban area, and it is
assigned zero otherwise.)

The Variables

The model is estimated through linear
regression. Here admissions represent
volume of production. A positive relationship between the dependent variable,
cost per admission and admissions suggests the larger the hospital, the more
costly the hospital. The case flow variable is included to adjust for the effect of
capacity utilization on costs. Service mix
and case mix variables are included to
account for the effect of service capability and diagnostic mix on costs. The
dummy variable, indicating whether a

hospital is located in an urban area (Standard Metropolitan Statistical Area), is included to control for cost-influencing factors associated with location that are not reflected by service, patient mix or size. The major locational influence reflected in this variable is likely to be prevailing wage levels in urban versus rural labor markets.

THE DATA

The data used in this study were obtained from three sources: (1) American Hospital Association (AHA) Annual Survey, 1971, (2) California Health Data Corporation (CHDC), and (3) Professional Activities Study (PAS). The last two sources yielded data on diagnostic mix of patients.

Case Mix Variables

A common case mix data set was identified enabling the combining of PAS and CHDC records into one file. This file had as the unit of observation, the individual discharge (about one million discharges are on the file), while the AHA file (on costs, services and utilization) uses the hospital as the unit of observation. Diagnoses, originally coded according to four-digit ICDA-8, were aggregated into 45 categories (see Table 8-1). These data were then merged with the AHA file, providing the basic data base for the regressions.

Diagnostic information was retained in the form of proportions of patients in each of the 45 diagnosis categories in each hospital. Obviously, 45 case mix variables is an excessive number for use

TABLE 8-1

Aggregation of Four-Digit ICDA Categories Into 45 Groups

Diagnosis Group
Infective Diseases
Malignant Neoplasms
Benign Neoplasms
Metabolic Diseases
Diabetes
Other Endocrine Disorders
Hematology
Mental Disorders
Disease of Central Nervous System
Disease of Eye and Ear
Disease of Other Nervous System
Acute Coronary
Other Heart Disease
Hypertension
Vascular Disease
Acute Upper Respiratory Infection
Hypertrophy of Tonsils & Adenoids
Pneumonia & Bronchitis
Other Respiratory Disease
Dental Disorders
Disease of Mouth & Esophagus
Disease of Stomach and Duodenum
Appendicitis
Hernia
Other Disease of Intestine
Disease of Liver/Gallbladder/Pancreas
Genitourinary Diseases
Disease of Breast
Disease of Female Genital Organs
Complication of Pregnancy
Abortions
Normal Deliveries
Complicated Deliveries
Complications of Puerperium
Diseases of Skin
Disease of Muscular/Skeletal System
Congenital Anomalies
Diseases of Infancy
Symptoms & Signs
Fractures
Other Trauma
Adverse Effects
Special Services
Births
Miscellaneous

n a regression equation, regardless of legrees of freedom, due to multicollinarity and the resulting (impossible) task f interpreting the coefficients. (Multiollinearity occurs when two or more of he independent variables are highly correlated with each other. This creates piases in the resulting estimated oefficients.) Since the original 45 varibles consisted of proportions, 45 omponents could not be obtained as the 5th proportion is a linear function of the ther 44 proportions. (Principal components are linear combinations of a set f variables calculated in a manner to xplain as much variation in these varibles as possible with as few components—linear combination—as possible.)[7,8] Therefore, the 45 case mix proortions were converted to 44 principal omponents, each with a mean of zero, ariance of unity and orthogonal to (not orrelated with) each of the other 43 omponents.

Had we only been concerned with the ffects of case mix on cost per case, all 4 components could have been retained nd used in a regression of cost per case n the 44 components. Since the omponents are orthogonal, multicollinarity would not be a problem. However, he emphasis here is on estimating the ost function, using the components to orrect for case mix variation across hositals. Multicollinearity is expected etween the components and the econ019omic variables; hence, it is desirable to estrict the number of components to be sed as independent variables in the egression.

Using a pragmatic approach, which involves extracting components up to the point where the associated eigenvalue falls below unity, the first 12 components were retained, explaining 69 percent of the variance in all 44 components. Thus, the cost functions include 12 principal components as independent variables.

For the project, the components were viewed as composite variables included in the cost function to account for the aggregate effect of patient mix on hospital costs. Rather than analyzing the cost effects of particular diagnoses, the project accounted for case mix effects so that the estimated relationship between cost and volume, for example, was not biased, and to explore methods to equitably compare costs and productivity among hospitals.

In addition to the diagnosis variables, a dummy variable was included indicating whether the hospital was located in a metropolitan area (Standard Metropolitan Statistical Area). This variable partially reflects socioeconomic characteristics of the hospital's service area and also reflects labor market conditions (i.e., average wage level).

Service Mix Variables

The literature on hospital cost analysis which attempts to account for service mix variation is abundant. From this literature, two methods were selected for their ability to condense service mix data into few variables.

THE GUTTMAN SCALE APPROACH

The first approach involved a Guttman scale developed by Edwards et al. in 1972.[9] Using data reported in the AHA Annual Survey on service capability

TABLE 8-2

Services Composing Service Mix Index, in Guttman Scale Order
1. Pharmacy
2. Postoperative Recovery
3. Physical Therapy
4. Inhalation Therapy
5. Intensive Care
6. Histopathology
7. Intensive Cardiac Care
8. X-ray Therapy
9. Radioisotope Laboratory
10. Electroencephalography
11. Radium Therapy
12. Social Work
13. Emergency Psychiatry
14. Inpatient Psychiatry
15. Occupational Therapy
16. Inpatient Renal Dialysis
17. Cobalt Therapy
18. Open-Heart Surgery
19. Organ Bank

Source: M. Edwards, J. D. Miller, and R. Schumacher, "Classification of Community Hospitals by Scope of Service: Four Indexes," Health Services Research, 7 (Winter 1972) p. 301–313.

(offer or do not offer particular services), an index was created on the principle of cumulative scaling (i.e., services are assumed to be acquired in order of increasing sophistication, and the later acquisitions represent a greater scope of service than earlier acquisitions). Table 8-2 shows the general index of services developed by Edwards et al.[10] If a hospital has occupational therapy but does not have any of the services "above" (e.g., renal dialysis, cobalt therapy), the assumption is the hospital offers all services "below" it (e.g., inpatient psychiatry, emergency psychiatry). This index results in one variable with a range from one to 19.

A GROUPING STRATEGY APPROACH

An alternative approach involved using a grouping strategy developed by Berry in 1973.[11] The principle behind both approaches is similar. That is, hospitals go through certain stages of "growth." At first, a given institution offers only basic services. Additions to these services become more and more sophisticated. Again, an assumption is made that if a hospital offers certain

TABLE 8-3
Facilities and Services Composing Berry Groups

Berry Group	Services
Basic	Clinical Laboratory
	Emergency Room
	Operating Room
	Delivery Room
	X-ray, Diagnostic
Quality Enhancing	Blood Bank
	Pathology Laboratory
	Pharmacy with Pharmacist
	Premature Nursery
	Postoperative Recovery Unit
Complex	Electroencephalography
	Dental Facilities
	Physical Therapy
	Intensive Care Unit
	X-ray, Therapeutic
	Radioisotope Therapy
	Psychiatric Inpatient Unit
	Cobalt Therapy
	Radium Therapy
Community	Occupational Therapy
	Outpatient Department
	Home Care Program
	Social Work Department
	Rehabilitation Unit
	Family Planning Service

Source: Berry, Ralph E., Jr., "On Grouping Hospitals for Economic Analysis," Inquiry, Volume X (December 1973) p. 5–12.

ervices at a given level of sophistication or scope, it offers all services of a lesser level.

Through extensive analysis of AHA Annual Survey data, Berry was able to group hospitals into five general categories (see Table 8-3). The first category—basic services—is composed of the services a small (new) institution would have to offer to be an acute care institution. As the hospital "grows" beyond this basic capability, it goes through a "quality enhancing" stage where additional services represent enhancements in quality (depth) rather than expansion in scope (breadth). The next additions involve complex services, adding to the hospital's capacity to treat a wider variety of medical conditions.

The "final stage" is encountered when a hospital becomes a community medical center (full service institution) offering outpatient care, home care, social work and so on. Another category, "special services," was identified but it did not represent an expansion of service so it was ignored in the analysis. Hospitals are assigned to one of the four groups based on a simple algorithm, where if a hospital has four or more of the community services it is assigned to that group, and so on for the other groups.[12] ("Three or more" services was the criterion for the quality-enhancing group.)

Dummy variables based on three of the four groups were included as regressors. (Four dummy variables were not included as each regression had a separate intercept term.) Alternatively, the Guttman index was included as a regressor.

While it would have been preferable to group hospitals according to Berry's criteria prior to running the regressions, i.e., let the slopes vary among groups instead of only the intercept, the large number of case mix variables creates too severe a constraint on available degrees of freedom.

Economic Variables

OUTPUT

In hospital cost studies, output measures alternate between inpatient days and cases (admissions or discharges). The major argument in favor of the former is that cost per case is very much dependent on length of stay, which is in turn a reflection, at least in part, of case mix.[13] The natural measure of

---

Hospitals should be free to select the "optimal" combination of length of stay and cost per day and should be evaluated on the resulting cost per case.

---

output seems to be the case, which allows one to recognize the trade-off between length of stay and cost per day (i.e., relatively more intense care can substitute for longer, less intensive stays). Thus, hospitals should be free to select the "optimal" combination of length of stay and cost per day and should be evaluated on the resulting cost per case. If one is able to control for case mix variation, use of cost per case is clearly preferred.

ADJUSTED PATIENT DAYS

Since many hospitals treat patients on both an inpatient and outpatient basis, admissions as an output measure is downward biased. Moreover, hospital cost data are not broken down by inpatient and outpatient, thus inhibiting estimation of an inpatient cost curve. A commonly used approach to adjust for this deficiency is "adjusted patient days" rather than actual patient days. The former is the product of patient days and the ratio of total revenue to inpatient revenue.

The project used adjusted admissions, obtained from the AHA tape by multiplying admissions by the ratio of adjusted patient days to patient days. The implicit assumption here is that outpatient charges and inpatient charges are based strictly on costs (since "adjusted patient days" is calculated by the ratio of charges to charges). It is widely believed that this assumption does not hold in practice. While there are little data available for testing this assumption, analysis of departmental data from 38 hospitals indicates, on the average, hospitals incur negative profits in daily hospital services and positive profits in most ancillary services (with the exception of emergency room).[14] Thus, while most likely biased, the adjusted measures are preferable to the unadjusted measures.

SCALE

As a scale measure, number of beds appears to be the most appropriate. Number of beds is the "most fixed" factor in the short run on which data are available. (Scale could alternatively be measured by value of the hospital's assets, but given various depreciation methods and differences in vintages of equipment, reported assets are likely to be highly unreliable for our use.) Use of output as a scale proxy is valid when a long-run cost function is being estimated since it implies all factors are variable. Cost functions using both measures of scale were estimated; however, only the equations based on output (admissions) are reported here. (Results were similar for both measures.)

COSTS

The cost variable is total hospital expenses for the 12-month period reported on the AHA 1971 Annual Survey. The reporting period for most reporting hospitals is October 1, 1970 to September 30, 1971, although some institutions used their last fiscal year. Total expenses include payroll expenses, employee benefits, professional fees and other expenses, including supplies, purchased services, depreciation and interest.

Obviously, there are many shortcomings in the cost data, but these are common to cost data employed in many cost function studies. An exception is found in cost studies of regulated industries since these firms are required to file uniform accounting reports with their regulatory agencies. However, this only solves the problem of uniformity. The problem of reconciling accountants' and economists' definitions of cost still remains. In particular, the economists' definition of production cost includes capital costs composed of depreciation, interest, insurance, rent and an implicit rental charge for owned assets (opportunity costs). The latter measure is not included n the accounting definition. Moreover, depreciation calculations are arbitrary and inconsistent across firms.

In general, economic theory defines costs to the firm as those payments necessary to induce factors of production (labor and capital) to continue their employment with the firm. Economic theory further divides cost into variable and fixed. This division is dependent on the reporting period. Costs of fixed factors should not enter into short-run decisions. A useful and succinct discussion of problems in using accounting data is presented by Walters.[15]

Another problem with the AHA data is that the cost data cover expenses for all hospital operations, inpatient and outpatient. Our adjustment is made on the output variable (adjusted admissions) rather than the cost variable.

Short-Run Capacity Utilization

As it is widely recognized that there is excess capacity in the hospital industry, which has an important effect on costs, short-run capacity utilization variables are often included in cost function models. (When the cost function specification includes both output and scale measures, effects of short-run variations can be obtained from the estimated coefficients and thus explicit utilization measures—e.g., occupancy—are not necessary.) Three utilization variables are employed here: (1) case flow (admissions per bed); (2) occupancy rate; and (3) average length of stay. Case flow is proportional to occupancy and inversely proportional to length of stay;

hence, when case flow is included in the regression, the other two variables are not: case flow = 365/LOS × occupancy.

The occupancy and length of stay variables are always included as a pair (with the coefficient of each unrestricted). Use of these utilization variables is questionable. For example, occupancy (average daily census/beds) is appropriate only if patient days is the output measure. It has no clear economic meaning if the case is considered the output. On the other hand, case flow, while an intuitively obvious measure of intensity of utilization of beds, is objected to since it masks the effects of offsetting changes in length of stay and occupancy. A problem common to case flow and occupancy when used as regressors in an average cost equation is that they are endogenous; that is, they have an effect on the system being studied and are also affected by the system being studied. Thus, their coefficients are biased and inconsistent.

EMPIRICAL RESULTS

The following cost functions were studied:
1. COST/ADM = f_1(ADM, FLOW, SERVICE, CASEM, URBAN)
2. COST/ADM = f_2(ADM, OCCUP, LOS, SERVICE, CASEM, URBAN),

where the variables are as defined above, and **OCCUP** represents occupancy rate and **LOS** represents length of stay. As mentioned above, two alternative service mix (SERVICE) proxies, a Guttman index and three dummy variables, were also included in the project. CASEM represents 12 principal components based on case mix proportions of patients.

The procedure used to estimate cost function specifications was ordinary least squares. (Obviously, many statistical and theoretical problems exist giving rise to possible statistical biases). For our purposes, it is preferable to view these cost function estimates as a convenient way to compare hospital costs in terms of size, service capability and case mix.[16]

Effects of Service Mix and Case Mix on Cost Function Specifications

The effect of inclusion of case mix and service mix variables on the cost function were determined, and the results are presented in Tables 8-5 and 8-6. To the extent that size (or output) is related to these "product dimension" variables, inclusion of the latter was expected to affect the estimated coefficient(s) of the size (or output) variable(s).

CASE MIX

Tables 8-5 and 8-6 present results of linear equations using alternative service mix variables, with and without the case mix variables. (Table 8-4 presents the sample means of the dependent and independent variables.) Note that when case mix is included, the output (admissions) coefficient in each equation is negative but not significant. Exclusion of the case mix principal components causes the output coefficient to be positive, and significant in the equations including length of stay and occupancy (see Table 8-6). Similar results are obtained when

TABLE 8-4

Sample Means and Standard Deviations of Variables Used in Cost Function Estimation

(n = 176)		
Variable	Mean	Standard Deviation
COST/ADM	735.45	233.25
ADM	7399.92	5604.43
OCCUP	0.67	0.14
LOS	6.37	2.12
FLOW	40.59	15.37
SERVICE$_1$ (Basic)	0.20	0.40
SERVICE$_2$ (Quality)	0.28	0.45
SERVICE$_3$ (Complex)	0.36	0.48
SERVICE$_4$ (Guttman)	13.31	4.62
URBAN	0.84	0.36
CASEM$_i$ (Principal Component$_i$)*	0	1

*CASEM$_1$ through CASEM$_{12}$ have means of zero and variances of unity.

number of beds is used as the scale variable.[17]

The implication of these results is that the positive (simple) correlation between unit cost and volume (size) is due to larger hospitals treating relatively more costly cases. Thus, failure to account for case mix differences leads to misleading inferences regarding returns to scale.

In all equations in Tables 8-5 and 8-6, the three service level dummy variables are negative and significant, suggesting that the omitted variable, Community Medical Center, significantly raises the intercept, as expected. It should also be noted that, as expected, the magnitudes

TABLE 8-5
Cost Function Estimates
(Standard Errors in Parentheses)

Independent Variables	Linear Equation			
	(1)	(2)	(3)	(4)
ADM	.0047	−.0053	.0056	−.0058
	(.0028)	(.0031)	(.0032)	(.0034)
FLOW	−6.6437**	−4.8662**	−7.9077**	−5.1900**
	(.8138)	(.9190)	(.8628)	(.9699)
SERVICE$_1$ (Basic)	−328.3520**	−248.1328**		
	(48.6617)	(48.8075)		
SERVICE$_2$ (Quality)	−292.3359**	−215.5719**		
	(43.4683)	(44.2670)		
SERVICE$_3$ (Complex)	−246.8356**	−180.6063**		
	(37.1920)	(37.8657)		
SERVICE$_4$ (Guttman)			15.4882**	10.5216**
			(3.7748)	(3.4334)
URBAN	105.4337**	100.0621**	119.1642**	122.2923**
	(35.7839)	(34.7446)	(37.6087)	(35.2060)
CASEM$_1$ (Principal component 1)		−33.5091**		−21.6935
		(11.1899)		(11.4129)
CASEM$_2$ (Principal component 2)		55.4870**		56.4527**
		(13.9545)		(14.5118)
CASEM$_3$ (Principal component 3)		−67.7004**		−90.7877**
		(13.4322)		(12.8789)
CASEM$_4$ (Principal component 4)		−16.9687		−11.0272
		(11.7080)		(12.1318)
CASEM$_5$ (Principal component 5)		−44.0417**		−54.6116**
		(11.7193)		(12.0045)
CASEM$_6$ (Principal component 6)		14.1172		14.9493
		(10.6344)		(11.3028)
CASEM$_7$ (Principal component 7)		25.7664*		26.3657
		(10.6251)		(11.2335)
CASEM$_8$ (Principal component 8)		8.1891		19.4866
		(11.1391)		(11.3755)
CASEM$_9$ (Principal component 9)		−6.5547		−10.0106
		(10.8513)		(11.2804)
CASEM$_{10}$ (Principal component 10)		***		14.7097
				(11.0529)
CASEM$_{11}$ (Principal component 11)		4.4811		10.4250
		(10.7475)		(11.0225)
CASEM$_{12}$ (Principal component 12)		−9.7361		−12.4263
		(10.3293)		(10.9667)
Constant	1119.0531	1063.3824	708.1334	746.0285
R^2	.5853	.6976	.4939	.6620
S.E.E.	152.8456	134.9945	167.8711	142.2578
N.	176	176	176	176

*Significant at the .05 level.
**Significant at the .01 level.
***Did not enter into equation due to insufficient E. level.

TABLE 8-6
Cost Function Estimates
(Standard Error in Parentheses)

Independent Variables	Linear Equation			
	(1)	(2)	(3)	(4)
ADM	.0054*	−.0033	.0064*	−.0031
	(.0027)	(.0030)	(.0029)	(.0031)
OCCUP	−232.3243*	−224.1216*	−346.1718**	−265.5317**
	(90.7261)	(87.9265)	(91.7562)	(88.8826)
LOS	63.6787**	52.2715**	72.7082**	56.5569**
	(5.8883)	(6.5164)	(5.5958)	(6.5562)
SERVICE₁ (Basic)	−216.4829**	−206.6240**		
	(47.2087)	(45.6178)		
SERVICE₂ (Quality)	−189.5172**	−167.5852**		
	(42.4023)	(42.4991)		
SERVICE₃ (Complex)	−164.1115**	−126.8893**		
	(36.3432)	(36.9616)		
SERVICE₄ (Guttman)			10.5092**	9.3874**
			(3.3659)	(3.1125)
URBAN	140.0613**	139.3256**	154.5971**	162.7209**
	(32.9389)	(32.4103)	(32.6503)	(31.9793)
CASEM₁ (Principal component 1)		−38.5415**		−28.2853**
		(9.8513)		(9.8537)
CASEM₂ (Principal component 2)		42.0115**		43.0027**
		(13.0563)		(13.2097)
CASEM₃ (Principal component 3)		−46.3254**		−58.4762**
		(13.1650)		(12.7242)
CASEM₄ (Principal component 4)		−6.7799		−2.7113
		(10.2660)		(10.3917)
CASEM₅ (Principal component 5)		−43.5328**		−50.0091*
		(10.8030)		(10.8269)
CASEM₆ (Principal component 6)		−9.9996		−11.4227
		(10.4989)		(10.8475)
CASEM₇ (Principal component 7)		16.7026		16.4290
		(9.8987)		(10.1964)
CASEM₈ (Principal component 8)		4.2966		10.5446
		(10.1899)		(10.1926)
CASEM₉ (Principal component 9)		20.3977*		18.5515
		(9.6848)		(9.8388)
CASEM₁₀ (Principal component 10)		2.6252		12.4044
		(10.0423)		(9.9706)
CASEM₁₁ (Principal component 11)		−1.9883		2.4849
		(9.6192)		(9.6934)
CASEM₁₂ (Principal component 12)		−4.3945		−6.7981
		(9.4198)		(9.7858)
Constant	482.4874	592.9658	185.1587	312.4477
R²	.6594	.7491	.6290	.7305
S.E.E.	138.9441	123.7401	144.1453	127.4384
N.	176	176	176	176

*Significant at the .05 level.
**Significant at the .01 level.

> *The positive (simple) correlation between unit cost and volume (size) is due to larger hospitals treating relatively more costly cases. Thus, failure to account for case mix differences leads to misleading inferences regarding returns to scale.*

of the three coefficients correspond to the relative complexities of the service groups; that is, the basic dummy has the largest negative coefficient (−248), followed by the quality (−216) and complex (−181) dummies, respectively.

The metropolitan coefficient is positive and significant. Since case mix and service mix are controlled, it is likely that the "net effect" of urban location is due to relative wage levels.

THE CASE FLOW VARIABLE

The case flow variable (Table 8-5) has, as expected, a negative (and significant) coefficient. A unit increase in case flow will decrease per admission cost in the case flow equation by $4.87, when case mix is controlled. This could take place through a reduction in length of stay, an increase in occupancy, or both. The following identity relates case flow to occupancy and length of stay:

$$\text{FLOW} = \frac{365}{\text{LOS}} \text{OCCUP}$$

If length of stay is held constant, it can be shown a ten-unit increase in case flow (resulting in a $48.70 reduction in cost per admission) would require an increase in occupancy of 0.175 to 0.845 at the mean. Thus, leaving length of stay unchanged, an 18 percentage point increase in average occupancy (to 85 percent) would be sufficient to decrease unit cost by about $50 (from $735, at the mean, to $685). This assumes no indirect effect on cost of providing other hospital services through increased occupancy.

Alternatively, holding occupancy constant, length of stay would have to decrease by 1.7 days, to 4.7 days at the mean, for an equivalent reduction in cost. This substantial decrease in average stay does not appear feasible. However, if length of stay were moderately decreased to six days (a decrease of 0.4 days), an increase in occupancy of 0.13, to 0.80 at the mean, would drop average cost $50. Given current levels of input prices, moderately increasing controls on length of stay while restricting future bed growth could pay substantial dividends in reducing the cost of a hospital stay. At the mean, this represents a seven percent savings for each admission. In 1977 dollars, this savings would be approximately $90 per admission, or about $290 million statewide (California) out of an aggregate $4.5 billion expenditure.

Obviously, it is quite unrealistic to vary such an important variable as length of stay while assuming other variables remain constant. Length of stay is an input into the patient's recovery, and is to some degree a substitute for other inputs (e.g., nursing care, certain ancillary services). Thus, cutting length of stay, *holding case mix constant,* would imply raising the input of other factors (e.g., nursing care) and would reduce occupancy. The numerical examples given here are given only to

---

> **Given current levels of input prices, moderately increasing controls on length of stay while restricting future bed growth could pay substantial dividends in reducing the cost of a hospital stay.**

---

illustrate uses of the cost function. (A more complete model would treat the relationships between length of stay and other inputs into the patient's recovery in the context of the production function for health.)[18]

LENGTH OF STAY AND OCCUPANCY VARIABLES

We now consider the equation treating length of stay and occupancy as separate variables (see Table 8-6). Both coefficients are significant. The occupancy coefficient (with case mix controlled) suggests an increase in occupancy of 0.1 (ten percentage points) will decrease average case cost by $22. An increase of 0.175, as in the case flow example, will decrease unit costs by $39, as opposed to the suggested $49 in the previous (case flow) equation. It should be noted that with length of stay held constant, there could be a relationship between case difficulty and occupancy, but this is not expected *a priori*.

The length of stay coefficient suggests a one-day decrease will decrease unit costs by $52. A 1.7-day decrease will decrease costs by $89, considerably more than implied by the case flow equation. To reduce costs per case by $49, occupancy would thus have to increase 12.5

percentage points, nearly identical to the 13 percentage points suggested in the case flow equation. Treating length of stay and occupancy as separate regressors, as opposed to including the case flow variable, has the effect of assigning relatively greater sensitivity to length of stay. This is consistent with Feldstein's observation.[19]

CASE FLOW VARIABLE PREFERRED

It is not clear which configuration should be preferred. The major argument against using the case flow variable as a regressor is that its numerator is the denominator of the dependent variable; thus, it is not exogenous. Recognizing that case flow is endogenous, Feldstein obtained instrumental variable estimates (which "correct" the endogenous variables for error).[20] These estimates were similar to his ordinary least squares estimates. These characteristics also apply to the individual occupancy and length of stay variables, with the additional problem that occupancy relates to patient days, while we are defining "output" as the case; occupancy would be more appropriate in a cost per patient day equation. Moreover, length of stay is definitionally related to the dependent variable. On the basis of these admittedly weak criteria, case flow is selected as the preferable capacity utilization variable. Moreover, case flow can be interpreted as "turnover" which has, *a priori*, a negative correlation with unit cost.

EFFECT OF CASE MIX ON ADMISSIONS COEFFICIENT

Four to five case mix components are significant in the equations in Tables 8-5 and 8-6. The underlying nature of each component is not known and requires further investigation. The most notable result is the effect of inclusion of the case mix components on the admissions coefficient. These variables have the effect of changing the admissions coefficient from positive (and significant in several cases) to essentially zero (and insignificant). The implication is larger hospitals treat relatively more complex and costly cases. Controlling for service mix alone is not sufficient to nullify the effect of size. (The admissions variable picks up correlation with the case mix variables, to the extent of making admissions insignificant.)

SERVICE MIX VARIABLES

A strong intuitive case could be advanced suggesting that large hospitals are more costly than small hospitals because they are *prepared* to offer more complex services. In fact, the service mix variables used here only measure what services hospitals are capable of providing, and not the volume of each service provided.

Berry suggested that the most important factor in hospital costliness is what hospitals gear up to produce and not what is actually produced. This is due to high fixed costs of most services and facilities. This suggestion resulted from alternatively fitting equations including case mix variables (and excluding service mix variables) and equations including service mix variables (and excluding case mix variables) to data from the same hospitals (57 New England hospitals). The equation including service mix variables had a higher R^2.[21]

On the basis of the "better explanatory power" of the equations using services, Berry concluded that what hospitals "gear up to do" is more important, with respect to costs, than what they actually "end up doing." Our results suggest that case mix, while not contributing substantially to explained variation, does have a profound effect on the cost model by eliminating the positive relationship between average cost and size (or output)—a positive relationship that holds when only service mix is controlled. In any event, these results indicate that controlling only for what hospitals are "geared up" to do is not sufficient.

EFFECT OF PATIENT MIX

Results of estimation of linear equations using the Guttman service index rather than the three Berry dummy variables, are similar (see Tables 8-5 and 8-6). The Guttman index is significant in both equations. In these equations, the same pattern emerges; inclusion of the patient mix components causes the admissions coefficient to fall to zero. In these equations the occupancy coefficient is slightly larger (266 versus 224) as is the length of stay coefficient (57 versus 52).

Table 8-7 presents estimates for the Table 8-5 equation, excluding the service mix variables. Note that in the first-step equation, the scale coefficient is highly significant, positive and relatively large (the equivalent scale coefficient in Table 8-5 when service mix and case mix are included is −.005), where service mix but not case mix is controlled. As the case mix components are added, the coefficient falls and becomes insignifi-

TABLE 8-7

Cost Function Estimates

(Standard Errors in Parentheses)

Independent Variables	Linear Equation	
	(1)	(2)
ADM	0.0142**	−0.0014
	(0.0025)	(0.0032)
FLOW	−8.7200**	−5.6016**
	(0.8775)	(0.9854)
URBAN	127.0578**	
	(39.2503)	
CASEM₁ (Principal component 1)		−21.4482
		(11.7081)
CASEM₂ (Principal component 2)		63.3989**
		(14.7047)
CASEM₃ (Principal component 3)		−97.3145**
		(13.0303)
CASEM₄ (Principal component 4)		−12.6949
		(12.4334)
CASEM₅ (Principal component 5)		−57.0423**
		(12.2884)
CASEM₆ (Principal component 6)		22.7203
		(11.2998)
CASEM₇ (Principal component 7)		31.0971**
		(11.4149)
CASEM₈ (Principal component 8)		17.0381
		(11.6411)
CASEM₉ (Principal component 9)		−11.7727
		(11.5574)
CASEM₁₀ (Principal component 10)		10.9288
		(11.2682)
CASEM₁₁ (Principal component 11)		10.3349
		(11.3079)
CASEM₁₂ (Principal component 12)		−8.1168
		(11.1578)
Constant	877.0274	864.6927
R²	0.4440	0.6421
S.E.E.	175.4285	145.9405
N.	176	176

**Significant at the .01 level.

cant. The size coefficient in the last-step equation is −0.001. If this is compared with the first-step equation admissions coefficient in Table 8-5, Column 1 (0.005), it is seen that patient mix is more effective than service mix in lowering the size coefficient. Thus, contrary to Berry's conclusion, what a hospital is geared up to do may not be more important in explaining average cost than what it actually does do; however, *both* effects must be considered. (The criterion adopted here for assessing the relative importance of the service mix and case mix variables is their effect on the admissions coefficient. *A priori,* it is suggested that average cost is positively related to output because larger hospitals treat more complex cases and if product dimension is sufficiently controlled, average cost should be constant, or even decrease with respect to output. It should also be noted that the equation in Table 8-7 including the case mix components has a standard error of 146, as opposed to 153 for the equation in Table 5, Column 1.

Quadratic average cost curves were estimated, yielding results that are reasonably consistent with the above. That is, when case mix is not controlled, linearly increasing costs throughout the sample are observed, but when case mix is controlled, costs are very slightly increasing for small- and medium-sized institutions but decreasing for large facilities.[22]

The results for all specifications are fairly consistent; that is: (1) when case mix is not controlled, unit costs appear to increase with size; (2) when case mix is controlled, unit cost appears to be unrelated to size, or at most, related through a primarily flat inverse U-shaped curve; and (3) service mix and case mix are highly significant and have separate effects that must be accounted for in cost function estimation.

Case mix and service mix have substantial and separate effects on the cost function; failure to control for both these factors yields estimates of returns to scale that may be biased toward decreasing returns (in our sample). Pre-vious studies do not account for case mix and service mix to the extent attempted in this study. In general, estimates obtained in previous studies, by not adequately controlling for product dimension, should be viewed as biased. Accounting for only one aspect of product dimension (e.g., case mix as opposed to service mix) is not sufficient; there still remains a substantial amount of unexplained variation in product dimension.

EFFECTS OF CONTROLLING FOR SERVICE AND CASE MIX

The cost function estimates described above suggest that when adjustments are made for service mix and case mix, size or volume does not greatly influence cost per case. Various specifications were estimated with results being fairly consistent. This research has shown that adjustments should be made for both service mix and case mix; adjusting for only one of these factors is not sufficient.

Adjusting for Service Mix Variation

Two alternative approaches were used to adjust for service mix variation. Three dummy variables indicating various levels of service, as developed by Berry, were included and performed well, in that: (1) their coefficients were significant at the 0.05 level; (2) their coefficients were negative, suggesting that the coefficient of the excluded variable (Community Medical Center) is positive; and (3) their inclusion caused the magnitude of the size coefficient to fall.[23] Moreover, these variables remained significant even after all 12 case mix components entered into the equation. The coefficients suggest the most complex institution (Community Medical Center) has the largest intercept.

The Guttman scale index also performed well, but was more sensitive to inclusion of the patient mix variables. Moreover, use of this type of variable in a regression is not as common as use of dummy variables, and scaling of qualitative variables is questionable.

Principal Components

The case mix principal components also performed well. At least four of the 12 components were statistically significant. Principal components have the advantage of being orthogonal to each other; thus, there is no multicollinearity between given components and certain independent variables. Inclusion of case mix components had the effect of offsetting the effect of scale or output, in some cases changing a positive scale coefficient to a negative one.

AN ALTERNATIVE APPROACH

Of the 44 principal components calculated, only the first 12, after which the eigenvalue drops below unity, were included in the regressions. An alternative approach would involve including all 44 components in a step-wise procedure, retaining only those that were statistically significant at, say, the 0.05 level. This approach, while no more arbitrary than the first, involves a process where different components would be included in different equations depending on the noncase mix variables included.

Moreover, in most cases no more than five components would be included and these components would account for less than 50 percent of the variation of all 44 components.

Principal components and factor analysis are exploratory techniques used when the researcher lacks a sound model of the structure under study. The economist justifies use of these techniques when the concern is with "noneconomic" variables about which an acceptable model is not expected to be formulated. Such is the case with medical variables. The approach used here seems to make statistical sense, but at this time the "structure" of each component defies explanation. Further work is necessary here. For example, medical experts could inspect each component for observable "clusters" of diagnoses.

THE INFORMATION THEORY INDEX

An interesting approach that should be further explored is the information theory index developed by Evans and Walker.[24] This technique enables summarization of diagnostic classifications into very few indexes, incorporating more information than can a small subset of principal components.

ECONOMIES OF SCALE

A review of the literature suggests that findings regarding possible economies of scale are inconsistent among the various studies. Our results, which are generally consistent across the different specifications estimated, suggest fairly constant returns to scale when account is taken of service mix *and* case mix. When case mix is not controlled, estimates suggest decreasing returns to scale.

COST FUNCTION AS A USEFUL TOOL

The cost function is a useful tool for evaluating hospital costs, considering a wide range of cost-influencing factors. It has particular value in forecasting unit costs, reviewing budgets, comparing costs among hospitals, establishing reimbursement rates, and so on. Moreover, the particular specification under consideration here allows determination of the effects of changes in diagnostic mix on cost per case.

While the exact composition of the case mix variables (principal components) is not immediately identifiable, they can be used in a straightforward manner to compare costs of hospitals with different mixes of patient types. This method of comparing hospital costs is more efficient than traditional methods of classifying hospitals into peer groups on the basis of, for example, size, location and teaching status. Although additional research on the cost model, as well as other grouping approaches, is necessary (i.e., cluster analysis), substantial use currently can be made of the cost function approach in comparing diverse institutions.

REFERENCES

1. Zaretsky, H. W. *Analysis of Hospital Costs Controlling for Service Mix and Case Mix.* (Sacramento, Ca.: California Hospital Association 1974b).

2. *Ibid.*

3. Feldstein, M. S. *Economic Analysis for Health Service Efficiency.* (Amsterdam: North Holland Publishing Company 1967).

4. Evans, R. G. " 'Behavioral' Cost Functions for Hospitals." *Canadian Journal of Economics,* 4 (May 1971) p. 148–215.

5. Lave, J. R., Lave, L. B. and Silverman, L. P. "Hospital Cost Estimation Controlling for Case Mix." *Applied Economics,* 4 (1972) p. 165–180.

6. Evans, R. G. and Walker, H. D. "Information Theory and the Analysis of Hospital Cost Structure." *Canadian Journal of Economics,* 5 (August 1972) p. 398–418.

7. Johnston, J. *Econometric Methods* (2nd ed. New York, N.Y.: McGraw-Hill 1972).

8. Harman, H. H. *Modern Factor Analysis* (Chicago, Ill.: University of Chicago Press 1960).

9. Edwards, M., Miller, J. D. and Schumacher, R. "Classification of Community Hospitals by Scope of Service: Four Indexes." *Health Services Research,* 7 (Winter 1972) p. 301–313.

10. *Ibid.*

11. Berry, R. E., Jr. "On Grouping of Hospitals for Economic Analysis." *Inquiry,* 10 (December 1973) p. 5–12.
12. *Ibid.*
13. Feldstein. *Economic Analysis for Health Service Efficiency.*
14. Zaretsky, H. W. *Development of a Financial Reporting System for Hospitals as a Basis for Regulation* (Sacramento, Ca.: California Hospital Association 1974a).
15. Walters, A. A. "Production and Cost Functions: an Econometric Survey." *Econometrica,* 31 (January–April 1963) p. 1–66.

16. Zaretsky, H. W. *Analysis of Hospital Costs.*
17. *Ibid.*
18. Grossman, M. *The Demand for Health: a Theoretical and Empirical Investigation* (New York, N.Y.: Columbia University Press 1972).
19. Feldstein. *Economic Analysis for Health Service.*
20. *Ibid.*
21. Berry, R. E., Jr. "Efficiency in the Production of Hospital Services: Progress Report." (March 25, 1970).
22. Zaretsky. *Analysis of Hospital Costs.*
23. Berry. "On Grouping of Hospitals."
24. Evans and Walker. "Information Theory."

15. HMO Performance: The Recent Evidence

MILTON I. ROEMER AND WILLIAM SHONICK

Reprinted with permission from *The Milbank Memorial Fund Quarterly/Health and Society* 51. Copyright © 1973, Milbank Memorial Fund 271-317.

Health maintenance organizations (HMOs) are being promoted as a strategy to modify the U.S. health care delivery system toward more economical patterns, encouraging preventive and ambulatory rather than costly hospital services. Evidence of HMO performance has accumulated over the years, much of it reviewed in 1969. Since then, additional evidence suggests that the "prepaid group practice" (PGP) model of HMO continues to yield lower hospital use, relatively more ambulatory and preventive service, and lower overall costs (counting both premiums and out-of-pocket expenditures) than conventional open-market fee-for-service patterns. Economies of scale in group practice per se are still not proved, but some evidence supports this theoretical hypothesis. New data point to reduced disability from the PGP model of HMO, as well as to more favorable consumer attitudes (based mainly on the economic advantages, in spite of certain impersonalities of clinics) than exist toward conventionally insured private solo practice. The medical care foundation (free choice of private practitioners with fee payments) model of HMO has yielded some evidence of economies in physician's care, but none in hospital use. HMOs entail hazards of underservicing and distorted risk-selection, but with appropriate public monitoring they constitute an approach to health planning, stressing local initiative, competition, and incentives to self-regulation.

Introduction

In a "health strategy" message of February, 1971, the President gave new prominence to an idea which had been evolving in the United States for half a century or more. Basically, the idea involves the assumption of responsibility for the health of a population by an organized entity, in consideration of a fixed, prepaid amount of money. Incentives to increase medical earnings through maximizing services are theoretically replaced by incentives to maximize earnings by prudent use of costly services. Initially a contentious deviance from the conventional open-market, fee-for-service concept of medical care, the idea gradually gained social acceptance in the 1950s and 1960s, as experience demonstrated that it could yield medical care of good quality at lower than prevailing average costs. By the 1970s, the spiraling of medical costs had become so alarming that a conservative federal administration decided to push the idea and to give it a glamorous new label: the "Health Maintenance Organization," or HMO.

Clearcut evidence of the effects of HMOs has not been abundant but it has gradually mounted. Avedis Donabedian (1969) published a comprehensive evaluation of the principal model of HMO—that based on group practice organization—and since that time additional evaluative evidence has accumulated. Most of this evidence compares the prepaid group practice (PGP) model with other patterns of health care delivery, but some of it concerns the model of the "medical care foundations," in which the key principles of HMOs are implemented under a pattern of physician's service offered through individual rather than group practices. This paper will review this recent evidence and offer interpretations of its meaning, with respect to social policy decisions on HMO strategy.

The definition of HMO applied here is an organization which:

(a) makes a contract with consumers (or employers on their behalf) to assure the delivery of stated health services of measurable quality;

(b) has an enrolled population;

(c) offers a stated broad range of personal health service benefits, including at least physician services and hospital care;

(d) is paid on an advance capitation basis.

Regarding element (c) in this definition, the investigations reviewed here have been applied to HMOs with rather widely varying scopes of benefits, not all of which offer protection for *all* physician and hospital services used or needed by a population. At this point, however, we believe there are lessons to be learned from study of some HMOs which may not fit perfectly under an ideal definition.

Since 1969, there have been published a number of other general review papers which examine the whole question of HMOs and their consequences: for health, economy, and other values. In offering this review we have naturally made use of these papers, in particular those by Herbert Klarman (1971), John Glasgow (1972), Merwyn Greenlick (1972), and Ira Greenberg and Michael Rodburg (1971) in the *Harvard Law Review*. We shall, of course, in addition review the main findings of several other studies reported separately.

The recent material has not only provided additional empirical evidence but has also extended and deepened our understanding of the various dimensions along which analysis must proceed if we are to infer, from the accumulated evidence, generalizations useful for social policy decisions.

Previous studies

Research on comparative performance under alternative forms of organization of medical care delivery had been going on with ever increasing frequency since the issuance of the final report of the Committee on the Costs of Medical Care (1932). Particular interest centered around the performance of prepaid group practice (PGP) as compared with other modalities for delivery of care. In attempting to design research which would provide information about these effects, the investigators were faced with evaluating a phenomenon whose input consisted of a number of different and perhaps separable factors and whose output similarly consisted of a number of separately identifiable elements.

On the *input side* have been included the factors of (a) prepayment by the subscriber, (b) practice in a group setting, (c) paying the physician by salary, and, in some cases, (d) owning or at least controlling the operation of the associated hospitals. Although each of these components was often present in the operation of a PGP, not all of them existed in "pure" form in every PGP studied. The degree to which each of these factors was present varied among the PGPs studied; attributing an appropriate aliquot part of the observed effect to these several input factors was often the aim of later research, using ever more refined designs.

Similarly, on the *output side,* the criteria to be applied in judging the effects produced by the PGP, as compared with alternative practice modalities, were increasingly broken down by researchers into more particular elements, such as patient satisfaction, effects on hospital use, and the like.

As the number of such studies proliferated, publications reporting their results began to be interspersed periodically with review articles summarizing and analyzing the current state of the findings on various facets of the question. In attempting to draw generalization about the performance of PGP from the published results, the several reviewers formulated various typologies for analysis.

The earlier reviews did not discuss in great detail the various components of PGP (noted above), in general considering all such organizations to be members of one generic group. These earlier evaluation articles each focused on some particular aspect of the performance results of PGP, as compared with alternative forms of organization of practice. Klarman's initial review (1963) addressed itself to the effects of the PGP and other practice modalities upon hospital utilization; Weinerman (1964) dealt mainly with patients' perception of the medical care provided in prepaid group practice.

Donabedian's 1969 review constituted a landmark in its attempt to analyze the research results according to a broad series of criteria, considering the entire spectrum as the necessary basis for evaluating medical care system performance. He grouped these criteria, and the parameters for measuring them, as follows:

1. Patient satisfaction:
   frequency with which consumers choose PGP, when this
       choice is available
   expressed opinions of subscribers
   frequency of out-of-plan use by PGP members

2. Opinions of participating physicians:
   concerning conditions of medical practice
   concerning the nature and behavior of subscribers

3. Health service utilization rates:
   from hospital and insurance records
   from survey questionnaires to subscribers

4. Costs to patients:
   premiums paid (from insurance records and surveys)
   out-of-plan expenditures from surveys

5. Economic productivity:
   theoretical analysis of expectations
   economic analysis of empirical data

6. Quality of medical care:
   influence of pattern on ways of using medical services
       (through survey questionnaires)
   qualifications of physicians and hospitals used (from rec-
       ords and surveys)
   physician performance (from direct observation and "au-
       dits" of medical records)

7. Ultimate health outcomes:
   mortality rates on matched samples

Format of the present study

While this Donabedian analysis, in its multifaceted approach to PGP performance, was the most comprehensive up to 1969, it was based entirely on the author's study of previous individual investigations which he had identified and considered relevant. Indeed, Donabedian specifically states that his "review was made without reference to Klarman's 1963 and Weinerman's 1964 reviews . . ." referred to earlier in this paper.

The present review will consider the evidence on HMO performance that has been newly accumulated since the Donabedian paper, along with material that he did not include, especially from the Klarman (1963) and the Weinerman (1964) papers. In the light of present-day perspectives on HMOs, our analysis will be classified along somewhat different evaluative categories, as follows:

1. Subscriber composition
2. Participation of physicians

3. Utilization rates
4. Quality assessments
5. Costs and productivity
6. Health status outcomes
7. Patient attitudes

With respect to each of these features, we will attempt to report empirical findings under both the PGP and the "medical care foundation" (MCF) models of HMO. Finally, we will offer a few interpretive comments about the apparent need for surveillance of HMOs, the implications for comprehensive health planning, and the indications for further required research.

Subscriber Composition

The performance of HMOs will naturally be influenced by the composition of their memberships. Rates of utilization, costs, health status outcomes, and other measures for evaluation are inevitably influenced by the demographic composition of HMO members, their pre-existing medical conditions, and related factors.

A. T. Moustafa et al. (1971) reported on the characteristics of persons choosing among a series of five health insurance plans, two of which represented the PGP model (Kaiser-Permanente Health Plan or Ross-Loos Medical Group Plan). They found that married persons with children, in contrast to single persons, were more likely to choose the more comprehensive HMO-type plans, but that, otherwise, educational or income levels showed no significant relationship to plan choice. When, for some reason, persons changed their plan affiliation (at an annual open-enrollment period), those in comprehensive benefit plans—whether HMO-type or commercial insurance with wide benefits—were most likely to shift to another plan of comprehensive benefit scope.

The social acceptance of the idea of group medical practice, in contrast to the traditional pattern of individual practice, was investigated over several years in three cities (Detroit, Cleveland, and Cincinnati) by C. A. Metzner et al. (1972). A substantial majority of persons surveyed expressed preference for the idea of getting their care through group practice arrangements, even though many had no actual experience with such arrangements. The preference tended to prevail for all demographic breakdowns but was somewhat stronger in persons of higher educational and middle income levels. While this study did not explore *prepaid* group practice, the findings would seem to have implications for the HMO model as well.

Virtually all the investigations cited in the review by E. R. Weinerman (1964) were included by Donabedian (1969), and we shall not repeat them here. However, Weinerman's own analytic contribution is worth noting. He drew these inferences on the initial choices, among different patterns of delivery, made by subscribers to health insurance plans (Weinerman, 1964: 882):

> The fee-for-service plans still attract a majority of workers in a dual choice situation, especially when their benefits are broad in scope. The advantages of initial enrollment have been indicated. Certainly, the organizational effort preceding the election date is of enormous impact. . . . The group practice method is still new and unfamiliar to most patients and to most doctors. . . . The comparative advantages of group practice health plan benefits are often complex and difficult for the average worker to decipher. Most significant is the repeated observation that enrollees respond primarily to the prospect of comprehensive benefits, and seem less concerned with the alternative of group versus solo practice.

It would seem to follow that greater familiarity with the PGP pattern is likely to increase the tendency of persons to like it, in spite of some of the impersonal "public clinic" connotations of *large* group practices.

In 1973, there were reported, for the first time, the actual characteristics of random samples of *total memberships* enrolled in various types of insurance organization, including HMO models. Studying health insurance plans in southern California in 1968, Roemer et al. (1973) found that significantly higher proportions of persons with generally greater risk of sickness were members of PGP organizations than were in commercial insurance or provider-sponsored (Blue Cross and Blue Shield) plans. This was reflected by slightly higher proportions of plan members aged 41 years and over, substantially higher proportions of families with a history of one or more chronic illnesses (60.6 percent in PGP plans, in contrast to 46.6 percent and 37.4 percent in the two open-market plan-types), and somewhat greater proportions of persons scoring high on a "symptom sensitivity" test. They also found a slightly greater proportion of foreign-born and nonwhite persons in the HMO-type plans, although the average family incomes in those plans, paradoxically, was slightly higher ($11,309 compared with $10,987 and $10,398 in the other two plan-types).

These studies suggest that any advantages that may be found for HMO-type plans, in terms of lower costs or better health status outcomes (as reflected in the pre-1969 research reports), cannot be attributed to their containing a smaller membership of high-risk persons, but would seem to be associated with the opposite.

With respect to the medical care foundation model of HMO, we have found, unfortunately, no documentation on the nature of its subscriber composition. We can only point out that the MCFs operate predominantly in relatively small counties of low urbanization. Moreover, as Richard H. Egdahl (1973) notes, a major share of member composition in many foundations has been derived from Medicare and Medicaid beneficiaries in recent years.

Participation of Physicians

The performance of HMOs is bound to be influenced by the qualifications of physicians as well as of other personnel entering this pattern of health service. It is also likely to be influenced by the satisfaction of professional personnel with their general conditions of work (including earnings) in this setting.

Prepaid group practice

Careful investigation of the qualifications of doctors in PGP (compared with others) has not been made, except for what may be inferred from the espoused policies of PGP organizations. The policies of large HMO models, like the Health Insurance Plan of Greater New York (HIP) and the Kaiser-Permanente Plan, are believed to result in careful selection of properly qualified specialists for all positions requiring specialty status (Greenberg and Rodburg, 1971). Insofar as general practitioners are selected for primary care, qualifications under the new specialty board in family medicine are encouraged. Similarly rigorous criteria for appointment, however, evidently do not apply to all HMOs, such as some of the new ones with small group practice units organized mainly to serve Medicaid beneficiaries in California (Nelson, 1973).

Empirical studies have recently been made regarding the satisfaction of physicians with the conditions of work in PGP. The earlier literature on group medical practice gave the impression that, with or without prepayment, difficulties and dissatisfactions were rampant (Dickinson and Bradley, 1952). D. M. Du Bois (1970) studied in 1966 a small series of private group practices that failed and disintegrated, comparing them with a series of private group practices that grew and prospered; he concluded that organizational failure was mainly associated with "policies in conflict with the professional role"—in a word, commercialization. Other relevant factors were a hostile professional environment and poor administrative management.

Based on a national survey in 1970 of private multispecialty medical group practices, Laurence D. Prybil (1971) found that the annual turnover rate—a long-used index of job dissatisfaction—was less than 5 percent. The respondents were from institutional members of the American Association of Medical Clinics $(N = 237)$, a series that might admittedly be expected to have especially high stability. Even this low rate of turnover, however, seemed to be declining; it involved physicians mainly under 45 years of age, and most of those who left went to other positions in organized settings rather than into solo practice. Low turnover was also confirmed by the study of Austin Ross (1969), who found problems of remuneration in group practices to be the major cause of departure. David Mechanic (1972) in a recent national survey also found high rates of satisfaction in group practice—95 percent were either "very" or "fairly" satisfied (over 50 percent were "very satisfied") —with no differences evident in comparison to satisfaction with solo practice. Of course, one may infer that only those physicians who like the concept enter group practice in the first place.

Focusing more specifically on *prepaid* group practice, Mechanic found these doctors most satisfied of all subgroups with opportunities for professional contacts, total time of work required, and leisure opportunities; they were least satisfied with respect to time available per patient, income level, office facilities, and community status. Nevertheless, in aggregate "general satisfaction with one's practice," the PGP physicians reported "very satisfied" in 52 percent of the cases, which was precisely the same percentage as reported by fee-for-service solo practitioners. A turnover study in the Northern California Kaiser-Permanente PGP over the period 1966–1970 by Wallace H. Cook (1971), reported under 10 percent departures per year for employed doctors and less than 2 percent for Permanente Group partners.

Considering the socially marginal character of prepaid group practice in American medical culture, the remarkable point would seem to be how little dissatisfaction is evident among physicians who have "bucked the tide" and engaged in this pattern of work. One can readily speculate that, with the steady growth of open-market private group practice (now up to about 20 percent of clinical physicians, according to the AMA Survey reported in 1972) and the general national promotion of the HMO idea, participation in PGP will become regarded as less and less "deviant," will attract more doctors, and will become associated with greater stability.

Medical care foundations

In regard to the medical care foundation HMO pattern, participation of physicians is, of course, open to all members of local medical societies. Except for young physicians-in-training, doctors in full-time research, education, or administration, and some physicians in full-time salaried hospital employment, one may assume that local medical societies (not necessarily the American Medical Association or the black physicians' National Medical Association) contain in their memberships virtually all private clinical practitioners in their areas. In the Physicians' Association of Clackamas County, Oregon, for example, it is reported (Bechtol, 1972) that all but two members of the County Medical Association participate in the foundation. Such widespread participation, of course, implies wide free choice for patients, but says nothing about the specialty or other technical qualifications of the physicians, beyond the licensure and "ethical" requirements for medical society membership.

Studies of the San Joaquin County Foundation for Medical Care by the UCLA School of Public Health cast some light on the participation of these physicians in the care of Medicaid beneficiaries. One study (Gartside and Proctor, 1970) found a higher proportion (85 percent versus 78 percent) of all physicians and particularly of certain qualified specialists (strikingly so in pediatrics and obstetrics) from the foundation area to be serving Medicaid patients than in a closely matched comparison county (Ventura) without a medical foundation. Another UCLA study (Roemer and Gartside, 1973) found that, in the performance of surgical operations, the work was more often done by properly qualified surgeons in the San Joaquin Foundation area than in the comparison county. These findings would suggest that, in the nonmetropolitan type of county where medical foundations have tended to develop, they exert a positive influence on the qualifications of doctors serving the poor; similar disciplinary influence might possibly apply to the care of all patients in foundation-type HMOs.

Utilization Rates

The data on differential utilization rates for health services under HMOs, compared with other medical care arrangements, have continued to accumulate. One of the principal advantages long claimed for the HMO model, of course, has been its association with relatively lower use of expensive hospital days, resulting in substantial cost savings. Before reviewing the recently produced data on this (and other) utilization features, we should consider some of the earlier interpretations of them not included in the benchmark Donabedian paper of 1969.

Hospital utilization

The Klarman review (1963) was one of the earlier assessments of the general influence of health insurance on hospital utilization. Some of his interpretations, not reported in the Donabedian review (1969), should be cited. Drawing upon the studies of Osler Peterson in the United States and of G. Forsythe and R. Logan in Great Britain, Klarman noted that the concern of the 1930s about underutilization of hospitals shifted, in the 1960s, to concern about overutilization. Which concern is "correct," he notes, cannot be determined, since no objective standards for "proper" utilization exist. This implies that lower hospital utilization rates cannot appropriately be used as evidence of good performance without reference to what type of utilization is being reduced—"necessary" or "excess." Donabedian (1969) attempted to address this question by pointing to studies which analyzed certain aspects of hospital utilization between different practice modalities, in particular the diagnostic composition of this differential. Although the final verdict is far from being rendered, the prevailing pattern in the various studies of admission rates for the Health Insurance Plan of New York (HIP), as compared with other types of practice organization in New York City, was substantially lower in precisely those diagnostic categories most often suspected to comprise unnecessary admissions—tonsillectomies and upper respiratory infections.

There are two additional analytic points covered by Klarman (1963) which were either omitted or skimmed over by Donabedian. One concerns the early findings of 1940–1946 that Blue Cross–insured persons had higher hospital admission rates and lower average lengths of stay than did the general United States population. The other was the finding that, although HIP subscribers experienced lower hospitalization rates than persons under Blue Shield–Blue Cross, they showed the same rates as persons who used a union self-insured plan for ambulatory care. In the latter comparison, both the HIP subscribers and the self-insured union members used a self-insured hospital plan, leading to a hypothesis that control, specifically, of hospital use is a deciding factor. This is an important point, since it represents an attempt at identifying which structural variables in PGP affected which output results.

M. I. Roemer and M. Shain (1959) had reviewed the available evidence up to that time on hospital utilization under insurance. They conceptualized the determinants both of rates of hospital admission and hospital days in an area as derived from three sets of influences operative under conditions of economic support through insurance:

1. Patient determinants:
    incidence and prevalence of illness
    attitudes towards illness
    cost of medical care to the patient
    marital status
    housing and social level

2. Hospital determinants:
    supply of beds
    efficiency of bed utilization
    mechanisms of hospital remuneration
    availability of alternative bed facilities
    outpatient services

3. Physician determinants:
    supply of physicians
    method of medical remuneration
    nature of community medical practice
    medical policies in the hospital
    level of medical alertness
    medical teaching needs

Roemer and Shain speculated that, while all these factors must theoretically exert an influence under the cost-easing operation of insurance (and there was support from empirical data for the influence of most of these factors), the most pragmatically effective mechanism of *control* was probably through constraints on the supply of hospital beds, that is, the bed-population ratio in an area. As we shall see, the subsequent findings on hospital utilization under the HMO models have continued to point to the bed supply as an important explanatory variable. The enactment of "certificate of need" laws on hospital construction in some 20 states, moreover, seems to reflect a growing consensus on the importance of the influence of bed supply on bed demand, with obvious implications for community costs (American Hospital Association, 1972).

Subsequent to the Donabedian review, additional publications dealing with hospital utilization levels of HMOs continued to accumulate. These consisted both of additional reports of empirical results and newer evaluative and analytic works.

Another Klarman paper (1970) concentrates its analysis upon "expected savings in health services expenditures" from the PGP pattern, thus again exploring the general criterion of his 1963 paper. Reviewing again the HIP studies summarized in the Donabedian review, Klarman clarifies certain aspects of the unavoidable confounding of the many causative (independent or input) variables in those studies that resulted from the special circumstances of the HIP structure and the New York City location. Included in these variables are group practice organization; prepayment by the subscriber; capitation payments to the 30-odd medical groups, accompanied by the diverse methods of payment by the groups to the physicians; the use of part-time as well as full-time physicians; the unique nature of the New York municipal hospital system; and the limited access which HIP physicians had to community hospital beds. From these studies, as well as others involving Kaiser-Permanente, Klarman concludes that the evidence indicates that limiting physicians' access to hospital beds has been an important factor in keeping the utilization of hospitals low under the PGP pattern.

Hill and Veney (1970) offer new empirical evidence from a Kansas Blue Cross–Blue Shield experiment on insured outpatient benefits. This experiment confirmed earlier evidence supporting the proposition that increased ambulatory insurance benefits per se for patients lead to no reduction in hospital use and, in fact, result in at least a temporary increase of such use. These findings, Klarman argues, effectively rule out the availability of ambulatory care benefits as an explanatory cause for the reduced hospital utilization generally experienced by PGP organizations.

Besides limiting access to beds, Klarman notes that the salary or capitation forms of paying the physician may reasonably be expected to contribute to decreased hospital utilization on theoretical economic grounds. He cites the work of Monsma (1970), who showed that fee-for-service physicians derive a marginal increment in earnings for the performance of additional service (surgery, for example) while capitation payments (and salary) do not offer such an increment. This theory fits the findings noted in Donabedian's review that the excess hospitalization of the fee-for-service arrangement over that of PGP care modalities is centered in surgical diagnoses, particularly in tonsillectomies, cholecystectomies, "female surgery," and appendectomies. It is also supported by Bunker's findings (1970) that surgery rates are much lower in England (where there are relatively fewer surgeons, most of whom are on salary) than in the United States.

Klarman's most recent review (1971) broadened the field surveyed from PGP to the generalized HMO concept. Thus, besides reporting on some additional research and giving further analysis of PGP experience, he considered the data on medical care foundations reported in the literature and analyzed the factors in the MCF form of organization which might affect performance. Dealing with savings on hospital utilization under PGP, Klarman has summarized some of these results in the following generalizations: (1) It has been widely held, based on the implications of two HIP studies conducted in the 1950s, that there is a saving of about 20 percent in patient days and admission rates under PGP plans, compared to other health insurance plans; and (2) These results have been "subsequently reinforced in several ways."

Most of the "reinforcing" studies discussed by Klarman were cited and described by Donabedian in 1969, but there have since been additional ones. Moreover, Shapiro (1971) estimated a 25 percent lower rate of hospital utilization for HIP compared with other matched subscribers.

The Social Security Administration (1971) reported that per capita medical *expenditures* for hospital use were, respectively, 18 percent and 11 percent lower in northern and in southern California for Kaiser-Permanente, compared with care under other auspices. While these differentials are for expenditures rather than for use, it is probably safe to assume that they reflect patient-days utilized as well as possible differences in per diem costs. In any case, Klarman discusses this finding under his "utilization" category. A surprising datum in this same report is that HIP per capita Medicare expenditures did not differ from those for care under other auspices. Klarman speculates that this may be due to unreported utilization by the over-65 age group in the New York City municipal hospital system. He also notes that the differential in hospital utilization between HIP subscribers and other persons, reported in the past, was always quite small in the over-65 age group. If the zero difference currently reported by the Social Security Administration (SSA) is not due to an easing of HIP physician accessibility to beds, then the possibility exists that the difference in under-65 hospital utilization has been considerably greater than 20 percent.

A newly issued and more complete report by George St. J. Perrott (1971), describing the experience of the Federal Employee Health Program for the years 1961 through 1968, focuses mainly on hospital utilization among 8,000,000 federal employees insured under different types of plans throughout the country. Over these years, the rates for both hospital admissions and aggregate patient-days in the prepaid group practice plans have consistently remained the lowest, compared with the open-market "Blue" or commercial indemnity plans. These variations have prevailed for each age-sex level examined separately; they are especially striking for elective surgical admissions (such as tonsillectomy, appendectomy, and gynecological surgery).

Klarman (1971:29) notes, as a conclusion of his overall studies, that increasingly he has "come to single out the control exercised through bed supply" as a potent determinant of hospital use in the observed experience of PGP models, compared with that of other modes of health care organization.

"Foundations" and hospital use

Turning to the medical care foundation form of HMO, Klarman in his 1971 review notes that savings from reduced hospital utilization should not be expected from this form of organization on both theoretical and empirical grounds, although thus far evidence for the latter is slim. Since the prevailing method of payment to the physician under the MCF type of HMO is fee-for-service, there remains the incentive for the physician of higher income for additional services, according to Monsma's type of analysis. While the MCF type of HMO does not alter the method of paying the physician, it does broaden the ambulatory service benefits available to the subscriber. Empirical results have failed to indicate that such a broadening lowers hospital utilization rates. In addition to the Kansas findings of the Hill and Veney study (1970), Klarman also reminds us of the Avnet study (1967) for Group Health Insurance (GHI) in New York and of the reported results from extended out-of-hospital Blue Shield benefits offered in Maryland and described by Kelly (1965). All of these substantiated the theoretical expectations of no decrease (and, indeed, an increase) in hospital utilization when "physician services are broadened in a solo practice fee-for-service setting." In the Saskatchewan setting, Roemer (1958) had reported the same finding—increased hospital use associated with prepaid comprehensive doctor's care, compared with no insurance for ambulatory care—as far back as the late 1950s.

In recent years, further data on hospital utilization continued to be reported. Another study of government employees (state, rather than federal) insured under different types of health plan was reported from California (Medical Advisory Council to the California Public Employees Retirement System, 1971). Hospital utilization findings in this PERS (Public Employees Retirement System) study corresponded generally with those found for federal employees, with aggregate days per 1,000 per year being much lower than PGP plans. Unlike the federal study, the California one also reported utilization under the medical care foundation plans, which are relatively numerous in this state. Interestingly, the utilization rates for both hospital days and ambulatory doctor visits were *higher* under the foundation-type plans than for any of the other plan-types. The experience applied to a 12-month period in 1962–1963.

Still another comparison of hospital utilization under the PGP type of HMO with other types of health insurance plan in California is given by Roemer et al. (1973). This study examined the experience of random samples of the total memberships of the three main types of plan, selecting two examples of each type. In contrast to some others, this study found the differential for hospital admission rates to be relatively small, but, because of a very short length of hospital stay under the PGP plans, the differential in aggregate hospital days was great—526 days per 1,000 per year in the PGP plans, compared to 864 and 1,109 days in the commercial and provider-sponsored plans, respectively. In this investigation, out-of-plan hospital use (determined through study of a subsample) was found to involve 7.2 percent of the admissions, many of them for maternity care (short-stay cases). These cases, unlike those in the earlier Densen studies of HIP experience, however, are included within the group practice hospitalization rates reported above.

Roemer et al. (1973) also analyzed hospital utilization according to several demographic breakdowns. It became evident that the low use rate (in days per 1,000 per year) of the group practice or HMO-type plans was largely referable to the experience of families with dependents and families of other than Protestant faith. With respect to social class (as measured by educational attainment and occupation), hospital day rates in all plan-types were consistently higher in the lower-class group, but the markedly lower rate under the HMO-type plans prevailed for both social classes. The same was true of families with and without a history of chronic illness—much greater hospital use in the "chronically ill" families, but markedly fewer days in the HMO-type plans for both types of families.

Interpretations of hospital experience

The total complex of causes contributing to the lower use rates of hospital days in the PGP type of HMO remains a matter for discussion and research. As noted earlier, the absence of fee incentives, especially for elective surgical operations, has been credited by much of the data (and theoretically justified by Monsma). Easier financial (if not geographic) accessibility to ambulatory care under these plans has also been considered causative, but both the findings of the California PERS study (Medical Advisory Council, 1971) and the numerous studies of ambulatory care insurance for private doctor's care in Kansas, Saskatchewan, Maryland, and elsewhere, reported above, would not seem to support this contention. The constraint exercised by a limited hospital bed–population ratio, however, in the PGP plans would seem to be clear. The less-than-average supply of hospital beds in the Kaiser-Permanente Health Plan (below 2.0 per 1,000 members) obviously places an upper limit on the number of hospital days of care that can be provided. Striking evidence of this influence of bed supply is furnished by the differentials noted earlier in this paper on hospital expenditures for Medicare beneficiaries in the Kaiser-Permanente Health Plan in 1971, compared with other California Medicare beneficiaries; on the other hand, in HIP of New York, where the Medicare members use ordinary community hospitals, their hospital use expenditures were just the same as those of non-HIP Medicare beneficiaries (Social Security Administration, 1971). The degree to which this latter finding is due to the "opening up" of HIP physician accessibility to community hospital beds in New York, or to the other factors which Klarman postulates, cannot be determined on the basis of available data.

The point is that PGP doctors can evidently "live with" a constrained bed supply; they adjust by being prudent on hospital admissions, doing the maximum diagnostic workups on an outpatient basis, and keeping patients hospitalized for relatively short stays. Whether this results in better or poorer health for the patient is a serious question yet to be answered (refer to the section on Health Outcomes). That it results in cost savings (refer to the section on Costs and Productivity) is beyond doubt.

Aside from the PERS study reviewed above, meaningful data on hospitalization under the medical care foundation model of HMO are sparse. The Physicians' Association of Clackamas County, Oregon (Haley, 1971), reported that for 1969–1970 the average length of stay of Clackamas County patients at one Portland hospital was 5.18 days, compared to 6.82 days for patients from metropolitan Portland. No other data about the characteristics of these patients or the rate of admissions are given; since Clackamas County is essentially suburban to Portland and since its population characteristics doubtless differ from those of the central city, it is difficult to interpret these figures.

A still unpublished study of the Clackamas County Foundation by the UCLA Survey Research Center (Berkanovic, 1973) gives other data on hospital utilization under this pattern. Based on 1971 experience of Medicaid beneficiaries enrolled in the Clackamas County foundation, the preliminary findings suggest a *higher* hospital utilization rate (by a factor of 1.5 to 2.0), in days per 1,000 persons covered per year compared with a Medicaid population in a neighboring county using open-market patterns without a foundation.

Ambulatory care utilization

Donabedian (1969) noted that the sparsely reported data on ambulatory care utilization tended to indicate that, in general, such utilization increased under plans which insured for out-of-hospital benefits. The increase, however, was no different under PGP than under fee-for-service private practice. Also, there seemed to be no evidence of flagrant or obvious overutilization of ambulatory services.

Klarman (1971) attempted to assess the import of various published reports on physician-population ratios, in an effort to arrive at generalizations about respective ambulatory care utilization rates in PGP and in other delivery forms. Physician-population ratios presumably give indirect evidence of patient-doctor contact rates—if productivity levels are assumed constant. Based on the reported evidence of physician-population ratios, Klarman noted the often contradictory results of published studies, beginning as far back as 1940. In some cases the savings, in terms of per capita expenditures for physician care, were found to be greater than the proportionately lower physician-population ratio, presumably because of lower rates of reimbursement of physicians in PGP plans.

The actual rate of physician visits per capita is estimated by Klarman to be 4.50 per year for Kaiser-Permanente, compared to 4.42 for the general California population, after adjustment for out-of-plan utilization as well as for telephone and other nonphysician contacts reported as visits in the California-wide data. These estimates are based on the report of the National Advisory Commission on Health Manpower (1967) and on the Columbia University survey of three plan-types in 1962. The greater number of visits and the generally lower physician-population ratio in Kaiser-Permanente implies a higher level of production for the latter's physicians, but Klarman believes the Manpower Commission's report overstates the general California physician-population ratio. Data (Social Security Administration, 1971) on ambulatory care from the Medicare program could be used without the dubious intervention of "adjustments," except that only expenditures, not medical visits, are reported. Per capita expenditures for physician's care were 7 percent less for Kaiser-Permanente, Northern California, the same as other sources for Southern California, and 35 percent higher for HIP, as reported by SSA in 1971. Expenditures may, indeed, reflect utilization differences, but the relationship can be confounded by different levels of earnings and different productivity rates of physicians. Thus, the picture presented by Klarman (1971) provides very little information on differentials in utilization rates for ambulatory services between PGP and other forms of medical care delivery.

The Roemer et al. study (1973) does provide some comparative data on ambulatory services. Basically, the findings showed much lesser differentials among the plan-types than for hospital days; the PGP-type plans had doctor-contacts at the rate of 3,324 per 1,000 persons per year, compared with 3,108 in the commercial and 3,984 in the "Blue" plans. A revealing categorization in which these relationships, however, did not prevail was by educational level of the family head. Among persons with college education, ambulatory care use was higher under the PGP plans than under either of the other two plan-types. It would appear that better educated and probably more sophisticated persons are able to make greater use of ambulatory care in the relatively complex framework of the large prepaid group practice plans found in California; this is less true under conventional conditions of private medical practice.

Another study in California (Kovner et al., 1969) examined the effect of family income on ambulatory care utilization under two HMO patterns: both the prepaid group practice (the Ross-Loos Medical Clinic Plan) and the medical care foundation (San Joaquin County) patterns. The study found that, in both these HMO patterns, the effect of income was virtually nil—eliminating the usual correlation between poverty and low utilization of outpatient services.

It has been shown both theoretically and empirically that merely extending insured ambulatory service benefits will not reduce hospital utilization under fee-for-service practice; the same economic theory indicates that there is reason to believe that paying the physician either by capitation or salary should lead to decreased hospital utilization. If one adds to this the influence of substantial ambulatory diagnostic and treatment facilities found in a group practice setting, as well as a restriction on available beds, one may expect a *relatively* higher level of ambulatory, compared with hospital, utilization under the PGP type of HMO.

A revealing demonstration of these dynamics is given in the ratios between doctor visits and hospital days reported by Roemer et al. (1973) in the three plan-types. These were as follows:

Plan-type	Doctor visits per 1000/year (a)	Hospital days per 1000/year (b)	Ratio (a):(b)
Commercial	3,104	864	3.6
"Blues"	3,984	1,109	3.6
Group practice	3,324	526	6.3

It is apparent that the PGP-type plan gives almost double the *relative* emphasis on ambulatory, compared with hospital bed service, as does either of the open-market plan-types.

Further evidence of the influence of the PGP model of HMO on the ratio between ambulatory and hospital services came from the Columbia (Maryland) Plan in 1969–1970. Malcolm Peterson(1971) reported that physicians' office visits were occurring at a rate of about 8.0 per person per year (of which 40 percent were for well-person care), compared with 4.6 nationally; hospital days, by contrast, were at a rate of 335 per 1,000 per year, compared with about 1,100 days nationally. Although these rough figures were not adjusted for age, socioeconomic status, etc., they are still striking.

Quality Assessments

Regarding the persistently difficult question of quality evaluations, an excellent review of all the methodologies was produced by Robert H. Brook (1972) as a doctoral dissertation at the Johns Hopkins School of Hygiene. Although the evaluation of HMOs, in comparison with other patterns of medical care, figures only tangentially in this work, Brook concludes that both "process" and "outcome" measures should ideally be used in combination. Among outcome measures, he advocates greater application of the so-called "tracer" technique, in which the incidence of morbid sequelae of specified pathological conditions (e.g., middle ear infection leading to deafness or hypertension leading to stroke) is traced under varying subsystems of medical care.

In the last several years, investigators do not seem to have devoted much effort to quality assessments of HMOs based simply on "structure" or the input of resources (personnel, equipment, etc.). The unitary medical record and the greater convenience of interspecialty consultations were emphasized as structural avenues to quality care in the *Harvard Law Review* paper by Greenberg and Rodburg (1971), but these factors in the PGP model have not been subjected to quantified comparisons with ordinary medical practice. Williamson (1971) has demonstrated the discrepancies between "input" measures of the qualifications of doctors, and "output" measures of the quality of their work, pointing further to the importance of using process and outcome measures in combination as a basis for quality evaluation.

With regard to "process" evaluations, the recent years also do not seem to have produced medical audit studies comparing HMO services with traditional patterns of medical care delivery. The belief continues to be widely held, nevertheless, that peer review—whether on a day-to-day basis or on the post-hoc basis of claims surveillance in medical foundation plans—helps to assure the quality of the doctor's work. Yet Weinerman (1969), commenting on group practice (whether prepaid or not) noted: "Group conferences, medical audits, and informal office consultations . . . are common in the descriptive literature but infrequent in daily practice."

The Roemer et al. study in California (1973), from its examination of samples of actual medical records in doctors' offices or clinics, developed a "rationality index" as an approach to quality evaluation. This index was based on such documentable criteria as completeness of the medical history, extent of physical examination, frequency of consultations, and other elements of service. With the use of "factor analysis" technique, the value of this index for the HMO model plans turned out to be 0.527, compared with 0.515 in the "Blue" plans and 0.503 in the commercial plans. The fallacies of medical record analysis as a reflection of the actual medical care process have long been recognized, yet there is no reason to expect less complete records in private medical offices than in prepaid group clinics, and it is the comparative values that the above indices reflect. In fact, one might suspect that in private offices, where fees are paid for each unit of service, records would be more nearly complete than in prepaid clinics where the doctors are on salary; if so, the differentials on "rationality" indicated above may understate the relative performance level under the HMO pattern.

Another dimension of the quality of medical care is often considered to be the degree to which preventive services are provided and used. Under HMOs, there has long been discussion of the effect of incentives to preventive service, aside from the influence of early, rather than late, attention to overt symptoms. Roemer et al. (1973) have produced some of the first hard data on this question through the examination of medical records (and hospital records) under the PGP versus open-market patterns. Indicators of prevention, identifiable in patient charts, were such items as "checkup" examinations of adults, well-child examinations, vaginal cytology tests, routine rectal examinations, chest x-rays, serological tests for syphilis, and immunizations. Summating these, by "factor analysis," a "preventive service index" was derived for the three types of health plan. It was computed as 0.452 in the HMO-type plan, compared to 0.404 in the "Blue" and 0.384 in the commercial insurance plans.

Another reflection of prevention in HMOs is given in data reported by Lester Breslow (1972), derived from 1965 studies in Alameda County, California. In the sample of the "Human Population Laboratory" in that county, those persons who were insured under the Kaiser-Permanente Health Plan had a "health maintenance examination" within the past year more frequently than those covered by open-market plans; the comparisons were, respectively, 58 percent versus 43–46 percent for men and 63 percent versus 49–57 percent for women.

A study of schoolchildren in whom physical defects had been detected was reported by Cauffman and Roemer (1967), with information on utilization under the different types of health insurance plans that covered the various children's families. They found that any type of health insurance coverage, compared with noninsurance, was more likely to be associated with treatment of the child's defect, but that children in families covered by PGP health insurance plans were more likely to have received a general "checkup" examination than children in families covered by open-market plans.

Costs and Productivity

The economic dimension of HMOs, compared with other modes of medical care delivery, must distinguish between the overall expenditures by the patient or the community, on the one hand, and the "costs of production" or the productivity of the subsystem, on the other, whether or not any productive efficiencies are "passed along" to the consumer in the form of lower prices. Each of these questions will be considered separately.

Expenditures by the consumer

With regard to expenditures by consumers or costs to patients, the Roemer et al. California study (1973) produced data on the PGP model of HMO, as compared with conventional patterns. It analyzed annual expenditures by family units for physician and hospital services in terms of (a) insurance premiums (whether or not paid partly or wholly by employers) and (b) out-of-pocket expenditures. The basic findings for families of all sizes in the three plan-types were as follows:

Plan-type	Average premium	Out-of-pocket expenditures	Total costs
Commercial	$208	$156	$364
"Blues"	257	190	447
Group practice	271	52	323

Thus, it is evident that the average family premiums of the PGP-type plans are higher, but that the out-of-pocket expenditures for medical and hospital services are so much lower than in the other two plan-types that the aggregate costs are the lowest among the three types of plan. When family size is held constant, the same general findings prevail. There are, however, different relationships by other demographic breakdowns. In families of three to four members defined as "lower income" (under $11,000 per year), the lowest aggregate expenditures occur in the commercial plans; they are $391 in the latter plans, compared with $417 in the PGP-type plans. These findings may reflect the lower illness risk composition in the enrollment of commercial plans (reported earlier) as well as the lower available family incomes (even in the "under $11,000" category), also reported earlier.

For the medical care foundation model of HMO, the available data are, again, confined largely to the experience of Medicaid beneficiaries on the California scene. In a comparison (Gartside,

1971) of the four-county area covered by the San Joaquin County foundation with a similar county lacking a foundation, the monthly costs per eligible person averaged $5.81 for physician services in the MCF area and $6.66 in the comparison traditional area; the state-wide average, adjusted for the mix of Medicaid categories, was $7.33. The overall average costs for all types of health service were actually higher in the MCF than in the comparison area ($10.43 versus $10.13), although this was due almost entirely to a higher expenditure for nursing-home services in the San Joaquin area.

The MCF of Clackamas County, Oregon (Haley, 1971), reported that "generally costs in Clackamas County, are 23 percent under the cost of service outside the county," but clear data in support of this statement have not been issued.

Production efficiencies

In considering the crucial question of production efficiencies under the HMO model, studies on economies of scale within prepaid group practice have figured prominently. Herbert Klarman, (1970; 1971) goes into this subject at some length. He notes at the outset that empirical results represent experience drawn entirely from fee-for-service practice since "little, if anything, has been published on variation in productivity among medical groups in the same prepayment plan" (Klarman, 1971:30). By implication at least, he minimizes the dangers of extrapolating conclusions, reached on the basis of findings from the fee-for-service group practice milieu, to the PGP model, asserting that the caveats of Roemer and Du Bois (1969) about the noncomparabilities of the two practice media "pertain to who gets the benefits of any savings, but do not appear to bear on the issue of variation in physician productivity by the size of the medical firm" (Klarman, 1971:30). Although this particular point is well taken, it would still seem that such extrapolation should be made with extreme caution.

First, much of the fee-for-service practice data have been obtained in single-specialty settings, and PGP is typically carried on in a multi-specialty setting. Second, in view of the important influence on other performance criteria believed to be associated with different methods of paying physicians, one would hesitate to assume that there is no impact on productivity just because one cannot at present make a clearcut case for it. After all, until Monsma's work (1970) articulated the issue, there was no commonly accepted theoretical explanation for the method of physician payment influencing HIP versus non-HIP hospitalization differentials in New York City. It may very well be, for example, that the management option of "pacing" physician visits, by control over the appointment system when the physician is on salary, can be more strongly asserted in large PGPs than in smaller ones. It may also be that substitution of lower-paid personnel for part of the physician's time is more feasible in the PGP model.

Many of the research findings cited by Klarman appeared in Donabedian (1969), but Klarman noted some additional works and further refined the economic analysis. The major studies again concern the work of Boan (1966), Bailey (1968), and Yett (1967). The study by Yankauer et al. (1970) is new. Klarman notes that theoretical considerations have led economists to expect returns to scale in medical care output on a priori grounds, and that Boan's and Yett's work seems to support this hypothesis. Bailey (1968), however, draws opposite conclusions. His findings (focused on specialists in internal medicine) lead him to infer that physicians in larger group practices earn more because of the profits earned on a proportionately higher rate of ancillary services performed in their establishments. The output, in terms of clinical visits per physician per unit time, was found to hold constant with increasing size of medical group. Bailey interpreted this to mean that the proportionately greater use of ancillary services by the larger groups of internists apparently did not represent a substitution of the time of allied health personnel for that of physicians, but could be viewed as merely incremental services delivered by larger groups.

Yankauer et al. (1970) reported a similar finding based on a nationwide survey of pediatric practices. This study also found the number of physician visits per unit time to be virtually constant with increase of size of the group practice. Delegation of tasks by the physician was generally in the administrative, technical, and clerical functions, but not in patient care functions. Where the latter type of delegation was found to occur, it was in response to relative local shortages of pediatricians, rather than in relation to the size of the medical group.

Klarman notes that the conflicting interpretations placed on these findings cannot be resolved by further analysis of existing data, but require additional research on medical care production, designed to answer the open questions. For the present, he concludes (1971:31) that "economies of scale have not yet been demonstrated empirically."

It should be noted that arguments which postulate a possibly greater willingness to delegate patient care tasks to ancillary personnel are related to the circumstances found more widely under large PGP conditions. These include the feasibility of close supervision of such tasks by the physician, a relative lack of concern by him that his income position may be eroded, and, in the case of large, self-sufficient PGPs, lessened fear of retaliation by competitors. Moreover, it is difficult to see why one could expect any increase in productivity, as measured solely by physician visits, under conditions which closely prescribe the tasks reserved for physician performance. In particular, in a PGP situation the number of visits to be handled by a physician per hour would largely be determined

by the scheduling mechanism, and could resemble the moving assembly line in industry.

It is also necessary to note that defining physician productivity
solely in terms of office visits, in fee-for-service private practice, can
be illusory. Since, in the American scheme of things, physicians
typically prescribe treatment for the same patient in the office and
in the hospital, it is not unreasonable to postulate that solo practitioners and small private groups run up physician visit "scores" by
hospitalizing freely. In that case, as Roemer and Shain (1959)
have pointed out, the private physician can ostensibly increase his
efficiency of practice by hospitalizing patients, passing along the
heavy diagnostic work to the hospital and the expense to insurance
plans. The larger, better equipped group practices may reasonably
be expected to handle more of these cases in the office—spending
more time with the patients, doing more tests, and hospitalizing less.
Bailey's (1968) data tends to support this hypothesis, at least for
solo as compared with group practice.

The important missing data in Bailey's study are the total utilization by and cost to the patients per year, per illness, etc. Lacking
a defined subscriber population, these data are virtually impossible
of meaningful interpretation. (If one wished to dramatize the deficiencies of these data, one could argue that all the data on visits to
a particular physician might pertain to two or three patients with
chronic illness making repeated visits, with astronomical cost to
themselves or their insurance carriers.)

Boan (1966) stated the conclusions from his research in Canada straightforwardly. He found that physicians in group practice,
compared to solo practice, had higher ratios of allied health personnel per physician, lower costs per physician for such personnel, and
lower costs of investment per physician. However, these results are
not strictly proof of economies of scale, since only the dichotomy between solo and group practice is examined. Furthermore, the applicability of nationwide Canadian results to the United States scene
remains open to question. Direct inferences on returns to scale can
be made only if one assumes that Boan's conclusions follow from
observation on two discrete points along the size-of-firm scale—
solo and larger than solo—and if one is further willing to assume
that his upward slope of the returns-to-scale line would hold if the
group practices were categorized along an increasing size scale.

Yett (1967) measured total tax-deductible expenses per physician as related to output (of computed patient visits) per physician,
and found definite economies of scale. The result would suggest
that practices in which the physicians were more productive, in
terms of visits produced, exhibited a smaller overhead cost per
physician visit. It would seem that a cost function analysis of this
type does not directly address the question of economies of scale in
terms of larger versus smaller group practices, and, a fortiori, does
not shed light on what one might expect in an HMO situation.

Furthermore, it does not directly address the problem of physician output as a function of size of practice (measured by number of physicians involved), which was Bailey's concern.

However, subsequent work by Reinhardt and Yett (1972), at the University of Southern California has produced insight on this crucial subject. The published work concentrates on fitting production functions to national data reported to the magazine *Medical Economics* (MEDEC). These investigators are now tackling the question of the output of physicians (measured in patient visits per physician per week and, separately, by annual gross patient billings per physician) as a function of inputs. The latter consist of the services of medical auxiliary personnel, cost of plant and medical equipment, medical supplies used up in the conduct of practice, and the amount of physician's time (hours per week) occupied "strictly on practice-related activities." Physicians' visits are totaled over three sites: office, home, and hospital. The Reinhardt-Yett study defined "returns to scale" as the relative increase in number of visits per physician associated with the same percentage increase applied to all input factors.

Without reference to mode of practice, their results were that the output (visits per week) of the individual physician showed the expected increasing returns to scale, if inputs were to be increased in relatively small private practices. Comparing solo practices to single-specialty group practices, they found that the latter produce "between 4 and 13 percent more patient visits than do solo practitioners at any given level of factor input." The report cautions that these results may be flawed because of the lack of data on total medical group output, instead of output of individual physicians. So little data were available on mixed-specialty groups that they decided to exclude all multi-specialty group data from the group-solo comparisons in this study. Furthermore, the preponderance of the single-specialty groups studied was very small, consisting of three to six physicians.

Included among the USC (1972) findings were these points: (a) "Solo practitioners tend to work fewer hours and employ fewer aides per physician than do their colleagues in groups or partnerships"; (b) quite apart from the longer hours worked, group practice physicians produced more visits per hour than those in solo practice—4.5 percent more for general practitioners, 6.2 percent for pediatricians, 13.8 percent for obstetricians-gynecologists, and 4.0 percent more for internists; (c) up to about four or five aides per physician, the total number of patient visits per week per physician increases with additional aides; and (d) adding more physician time as an input will increase patient units by a greater factor than an increase of proportionate size in any other input.

Another USC study by Kimbell and Lorant (c. 1970) used the responses to the Seventh Periodic Survey of Physicians by the American Medical Association as its data for analyzing production functions of solo physicians, and the data of the AMA's Survey of Medical Groups for analyzing group practice relationships. Economies of scale were measured in terms of *office* visits as a function of the inputs: physician time, number of allied personnel employed, and number of examining rooms (representing capital investment). Among their findings on solo practice were these: (a) an increase in physician time increases the number of office visits by a greater factor than an identical percentage increase of any of the other inputs— in fact, more than the increase in allied personnel and capital (examining rooms) combined (a given percentage increase in allied personnel will have a greater effect on office visits than the same percentage increase in examining rooms, although increases in the latter will also increase the output); (b) physicians who charge higher initial fees have a lower output of office visits; and (c) the total R^2 (the proportion of the total variation due to the "explanatory" variables) is only 0.13, so that other factors not in the analysis explain much more of the production than those included.

Regarding group practices, Kimbell and Lorant found that: (a) the most important factor in increasing office (as well as total) patient visits by far is still physician time input; (b) there are decreasing returns to scale in office visits (and total visits) for an increasing size of output (i.e., an increase of about 10 percent in input factors will increase output by only about 8 percent, although, for gross revenues, the return to scale is almost constant, tending to agree with Bailey's findings); and (c) practices using an incentive plan for income distribution "had 10 percent greater apparent efficiency" than practices applying completely equal sharing or salaries. "Efficiency" was measured by the degree to which the group practices produce above or below the output predicted by the model. The R^2 achieved by this analysis of group practices was about 0.80, so that the explanation of output by the input variables was much better than for solo physicians.

Another recently reported study on medical care productivity is that of Newhouse (1973). This paper addresses the question of costs per physician visit in different practice patterns, and a principal determinant was found to be whether or not the practice shared income equally or divided it among the members of the practice in proportion to the number of visits each doctor produced. It followed that solo, fee-for-service practice was found to yield the lowest overhead costs per visit, since this form of organization represents the most direct relationship between the income received by the physician and the visits produced by him. The sample studied comprised 20 practices, varying from 11 solo practices to two 5-physician groups, and three outpatient clinics of hospitals. Newhouse states "there is the obvious qualification that the sample is extremely small," and much of the paper is devoted to showing that equal income-sharing should theoretically lead to increased unit costs per visit.

Effects of size

In concluding this section on the literature dealing with economies of scale, a number of points must be noted. In using production functions in private fee-for-service practice, investigators have often considered patient visits as the key output measure. It would seem to be a questionable assumption, however, that more visits per hour are uniformly desirable. Clearly, the desirable number depends on patient care considerations, and flatly to equate an increasing number of visits per hour with greater efficiency cannot be excused by appealing to the assumption of "other things being equal." Studies of productivity which do not include some simultaneous observations on the content or quality of care are of doubtful usefulness at best, and may even be misleading.

Similar considerations hold in studying *economies of scale* in private fee-for-service practice. Assuming that physicians will keep unit (per visit) overhead costs down, if their income is directly tied to the net earnings of the visits they produce, might also imply that doctors would do almost anything they can "get away with" to maximize their net incomes. In a period of physician shortage, and in consideration of legal restrictions on competition entering the field, it would again seem to be questionable whether this type of motivation is widely operative.

Finally, with the preceding two points in mind, it might be germane to restate Klarman's 1972 summary on the research to date in the following manner: General economic theory, as outlined by Boan, Fein, and others, indicates that group practice should be more efficient than solo practice, all other things being equal, in terms of productivity. Monsma's theoretic formulation indicates that *prepaid* practice is expected to be more efficient than fee-for-service practice, in terms of avoidance of unnecessary utilization of expensive procedures. Research to date has not effectively proven these reasonable hypotheses false. In any event, the entire question of production efficiencies touches only one aspect of the HMO concept; other aspects of incentives to economy, when a fixed annual premium is paid for a broad scope of services, will be considered in the following sections.

Health Outcomes

PGP and health outcomes

The ultimate measure of HMO performance, as suggested earlier, is how healthy these organizations keep their members, compared with other patterns of medical care delivery. The sparsity of data on this crucial question, up to 1969, was evident in the review by Donabedian. It had been largely confined to the experience of the

Health Insurance Plan of Greater New York and focused on mortality in the very young and the very old.

Since then, some little additional outcome data have been produced on this key question, but not always with conclusive results. A study by William I. Barton (1972), though based on a nationwide mortality study in 1964–1966, provides the first such nationwide data on infant mortality in relation to health insurance coverage. After adjustment for race, region, parental education, and live-birth order, the mothers with some health insurance coverage had significantly lower infant mortality rates than those not insured; when adjustment was made for family income, the infant mortality rate was still slightly lower for the insured childbirth cases (23.3 per 1,000 live births compared with 24.5), but the difference was not statistically significant. This study, unfortunately, does not come to grips with the HMO question. In fact, it was found, paradoxically, that mothers with more comprehensive health insurance coverage actually had *higher* infant mortality rates than those with more limited coverage; the author, however, speculates that this unexpected finding reflected characteristics of the mothers, rather than being attributable to the extent of insurance protection. He postulates that women with more complete insurance coverage were probably higher-risk mothers in the first place—in other words, a previous pregnancy complication had induced them to secure broader insurance protection.

The first American report applying sickness absenteeism as an outcome measure for comparing prepaid group practice with other patterns appeared in 1971. Robert L. Robertson (1971) studied work loss in 1966–1967 among schoolteachers covered under a PGP-type of HMO, compared with teachers covered under a "Blue" plan. Although in this, as in other comparative studies, the effects of self-selection could not be completely eliminated (since membership in either type of insurance plan is the individual's own decision), the findings suggests a slightly lower råte of "work-loss from sickness or injury" for both men and women teachers covered by the HMO-type plan. The size of the differences varied with age level, and the greatest different characterized younger females. The overall age-standardized mean days of work loss were 3.88 days per year in the HMO-type plan for males compared with 4.01 days in the "Blue" plan; the parallel figures for females were 5.93 days compared to 6.41 days.

"Foundations" and health outcomes

With respect to the medical care foundation pattern of HMO, an as yet unpublished study from the UCLA School of Public Health (Newport and Roemer, 1973) examined perinatal mortality among mothers covered by Medicaid through the San Joaquin Foundation for Medical Care, compared with a closely matched county (Ventura) lacking a foundation and using traditional methods. Newport and Roemer found that, excluding county hospital births which are not influenced by MCF procedures, the perinatal death rates were lower in the foundation area for "white Anglo" childbirths, but higher for childbirths in black and Spanish-surname families. When ethnically standardized for the mix of these groups in the state-wide Medicaid population, the perinatal death rates in the foundation and matched comparison areas were virtually identical: 29.6 deaths per 1,000 total births in the former group and 30.1 in the latter. More interesting, perhaps, was the finding that in a third area, admittedly not matched to the foundation county, but lacking a foundation and having a strong county health department (with an active maternal and child health program), the perinatal death rate was *half* of that in either of the study counties, at 15.5 deaths per 1,000 births.

While these were the only recent health outcome studies with a direct bearing on evaluation of HMO performance, other investigations have been providing new approaches to the use of adjusted mortality data for evaluating the performance of complex organizations. Moses and Mosteller (1968) revealed large differences in the death rates for specified surgical operations made in large teaching hospitals throughout the country, even after adjustments for various patient characteristics. Roemer et al. (1968) developed a formula by which crude hospital death rates could be adjusted for average case-severity, so that adjusted death rates could serve as a basis for evaluating the overall quality of hospital performance. These methodologic studies may provide clues for evaluation of HMO performance on the basis of mortality outcomes.

Patient Attitudes

While more substantial data on health status outcomes is awaited, some idea of the quality of service in a medical care program may be validly inferred from the attitudes expressed by consumers or patients. Although consumer attitudes may be influenced by many factors in health service delivery unrelated to technical excellence, it is reasonable to consider that the speed and degree with which the service helps a person to recover from illness or to maintain his health is an important determinant of attitudes. This becomes more plausible as patients become better educated about health care requirements.

Since the Donabedian review, additional studies have reported relatively high degrees of satisfaction with health services associated with HMO patterns. The favorable population attitudes toward group practice in general, even when experience with such clinics was lacking, were noted earlier from the study by Metzner et al. (1972). Weinerman's paper (1964) on patient attitudes toward prepaid group practice plans showed a high degree of overall satisfaction in spite of many complaints about the impersonality of the doctor-patient relationship in a "clinic setting." His general summary of numerous studies up to 1964 is worth quoting (Weinerman, 1964:886):

> In general, the various investigations of attitudes of group health members suggest much appreciation for the technical standards of group health care, but less satisfaction with the doctor-patient relationship itself. In one way or another patients report disappointment with the degree of personal interest shown by the doctor and with the availability of his services when requested. Much more rarely is there criticism of the quality or the economics of group health care.

The dynamics of a sort of psychological trade-off—that is, tolerance of unsatisfactory doctor-patient relationships in return for judgment of good technical service and a "good buy" financially—in patient acceptance of the PGP pattern are reflected in the findings of Roemer et al. (reported in 1973, although based on a 1968 investigation). This study solicited the attitudes of health plan members along two dimensions: satisfaction with financial protection and with medical care received. Regarding financial protection, the preference for the PGP pattern, compared with open market plans, was overwhelming, prevailing in all types of family (large and small), in all religious categories, in all social classes, in families of either high or low geographic mobility, and whether or not the family had a history of chronic illness.

With respect to satisfaction of plan members with "the medical care received," the positive attributes of the PGP plans were not so impressive, although the occurrence of frank dissatisfaction was substantially *lower* in those plans, compared with private medical practice patterns. Definite dissatisfaction was reported by 8.6 percent of PGP plan families, compared to 17.4 and 20.3 percent in the commercial and "Blue" plan-types.

When these responses are analyzed by social groupings, some interesting differentials become evident. The low level of frank dissatisfaction with the PGP-type patterns, compared with the others, prevails in all social subgroups. For certain subgroups, however, the HMO-type plans also show the highest level of "very satisfied" members: these include (a) single-person family units (compared with larger units), (b) Protestants (compared with other faiths), (c) families with no history of chronic illness (compared with sicklier families), (d) adult men alone (compared with adult women), and (e) geographically mobile families (compared with relatively stable ones).

Similar general findings were reported by Greenlick (1972) regarding the Kaiser-Permanente Health Plan in Portland, Oregon. While his respondents indicated substantial general satisfaction with the plan, that satisfaction was most often attributed to the financial advantages ("reasonable premiums" for the benefits offered) and to the actual care received after the doctor was reached, but over 50 percent of the respondents complained about the time it took before they got an appointment—in other words, access to the doctor.

Another study of patient satisfaction (Leyhe and Procter, 1971) was focused on Medicaid recipients enrolled in a PGP plan in California, compared with other such persons getting care through traditional private doctor mechanisms. The investigators in that study concluded (Leyhe and Procter, 1971:II) that:

> No appreciable differences were found between responses of . . . [the PGP] enrollees and of those who used individual practitioners. . . . Medi-Cal enrollees of this private group practice apparently appraised their medical care as equivalent in almost all respects to that received from individual practitioners. This private (prepaid) group practice was not seen by the majority of the enrollees as having the objectionable features often attributed to public clinics.

Of the 51 questions used in this patient attitude survey, only four yielded significant differences between PGP and non-PGP respondents. In three of these questions, OAS (old-age security) Medicaid patients expressed the familiar objection that they had difficulty reaching a physician by telephone, could not see the same physician continuously, and did not get house call service. In the remaining question of these four, the *non-PGP* sample of AFDC (aid to families with dependent children) clients complained that they had difficulty obtaining ambulatory care because of problems with transportation—a service the PGP plan provided for its members.

One other conclusion of this study worth citing is that ". . . it became evident that patient education pertaining to the current source of care is extremely important." Since about 20 percent of the respondents reported that they had had no identifiable source for medical care before being accepted into the Medicaid program, this conclusion seems to suggest that a pattern of delivery with a clearly identified, physically accessible source for primary care is likely to be more successful in reaching previously underserviced populations with medical service.

Meaning of attitudes

Several comments are in order about patient attitudes toward prepaid group practice, typically associated with HMOs, as compared with traditional patterns. First, the policy of "dual" or "multiple choice" among plan types, always followed by the Kaiser-Permanente Plan and increasingly followed by other HMO-type plans, helps to assure that only persons willing to accept the "clinic pattern" of service will join such plans in the first place. Second, on the other hand, the clinic pattern clearly departs from traditional custom and experience among self-supporting families, and it is small wonder if the inevitable impersonalities, especially if the clinic is a

large one, cause irritations or, at least, require psychological adjustment. Third, it must be realized that some of the dissatisfactions
with PGP patterns are basically a result of the insufficient numbers
of doctors in those programs—a situation which, in turn, relates to
nationwide shortages; in light of the high incomes attainable in private practice, the PGP plans have understandably had difficulties in
recruiting qualified physicians to fill all their posts.

Finally, it must be recognized that managerial problems are
far from solved in most large-scale medical care organizations,
whether for ambulatory or for impatient service. The hospital literature is full of reports about the "insensitivities" of patient care in
large hospitals, whether or not prepayment is in the picture. There
are obviously improvements needed in the efficiency of managing
patient flow in organized medical care systems. In a sense, the most
remarkable fact is the increasing degree of satisfaction that seems to
be characterizing clinic services in spite of their departure from traditional patterns.

In regard to patient attitudes toward the medical care foundation pattern of HMO, compared with conventional private practice,
there is little reason to expect much difference since conventional
patterns of medical care are indeed applied by the foundations. The
California PERS study (Medical Advisory Council, 1971) did,
however, solicit three levels of satisfaction ("satisfied", "not entirely satisfied", or "dissatisfied") toward different aspects of the
four plan-types used by these state government employees. The responses showed overwhelmingly high "satisfaction" in all plan-types
across the three dimensions: plan administration, doctor's care, and
hospitalization.

The differences were all very small, by these measures; but for
the foundation plans, compared with the PGP model of HMOs, satisfaction levels appeared to be slightly higher for doctor's and hospital care, and slightly lower for plan administration. It is doubtful
if these figures have any statistical significance. More important,
they are bound to be strongly influenced by the general social
settings, since, in California, the medical foundations operate in
the smaller and more rural counties, while the PGP plans are largely concentrated in metropolitan counties.

Out-of-plan use

A reflection of patient attitudes toward the PGP pattern of HMO is
bound to be given by the extent of out-of-plan use. Since the Donabedian review, the new data seem to suggest that this use is somewhat lower than reported in the earlier studies. Greenlick's report
(1972) on the Portland branch of the Kaiser-Permanente Plan
found that about 10 percent of persons had some out-of-plan use
during the previous 12 months, but since this might have ranged
from little to much service for these persons, he estimates that it
would amount to under 10 percent of the total services.

Roemer et al. (1973) analyzed out-of-plan use separately for ambulatory doctor and hospital services. They found, through examination of medical records, that 12 percent of the ambulatory doctor contacts of PGP plan members during one year occurred with private doctors outside the plan; for hospitalizations, the out-of-plan admissions were 7.2 percent of the total. The relative lowness of these figures suggests that, in spite of some dissatisfactions, a decision of PGP plan members to seek care elsewhere (and pay privately—which may not be such a hardship, when premiums have been paid by employers, as is commonly true) is made relatively rarely. Moreover, even these low figures may be an overstatement, since the questionnaire used did not distinguish between outside care sought because of dissatisfaction (impatience for an appointment or the like) and such care sought in an emergency occurring outside the plan's geographic area—a type of care financially covered by "out-of-area" indemnity benefits.

In the previous section, it was noted that out-of-pocket outlays for doctor's and hospital services by PGP plan members were strikingly low, even though these figures included certain small in-plan copayments that are levied on certain membership groups in the HMO-type plans of the RHH study (Roemer et al., 1973). The general extent of out-of-plan use in PGP plans, by various measures of services or expenditures, would seem to be lower than in the earlier studies summarized by Donabedian (1969). It would seem reasonable to conclude that, as people have become more accustomed to the PGP model of medical care, they have been more inclined to stay with it, in spite of some difficulties; perhaps over the years there has also been improved efficiency in PGP operations. There still remain, nevertheless, obvious problems to solve in the sphere of plan-patient relationships within the HMO model.

HMOs and Planning

The whole HMO strategy has important implications for planning. In a sense, it shifts planning responsibilities from central governmental authorities to local voluntary bodies, within certain ground rules. It says that for a fixed monetary sum, the HMO must keep its customers happy, or at least sufficiently satisfied to stay with that HMO and not to leave it for the open market or to join another one. Within the constraints of money and membership expectations, the HMO would have wide leeway to provide health services in a variety of ways. The evidence so far suggests that, given a promotional boost by government "seed" grants, the potentials of HMOs, based on the PGP model, to provide good health service at relatively lower costs than the traditional open-market private medicine model are substantial. Reasonable interpretation, however, of the evaluative data on HMO performance, summarized above, requires certain "caveats."

Nearly all of the studies on effects, whether based on structure, process, or outcome, have been made on relatively large, stable, and well-established HMO models. It is altogether possible—and some of the recent California experience mentioned (Nelson, 1973) underscores the hazards—that some HMOs, especially the newer ones, may yield a very different performance record. As the American Public Health Association (1971) pointed out in an official policy statement, there are two principal hazards in the HMO concept: inequitable "risk" selection among enrollees and poor-quality care through underservicing.

Safeguards against both of these hazards are feasible through a process of public surveillance. Regarding risk selection or, more accurately, membership composition, standards with respect to age, sex, socioeconomic status, and past illness history could be set and applied to the actual enrollees of each HMO. Recurrent "open enrollment periods" are another device to help assure that every HMO is serving its fair share of high- and low-risk persons. Without such procedures, one or another HMO could offer competitively wider benefits or particularly low premiums simply by excluding or reducing its load of high-risk members.

Regarding the hazard of underservicing or other strategies for cutting HMO costs at the expense of quality, the surveillance procedures are more difficult and complex. There seems to be an increasing consensus that monitoring would be required along all principal channels of evaluation: input, process, and health outcomes. In January, 1972, a conference was sponsored by InterStudy and headed by Paul M. Ellwood (1973), who has done so much to promote the HMO concept, in order to grapple specifically with the problems of quality assurance under HMOs. The report of this conference suggests that the main emphasis was on the importance of developing sharpened measures of "clinical outcomes," as essential tools of a "Health Outcomes Commission" (in government) to promote quality assurance.

The general question of quality assurance has, of course, acquired greater national importance as collective financing of medical care (both through government and voluntary insurance) has increased—quite aside from the issue of HMOs. In January of 1973, still another major national conference was held on this question (U.S. Department of Health, Education, and Welfare, 1973), again stressing the importance of developing reliable measurements of both medical care process and outcome. The enactment of P.L. 92–603, the 1972 amendments to Medicare and Medicaid, adds further impetus to the need for quality criteria, with the new legal requirement of "professional standard review organizations" (PSROs) to blanket the nation. More research on formulating readily applicable measurements of both medical care process and outcome is obviously needed.

With several bills pending in the U.S. Congress for promotion of HMOs, including versions backed by both major political parties, it is a fair guess that the future holds expansion of HMO patterns of both major types—the PGP and the medical care foundation models. In the light of both continuously rising health care costs and the agreed-upon persistent need for comprehensive health planning (one item in the 1973–1974 Presidential budget contemplated for expansion, in contrast to the cutbacks in so many other sectors of the health field), one may reasonably look upon the HMO strategy as a peculiarly American approach to planning, in which responsibilities are delegated to numerous local mini-systems, in contrast to the usual European strategy of centralized controls. The private sector, through HMO development, would be vested with responsibilities and incentives to regulate itself and to meet the health needs of the population. As we have seen from the accumulated evidence, there is much reason to have confidence in the soundness of this strategy. Yet, as we have also seen, when and if HMOs become more a "mainstream" than a "vanguard" phenomenon, there will be enormous needs for continuing vigilance to protect the interests of consumers both inside and outside of health maintenance organizations.

Milton I. Roemer, M.D.
University of California
School of Public Health
405 Hilgard Ave.
Los Angeles, California 90024

William Shonick, PH.D.
University of California
School of Public Health
405 Hilgard Ave.
Los Angeles, California 90024

Prepared at the invitation of the National Academy of Sciences, Institute of Medicine (Washington, D.C.).

References

American Hospital Association
    1972   Review of 1971 Certificate-of-Need Legislation. Survey report. Chicago: American Hospital Association.

American Public Health Association
    1971   "Health maintenance organizations: a policy paper." American Journal of Public Health 61 (December): 2528–2536.

Avnet, Helen H.
   1967   Physician Service Patterns and Illness Rates. New York: Group
           Health Insurance.

Bailey, Richard M.
   1968   "A comparison of internists in solo and fee-for-service group
           practice in the San Francisco Bay area." Bulletin of the New
           York Academy of Medicine 44 (November): 1293–1303.

Barton, William I.
   1972   "Infant mortality and health insurance coverage for maternity
           care." Inquiry 9 (September): 16–29.

Bechtol, Thomas A.
   1972   (General manager of the Physicians' Association of Clackamas
           County, Oregon) Personal communication, July 10.

Berkanovic, Emil
   1973   Prepayment vs. Fee-for-Service for Medicaid Recipients. Unpub-
           lished data, University of California Survey Research Center.

Boan, J. A.
   1966   Group Practice. Ottawa: Royal Commission on Health Services,
           Queen's Printer.

Breslow, Lester
   1972   "Health maintenance services in health maintenance organiza-
           tions." Association of Teachers of Preventive Medicine Newslet-
           ter 19 (Winter): 2.

Brook, Robert H.
   1972   A Study of Methodologic Problems Associated with Assessment
           of Quality of Care. Doctoral dissertation, Johns Hopkins School
           of Hygiene (May, processed).

Bunker, John P.
   1970   "Surgical manpower: a comparison of operations and surgeons in
           the United States and in England and Wales." New England
           Journal of Medicine 282 (January 15): 135–144.

Cauffman, Joy G., and Milton I. Roemer
   1967   "The impact of health insurance coverage on health care of
           school children." Public Health Reports 82 (April): 323–328.

Committee on the Costs of Medical Care
   1932   Medical Care for the American People. Chicago: University of
           Chicago Press.

Cook, Wallace H.
   1971   "Profile of the Permanente physician." P. 104 in Somers, Anne R.
           (ed.), The Kaiser-Permanente Medical Care Program. New York:
           Commonwealth Fund.

Dickinson, Frank G., and C. E. Bradley
  1952   Discontinuance of Medical Groups 1940–49, Bulletin No. 90. Chicago: American Medical Association, Bureau of Economic Research.

Donabedian, Avedis
  1969   "An evaluation of prepaid group practice." Inquiry 6 (September): 3–27.

Du Bois, Donald M.
  1970   "Organizational viability of group practice." Pp. 378–414 in Roemer, Milton I., Donald M. Du Bois, and Shirley W. Rich (eds.), Health Insurance Plans: Studies in Organizational Diversity. Los Angeles: University of California School of Public Health.

Egdahl, Richard E.
  1973   "Foundations for medical care." New England Journal of Medicine 288 (March 8): 491–498.

Ellwood, Paul M., et al.
  1973   Assuring the Quality of Health Care. Minneapolis: InterStudy.

Gartside, Foline E.
  1971   The Utilization and Costs of Services in the San Joaquin Prepayment Project. Los Angeles: University of California School of Public Health (January, processed).

Gartside, Foline E., and Donald M. Procter
  1970   Medicaid Services in California under Different Organizational Modes: Physician Participation in the San Joaquin Prepayment Project. Los Angeles: University of California School of Public Health (January, processed).

Glasgow, John M.
  1972   "Prepaid group practice as a national health policy: problems and perspectives." Inquiry 9 (March): 3–15.

Greenberg, Ira G., and Michael L. Rodburg
  1971   "The role of prepaid group practice in relieving the medical care crisis." Harvard Law Review 84 (February): 887–1001.

Greenlick, Merwyn
  1972   "The impact of prepaid group practice on American medical care: a critical evaluation." The Annals of the American Academy of Political and Social Science 399 (January): 100–113.

Haley, Thomas W.
  1971   "Physicians' Association of Clackamas County." Hospitals 45 (March): 8.

Hill, Daniel B., and James E. Veney
  1970   "Kansas Blue Cross–Blue Shield out-patient benefits experiment." Medical Care 8 (March–April): 143–158.

Kelly, Denwood N.
    1965   "Experience with a program of coverage for diagnostic proce-
            dures provided in physicians' offices and hospital out-patient de-
            partments—Maryland Blue Cross and Blue Shield plans
            (1957–1964)." Inquiry 2 (November): 28–44.

Kimbell, Larry J., and John H. Lorant
    c.1970 Production Functions for Physician Services. Los Angeles: Uni-
            versity of Southern California, Human Resources Research Cen-
            ter (undated, processed).

Klarman, Herbert E.
    1963   "The effect of prepaid group practice on hospital use." Public
            Health Reports 78 (November): 955–965.

    1970   "Economic research in group medicine." Pp. 178–193 in Beamish,
            R. E. (ed.), New Horizons in Health Care. Winnipeg, Canada:
            First International Congress on Group Medicine.

    1971   "Analysis of the HMO proposal—its assumptions, implications,
            and prospects." Pp. 24–38 in Health Maintenance Organizations:
            A Reconfiguration of the Health Services System. Chicago: Uni-
            versity of Chicago Center for Health Administration Studies.

Kovner, Joel W., L. Brian Browne, and Arnold I. Kisch
    1969   "Income and use of outpatient medical care by the insured." In-
            quiry 6 (June): 27–34.

Leyhe, Dixie L., and D. M. Procter
    1971   Medi-Cal Patient Satisfaction under a Prepaid Group Practice
            and Individual Fee-for-Service Practice. Los Angeles: University
            of California School of Public Health (June, processed).

Mechanic, David
    c.1972 Physician Satisfaction in Varying Settings. University of Wiscon-
            sin (mimeographed, undated).

Medical Advisory Council to the California Public Employees Retirement System
    1971   Final Report on the Survey of Consumer Experience under the
            State of California Employees Hospital and Medical Care Act.
            Sacramento: Medical Advisory Council, California Public Em-
            ployees Retirement System.

Metzner, Charles A., Rashid L. Bashshur, and Gary W. Shannon
    1972   "Differential public acceptance of group medical practice." Medi-
            cal Care 10 (July–August): 279–287.

Monsma, George N.
    1970   "Marginal revenue and demand for physicians' services." Pp.
            145–160 in Klarman, Herbert E. (ed.), Empirical Studies in
            Health Economics. Baltimore: Johns Hopkins Press.

Moses, Lincoln E., and Frederick Mosteller
    1968   "Institutional differences in post-operative death rates: commen-
            tary on some findings of the National Halothane Study." Journal
            of the American Medical Association 203 (February 12): 7.

Moustafa, A. Taher, Carl E. Hopkins, and Bonnie Klein
    1971   "Determinants of choice and change of health insurance plan."
            Medical Care 9 (January–February): 32–41.

National Advisory Commission on Health Manpower
    1967   Report. Vol. 11:197–228. Washington: Government Printing Of-
            fice.

Nelson, Harry
    1973   "Investigation of prepaid health programs asked: possible fraud
            in some cases hinted by L.A. County unit." Los Angeles Times,
            February 24:1.

Newhouse, Joseph P.
    1973   "The economics of group practice." The Journal of Human Re-
            sources 8 (Winter): 37–56.

Newport, John, and Milton I. Roemer
    1973   "Health service outcome under medical care foundations: perina-
            tal mortality in Medicaid childbirths covered by a county medical
            foundation compared to other delivery models." Publication
            pending.

Perrott, George St. J.
    1971   Federal Employees Health Benefit Program: Enrollment and Uti-
            lization of Health Services 1961–1968. Washington: Department
            of Health, Education, and Welfare, Public Health Service.

Peterson, Malcolm L.
    1971   "The first year in Columbia: assessments of low hospitalization
            and high office use." Johns Hopkins Medical Journal 128 (Janu-
            ary): 15–23.

Prybil, Lawrence D.
    1971   "Physician terminations in large multi-specialty groups." Medical
            Group Management 18 (September): 4–6, 23–25.

Reinhardt, Uwe E., and Donald E. Yett
    1972   Physician Production Functions under Varying Practice Ar-
            rangements. Technical Paper Series No. 1. Washington: U. S. De-
            partment of Health, Education, and Welfare, Community Health
            Service.

Robertson, Robert L.
    1971   "Economic effects of personal health services: work loss in a
            public school teacher population." American Journal of Public
            Health 61 (January): 30–45.

Roemer, Milton I.
   1958   "The influence of prepaid physician's service on hospital utiliza-
           tion." Hospitals 16 (October): 48–52.

Roemer, Milton I., and Donald M. Du Bois
   1969   "Medical costs in relation to the organization of ambulatory
           care." New England Journal of Medicine 280 (May): 988–993.

Roemer, Milton I., and Foline E. Gartside
   1973   "Peer review in medical foundations: its effect on qualifications
           of surgeons." Health Services Reports. University of California
           School of Public Health (December).

Roemer, Milton I., Robert W. Hetherington, Carl E. Hopkins, Arthur
E. Gerst, Eleanor Parsons, and Donald M. Long
   1973   Health Insurance Effects: Services, Expenditures, and Attitudes
           under Three Types of Plan. Ann Arbor: University of Michigan
           School of Public Health.

Roemer, Milton I., A. Taher Moustafa, and Carl E. Hopkins
   1968   "A proposed hospital quality index: hospital death rates adjusted
           for case severity." Health Services Research 3 (Summer):
           96–118.

Roemer, Milton I., and Max Shain
   1959   Hospital Utilization under Insurance, Monograph Series No. 6.
           Chicago: American Hospital Association.

Ross, Austin, Jr.
   1969   "A report on physician terminations in group practice." Medical
           Group Management 16: 15–21.

Shapiro, Sam
   1971   "Role of hospitals in the changing health insurance plan of
           Greater New York." Bulletin of the New York Academy of Med-
           icine 74 (April): 374–381.

Social Security Administration
   1971   Medicare Experience with Prepaid Group Practice Enrollees.
           Washington: Social Security Administration Office of Research
           and Statistics (March, processed).

U. S. Department of Health, Education, and Welfare
   1973   Quality Assurance of Medical Care. Monograph. Washington:
           Regional Medical Programs Service (February, processed).

Weinerman, E. Richard
   1964   "Patients' perceptions of group medical care." American Journal
           of Public Health 54 (June): 880–889.

   1969   "Problems and perspectives in group practice." Group Practice 18
           (April): 30.

Williamson, John W.
   1971   "Evaluating quality of patient care." Journal of the American
           Medical Association 218 (October 25): 4.

Yankauer, Alfred, John P. Connelly, and Jacob J. Feldman
  1970   "Physician productivity and delivery of ambulatory care: some
          findings from a survey of pediatricians." Medical Care 8 (January–February): 35–46.

Yett, Donald E.
  1967   "An evaluation of alternative methods of estimating physicians'
          expenses relative to output." Inquiry 4 (March): 3–27.

16. Medical Manpower Models: Needs, Demand and Supply

JUDITH R. LAVE, LESTER B. LAVE, AND SAMUEL LEINHARDT

Reprinted with permission of the Blue Cross Association, from Inquiry, Vol. XII, No. 2 (June 1975), pp. 97-125. Copyright © 1975 by the Blue Cross Association. All rights reserved.

As planning has moved into center stage in health care delivery, Comprehensive Health Planning and other agencies have sought advice in estimating the extent of manpower shortages and in finding policies to remedy existing ones. We propose a framework for examining these questions and summarize the literature that bears on them.

We begin by looking at expectations of the medical care delivery system and at what it can provide. We then discuss a range of models used to forecast physician requirements, demand for physicians, and the distribution of physicians, and examine their implications for the formulation of public policy. Given the nature of the topic, more questions are raised than answers provided.

Some Issues in Health Care Delivery

The goal of a medical care system is to improve the health status of the population served. One of the first questions that results from this assumption is: What is the effect on the health of the population of having more physicians? In other words, what is the health effect of an increase in the physician/population ratio?

Judith R. Lave, Ph.D. is Associate Professor of Economics and Urban Affairs, School of Urban and Public Affairs; Lester B. Lave, Ph.D. is Professor and Head, Department of Economics, Graduate School of Industrial Administration; and Samuel Leinhardt, Ph.D. is Associate Professor of Sociology, School of Urban and Public Affairs, Carnegie-Mellon University (Pittsburgh, PA 15213). Their names appear in alphabetical order.

Financial support for this study was provided by the Department of Health, State of California, through a contract with the Rand Corporation, and by grant #1 R01 HS01529-01 from the National Center for Health Services Research, DHEW.

But this question contains a question: How should health be measured?[1] Health status encompasses mortality, morbidity, disability, restricted activity, bed-days, hospital days, patient anxiety, and the level of satisfaction with the medical care delivery system. There are conceptual difficulties in formulating what is to be measured; and there are methodological difficulties in measuring and combining each of the components so that an acceptable, reliable health status index results. Yet, as we argue in more detail later, there is no reasonable alternative to using a quantitative output measure of the medical care delivery system. The major policy issues require such measures as inputs in the search for a solution.

Suppose there were a health index, the next question that arises is: What is the most effective way of improving the health status of a population? Is it through personal health services, through public health services, through educational programs aimed at altering personal habits with respect to diet, exercise, and smoking? A fundamental paradox in the development of public medical care policy is that medical care obviously does save specific lives, it does lessen disease, and it does prevent or repair disability; yet, it appears that increases in medical care expenditures have little effect on overall mortality rates[2]—the whole is less than the sum of the parts due to competing risks or simply aging. Indeed, more of a good thing can be harmful if iatrogenic disease—that due to drug reactions, mistaken therapies and unnecessary surgery—is considered. It is difficult to get the right mix and amount of medical care to all groups, especially those most in "need" of care—the poor and other disadvantaged groups. Although additional personal health services do not seem to improve health, save for those most in need of care, additional expenditures on public health and improved personal habits do improve health.

If we knew which health services were efficacious, we would have to raise another question: What is the most effective way of producing them? Traditionally, a physician visit has required a physician, a secretary, and possibly an office nurse. A richer set of resources can be used. For example, paraprofessionals working under a physician's direction can handle a great part of the traditional patient visit. In particular, patients with chronic diseases can be monitored without routine involvement of the physician.[3]

Assuming we knew the "right" way to produce physician services, we would then want to know how physicians should be distributed geographically. Equally distributed, physicians in urban areas would probably be much busier than those in rural areas, both because urban residents would find it easier to get to physicians and because they have different perceptions about when care is needed. Those physicians in areas with a heavy concentration of older residents would be busier because the aged seek more care than the young.

Do remote areas, those with low population density, have unique problems? An area with a population density of less than one person per square mile, located far from a metropolitan area, is extremely difficult and costly to serve. Non-acute care can be provided by transporting the patient to the physician or vice versa, but providing emergency care is difficult. Given threshold requirements for practices, can one expect a "sufficient" number and diversity of physicians to choose to locate in these areas? The problem of serving remote and highly dispersed populations is probably the most difficult one in health care delivery, and is not likely to be handled by policies that provide financial incentives for relocation.

Such questions are usually raised individually and, in effect, we examine demand and supply independently; but we must also look at their interaction. To what extent is the demand for medical care amenable to manipulation by physicians; that is, to what extent can physicians increase or decrease the demand for their services?

One of the most important public policy trends has been to lessen or remove price as a mechanism for rationing the allocation of care. This trend has made the monetary cost of care zero or very small for a significant proportion of the population (because of government programs or insurance). As a result, access costs (travel time, waiting time, transportation cost, etc.) have become one of the most important means of rationing care. We can expect this trend to continue since an increased proportion of the population will soon be facing a negligible price for medical services. Thus, in the future, access costs will increase in importance.

We raise these general issues to provide a framework within which to consider demand and supply models. If the reader has a feeling of unease or dissatisfaction, we have no immediate antidote to offer. Later in this paper we will provide a more structured framework for handling these issues and then examine policy issues.

Models Used to Forecast Physician Requirements

What will be the *demand* for, the *need* for, and the *supply* of physicians at a given time and place? What is the gap (if any) between estimated requirements and estimated supplies? What actions, if any, does a gap suggest? The concepts of need and demand are quite different and are often confused. Since they play an important role in motivating the development of forecasts, we discuss them briefly before considering various approaches.

A population's *need for medical services* has been defined by Jeffers, *et al.*, as "that quantity of medical services which expert medical opinion believes ought to be consumed over a relevant time period in order for its members to remain or become as 'healthy' as is permitted by existing medical knowledge."[4] Need is thus a "normative" concept and is identified with the amount of preventive care medical professionals believe the population should have, as well as the amount of care they believe will bring the best medical knowledge to bear on the population's illness problems. These standards are flexible, and as Hiestand has pointed out: "Such standards will always advance in front of what can exist in fact. In a progressive, increasingly affluent society this is perfectly reasonable."[5]

A related concept is "wants." According to Jeffers, *et al.*, a population's *wants for medical services* may be defined as "that quantity of medical services which its members feel they ought to consume (at zero price, zero lost wages, zero waiting time, zero access constraints, etc.) over a relevant time period based on their own psychic perceptions of their health needs." Thus, wants are quite distinct from needs and vary among different groups. Some care that may be deemed "needed" by professionals may not be "wanted" by the population; preventive medical care and, especially, preventive dental care are examples. Other care, such as visits for the common cold, may be "wanted" by the lay population, but not deemed "needed" by physicians.

Demand is yet another related concept. Jeffers defines *the demand for medical services* as the "multivariate functional relationship between the quantities of medical services that its members desire to consume over a relevant time period at given levels of prices of goods and services, financial resources, size and psychological wants of the population as reflected by consumer tastes and preferences for (all) goods and services." Thus, the demand for medical care will depend on the underlying health status, perceptions of the efficacy of medical care, and the cost of medical care. "Demand" will be less than "need" because seeking care involves out-of-pocket costs, travel and waiting time, lost wages, discomfort, and emotional or psychic costs.

There are, therefore, important differences between need and demand: A person may not demand needed medical care because it is not perceived to be effective (not wanted or demanded at a zero price) or because, relative to the desirability of other goods and services (which compete for the individual's scarce money, income and time), it is not valued highly. In addition, price, waiting time, travel cost, or psychic costs may be so high that the

individual demands no care, even though physicians believe it is needed and the individual wants it.

We consider next some of the approaches developed for forecasting manpower requirements and indicate the strengths and weaknesses of each approach. It should be clear that this analysis is closely related to the analysis of the concept of "physician shortage," which will be discussed in a later section. Note that here we are considering how to forecast future physician requirements; we are not concerned with the precision of the forecasts, an issue that will also be discussed later.

Approaches Based on Professionally Defined Standards

The classic approach to developing manpower estimates based on professional standards or estimates of a population's medical *needs* was developed by Lee and Jones in 1933.[6] The approach consists of four steps: 1) determining the frequency of occurrence of illness by type in a population; 2) polling experts to determine the amount of services required to diagnose and treat each illness type; 3) estimating the average number of services rendered per hour by a provider; and 4) securing professional opinion on the average number of hours that a provider spends per year in caring for patients. Applying their method, Lee and Jones estimated that the need for individual preventive services and the need for the diagnosis and treatment of diseases and defects— i.e., all medical services—required 135 physicians per 100,000 population instead of the 126 per 100,000 existing when the study was performed.[7]

The Lee and Jones study was not replicated until the study by Schonfeld, *et al.* in 1972.[8] They interviewed practicing internists and pediatricians and determined what these professionals thought constituted good primary care. They then collected morbidity data from the National Health Survey, and, assuming that pediatricians worked 2,227 hours and internists 2,198 hours per year, they estimated that 133 physicians per 100,000 population were required to give good *primary* care (not including dental, mental health and obstetric care, nor routine physical examinations for adults). This estimate implies that a substantially greater gap between need and supply exists in the 1970s than Lee and Jones estimated existed in 1933, since it reflects only a portion of primary care, whereas the Lee and Jones estimate was for total medical care.

Even if we accept the concept of need as the relevant criterion, these estimates suffer from many drawbacks. We detail some of these here:

1 The standards used represent only averages. Neither Lee and Jones nor Schonfeld, et al., indicated the range of appropriate treatment patterns identified by physicians. If there is little agreement among professionals, so that the variation in individual estimates is large, then the need concept is not very meaningful for policy purposes.

Another difficulty derives from the fact that the approach does not take account of substitution for physician services in the delivery of primary care. Although independent "practice" for paramedics and nurse practitioners is still being debated, few would argue that they cannot perform, under supervision, many of the services currently performed by physicians.[9] It would thus appear, as Huebscher notes, that the number of physicians required to render primary medical care is "fluid."[10]

2 This approach does not include an evaluation of the health outcomes implied by the standards. How do morbidity and mortality rates compare between groups receiving care at the professional standards level and groups receiving much less care? Is there a noticeable difference, and can it be attributed to the level of care? Evidence indicates that the relationship is far from straightforward. For example, the Kaiser Health Plan (which is often cited as an ideal health plan where high quality medical care is believed to be provided) has less than half the number of "needed" primary care physicians (34 internists, 10 generalists and 16 pediatricians) available per 100,000 subscribers.[11] These questions must be considered if the standards approach is to be taken seriously.

3 The approach is excessively narrow because it regards "need" strictly from a professional viewpoint. Do people demand this much medical care? It is not altogether clear that, under the best circumstances, patients behave as physicians would have them. For example, Jacobs,[12] in criticizing the Schonfeld, et al., study, noted that in his community of 200,000 there were 122 primary care physicians (less than half the standard). He pointed out that although these doctors provided more inclusive care (e.g., routine medical examinations) and the community was very wealthy, the physicians were underemployed. Should the patients be "educated" to demand more care? Surely that depends on the answer given to the question of the preceding paragraph.

4 The approach fails to consider alternatives. It emphasizes physician-based personal medical services, but what priority should the government place on the provision of personal medical services? If resources were available to provide medical care meeting professional standards, then surely the share of national income going to personal medical services would increase enormously. Should such an allocation of national income be preferred to one of more recreation, books, housing, and the like? If the goal of public policy is to improve health, we must determine—or at least consider—whether that goal will be better met by providing enough personal medical services to meet professionally determined standards or by the provision of other services such as nutritional programs or education?[13]

These criticisms are quite general and apply equally well to other studies where the estimates of need are based on professional standards. Professional standards and, indeed, all normative approaches should be used for manpower planning purposes only after careful evaluation of alternative approaches.

Approaches Based on Evidence in Comprehensive Prepaid Group Practice

A number of observers have argued that the observed demand for manpower in specific

Table 1. Average number of physicians per 100,000 population served in six medical groups providing prepaid medical services, by specialty

Specialty	Average number of physicians	
	Mean	Median
Internal medicine	45.2	44.9
Allergy	1.6	1.4
Dermatology	2.8	2.5
Pediatrics	18.0	15.8
Obstetrics	9.1	8.0
Orthopedics	3.2	3.0
Ophthalmology	3.7	3.3
Otolaryngology	4.6	3.5
Surgery	6.5	6.7
Urology	1.9	1.5
Radiology	4.4	4.0
Physical medicine*	1.3	1.0
Anesthesiology*	1.5	1.5
Pathology*	1.8	1.6
Neurology*	1.0	1.0
Psychiatry	2.8	1.5
Total**	109.4	....

* Physical medicine based on three groups; anesthesiology based on two groups; pathology and neurology based on four groups. These services are provided in the remaining groups in other ways.
** Exclusive of interns and residents in hospitals.
Source: *Health Manpower Perspective*, 1967. U.S. Public Health Service, Bureau of Health Manpower, Washington, D.C., 1967, Appendix Table 6, p. 75.

prepaid group practice plans is the best guide for general manpower planning. They have argued that this mode of practice is ideal (supporters of prepaid medical practice often ignore the effect of access costs). It is presumed that the plan provides members with all needed medical care and that this care is of high quality. Whatever one's beliefs about prepaid group practice, we doubt that the staffing ratios observed in these groups could serve to forecast the need for specialist or primary care manpower.

In Table 1 we show the distribution of physicians by specialty averaged across six prepaid group practices. In interpreting the data presented in the table, one should note that the numerator includes only active physicians engaged primarily in clinical care and that the average masks a considerable amount of variation.

The Kaiser System, for example, is composed of numerous different local plans. The number of physicians per 100,000 members varies across the different plans. There were 96.6 physicians per 100,000 Kaiser member in 1970. This ranged from 76 in the Colorado plan to 105 in the Northern California plan. In plans with over 100,000 members, the range was from 82 to 105.[14] Before one uses estimates derived from such prepaid group practice programs, several questions must be answered. For example: What factors generated the between-plan manpower ratio differences? Are the populations served different? Is more use made of outside physicians in some plans? Are there more paramedical personnel in some plans? Are the health levels of the groups different? These questions have not been answered, but the variability across plans is striking. This variability is strong evidence that fixed manpower ratios make little sense.

Even if these questions are answered, it is still not clear whether these prepaid comprehensive group ratios should be used in determining manpower requirements for the nation. The data are of doubtful relevance and are likely to underestimate the physicians needed for the following reasons:

1 The plans in the Kaiser System are tightly administered. The total number of physicians is administratively determined and does not necessarily represent a physician/population ratio that would be observed in fee-for-service practice. The number of patients to be seen per hour and the length of the work week are defined; physicians are closely monitored for such aspects of care as ordering lab tests and hospitalization of patients; patients must often wait substantial periods to have a scheduled visit with their physician.

2 The distribution of physicians by specialty type is determined administratively. Supposedly, intensive peer review is practiced, and referral and hospitalization rates are closely monitored, resulting in lower rates than in fee-for-service practice. Without the organization of the prepaid comprehensive plan, it is hard to see why their utilization patterns would generalize. Note also that this kind of medical system represents a

Table 2. Non-federal physicians by census region and activity, December 31, 1970

Census region	Total physicians*		Patient care	
	Number	Percent	Number	Percent
Total non-federal	281,344	100.0	255,027	100.0
Northeast	87,641	31.2	77,928	30.6
New England	20,391	7.2	17,802	7.0
Middle Atlantic	67,250	23.9	60,126	23.6
North Central	66,993	23.8	61,451	24.1
East North Central	48,162	17.1	44,281	17.4
West North Central	18,831	6.7	17,170	6.7
South	70,178	24.9	64,031	25.1
South Atlantic	37,560	13.4	33,871	13.3
East South Central	12,155	4.3	11,200	4.4
West South Central	20,463	7.3	18,960	7.4
West	54,043	19.2	49,368	19.4
Mountain	10,368	3.7	9,500	3.7
Pacific	43,675	15.5	39,868	15.6
Possessions	2,489	0.9	2,249	0.9

* Excludes 19,621 inactive physicians and 358 not classified.
Note: Percentages may not add due to rounding.
Source: Haug, J. N.; Roback, G. A.; and Martin, B. C. "Distribution of Physicians in the United States, 1970," (Chicago, American Medical Association, 1971).

type of practice that currently serves only 5 percent of the population. The members themselves selected this type of system (all had a fee-for-service alternative) and are not a representative subsample of the national population. They tend to be actively employed, middle-class individuals whose level of income and knowledge leads to better health, less need for prolonged hospitalization, and fewer complicated illnesses. In 1970, for example, about 4.5 percent of the members of the Kaiser plans were over 65 and 1.5 percent were on Medicaid. To put these figures in perspective, in 1970, 9.8 percent of the United States population was over 65 and about 10 percent had incomes below the poverty level.

3 At least in the past, Kaiser patients had incentives quite different from those of other patients; monetary costs were low and access costs could be substantial. Indeed, many patients sought care outside the system at a substantial monetary cost rather than accept the nonmonetary costs within the system. Subtle rationing is associated with the centralized clinic ambulatory practice which leads to greater travel time and cost. A final factor is the emphasis placed on educating subscribers to recognize disease that

is not helped by medical care and to improve personal habits, such as not smoking, getting exercise, and avoiding obesity.

Although the data from the Kaiser System do provide a minimum reference point, they are unlikely to be of direct relevance for planning in the absence of significant structural change in the nation's medical care delivery system.

Manpower Planning Using the Ratio Approach

There is considerable variation in the ratio of physicians to population among various geographic regions. In Table 2, the 1970 distribution of M.D.s by region is presented. The Northeast and West have proportionately more physicians per capita than the South and North Central regions; the variation among states is much greater than that among regions. For example, in 1970 for the country as a whole, there were 171 physicians per 100,000 population, with a range of 83 per 100,000 in Mississippi to 238 per 100,000 in New York. The District of Columbia had 385 physicians per 100,000. There is some indication that these regional differences are becoming larger. In 1950, Mississippi had 66 physicians per 100,000 and New York had 201; thus, between 1950 and 1970, the gap between the state with the highest and lowest number of physicians per 100,000 population rose from 135 to 155. There is also some evidence that these trends favor the coastal states at the expense of those that are more inland.

Within states there are great differences between rural and urban physician/population ratios. In 1970, there were 173 physicians per 100,000 population in the urban areas, but only 80 physicians per 100,000 in rural areas. Within the state of California, physician/population ratios across the planning areas ranged from 220 per 100,000 in the San Francisco Bay area to 99 per 100,000 in Superior, California. Even within urban areas, the variability in the local supply of physicians is great. Physicians are usually concentrated in only a few census tracts, while most census tracts have none.

We explore spatial distribution of physician manpower more extensively in the next section. Here, we consider an approach to planning for medical manpower that makes use of physician/population ratios. In it, some present physician/population ratio is considered a minimum requirement for the future. This approach has a number of variations involving the selection of the ratios:

☐ The minimum required physician/population ratio at some future time is taken as the average ratio existing now in the United States.

☐ The minimum required physician/population ratio at some future time is taken as that now existing in the states with the highest physician/population ratios (the criterion ratio).

☐ The minimum required physician/population ratio is calculated for each demographic group in a place where the population is deemed to be "adequately" served. To determine the number of physicians required, it is then necessary to forecast the expected population growth and the future demographic characteristics of the population. For example, if the aged need more physicians and if the mean age in the population is rising, then to ensure continued access to physicians similar to that of today, the overall physician/population ratio will have to rise.

Ignoring for the moment the problems that can arise in forecasting, we address the strengths and weaknesses of forecasting requirements on the basis of existing physician/population ratios.

1 Of these planning techniques, the first ratio approach seems to require the least information. Projections that incorporate expected changes in the demographic composition of the population (the third method) will provide more reliable insight than projections based simply on total population.

2 There is an implicit, but untested, assumption that the base ratio is adequate and needed; that is, a reduction in the ratio would be adverse. It is often assumed that the more physicians, the better. However, there is evidence that adding physicians to an area may simply lead to unnecessary medical care or to underemployment of physicians. Thus, the criterion ratio approach (second method) is likely to set future requirements too high.

3 In the absence of structural changes in the delivery system, the ratio approach will provide reasonable forecasts of *demand* over the short term. Changes in organization, medical technology, immunology, treatment, financing and payment mechanisms, or mode of practice, for example, are likely to invalidate manpower projections based on current utilization patterns.

4 Using national ratios hides a great deal, e.g., variability in physician distribution by state, county, and type of practice. The wide variation in local physician/population ratios is shown in Table 2. Suppose, for example, that enough physicians are trained to raise the United States physician/population ratio to the level of the highest 10 states (as of 1975). There is little reason to believe that these newly produced physicians will choose to concentrate in states with relatively fewer physicians, or in areas within states that have the lowest ratios. Indeed, we would predict that the difference between areas would increase as a result of training these additional physicians, as it did between 1950 and 1970. However, all states had more physicians per capita in 1970 than in 1950; thus, the

poorer states were better off in absolute terms, even though they were worse off in relative terms.

5 If the numerator is to indicate the availability of physician services, it should be derived with respect to full-time-equivalent active physicians engaged in providing clinical services as opposed to teaching, research, public health, and other activities, and it should take account of physicians who work part time.

6 The ratio approach ignores all changes in physician productivity and assumes that physicians are used in fixed proportions in delivering medical services. Existing data indicate that the way in which physicians allocate their services to patients is predictable; for example, more tasks are delegated to allied health personnel when the physician/population ratio is low.[15] The volume of services provided by physicians is not fixed and physician productivity has been increasing over time. Klarman[16] presents a number of estimates of increases in physician productivity; the mean estimated increase is about 3 percent per year. The ratio approach also takes no account of changes in medical technology and public health practice or the introduction of new health manpower.

In all fairness, it should be pointed out that these criticisms are acknowledged by researchers who have used this approach. It should also be pointed out that without a good deal of clairvoyance it is impossible to forecast some of these trends. However, these arguments suggest that the system is more fluid than the ratio approach implies and that policies should encourage flexibility, not fixed ratios.

Economic Models

In developing an economic model of demand, the question is: What will utilization (use of physicians' services or other aspects of medical care) be at some future time? This question is approached by estimating a demand function, a relationship between the amount of care sought and its cost, access constraints, and other factors. To predict the future level of services that will be sought, the future value of each factor in the demand function is estimated and the estimated parameters are used to predict future utilization.

Economists have tended to neglect access costs, which are becoming more important than direct payment to the provider. Acton and Richardson[17] have investigated some of the effects of access costs. Costs due to scarcities in rural areas were investigated by Marshall, et al.[18] Their finding—that dissatisfaction over travel time to get to a physician in rural Kansas was great and was likely to have adverse effects on patient behavior—is corroborated in a study by Weiss and Greenlick,[19] who analyzed the behavior of urban and suburban patients in the Kaiser program. However, Weiss and Greenlick noticed that distance did not have a constant effect on all types of patients. Instead, they detected an interaction effect, which led them to conclude that patients in upper socioeconomic status (SES) groups were little affected by distance, while lower SES groups were led either to delay seeking care until symptoms became quite severe or to substitute emergency room encounters for routine appointments with medical staff. Such findings have been reported elsewhere[20] and have been incorporated into most current theories of patient illness behavior.[21]

The demand for medical care (and physician services) is derived from the demand for health.[22] Medical care is a service than can be bought to improve or maintain health "stock." The demand for medical care is thus dependent upon an individual's underlying health status, perception of the efficacy of medical care, and cost of getting medical care, where cost is a vector consisting of time costs, money costs, and psychological costs. To determine the demand relationship, this theoretical formulation must be made specific and then estimated with empirical data.

Investigators may use age as a surrogate for underlying health status, education as a measure of awareness, reported money income as a measure of both earned and unearned income, sex as another indication of the underlying health status, distance to facilities as a measure of time cost, and insurance and Medicaid coverage as a measure of the difference between the "market" price and actual price to the individual. Demand functions have been estimated using individuals, groups of individuals, and states as the basic unit of observation.[23] Single equation demand models have been estimated as have general systems (with demand as one part).

Economists have focused their attention on determining the income and price elasticities of the demand for medical care and physician services. Income elasticity is defined as the percentage change in quantity bought due to a 1 percent change in income, and price elasticity is defined as the percentage change in quantity bought due to a 1 percent change in price. The former is a measure of the responsiveness of demand to a change in income, and the latter is a measure of responsiveness of demand to a change in price.

In estimating income elasticities, economists distinguish between earnings and wealth. Separating earned income from unearned income is particularly important where the time price is high, such as in medical care. As earnings rise, other things equal, the value of time rises, and it is assumed that people are willing to substitute money for time. This may explain why employed men and women are more alike in their demands for care than employed women and homemakers, income level held constant.[24]

The empirical estimates of income elasticity have been varied. The range of these estimates is presented in Table 3. The Fein estimate indicates that a 1 percent increase in income will generate at .21 percent increase in physician visits.

The price elasticity of the demand for physician care has also been estimated. The estimates range from −.1 to −.36.[25] Some recent attention has been directed to estimating nonprice costs and their effect on services demanded. Both waiting time and travel time are shown to have high elasticities.[26]

These results indicate that as the monetary price (to consumers) of medical care falls and as income rises, the quantity of medical services demanded will also increase. As access costs to medical care drop, demand will also rise.

Table 3. Several measures of income elasticity of demand for physician expenditures or services[*]

Source	Income elasticity
Fein[1] (visits)	.21
Feldstein, P.[2]	
visits	.62
expenditures	.56
Gorham[3] (expenditures)	.33
Andersen and Benham[4]	
visits (observed income)	n.v.
visits (permanent income)	.01
expenditures (observed income)	.41
expenditures (permanent income)	.63
Fuchs and Kramer[5] (visits)	.04–.57

[*] This table is adapted from Klarman, H. E. "Economic Aspects of Projecting Requirements for Health Manpower," *The Journal of Human Resources* 4:360–376 (1969).

[1] Fein, R. *The Doctor Shortage* (Washington, D.C.: The Brookings Institution, 1967).
[2] Feldstein, P. J. "The Demand for Medical Care," in: Commission on the Cost of Medical Care. *General Report*, Vol. I (Chicago: American Medical Association, 1964).
[3] Gorham, W. "A Report to the President on Medical Care Prices," (Washington, D.C.: U.S Department of Health, Education and Welfare, 1967).
[4] Andersen, R. and Benham, L. "Factors Affecting the Relationship between Family Income and Medical Care Consumption," in: Klarman, H. E. (ed.) *Empirical Studies in Health Economics* (Baltimore: The Johns Hopkins Press, 1970).
[5] Fuchs, V. R. and Kramer, M. J. *Determinants of Expenditures for Physicians' Services in the United States 1948–1968*, DHEW Publication No. (HSM) 73-3013 (Washington, D.C.: DHEW, HSMHA, December 1972).

However, if the time costs of medical care rise, the number of services demanded will fall, particularly for those with a high opportunity cost for time.

Some investigators have argued that the demand curve may be affected by the supply of physicians.[27] In this conceptualization, the physicians themselves are thought to influence the number of visits people make by suggesting patterns of care (which include revisits) through follow-up recommendations, and by lobbying for the construction of medical institutions. The crux of the physician-induced demand argument is that the pattern of recommended care may vary with the physician load. That is, in areas with many physicians, physicians can maintain their income by recommending more visits—visits that may be of marginal medical efficacy.

Some major work on the demand for and supply of physicians has been done by Fuchs and Kramer.[28] They estimated a five equation model using state data that contained a demand function (number of visits per capita), a supply function (number of doctors per 100,000 population), an output per physician function (number of visits per thousand), an insurance benefits function, and two identities—the quantity demanded of physician services equals the quantity supplied, and one defining net price. Since it is a simultaneous system, two stage least squares was used to estimate the parameters.

Fuchs and Kramer hypothesized that one of the factors affecting the number of visits demanded per capita was the number of M.D.s per capita. This variable was included because it was argued that physicians were able to generate a demand for their services without lowering price. Fuchs and Kramer suggest that when physicians are abundant, they may order care that is not medically indicated (unnecessary surgery), or of marginal importance (numerous post-operative visits, follow-up visits, or overzealous well-baby care); when physicians are scarce, patients may lower their expectations and handle minor complaints themselves. They also suggested that when physicians are plentiful, the nonmonetary costs of care (waiting time, time to get an appointment, and travel costs) are likely to be lower. In the statistical results, the M.D. variable (physicians per capita) was the one with the highest elasticity and with the highest level of significance, presumably indicating that the supply of physicians had the most influence on the demand for care.

Although the number of M.D.s per capita may be a surrogate for nonmonetary costs, Fuchs and Kramer believe that the importance of the variable stems from physicians' ability to control demand. They quote Ginzberg:[29]

The supply of medical resources has thus far effectively generated its own demand. Much unnecessary surgery continues to be performed. . . . There is substantial over-doctoring for a host of diseases, including, in

particular, infections of the upper respiratory tract. . . . [Physicians] usually have wide margins of discretion about whether to recommend that a patient return to the office for one or more follow-up visits.

It could be argued that Fuchs and Kramer have uncovered a simultaneous equation problem rather than physician-induced demand. If physicians moved their practice to areas where the most care was needed, the data would show a close association between supply and demand. Although many of the characteristics expected to lead to increased need are included in the analysis, the possibility remains that the result reflects the altruistic nature of physicians rather than their artificially induced demand. Results similar to those obtained by Fuchs and Kramer were found in a study in Canada. Examining physicians in British Columbia, Evans[30] argued that a strong case could be made for supplier-induced demand. These results are open to question (and have been questioned). Nonetheless, they do have very important implications for manpower planning.

Systems Models of Health Care

A number of theoretical systems models of health care delivery have been proposed, but only two have been fully specified and estimated. The first is actually a series of models developed by Martin Feldstein.[31] These are econometric models with about half a dozen equations (and endogenous variables). For example, in his analysis of the effects of Medicare, the endogenous variables are the proportion of enrollees with supplementary insurance, the hospital admissions rate, the rate of extended care admissions per hospital admission, and the hospital insurance benefits per hospital episode. These variables are modeled as being determined by demographic variables, such as the proportions of white enrollees, male enrollees, those living in large cities, the ratio of enrollees over 75 to total enrollees, and per capita income. Other variables include the proportion of the population under 65 with health insurance, the proportion of enrollees for which the state government declines to pay premiums (and who are indigent), short-term beds per capita, private physicians per capita, per capita state expenditure for the aged on health, the number of months the state had participated in Medicaid, extended care beds per capita, and hospital cost per patient day. The equations were estimated by an instrumental variables technique (similar to two stage least squares) on observations for each state. Since the model was designed to explain the variation among states in the dependent variables, it has little to do with the sort of behavior one would expect to observe in individual patients, physicians, and hospitals. In this sense, it is a "macro" model and ignores the details of an individual's behavior, assuming it to be unaffected by the policy variables except as summarized in the macro variables. The other conceptual difficulty is the lack of an output measure, but we return to this difficulty after discussing the second model.

Yett, *et al.*,[32] have developed an elaborate model of the medical care sector that uses more than 100 equations (and endogenous variables) to characterize almost every aspect of the system. There are a number of submodels, concerned with manpower, hospitals, and so on, that are joined by some interaction equations. The rationale given for each of the behavioral equations is that of the decisions to be made by an individual and the factors affecting them. Thus, the Yett, *et al.*, model is different in orientation, as well as in complexity, from the Feldstein models, but data are not available to estimate the relations. The best that Yett, *et al.*, can do is to use state observations to get most of the variables. Even so, it is impossible to obtain the relevant measures of insurance coverage and other factors. Given the size of the model and the quality of the data, the authors choose to estimate the equations individually, using ordinary least squares. This means that the parameter estimates are inconsistent compared with estimates generated by, for example, two stage least squares, although, given the quality of the data, their choice of an estimating technique is appropriate. Unfortunately, the good intentions of constructing a model to reflect individual behavior are not realized because of the lack of data for estimating the model.

Yett, *et al.*, have attempted to spell out the implications of their model using simulation techniques. Using the parameter estimates gained from ordinary least squares regression on state data, the authors vary one or another parameter and use simulation to explore the resulting change in the equilibrium of the model. For a model of this size, there is no alternative way of investigating the system influences of a change in a set of parameter values. For example, their manpower planning subsystem uses the forecast demand for services, the production relations for these services and the equations determining the supply of manpower. The output is then a forecast of the number of physicians that would be required to meet the demand, as well as an estimate of the number of hours per week they would work and their income.

The Feldstein and Yett, *et al.*, models share the problem of not having a measure of the output of the medical care sector. They determine the conventional measures of utilization, available manpower, and cost, but have no explicit measure of output. One might continue to use utilization and input measures (number of patient visits, inpatient days, etc.) as surrogates for output, but the implications in a model of this sort would be that more and more resources should be put into medical care delivery. Although these models can be helpful in exploring the structure of the medical care system, they are inherently limited by their lack of an output measure. Policy implications must be drawn cautiously from a model when it cannot be known whether increasing the number of patient visits will have a positive or negative effect on health (much less on social welfare). The models do tell us the implications of parameter changes, such as those that might result from a particular type of national health insurance. If one knew whether an increase in one aspect of utilization was good or bad, such models might be used to determine what parameters ought to be altered to achieve a desirable result.

We have constructed a model with these properties[33] and are currently attempting to estimate its parameters. Summary inputs and outcomes in the model consist of physician hours, hospital days, physician visits, total cost, and several health status measures. The underlying health status of the population and an individual's health status at any point is the primary factor determining whether care will be sought or prescribed treatment compliance will occur. Since health status is treated explicitly in the model, there is no alternative to specifying spontaneous rates of improvement or deterioration in health, and the efficacy of some contact with the health care system in improving health status. We regard the model as giving many insights, but we must stress the obvious difficulties in getting health status measures and in estimating how these change spontaneously or with medical care.

Summary and Critique of the Models

The ratio model has the advantage of being simple and will predict utilization accurately insofar as the underlying conditions determining demand and supply do not change (no major changes in medical knowledge, organization, or financing of medical care). However, since the ratios reflect the current system, their use presupposes a future system where utilization is similar to the current one. In contrast, the Lee and Jones[34] approach is more of an attempt to get at ideal requirements. Its principal problem is that the actual level of medical care demanded is far less than that predicted by the model (since not everyone who needs care seeks it, nor do people adhere to their prescribed regimen). Thus, manpower policies based on the ratio approach will tend to preserve the current system, while policies based on the Lee and Jones approach would lead to an oversupply of physicians. Both approaches ignore the substitution possibilities in producing care and increasing productivity.

The simple economic models go far in allowing one to gain insight into the factors that affect physician utilization. They allow one to predict what effect changing socioeconomic or demographic characteristics of the population will have on the demand for medical care and what the effects will be of increasing population or the amount of insurance. However, many of the crucial variables, such as travel time and waiting time, are necessarily the result of inter-actions between supply and demand. Since these models look only at the demand side of the picture, they cannot determine the level of these access variables and so are conceptually incomplete (although one might guess at future values of these parameters).

Two models of medical care delivery that look at the simultaneous interaction of supply and demand have been described briefly. However, they are unsatisfactory in two important ways. First, they were estimated using aggregate (state level) observations. Second, they had no output measures associated with them. Thus, one knows only that by manipulating the system one can change the number of patient visits or hospital visits, but one cannot know whether these changes increase or decrease the public welfare.

To construct a model capable of predicting demand after a structural change (such as that represented by national health insurance or reorganization into health maintenance organizations), to take account of the simultaneity of supply and demand, and to estimate the social welfare implications of changes, one must have a model of the health care system like the two presented, but having the additional property that output is included directly. This is the crucial issue; however, in addition, the system must be estimated using disaggregated data so that it reflects individual consumer and physician preferences while acknowledging that there are other ways of providing care.

Models of the Supply of Physician Services

Physician services might be measured by the number of hours of service by physician specialty and location. Thus, one must know the current stock of physicians; changes in the stock due to deaths, retirements, and new graduates; factors affecting choice of specialty; factors affecting the number of hours a physician devotes to medical care; and factors affecting geographical location (by region, by rural versus urban area, and by location within an urban area). While there have been insightful discussion of these issues,[35] there has been little formal modeling and empirical investigation.

In this section we examine research findings

that bear on physician supply. These studies have focused predominantly on the maldistribution of physician services. Determining maldistributions, measuring their extent, and studying the factors associated with them are central policy issues since many government agencies have reacted to perceived local scarcities by elaborate, and often expensive, intervention into the local delivery system. Unfortunately, this research area is filled with contradictory results; thus, one must look carefully at the underlying data base and analytical methods to resolve the contradictions.

Approaches to Studying Physician Supply

Three techniques have been most commonly used to study maldistribution and the factors causing it. By far the most common involves a simple tabular comparison of physician/population ratios. Variability across the units of analysis is often presumed to be sufficient evidence of a maldistribution of physicians. The extent of this maldistribution is identified with the range of the ratios. Thus, DeVise[36] argues that coastal regions have a comparative advantage over inland regions; and Fahs, et al.,[37] argue that the central states lose medical graduates to the western states. Comparisons of this sort inevitably show that the more heavily urbanized states have more physicians than the rural states, and, within the states, urban counties have more physicians than rural counties. However, these findings while suggestive are not definitive. The studies suffer from an absence of control for other factors known to be important determinants of physician location. For example, the coastal states with the greatest number of physicians are also highly urbanized states; is the coastal location or the urbanization the true cause of the movement? What aspects of urban or coastal environments attract physicians? What qualities of rural communities repel them? For purposes of policy formulation, such simple comparisons represent only first steps.

The second most common approach employs multivariate statistical analysis and represents an improvement over tabular comparisons. Studies using these methods attempt (at levels of aggregation such as regional, state, county,

or census tract) to relate the physician population of a locality to qualities of the locality that are presumed to act as positive or negative inducements to physicians. These studies are often predicated on a well-formulated model of physician spatial behavior. Typically some form of regression is used to estimate the relation. In their classic study, Rimlinger and Steele[38] used least squares techniques to estimate a linear model relating physician/population ratios for 200 county groups that constituted the United States to characteristics of these areas in 1959. Their findings indicated that income, leisure, and mobility were significant explanatory variables; and they argued that such factors are positively associated with urbanization. The power of the multivariate approach is that it has the potential of allowing the investigator to examine the influence of a host of variables simultaneously and to estimate the individual effect of each. Since some of these variables are amenable to policy manipulation, the technique can provide a basis for choosing among alternative policies.

Although this approach is superior to cross tabulations, it has many pitfalls. Ordinary least squares (OLS) has predominated in these analyses, but it may not be an appropriate estimation technique because of multicollinearity or simultaneous influences among the variables. This is often the case when ratios are used as dependent variables.[39] Often the relevant variables are so closely associated in the observed data that it is impossible to distinguish among them.[40] Other problems in the applicability of OLS lie in the assumptions that must be made concerning independence and normality in the distribution of errors and linearity of the equation. Thus, estimation techniques such as two stage least squares, ridge, Tobit, and Poisson regression may be required to give accurate estimates of relationships.

The third approach, and one that is becoming more common, involves surveying physician opinion. Here, researchers attempt to ascertain from physicians themselves the factors regarded as most important in the choice of a practice location. This approach has the potential of uncovering factors that may be neglected by analysts who have little personal experience with the practice location decision. Clearly, the outcome of such studies may be input to more elaborate econometric analyses of aggregate data. For example, Cooper, *et al.*,[41] report the results of a survey conducted by the American Medical Association in an attempt to ascertain the conditions under which particular physicians decide to locate in rural or urban areas. Attitudinal surveys focus on preferential differences among physicians, whereas spatial models focus on extant differences among localities. Both are useful for policy formulation. On the one hand, surveys help determine which background qualities of physicians make them better long-term choices for rural locations. On the other hand, spatial models may reveal whether professional amenities lead more physicians on average to choose a particular type of locale.

These three approaches are not exhaustive of those used to investigate physician distribution but they do typify the bulk of the reported research. In general, the questions that have been phrased are these: Where are the physicians? What are the characteristics of the areas they favor and of those they shun? What are the characteristics of physicians in areas where there are scarcities? The underlying assumption of the research is that by understanding the attractive factors or the personal predispositions of physicians, policies can be instituted to modify or equalize the availability of medical care. We proceed to review this literature first in terms of the choice between urban and rural settings and then between sites within cities; we consider the role of the foreign medical graduate; and last, we examine what has been learned regarding the initial location decisions of recent medical graduates.

In Table 4 we have categorized factors that have been the subject of research and indicated the direction of their apparent influence on physicians. Some effects, such as that of loan forgiveness programs, are debatable. But in the absence of further research the displayed effects seem reasonable. The results emphasize the attractive nature of urban areas and the physician's personal acquaintance with a particular area or type of area. Although the table summarizes the most relevant research, we shall briefly consider some of the studies from which it was constructed.

The Rural-Urban Choice

The discussion of rural-urban differences in physician manpower is commonplace in state medical journals.[42] Generally, the opinion surveys indicate that those physicians who chose to locate in small communities did so simply because they or their spouses like these locales. Yett and Sloan[43] report that physicians tend to set up practice in areas near their place of rearing or medical training. These findings and the associated finding that most small town practitioners were reared in small towns suggest that, of those physicians practicing in small towns, personal life-style preferences rather than professional issues predominate.[44] Physicians who report that professional considerations predominate find urban locations most attractive. These physicians give a high priority to proximity to colleagues and supporting medical facilities, the ability to have a varied practice, and the possibility of joining a group practice—qualities associated with urban locations. Non-urban physicians report heavy workloads, while higher pay scales and more readily scheduled activities are reported by urban physicians. The surveys also indicate that young physicians are more anxious than older physicians to join group practices and that they are tending more often to choose financially secure and readily scheduled positions on academic or medical staffs and in other institutional settings. These findings imply that extant urban-rural differences are likely to increase as older physicians are replaced.

The regression studies have addressed the issue of life-style variables and urban versus rural location at many levels of data aggregation. In their analysis of state level data, Fuchs and Kramer[45] used two stage least squares techniques to estimate a model of physician distribution for 33 states in 1966. The most important variables they identified were per capita income, the presence of medical schools, the price of care, and the number of hospital beds. However, the relevant variables were so closely associated that they could not separate the various hypotheses. They concluded by

Table 4. Factors affecting physician location*

Dependent variable	Relationship	Independent variable
Number of physicians	+	Per capita income in state
	+	State educational expenditures
	+	Per capita income in county
	+	Construction of hospital in community
	+	Median income in community
	+	Population of area
	+	Physicians' price practices, based on per capita income of area
	+	Failure rate of licensing examination
	+	Physician income in state
	−	Lack of recreational facilities
	−	Contruction of hospital in rural county
	−	Cyclic variations in income levels in area
	+	Presence of commercial activity
Practice in urban areas	+	Graduation from certain medical schools
	+	Graduation from urban medical school
Practice in rural areas	+	Rural background
	+	Participation in loan forgiveness program
Practice in same state	+	Internship and residency training in state
Ability to attract physicians	+	Mobility of community residents
	+	Educational level of population
	−	Percent population in agriculture
Number of primary care physicians	+	Percent population white
	+	Percent population 0–5 years old and 65+ years old
	−	Inadequate cultural and recreational resources in community
Number of specialists	+	Educational level of population
	+	Number of supportive institutions
	+	Number of general hospital beds per 1000 population
	+	Medical school in community
	+	Presence of high concentrations of commercial activity
	+	Presence of university medical facility
Presence of physician	+	Economic growth rate of town

* This table is adapted from Cooper, J. K.; Heald, K,; and Samuels, M. "The Decision for Rural Practice," *Journal of Medical Education* 47:939–944 (December 1972).

suggesting that, in general, professional convenience and urban "life-style" factors were attractive to most physicians. Lave and Lave[46] performed a similar analysis on 1950 and 1970 state data in which they included variables meant to characterize urban qualities more precisely. The urbanization effect was strong in both 1950 and 1970. In a follow-up study to their 1963 report, Steele and Rimlinger[47] reported the results of county level analyses for 1949 and 1959. Although some specific results seemed at odds with their earlier findings, the general results from both studies were similar. Family income was less important as an explanatory variable in 1959 than in 1949, while the amenities that the authors associated with an "urban environment" became more important over time.

Marden's[48] study of physician location in 369 metropolitan counties was particularly important because he grouped physicians as either specialists or general practitioners. The following characteristics of the metropolitan areas were included: educational attainment, age composition, racial composition, and number of hospital beds in the counties. Race and age composition were found to be the most important explanatory variables, with hospital beds important only for the smallest cities. However, Marden's analysis was replicated by Joroff and Navarro[49] with contradictory results. Examining 299 cities and using 10 independent variables, they did not find race to be important once the presence of a medical school and the population's educational attainment were taken into account. Additional important factors were hospital beds and the population's age distribution. Lankford's[50] analysis supported the predominance of population as a determinant of physician location.

Further support for the role played by medical facilities or professional amenities is provided in two Ph.D. dissertations using state level data. Weiss[51] reported that physicians were attracted to states in proportion to the number of medical centers they contained; and Sloan[52] reported that high physician/population ratios were associated with high income, low cyclical economic variability, high capital stock, and high numbers of medical students (a likely surrogate for the medical center effect detected by Weiss). Finally, Benham, et al.,[53] performed analyses on 1930, 1940, 1950, and 1960 levels of physicians and dentists in the states and found that, over time, increasing importance was being placed on high per capita income, population, and medical training facilities.

These results for the effects of population and medical facilities on physician distribution have received widespread support. Income seems no longer to be the most important factor.[54] Instead, it would appear that physician salaries are currently so high that the lure of still higher income influences few. Physicians seem now to be more concerned with cultural, environmental and professional amenities. These include leisure time (attained by

a not overly-demanding practice and the effectiveness of non-price rationing procedures[55]), medical resources, interesting case variety, income security, colleagues, and other qualities associated with large populations or dense urban areas. In this vein, Parker, et al.,[56] found that most physicians who chose to practice in small towns could be readily distinguished from other physicians in that they did not share the views about urban and professional qualities. Instead, they were often originally from small towns, had a preference for this life-style, and claimed to be unconcerned about urban-rural physician income differentials.[57] These findings indicate that as the bulk of physicians come from urban backgrounds and as they pass through the medical education system, they acquire a set of values that reinforces their predisposition to choose an urban location for their practice. Thus, urbanization, medical specialization (leading to greater dependence among physicians on cooperative activities), dependence on hospital-based technological care, and the rise of staff positions in institutional medicine seem to be the primary processes influencing the contemporary national spatial distribution of physicians.

Intra-Urban Location Decisions

The state, metropolitan, and county level studies provide some information on the factors affecting the spatial distribution of physicians in the United States. They also suggest variables that may be relevant to intra-urban spatial research. The research we have reviewed indicates that physicians tend to gravitate toward areas that satisfy their own personal objectives in terms of life-style and professional behavior, and that factors such as the racial composition of the population do not appear to be very important.

The processes affecting regional distribution seem readily understood, although precision and knowledge of interactions need to be improved. On the local level, however, the situation is not as clear-cut. Because of the affected urban population groups—the poor, the aged, and the nonwhite—local maldistributions may be as significant as regional maldistribution. Adverse conditions are likely to lead here to patterns of behavior accentuating the severity of an illness episode and frustrating the efficient delivery of therapeutic medical services.[58]

There is a copious literature bearing on local distribution. Chicago, New York, and Boston have been the sites of extensive investigations. Some other cities have been studied.[59] We concentrate on recent studies of the three major sites, detailing others only when relevant.

Lepper, *et al.*,[60] performed a study of physician/population ratios in Chicago's OEO-defined poverty areas. Their conclusion that physicians were fairly scarce in these locales was also reached by Rees, by DeVise and Dewey, and by Dewey.[61] In his two studies, Rees examined the exodus of physicians from Chicago to the surrounding suburbs. He chose an extremely gross unit of analysis (three concentric zones or a few neighborhoods) and, consequently, only vague conclusions could be drawn. Thus, he could only determine that the numbers of physicians setting up practice in the Chicago suburbs appeared to outpace those starting up in the city. DeVise and Dewey summarize the Dewey study. Decennial data on physician/population ratios for 1950, 1960, and 1970 were contrasted with data on race, population, retail buying power, and hospitals. Again, physicians were found to be fleeing the inner city for the more affluent white suburbs; physicians were seen to seek office locations near expensive residential tracts so as to minimize their own travel time to the office; socioeconomic levels were the most influential qualities of a locale; suburban shopping centers and office buildings were observed to have high attractive potential for physicians. Unfortunately, these conclusions must be viewed cautiously because the coarse nature of the zone boundaries used in the analysis confuses the influence of many variables, some of which may be important and unrelated to locale, affluence, or racial characteristics.

Elesh and Schollaert[62] used data describing conditions in Chicago census tracts in 1960. In this study, general categories of physicians were regressed on population, commercial activity, hospitals, age distribution, education, and racial composition. The results indicated that physicians avoid black areas, are attracted to populated areas, commercial activity, hospitals, the central business district (CBD), older populations, educated populations, and high income areas. However, the explanatory power of the models was low (R^2 never exceeded .4), indicating that important variables influencing physician distribution had not been included in the models. Furthermore, several variables were entered in the analysis (such as hospitals) in a questionable fashion.

In a similar though less ambitious study, May[63] analyzed the distribution of physicians in Brooklyn, New York, in 1960. In contrast with Elesh and Schollaert, May did not find that race was important. Using both ratios and counts of physicians in tracts, he found median years of education to be the only important socioeconomic variable, while population size and hospitals were other crucial variables. May's findings also contradict the observation of Piore and Sokal[64] that New York City physicians avoid low income areas because of their obvious poverty-stricken character. Roemer[65] also drew this conclusion in his description of conditions in Los Angeles—and, regardless of the publication of seemingly contradictory evidence, it is the viewpoint most often represented when local "doctor shortages" or "physician maldistributions" are discussed.[66]

The true complexity of the situation, though, is best illustrated by the work reported by Dorsey and by Robertson on conditions in Boston, and by Hambleton's analysis of 15 SMSAs.[67] Dorsey examined data for census tracts in Boston and Brookline between 1940–1961. He observed the growth of an increasingly specialized population of physicians. Using income, occupation, and education in a composite indicator of socioeconomic status (SES), he determined that the changing physician mix over time had left low SES tracts with few primary care physicians. However, Robertson drew quite different conclusions in a study of Boston census tracts covering the same period, 1940–1960. He observed that because of a tendency for physicians to cluster together, simple longitudinal analyses are likely to be erroneous. This would be due to any lagged effect introduced by clusters of physicians attracting physicians. To avoid this problem he used a differential equation model of change originally described by Coleman.[68] Socioeconomic status was found not to be important for the location of general practitioners, but it was related to the distribution of internists and pediatricians. All three types of physicians tended to concentrate in areas characteristically high in a factor identified with low owner-occupied housing and low median income. Robertson concluded that in Boston between 1940 and 1960, medical practice had become more specialized and physicians had clustered into a few locales that were characterized by office buildings and proximity to hospitals. This clustering had proceeded with little regard to changes in other local conditions. The result was that although some few areas were well served by locally available primary physicians, this was generally accidental. Because of clustering, physicians were located near only a small portion of the population.

Hambleton's study[69] is in accord with these conclusions. Studying local distribution in 15 SMSAs in 1960, he found that clusters of physicians in the central business districts and in other inner city areas left predominantly poor or nonwhite groups with locational advantages over other areas. This was especially true for specialists, who, he argued, tend to cluster in the central business district more than do general practitioners because they have a city-wide market orientation. Poor and black residents near business districts were close to medical offices, which, it appeared, had been located without regard to neighborhood, race or income characteristics. However, Hambleton raised the cautionary note that proximity did not guarantee accessibility. Hambleton's conclusions were similar to those drawn by Kaplan and Leinhardt[70] in a multivariate study of physician location in Pittsburgh. Census tract data on commercial activity, hospital beds, and socioeconomic and demographic composition were used; and physicians were found to be attracted to professional facilities, giving little regard to local socioeconomic or racial conditions.

The importance of professional factors seems well documented. Physicians are not uniformly distributed within cities but instead are concentrated in areas that can provide professional amenities. Although this provides no overt advantage to the middle class, there are subtle advantages. The middle class can more easily travel the distances and deal with the centralized medical system than can the poor.

The Role of the Foreign Medical Graduate

A large portion of the current physician supply in the United States and the one most amenable to short-term policy-induced variation is the group that has received training outside of the United States. Some of these foreign medical graduates (FMGs) are U.S. citizens who sought · training in foreign countries. Most, however, are foreign citizens who have come to the United States for a period of years to improve their training or to immigrate. These FMGs represented approximately 20 percent of the active physicians and about 33 percent of the hospital interns and residents in 1970[71]. Between 1960 and 1970 the influx of FMGs increased at a faster rate than the domestic production of new physicians. In 1968–1970, FMGs made up 29 percent of newly-licensed physicians. Of all physicians admitted as immigrants in 1970, 70 percent (approximately 6,300 physicians) came from Central and South America, Asia, and Africa. Between 1962 and 1971, nearly 29,000 FMGs immigrated to the United States. During the same period, 46,812 FMGs came to the United States under the two-year exchange visitor physician program, and most of these have stayed.

This flow of skilled manpower from underdeveloped areas to the United States poses important questions for international relations and represents a form of reverse foreign aid that may be quite detrimental to the source countries.[72] However, United States policymakers view FMGs as a significant aid in alleviating the presumed physician shortage. Indeed, such thoughts led, in 1970, to legislation making it fairly simple for an FMG to convert a visitor visa to permanent-resident status. But the growing dependence of the United States on a manpower source over which U.S. policymakers have little control should not be accepted without question. Although, by evidence of their increasing numbers of applications, there is currently a large and anxious stock of FMGs seeking entrance to the United States, there is no way of assuring continuity in this supply. The health needs of other nations are certainly as great as those of the United States, and it is unclear how long these nations will permit skilled manpower to be drained off by the incentives of the U.S. market for physicians.

Another issue concerns the effect of this increasing supply of FMGs on the general distribution and availability of physicians within the United States. If one assumes that a non-uniform distribution of physicians is detrimental, then, clearly, the initial locational choice decisions of FMGs and their migratory propensities within the United States can work either to alleviate or to aggravate this maldistribution. Although important research on this topic is limited, Marguiles and Bloch[73] indicate that, at the state level, FMGs tend to concentrate in urbanized areas. An extensive investigation of FMGs has been performed by Butter and Schaffner.[74] Addressing spatial distributional effects, they used 1968 data from the AMA giving physician/population ratios for states and counties. They compared deviations from a uniform distribution of physicians first excluding FMGs and then including FMGs. They argued that state and urban-rural differences in physician/population ratios were exacerbated by the addition of FMGs.

FMGs appear to distribute themselves selectively, and although they add to the aggregate physician supply, they probably increase the disparity between states and between urban and rural areas. Several factors may explain this finding. FMGs may be dependent on institutional support, probably desire cosmopolitan environments, are likely to have urban backgrounds, and may desire to serve urbanized ethnic groups. Unless urban FMGs are viewed as replacements for U.S. trained physicians who are thus freed to serve rural communities (an unlikely assumption), they should not be considered as a force with which to arrest the growing rural-urban disparity in physicians.

In a second study, Schaffner and Butter[75] examined the interstate geographic mobility of FMGs. They questioned whether the regional mobility of FMGs would act to equalize the selectivity of their initial locational decisions. Using data from the AMA's 1966 and 1968 physician census, they computed FMG in- and out-migration rates for 36 states (95.4 percent of all FMGs). As surrogate measures for determining the relative physician shortage in a given state, they used the physician/population ratio, the five-year rate of change of physician income, and the state level of physician income (this assumes that physician income is responsive to demand and that relative increases in income indicate increases in demand without concomitant increases in supply, i.e., shortage). Only 8 percent of all FMGs moved between states during the period and the mobile FMGs tended to move to only those states that ranked low in terms of their measures of medical manpower shortage. Thus, the mobility of FMGs appeared to add to the disparity between the states. However, these conclusions must be viewed with caution. Only 36 states were included in the study, a period of only two years was analyzed, and the AMA records on FGMs are likely to be incomplete. An adequate study of initial locational propensities of FMGs, their migratory patterns, and the factors influencing their local spatial distribution would require a longer time span, a lower level of aggregation, controls for factors likely to attract or repel FMGs, and data detailing residency location, specialty, and subjective characteristics. Nonetheless, informed planning must take into consideration the large and increasing FMG physician population.

New Physicians

Understanding the locational decisions of physicians can be decomposed into two related issues: 1) the decision to locate and initiate a practice, and 2) the decision to move a practice. Presumably, different factors influence these decisions. Physicians making their initial locational decisions will be younger and less experienced, and their families will be at a different stage of development than physicians considering a move from one locale to another. This latter decision is often tied to the issue of changes in type of practice or specialty type.[76] Although an important distinction, few analyses of physician location or migration have attempted to distinguish between physicians who have relocated and those who are locating practices for the first time.[77] Clearly, just as with FMGs, if different concerns motivate these two groups of physicians, specific policies to take advantage of them might be formulated. The works that have made this distinction have focused on the behavior of new physicians. These studies detail the effectiveness of programs that have been instituted during residency to alter the specialty and geographic distribution of physicians.

Sloan and Yett have performed several studies investigating the behavior of recent medical school graduates. Sloan has examined choice of specialty and practice mode, and Yett and Sloan have modeled spatial distribution.[78] Their findings suggest that earnings differentials do not account for the strong trends away from general practice in favor of careers in specialty medicine. Elasticities based on lifetime earnings coefficients for most specialties were near zero and, although there was a significant positive effect in some regression results, the effect of the income variable was always small. The number of FMGs in a specialty was significant in several estimates, but it always had a negative coefficient. In other words, medical students are attracted to those specialties that have higher relative lifetime incomes and fewer FMGs, but neither effect is very great. Indeed, the negative FMG coefficient may indicate that FMGs are allocated into residual categories, i.e., they fill up positions domestic medical graduates shun.

On choice of practice, Sloan's report[79] is descriptive, presenting the results of a survey of residents carried out by the *Hospital Physician*. Partnerships and groups were clearly preferred and even academic medicine was preferred to solo practice. Although practice mode decisions are made fairly late in the medical education process, the decision to engage in academic medicine seems to be made while the physician is still a medical student.

In an extensive investigation of a 1966 survey carried out by Medical Economics, Inc., Yett and Sloan[80] studied the effect of several variables on the spatial distribution of new

physicians across states. Variables describing the following general factors were included: previous attachment to the state, income, population growth, barriers to entry (using licensure failure rate as a proxy), opportunities for professional development, general environmental conditions, and level of effort required to establish a satisfactory practice. Previous attachment to a state (through birth or attendance at a medical school, internship, or residency program) was found to be an attractive factor. Income levels and environmental conditions were significant, too. But the only action a state could take to increase its physician supply (besides attachment) that is predicted to have a strong effect is to lower the failure rate on licensure examinations.

Summary of the Planning Implications of Current Supply

The supply of physician manpower seems best explained by behavioral theories that emphasize decision-making by individual physicians in which the role of pecuniary incentives has diminished over time. Although fee-setting by physicians may involve profit-maximizing behavior, locational and specialty choices do not. Instead, professional and personal amenities and conveniences seem most important, with income security rather than income maximization gaining in importance. These findings suggest that physicians will be more, rather than less, ready to accept staff positions in institutional facilities and they will become more, rather than less, ready to accept paraprofessional substitution. Increasing concentration in group practice also indicates that there is an increasing readiness for the individual physician to relinquish some control over decision-making.

Policies that aim at reducing distributional inequities must build on these results if they are to succeed. Other policy effects that can be manipulated are the propensity of physicians to delay decisions until the time of residency and to emphasize life-style qualities in the locale they choose. Possible alternatives include programs to reduce the difficulty of entering practice in locales that are attempting to gain physicians, to reduce the differentials in insurance programs that pay "prevailing rates," to promote the social and organizational integration of FMGs, to attempt to motivate residents to choose certain areas, and to entice students from areas with few physicians to choose medicine as a career and to take training in their own state.

Concept of a Physician Shortage

In preceding sections we examined models of the demand for physicians and looked at physician supply. Here, we consider the following questions: Under what conditions does the interaction of supply and demand factors lead to a condition requiring government intervention? How is a physician shortage to be detected? Answering these questions will require a recapitulation of some of our earlier arguments. The six most important criteria for a physician shortage are as follows:

1 Professional standards: A shortage is said to exist if the number of physicians available at a given place and at a given time is inadequate to meet some professionally defined standard of medical care. We noted a number of methods that had been used to develop professional standards and argued that such measures were unlikely to help policymakers determine whether action should be initiated to change a situation. We also noted that in almost all areas, the amount of manpower available will be much less than that necessary to meet professionally defined standards, and that, by these definitions, shortages are perpetual.

2 Comparative ratios: A shortage is said to exist in all those states (or counties) with a physician/population ratio lower than the mean ratio across states (or counties), or with a physician/population ratio lower than that of the "best" areas—defined, for example, by the areas with the highest ratios. Since it is extremely unlikely that physicians will be uniformly distributed across regions, such a definition will always imply a shortage in some areas. As noted earlier, these ratios make no sense unless the numerator is full-time-equivalent physicians providing patient care, and the denominator is adjusted for age, sex, and race. Consider, for example, a situation in which one county has a physician/population ratio of 75/100,000 and another has a physician/population ratio of 150/100,000. Assume that half the physicians in the latter county spend their time in teaching, research, and administration, and in staffing a hospital that provides specialty care to citizens of the entire state, while some of the remaining physicians are retired or treat patients living in other counties. If, in the former county, all physicians are engaged in full-time patient care, strict manpower ratios would grossly overestimate the differential availability of physician services.

These ratios suffer the same problems as the professional standards approach. There is little reason to believe that additional physician services would be used, no assurance that additional physician services would improve the health of the populace, and no reason to believe that additional physicians would choose to settle in "underserved" areas.

3 Demand/supply differential: A shortage is said to exist if, at current prices, the demand for medical care exceeds the supply of medical care. This is a strict economic definition of a shortage. Consider, for example, the market for rental apartments. An economist would argue that a well-functioning market would equate the quantity supplied to the quantity demanded (and determine an equilibrium price). If the demand for apartments suddenly expanded or some event curtailed the supply, the rental price might rise a great deal, but this would not be considered a shortage. According to this interpretation, a shortage is possible only if the market is not functioning. For instance, in the apartment rental example, if an apartment owner cannot or will not raise prices but customers want more apartments than the owner can supply, an economic shortage would be said to exist. However, from an economic viewpoint, this shortage is artificial and created by the constraint on price. As with rent control in New York City, the pernicious effects of keeping the market

from clearing include curtailing future supply, increased litigation, and immobility. When such constraints occur in the market for medical care, they give rise to economically defined shortages. In such situations, the rationing role played by price is replaced by nonmonetary rationing devices.

Constraints on the supply of physicians lead, in a well-functioning market for medical care, to a high price per patient visit and high incomes for physicians. If physicians cannot or will not raise prices then the market would tend to equilibrate (i.e., ration services among those demanding them) through the use of nonmarket rationing. In the delivery of physician services the most common rationing devices are: 1) service unavailability (physicians refuse to see a new patient); 2) long waits for service (a delay of several weeks for an appointment); 3) deterioration in the product or service itself (a long wait to see the physician once one arrives, a small amount of time with the physician, a less than thorough examination, and perhaps little effort by the physician to be reassuring and friendly); and 4) other increased difficulties in gaining access (such as a greater distance to travel, less convenient office hours, and a general way of putting more burden on the patient and having the service take more of the patient's time and effort).

Much current evidence indicates that such shortages for some kinds of physicians exist. The market for medical care is not well functioning, since numerous factors prevent price from playing a rationing role. Some institutions commit themselves to deliver care at zero price to the patient, but they do not hire the manpower necessary to deliver that care. Physicians traditionally take an oath not to deny care to those who cannot pay for it; Blue Shield and other review mechanisms often set an effective upper bound on the price that physicians can charge (to specified groups); the welfare associated with medical care tends to induce strong expectations in the physician and patient that the price of care be related to the ability of each individual patient to af-

ford it. Thus, high prices are not considered a socially acceptable way of rationing medical care. Nonetheless, price may have an important role to play as an incentive.

4 Rate of return: A related way of detecting a physician shortage is to determine whether there is a high rate of return to physicians at a given time or place. A high rate of return across regions could indicate that physicians were able to create an artificially high demand for their services or that supply constraints existed. The latter is a market signal to attract more people into medical professions. Thus one could determine the rate of return to physician education at different locations (or equivalently, look at physician incomes and education costs at different places). This technique is likely to yield evidence that is contrary to the assumption of a general shortage. In addition, urban areas, which have the highest physician/population ratios and, therefore, should have relatively low prices and low physician incomes, have the highest prices and highest (hourly) incomes.

5 Health levels: A more difficult (but more objective) way of determining the existence of a shortage involves surveying the health of a population. Correcting for age, race, sex, and income, such a survey would determine the rates of mortality, acute disease, chronic disease, disability, and bed days. If one assumes that medical care is a principal factor influencing health, this approach could be used to identify the need for more physicians.

An alternative to a health survey is based on the assumption that a shortage of physicians leads individuals to seek care only when they are very ill. If so, looking at the mortality rate and at the severity of patient presentations to physicians in an area would provide an estimate of the population's health status.

6 Community satisfaction: A final measure of shortage involves surveying a population to determine whether there is general satisfaction with local medical services. The level of satisfaction need have little correspondence to the physician/population ratio. If

the health status indices indicate a shortage of physicians, but people are satisfied with the level of service and there is no indication of nonmarket rationing, it would make little sense to provide additional service since it would go unused. Alternative policies are required in this instance to motivate the use of extant supply. Note that if nonmarket rationing is important, the provision of extra services would be reasonable and the services would probably be used (since nonmarket rationing is an indication that current demand exceeds current supply at current price).

Discussion

We have described six methods of determining whether a physician shortage exists. Professional standards and ratios have little to recommend them other than their simplicity; there is no guarantee that additional services would be used or, if they were, that they would be efficacious. Examining the existence of nonmarket rationing of physician services is relevant because of the many constraints that prevent price from equilibrating supply and demand. This approach has the virtue of indicating that at current prices people desire more medical services than are being supplied. A similar approach, although a more costly one, is to survey the population regarding the satisfaction with the medical care system. Clearly, the best approach is to survey the health status of a population and determine whether additional physicians would be efficacious. This approach, together with one indicating unsatisfied demand, would indicate not only that additional physicians would be used, but that the additional services would be efficacious.

Accuracy of Forecasts

The demand and supply models described earlier imply that there is a physician shortage. Even more important, they indicate that this shortage is likely to become worse over time. Analysts have forecast population, number of physicians, and the requirement for physicians. On the basis of forecasts that we are in the midst of a worsening shortage, it has been argued that government policies influencing the supply of physician services must be rethought and that new policies, such as expanding the number and size of medical schools, must be established. However, as indicated in the earlier sections, we do not accept the conclusions that derive from the models that have been used to estimate physician requirements or supply. In this section we detail why we lack confidence in these estimates. Table 5 presents selected forecasts that have been made in the past for population, physician supply, and physician requirements. The notes to the table spell out the assumptions underlying each forecast. The table shows the shortages that were expected and the actual population and physician levels.

In general, these results indicate that: 1) the population estimates covered a wide range, and the smallest estimate exceeded the actual population of the United States (and its outlying territories) in 1970; and 2) the estimates of physician supply covered a wide range with the highest estimate lower than the actual number of physicians existing in 1970. Clearly, forecasting is not a science and is subject to considerable error. The table indicates that forecasters should make their assumptions clear, and instead of generating a single estimate they should present a range of possibilities.

In Table 6, we present some estimates that have been made for 1975 (in the notes to the table, the assumptions underlying the projections are given). The projections, made in 1966, indicate that, once again, a large doctor shortage is expected.

The forecasts of both physician supplies and population are poor. By 1970, we had more physicians than were predicted by the Bane Committee Report for 1975. By 1971 (according to the AMA), there were 344,823 physicians. Little has changed in forecasting techniques and it is very likely that again all forecasts of physician supplies will be underestimates.

It should also be noted that these forecasts do not take increases in productivity into account. If one assumed that physician productivity were to increase at 4 percent per year, the available "effective" supply in 1975 would be

Table 5. Projections from various sources of physician supplies and requirements for 1970*

Sources	Date of projection	Population (in thousands)	Supply M.D.s and osteopaths (active and inactive)	Supply M.D.s only	Requirement M.D.s and osteopaths	Difference
A	1958	209,380		273,474	276,458 (b) (c)	2,984
				274,469 (b)	286,938 (d)	12,469
B	1959	213,810	294,900 (a)		299,000 (e)	4,100
			296,500 (f)			2,500
C	1959					
		213,810		279,000 (g)	283,000 (h)	
D	1960					
E	1964	214,570	327,900 (j)			
			324,900 (k)			
			319,900 (m·)			
F	1966	212,683	335,000 (n)			
			340,000 (p)			
G	1966		306,954 (q)			
			326,915 (r)			
H	1966	208,576	332,700			
Actual	1970	207,976	348,300			

*Butter, I. "Health Manpower Research: A Survey," Table #4. Reprinted, with permission of the Blue Cross Association, from *Inquiry*, Vol. IV, No. 4 (December 1967), p. 21. Copyright © 1967 by the Blue Cross Association. All rights reserved.
(a) Present production rate. (b) Increase graduates of U.S. schools. (c) Maintaining 1955 physician/population ratio. (d) Increase graduates sufficiently to maintain 1955 ratio of graduates to population. (e) To maintain 1959 ratio. (f) Recent growth rate. (g) Graduates at levels currently predicted. (h) Increase graduates to maintain 1957 ratio. (j) At current planned growth, increase graduates (1,600 foreign graduates licensed annually). (k) 1,000 foreign graduates annually. (m) No foreign graduates licensed after 1965. (n) Low estimates of U.S. graduates and new foreign unlicensed, stable new foreign licenciates. (p) High estimates of graduates and foreign unlicensed, stable new foreign licenciates. (q) Based on HMP growth in 1950–60, 4½ percent per year. (r) HMP growth rate, 5½ percent per year.
Sources:
A Perrott, G. S. and Pennell, M. Y. "Physicians in the United States: Projections 1955–1975," *Journal of Medical Education* 33:638–644 (September 1958).
B U.S. Surgeon General's Consultant Group on Medical Education. "Physicians for a Growing America," USPHS Publication 709, Washington, D.C., 1959.
C *Health Manpower Source Book*, Section 9, "Physicians, Dentists, Nurses," (Washington, D.C.: DHEW, Manpower Analysis Branch, 1959).
D Stewart, W. H. and Pennell, M. Y. "Health Manpower, 1930–75," *Public Health Reports* 75:274–280 (March 1960).
E *Health Manpower Source Book*, Section 18, "Manpower in the 1960's," (Washington, D.C.: DHEW, Manpower Analysis Branch, 1964).
F Ruhe, C. H. W. "Present Projections of Physician Production," *Journal of the American Medical Association* 198:168–174 (December 1966).
G Weiss, J. H. "The Changing Job Structure of Health Manpower," Ph.D. dissertation, Harvard University, Cambridge, July 1966.
H Fein, R. *The Doctor Shortage* (Washington, D.C.: The Brookings Institution, 1967).

about 390,000, and the projected deficit would disappear.

Concluding Comments

Government agencies have taken on the role of planning the delivery of health care and consequently find themselves confronted with defining "need." How many physicians, hospital beds, ancillary health personnel and other health facilities are needed in an area? What policies will serve to increase the supply of these health resources when they are needed? An earlier paper[81] examines this set of questions for hospitals, focusing on the financing of new facilities. This study attempted to answer these questions for physicians.

Based on the criteria in the literature discussed, there is contradictory evidence on the overall shortage of physicians. There are significant problems with maldistribution of phy-

Table 6.   Summary of physician projections for 1975*

Projection study	Requirements (I)	Supplies (II)	(−) Deficit (+) Surplus (III)
Bane Committee Report[1]	30,000 (minimum)	(i) 312,800	−17,200
		(ii) 318,400	−11,600
Fein[2]	(i) 340,000 to 350,000	361,700	+21,700 to +11,700
	(ii) 372,000 to 385,000		−10,300 to −23,300
U.S. National Advisory Commission on Health Manpower[3]	(i) 346,000 (minimum)	360,000	+14,000
U.S. Bureau of Labor Statistics[4]	390,000	360,000	−30,000
U.S. Public Health Service[5]	(i) 400,000	360,000	−40,000
	(ii) 425,000		−65,000

*Hansen, W.L. "An appraisal of Physician Manpower Projections," Table #1. Reprinted, with permission of the Blue Cross Association, from *Inquiry*, Vol. VII, No. 1 (March 1970), p. 107. Copyright © 1970 by the Blue Cross Association. All rights reserved.

Notes: Physicians include both M.D.s and D.O.s, except for Line 2, which excludes D.O.s. Column III equals column II minus Column I.

Sources:

[1] U.S. Surgeon General's Consultant Group on Medical Education. "Physicians for a Growing America," USPHS Publication 709, Washington, D. C., 1959.
   Column (I) Table 2, p. 3.
   Column (II) Table 2, p. 3.
   Column (III) Calculated.
Requirements based on assumption that 1959 represents minimum rates to maintain health of population.
Supply: Continuation of physician growth rate.

[2] Fein, R. *The Doctor Shortage* (Washington, D.C.: The Brookings Institution, 1967).
   Column (I) (i) Based on 12–15 percent increase due to population growth above.
   (ii) Based on 22–26 percent increase due to all factors. See pp. 134–135.
   Column (II) Table III-9, p. 87.
   Column (III) Calculated.
Requirements based on the demand for physician services at 1965 prices given anticipated changes in population composition expected by 1975. (i) shows estimated effect only accounting for population change; (ii) shows the effect of a whole range of factors.
Supply takes into account expected increase in medical school graduates as well as the immigration of foreign trained physicians.

[3] U.S. National Advisory Commission on Health Manpower. *Report*, Vol. 1 (Washington, D.C.: GPO, 1967).
   Column (I) (i) Based on 13.5 percent increase in total visits by 1975. See p. 243.
   Column (II) Table 4, p. 235.
   Column (III) Calculated.
Methodology for determining requirements and supply similar to Fein.

[4] U.S. Bureau of Labor Statistics. *Health Manpower 1966–1975, A Study of Requirements and Supply* (Washington, D.C.: GPO, 1967).
   Column (I) Page 18.
   Column (II) No figure is given. We assume National Advisory Commission on Health Manpower Supply figure of 360,000 is appropriate to use.
   Column (III) Calculated.
Requirements taken into consideration: population changes, increased demand for services across all age groups and need for an expansion of physicians engaged in research.

[5] U.S. Public Health Service, "Health Manpower Perspective: 1967," USPHS Publication 1667, Washington, D.C., 1967.
   Column (I) (i) and (ii), Table 8, p. 15, and accompanying text.
   Column (II) Same as Column II, line 4.
   Column (III) Calculated.
Requirements: (i) is based on the application of "professional standards"; namely, the utilization rate for members of prepayment group practice plans to the entire 1975 population; and estimate (ii) applies the highest physician utilization rate among the four major regions of the United States to the entire 1975 population.

sicians, both by geographic area and by specialty. No simple policies to equalize the distribution of physicians are likely to be successful. However, it is not reasonable to assume that an area has a physician shortage just because some other area has a higher physician/population ratio. Instead, one must gather evidence of non-price rationing or of unsatisfactory health indices (mortality ratio, morbidity ratio, or disability days).

Although the overall number of physicians does not seem to warrant changes in government policy, locational problems are important. The research has implications for determining whether an area is underserved and what might be done to increase the supply of physicians. A major unsolved problem is the provision of services to rural areas distant from major cities.

In view of past attempts to solve medical care delivery problems by intervention, we would caution that good intentions are not enough. If funds are not to be wasted or to have a pernicious effect, careful data collection and analysis are necessary.

References and Notes

1 Berg, R. L. *Health Status Indexes* (Chicago: Hospital Research and Educational Trust, 1973).

2 See: Auster, R.; Leveson, I.; and Sarachek, D. "The Production of Health: An Exploratory Study," *The Journal of Human Resources* 4:411–436 (Fall 1969); and Stewart, C. T. Jr. "Allocation of Resources to Health," *The Journal of Human Resources* 6:101–122 (Winter 1971).

3 See: Lave, J. R.; Lave, L. B.; and Morton, T. E. "Paramedics: A Survey of the Issues," in: Stein, B. and Miller, S. M. (eds.) *Incentives and Planning in Social Policy* (Chicago: Aldine Publishing Co., 1973) and "The Physician's Assistant—Exploration of the Concept," *Hospitals* 45:42–51 (June 1, 1971). Also see: Sadler, A. M.; Sadler, B. L.; and Bliss, A. A. *The Physician's Assistant Today and Tomorrow* (New Haven: Yale University Press, 1972).

4 Jeffers, J. R.; Bognanno, M. F.; and Bartlett, J. C. "On the Demand versus Need for Medical Services and the Concept of 'Shortage'," *American Journal of Public Health* 61:46–63, Part 1 (January 1971).

5 Hiestand, D. L. "Research Into Manpower for Health Service," *Milbank Memorial Fund Quarterly* 44:146–179, Part 2 (October 1966).

6 Lee, R. I. and Jones, L. W. *The Fundamentals of Good Medical Care* (Chicago: University of Chicago Press, 1933).

7 Lee and Jones were aware of the difference between need and demand. They noted that people were not aware of the need for preventive care. In addition, they pointed to the fact that there was a wide distribution in the physician/population ratios across the states and emphasized that if the supply of physicians were increased the new doctors would probably locate in doctor "surplus" areas. They stressed the need for education and for changes in in the way medical care was financed and organized.

8 Schonfeld, H.; Heston, J.; and Falk, I. "Numbers of Physicians Required for Primary Medical Care," *The New England Journal of Medicine* 286:571–576 (March 16, 1972).

9 See: Lave, Lave, and Morton, "Paramedics," *op. cit.*, and "The Physician's Assistant," *op. cit.*

10 Huebscher, J. "Letter to the Editor," *The New England Journal of Medicine* 286:1164 (May 25, 1972).

11 Somers, A. R. *The Kaiser-Permanente Medical Care Program* (New York, The Commonwealth Fund, 1971).

12 Jacobs, G. "Letter to the Editor," *The New England Journal of Medicine* 286:1164 (May 25, 1972).

13 Other studies following the Lee and Jones method have been reported. Daitz [Daitz, B. D. "The Challenge of Disability," *American Journal of Public Health* 55:528–534 (April 1964)] proceeds by estimating that 74 million people had a chronic condition in 1960; of those, 10 million people had an incipient or manifest functional impairment associated with chronic disease, injury or congenital defects that require medical care to prevent further deterioration of functional capacity or to restore functional capacity. He then assumes that each of these 10 million people requires a minimum of 40 hours of professional care services per year, of which five should be physician time. This leads to an estimated need of 25,000 physicians to care for chronically ill patients. Knowles [Knowles, J. H. "The Quantity and Quality of Medical Manpower: A Review of Medicine's Current Efforts," *Journal of Medical Education* 44:81–118 (February 1969)] reports on responses he received from letters sent to the executive secretaries of the various specialty boards to determine what they thought the manpower needs were in their respective specialty. One executive secretary assumed that there would be one operation per 13 people per year and that the annual caseload of an anesthesiologist could be 800; he estimated that 37,000 anesthesiologists were needed. There are only 7,011 in practice. The estimate of needed anesthesiologists is based on what seems to be a small caseload (about four operations per day for a 200 day work year), and it neglects the fact that many anesthetics are given by nurse anesthetists. In addition, since Americans have many more operations (per person per year) than Western Europeans (or even Americans enrolled in prepaid group practices),

one may also want to question the assumed rate of surgical procedures.

4 Williams, G. *Kaiser-Permanente Health Plan—Why it Works* (Oakland, California: Henry J. Kaiser Foundation, 1971).

5 Riddick, F. A.; Bryan, J. B.; Gershenson, M. I.; and Costello, A. C. "Use of Allied Health Professionals in Internists' Offices," *Archives of Internal Medicine* 127:924–931 (May 1971).

6 Klarman, H. E. "Economic Aspects of Projecting Requirements for Health Manpower," *The Journal of Human Resources* 4:360–376 (1969).

7 See: Acton, J. P. "Demand for Health Care Among the Urban Poor with Special Emphasis on the Role of Time," (New York: The Rand Corporation, April 1973); and Richardson, W. C. "Ambulatory Use of Physicians' Services in Response to Illness Episodes in a Low Income Neighborhood," Center for Health Administration Studies Research Series 29 (Chicago: University of Chicago Press, 1971).

8 Marshall, C. L.; Hassanein, K. M.; Hassanein, R. S.; and Paul, C. L. "Time and Distance—Rural Practice: Dissatisfaction with Travel Distance to the Physician in a Rural Area," *Journal of the Kansas Medical Society* 70:93–96 (March 1969).

9 Weiss, J. E. and Greenlick, M. R. "Determinants of Medical Care Utilization: The Effect of Social Class and Distance on Contacts with the Medical Care System," *Medical Care* 8:456–462 (November–December 1970).

20 Lave, J. R. and Leinhardt, S. "The Delivery of Ambulatory Care to the Poor: A Literature Review," *Management Science* 19:78–99, Part 2 (December 1972).

21 Shannon, G. W.; Bashshur, R. L.; and Metzner, C. A. "The Concept of Distance as a Factor in Accessibility and Utilization of Health Care," *Medical Care Review* 26:143–161 (1969).

22 See: Grossman, M. "The Demand for Health: A Theoretical and Empirical Investigation," Occasional Paper 119 (New York: National Bureau of Economic Research, 1972) and "On the Concept of Health Capital and the Demand for Health," *Journal of Political Economy* 80:223–255 (March–April 1972).

23 The ratio model that projects current utilization ratios into the future, keeping them constant for each socioeconomic demographic group [an approach explored by: Fein, R. *The Doctor Shortage.* (Washington, D.C.: The Brookings Institution, 1967)] is a variant of this approach.

24 Newhouse, J. P. and Phelps, C. E. "Price and Income Elasticities for Medical Care Services," (Santa Monica: The Rand Corporation, R-1197-NC, 1972).

25 Fuchs, V. R. and Kramer, M. J. *Determinants of Expenditures for Physicians' Services in the United States 1948–1968*, DHEW Publication No. (HSM) 73-3013 (DHEW, HSMHA, December 1972).

26 See: Acton, J. P. "Demand for Health Care When Time Prices Vary More than Money Prices," (New York: The Rand Corporation, May 1973) and "Demand for Health Care Among the Urban Poor," *op. cit.* Also see: Weiss, J. E.; Greenlick, M. R.; and Jones, J. F. "Determinants of Medical Care Utilization: The Impact of Spatial Factors," *Inquiry*

8:50–57 (December 1971); and Richardson, "Ambulatory Use of Physicians' Services," *op. cit.*

27 See: Ginzberg, E. *Urban Health Services* (New York: Columbia University Press, 1971); Fuchs and Kramer, *Determinants of Expenditures for Physicians' Services, op. cit.*; Evans, R. G. "Supplier Induced Demand: Some Empirical Evidence and Implications," paper prepared for the International Economic Association Tokyo Conference on Economics of Health and Medical Care, April 1973; and Stevens, C. M. and Brown, G. D. "Market Structure Approach to Health-Manpower 'Planning'," *American Journal of Public Health* 61:1988–1995 (October 1971).

28 Fuchs and Kramer, *op. cit.*

29 Ginzberg, E. *Men, Money and Medicine* (New York: Columbia University Press, 1969).

30 Evans, R. G. "Supplier Induced Demand," *op. cit.*

31 See the following works of Feldstein, M. S. "An Aggregate Planning Model of the Health Care Sector," in: Paelink, J. (ed.) *Programming for Europe's Collective Needs* (Amsterdam: North Holland Publishing Co., 1970); "An Econometric Model of the Medicare System," *The Quarterly Journal of Economics* 85:1–20 (February 1971) and "Hospital Cost Inflation: A Study of Nonprofit Price Dynamics," *American Economic Review* 61:853–872 (December 1971).

32 See the following works of: Yett, D. E.; Drabek, L.; Kimbell, L.; and Intriligator, M. "The Development of a Micro-Simulation Model of Health Manpower Supply and Demand," in: *Proceedings and Report of Conference on a Health Manpower Simulation Model* (Washington, D.C.: U.S. Public Health Service, Bureau of Health Manpower Education, December 1970); "A Macroeconometric Model for Regional Health Planning," *Economic and Business Bulletin* 24: 1–21 (Fall 1971) and "Health Manpower Planning: An Econometric Approach," *Health Services Research* 7:134–147 (Summer 1972).

33 Lave, J. R.; Lave, L. B.; and Leinhardt, S. "A Model of Medical Care Delivery," in: Perlman, M. (ed.) *The Economics of Health and Medical Care* (London: The Macmillan Co., 1974).

34 Lee and Jones, *The Fundamentals of Good Medical Care, op. cit.*

35 Fein, *The Doctor Shortage, op. cit.*

36 DeVise, P. "Physician Migration from Inland to Coastal States: Antipodal Examples of Illinois and California," *Journal of Medical Education* 48:141–151 (February 1973).

37 Fahs, I. J.; Ingalls, K.; and Miller, W. R. "Physician Migration: A Problem in the Upper Midwest," *Journal of Medical Education* 43:735–740 (1968).

38 Rimlinger, G. V. and Steele, H. B. "An Economic Interpretation of the Spatial Distribution of Physicians in the U.S.," *The Southern Economic Journal* 30:1–12 (July 1963).

39 Lankford, P. M. "Physician Location Factors and Public Policy," *Economic Geography* 244–255 (July 1974).

40 Fuchs and Kramer, *Determinants of Expenditures for Physicians' Services, op. cit.*

41 See: Cooper, J. K.; Heald, K.; and Samuels, M. "The Decision for Rural Practice," *Journal of Medical Education* 47:939–944 (December 1972). A

more recent analysis is found in: Cooper, J. K.; Heald, K.; Samuels, M.; and Coleman, S. "Rural or Urban Practice: Factors Influencing the Location Decision of Primary Care Physicians," *Inquiry* 12: 18–25 (March 1975).

42 See: Stine, O. C. "Changes in the Supply of Physicians Giving Office Medical Care to Children," *Maryland State Medical Journal* 17:66–69 (January 1968) and "The Number of Children and the Supply of Physicians in Maryland Since 1940," *Maryland State Medical Journal* 19:51–55 (June 1970); Reas, H. W. "The Distribution of Physicians in Northwestern Ohio: 30 Years' Trends," *The Ohio State Medical Journal* 68:524–527 (June 1972); Mac-Queen, J. C. "A Study of Iowa Medical Physicians," *Journal of the Iowa Medical Society* 58:1129–1135 (November 1968); Baker, A. S.; Bishop, F. M.; Hassinger, E. W.; and Hobbs, D. J. "Distribution of Health Services in Missouri," *Missouri Medicine* 64: 925–926, 929 (November 1967); Martin, E. D.; Moffat, R. E.; Falter, R. T.; and Walker, J. D. "Where Graduates Go," *The Journal of the Kansas Medical Society* 69:84–89 (March 1968); Royce, P. C. "Can Rural Health Education Centers Influence Physician Distribution?" *Journal of the American Medical Association* 220:847–849 (May 1972); and Matthews, H. A. "The State of Franklin: A Physician Opinion Survey," *North Carolina Medical Journal* 32:242–246 (June 1971).

43 Yett, D. E. and Sloan, F. A. "Migration Patterns of Recent Medical School Graduates," *Inquiry* 11: 125–142 (June 1974).

44 Parker, R. C.; Rix, R. A.; and Tuxill, T. G. "Social, Economic and Demographic Factors Affecting Physician Population in Upstate New York," *New York State Journal of Medicine* 69:706–712 (March 1969).

45 Fuchs and Kramer, *Determinants of Expenditures for Physicians' Services, op. cit.*

46 Lave, J. R. and Lave, L. B. "The Hospital Construction Act: An Evaluation of the Hill-Burton Program, 1948–1973," (Washington, D.C.: American Enterprise Institute for Public Policy Research, 1974).

47 Steele, H. B. and Rimlinger, G. V. "Income Opportunities and Physician Location Trends in the United States," *Western Economic Journal* 3:182–194 (Spring 1965).

48 Marden, P. G. "A Demographic and Ecological Analysis of the Distribution of Physicians in Metropolitan America, 1960," *American Journal of Sociology* 72:290–300 (1966).

49 Joroff, S. and Navarro, V. "Medical Manpower: A Multivariate Analysis of the Distribution of Physicians in Urban United States," *Medical Care* 9:428–438 (September–October 1971).

50 Lankford, "Physician Location Factors," *op. cit.*

51 Weiss, J. E. "The Effect of Medical Centers on the Distribution of Physicians in the U.S.," Ph.D. dissertation, University of Michigan, Ann Arbor, 1968.

52 Sloan, F. "Economic Models of Physician Supply," Ph.D. dissertation, Harvard University, Cambridge, 1968.

53 Benham, L.; Maurizi, A.; and Reder, M. W. "Migration, Location, and Remuneration of Medical Personnel: Physicians and Dentists," *Review of Economics and Statistics* 50:332–341 (August 1968).

54 See: Marshall, C. L.; Hassanein, K. M.; Hassanein R. S.; and Marshall, C. L. "Principal Components Analysis of the Distribution of Physicians, Dentists and Osteopaths in a Midwestern State," *American Journal of Public Health* 61:1556–1564 (August 1971); and Terris, M. and Monk, M. A. "Recent Trends in the Distribution of Physicians in Upstate New York," *American Journal of Public Health* 46: 585–591 (May 1956).

55 Sloan, F. A.; Cleckner, J. E.; and Wayne, J. B. "Non-Price Rationing of Physicians' Services," University of Florida, Gainesville, September 1973.

56 Parker, R. C., *et al.*, "Social, Economic and Demographic Factors," *op. cit.*

57 Nonetheless, Steinwald and Sloan (Steinwald, B. and Sloan, F. A. "Determinants of Physicians' Fees," American Medical Association, Chicago, and University of Florida, Gainesville, July 1973) argue that income is still important since a profit-maximizing model of physician fee-setting dominates alternative models. But this conclusion does not conflict with individual location choice based on non-income considerations.

58 Shannon, G. W., *et al.*, "The Concept of Distance," *op. cit.*

59 See the following: Kaplan, R. S. and Leinhardt, S. "Determinants of Physician Office Location," *Medical Care* 11:406–415 (September–October 1973); McMillan, A. W.; Gornick, M. E.; Rogers, R. R.; and Gorten, M. K. "Assessing the Balance of Physician Manpower in a Metropolitan Area," *Public Health Reports* 85:1001–1011 (November 1970); Fine, E. M. "Urban Health Challenge: Survey of Physician Manpower in Metropolitan Baltimore," *Maryland State Medical Journal* 20:67–71 (October 1971); and Terris and Monk, "Recent Trends in the Distribution of Physicians," *op. cit.*

60 Lepper, M. H.; Lashof, J. C.; Lerner, M.; German, J.; and Andelman, S. L. "Approaches to Meeting Health Needs of Large Poverty Populations," *American Journal of Public Health* 57:1153–1157, Part 2 (July 1967).

61 See: Rees, P. H. "Movement and Distribution of Physicians in Metropolitan Chicago," Chicago Regional Hospital Study, Working Paper I.12, June 1967, and "Numbers and Movement of Physicians in Southeast Chicago: 1953–1965," Chicago Regional Hospital Study, Working Paper I.13, July 1967; De Vise, P. and Dewey, D. "More Money, More Doctors, Less Care," Chicago Regional Hospital Study, Working Paper I.19, March 1972; and Dewey, D. "Where the Doctors Have Gone," Illinois Regional Medical Program, Chicago Regional Hospital Study, Research Paper, 1973.

62 Elesh, D. and Schollaert, P. T. "Race and Urban Medicine: Factors Affecting the Distribution of Physicians in Chicago," *Journal of Health and Social Behavior* 13:236–250 (September 1972).

63 May, L. A. "The Spatial Distribution of Physicians —The Special Case of the City," B.A. Honors Thesis, Harvard University, Cambridge, March 1970.

64 Piore, N. and Sokal, S. "A Profile of Physicians in the City of New York Before Medicare and Mericaid," (New York: Urban Research Center, 1968).

65 Roemer, M. I. "Health Resources and Services in

the Watts Area of Los Angeles," *California's Health* 23:123–143 (February–March 1966).

66 Lave, J. R. and Leinhardt, "The Delivery of Ambulatory Care to the Poor," *op. cit.*

67 See the following: Dorsey, J. L. "Physician Distribution in Boston and Brookline, 1940 and 1961," *Medical Care* 7:429–440 (November–December 1969); Robertson, L. S. "On the Intraurban Ecology of Primary Care Physicians," *Social Science and Medicine* 4:227–238 (1970); and Hambleton, J. W. "Determinants of Geographical Differences in the Supply of Physician Services," Ph.D. dissertation, University of Wisconsin, Madison, 1971.

58 Coleman, J. E. "The Mathematical Study of Change," in: Blalock, H. M. Jr. and Blalock, A. B. (eds.) *Methodology in Social Research* (New York: McGraw-Hill, 1968) pp. 428–478.

59 Hambleton, J. W. "Determinants of Geographical Differences in the Supply of Physician Services," *op. cit.*

70 Kaplan and Leinhardt, "Determinants of Physician Office Location," *op. cit.*

71 Dublin, T. D. "The Migration of Physicians to the United States," *The New England Journal of Medicine* 286:870–877 (April 1972).

72 Bowers, J. Z. and Rosenheim, L. "Migration of Medical Manpower," *Journal of the American Medical Association* 214:2039 (December 1970).

73 Marguiles, H. and Bloch, L. S. *Foreign Medical Graduates in the United States* (Cambridge: Harvard University Press, 1969).

74 Butter, I. and Schaffner, R. "Foreign Medical Graduates and Equal Access to Medical Care," *Medical Care* 9:136–141 (March–April 1971).

75 Schaffner, R. and Butter, I. "Geographic Mobility of Foreign Medical Graduates and the Doctor Shortage: A Longitudinal Analysis," *Inquiry* 9:24–32 (March 1972).

76 Crawford, R. L. and McCormack, R. C. "Reasons Physicians Leave Primary Practice," *Journal of Medical Education* 46:263–268 (April 1971).

77 Although there are several surveys of medical school graduates [Martin, *et al.*, "Where Graduates Go," *op. cit.*, and Weiskotten, H. G.; Wiggins, W. S.; Altenderfer, M. E.; Gooch, M.; and Tipner, A. "Trends in Medical Practice. An Analysis of the Distribution and Characteristics of Medical College Graduates, 1915–1950," *The Journal of Medical Education* 35:1071–1121 (December 1960)], these are usually descriptive studies of the current character of various past graduating classes. They typically fail to distinguish initial from subsequent decisions or to look closely at the behavior of recent graduates.

78 See: Sloan, F. A. "Lifetime Earnings and Physicians' Choice of Specialty," *Industrial and Labor Relations Review* 24:47–56 (1970) and "Supply Responses of Young Physicians: An Analysis of Physicians in Residency Programs," (Santa Monica: The Rand Corporation, R-1131-OEO, March 1973); and Yett and Sloan, "Migration Patterns," *op. cit.*

79 Sloan, "Supply Responses of Young Physicians," *op. cit.*

80 Yett and Sloan, "Migration Patterns," *op. cit.*

81 Lave and Lave, *The Hospital Construction Act, op. cit.*

SECTION IV

INFLATION

17. Increasing Demand: The Driving Force of Hospital Inflation

MARTIN S. FELDSTEIN

Reprinted from THE RISING COST OF HOSPITAL CARE by Martin S. Feldstein by permission of Information Resources Press, Arlington, Virginia, © December 1971.

Previous discussions of hospital cost inflation have generally focused on *how* inflation has occurred (e.g., more staff, higher wages, more equipment, etc.) rather than on *why* it has. In contrast, the primary purpose of this essay is to explain why cost per patient day has risen so much faster than other prices in our economy. The explanation that is presented here emphasizes the role of increasing demand for hospital services. As will be clear, however, it differs substantially from the traditional economic models in which price rises are induced by shifting demand. Unlike these models, it introduces the notion that increasing demand causes hospitals to change the nature of the product itself. It also develops the ideas that technical progress in hospitals generally increases cost and that, because of the special characteristics of the hospital industry, increasing demand raises wages in an unusual way.

This chapter concentrates on the nature and origins of the increasing demand for hospital care and the general character of the hospitals' response. Discussion of the impact of scientific progress is postponed until Chapter 4; in this chapter it is assumed that hospitals choose from a range of possible techniques of care and standards of comfort that is known and constant through time. As a second simplification, the wage rates paid by hospitals are assumed to change independently through time and not to reflect changes in the demand for hospital services. This assumption will be dropped in the discussion of wage changes in Chapter 5.

Before the sources of increased demand can be discussed, it is necessary to be clear about the meaning of "a change in demand" for so complex a product as hospital care. An increase in demand must of course be defined to include the usual notion that the population would be willing to pay a higher price (i.e., charge per patient day) for the current amount of care and, at the current price, would want to purchase a greater number of hospital days. If hospitals are operating close to effective capacity, such an increase in demand would lead to a perceived "shortage" of hospital beds until more beds are acquired or the price is raised. This is the traditional way in which economic analysis defines an increase in demand. A discussion of hospital cost inflation requires a broader definition. An increase in demand must also be defined to include a willingness to pay more for a given improvement in "perceived quality." [1] The term "perceived quality" is intended to convey increases in the efficacy of medical care, increases in the comfort of hospital stay, and changes in medical practice that patients *believe* increase the efficacy of care, even if they do not in fact. For example, we shall say that demand has increased when, for any given length of stay, patients who would previously have paid five dollars more per day for a semiprivate room than for a bed in a ward become willing to pay ten dollars more. Other examples include an increase in the amount patients would pay for a bed in an intensive care unit, for a greater availability of nursing staff, or for more complete laboratory tests.

3.1 Sources of Increased Demand

The information presented in Section 2.2 identified three of the main reasons why the demand for hospital care has increased: the higher prices of other goods and services, rising personal incomes, and the growth of insurance. After considering these, the current section discusses several other noneconomic factors that have contributed to increasing demand.

Economic Factors.   Absolute money prices as such do not determine the demand for any product. Rather, it is the price of that

---

[1] Although one could incorporate this "quality" aspect of increasing demand into the usual framework of economic analysis by defining each of the quality differentials as a completely different product with a separate demand curve, it is more fruitful in the current context to think of a single "two-dimensional" (quantity and quality) product.

product *relative* to the prices of other goods and services that determines demand. The general level of consumer prices as measured by the CPI has risen almost continuously, although at very different rates, throughout the entire period since 1950. On average it rose 2.1% annually between 1950 and 1968. If hospital charges had remained constant, hospital care would have become less expensive relative to the other goods and services that consumers purchase even if there had been no change in insurance, and the demand for care would therefore have increased. Stated somewhat differently, if there had been no change in the nature or availability of hospital services or other factors influencing demand, the demand for hospital care would have exceeded supply, unless the average charge rose some 2.1% a year.

The mean per capita real disposable income rose 47% from 1950 to 1968. The tendency of economists to classify hospital care as a "necessity," implying that the demand for care rises little as income increases, is misleading. Although there is a substantial amount of survey evidence that admission rates and patient days per year do not rise with income, that evidence also indicates that the demand for higher "quality" care is quite sensitive to income. Table 3.1 presents estimates, based on the 1963-64 survey of hospital discharges conducted by the National Center for Health Statistics (1966b), that show generally lower admission rates and shorter average durations of stay for persons in higher income families.[2] Although expenditure data are not available in the 1963-64 survey, a similar study for 1962 (National Center for Health Statistics, 1966a) does provide estimates of per capita expenditure on hospital care; this is reported in column 4 of Table 3.1. There is a clear increase in this expenditure as income rises. The final column of Table 3.1 combines these expenditure data with the inverse relation between income and bed days in 1963-64 to estimate per patient day expenditures by income class for 1962. The results are striking: expenditure per patient day rises from

---

[2] The data in Table 3.1 have been adjusted for differences in the age composition of the income classes. More detailed data by age and sex generally repeat this pattern; the one exception is that, among persons over 65, those with family incomes exceeding $10,000 had higher per capita patient days than those with lower incomes.

Table 3.1
Income and Demand for Hospital Care*

Family income ($)	(1) Discharges per 1000 population	(2) Mean stay (days)	(3) Patient days per 1000 population	(4) Expenditures per capita	(5) Expenditures per patient day
Under 2000	123.5	9.5	117.3	$24	$20
2000-3999	141.7	9.3	131.8	29	22
4000-6999	132.6	7.4	98.1	31	32
7000-9999	124.9	7.2	89.9	32	36
10,000 and over	119.8	6.9	82.7	35	42

* All figures age-adjusted.
Source: Columns (1) and (2): National Center for Health Statistics, 1966b
Column (4):   National Center for Health Statistics, 1966a

$21 in families with incomes under $4,000 to $42 in families with incomes over $10,000.[3,4]

The growth of private and public insurance coverage has no doubt been the single greatest cause of increased demand.[5] The direct effect of insurance is to lower the *net* price paid by the patient at the time he decides how much care to consume and therefore to raise his demand for hospital care.[6] In practice, insurance pays not merely a fixed proportion of hospital bills but some complex combination of proportional payments, fixed indemnities, and service benefits, subject to a variety of deductions, exclusions,

[3] Although price discrimination (i.e., charging different prices to different patients for the same service) has been common among physicians, hospitals do not follow such a policy. The disproportionately higher prices charged for private rooms and greater amenities do not constitute price discrimination. There may, however, be some element of price discrimination in hospital bill collection.
[4] This evidence should be regarded with some caution since the statistics are based primarily on interview surveys. Respondents are asked to state their expenditure on hospital care, including both that part paid directly and the part paid by insurance. Differences in the type of insurance coverage in different income classes may affect estimates of the amount paid by insurance. The data also omit the value of care paid for by government or nonprofit organizations.
[5] The growth of insurance coverage is not, of course, an independent (exogenous) factor like the rise in income but is in part a response to the rapid increase in hospital charges.
[6] It is also extremely important in this context that insurance carriers have not actively interfered with hospital costs. Insurers either pay the patient and have no direct dealing with hospitals or reimburse hospitals on the basis of cost.

and ceilings. However, treating insurance as a proportional price reduction underlines its primary effect and provides a useful approximation for discussing its overall impact on demand.[7] The portion of *private* hospital expenditure (i.e., excluding all government direct and indirect payments) paid by insurance rose from 34.6% in 1950 to 73.7% in 1968. If the average cost per patient day had remained at its 1950 level of $15.62, the average *net* cost to be paid by patients would have fallen from $10.22 (65.4% of $15.62) to $4.10 (26.3% of $15.62) in 1968. Even if the demand for hospital care were not very sensitive to price, such a large decrease in net price could have increased demand substantially. To keep the average net cost unchanged from 1950 to 1968 (i.e., to "neutralize" the effect on demand of the increased insurance), the gross cost would have had to rise 149% to $38.86.[8]

The growth of government payments for hospital care, both directly and through programs like Medicare and Medicaid, further increased demand. When government payments were included, the proportion of total short-term hospital expenditure paid by "third parties" rose from 51.4% in 1950 to 84.2% in 1968.

This discussion of the impact of increases in income and insurance has implicitly assumed that it is the patient, and not his doctor, who makes the decisions about the use of hospital care. In fact, the decisions are to an important extent made jointly.

---

[7] It is sometimes asserted that the effect of insurance is to lower the price elasticity of demand (i.e., the sensitivity of demand to price as measured by the absolute value of the ratio of the percentage change in quantity demanded to the percentage change in price). There is no reason to believe that this is generally true; it depends on both the nature of the insurance and the structure of patients' preferences. If insurance paid 100% of hospital bills, patients would of course be completely insensitive to hospital price changes (a zero price elasticity). Other types of insurance may leave the price elasticity constant or even increase it. The approximation that insurance pays a proportion of the hospital bill illustrates this. It is perfectly possible that such insurance has no effect on the elasticity of demand; if, in the absence of insurance, the demand function has constant elasticity, this elasticity will not be changed by proportional insurance. It is also easy to see how insurance might actually increase the price elasticity of demand: at a very high price and in the absence of insurance, only medically urgent care would be purchased, with the result that a small rise or fall in price would have no effect on the quantity consumed. The introduction of proportional insurance that substantially lowers the *net* price induces patients to purchase many optional items, with the result that they might be quite sensitive to net price changes.

[8] To the extent that the rise in demand induced an increase in the perceived quality of care, an even larger price increase was necessary to remove excess demand. See Section 4.2.

But the significance of the patient's preferences should not be underestimated. The patient takes the initiative in seeking the advice and care of the physician. In many cases, the patient may reject the physician's advice to enter hospital, preferring to "postpone" an elective operation or to seek additional medical opinions until one confirms his preference to avoid hospital care. If he does go into a hospital, the patient may influence the choice of institution and the length of stay. Even if the physician makes these choices, he is likely to take into account the patient's income and insurance coverage. Relatively little is known about physician behavior in these matters. If doctors are also influenced in their use of resources by the *gross* price of services as well as the net price, insurance will influence their decisions less than the decisions of patients.

Noneconomic Factors. Income, insurance, and the prices of other consumer goods and services are three basic "economic" variables that have increased the demand for hospital care since 1950. Three other types of variables may be distinguished: biological (demographic structure and disease incidence), attitudes, and the availability of beds.

Because hospital use varies substantially by age and sex, the changing demographic structure of the population can influence the demand for hospital care. From 1950 to 1968, several offsetting demographic changes were occurring. For example, persons over 65, who use many more bed days per capita than average, increased from 8 to 10% of the population. At the same time, persons under 25, whose per capita use of hospital beds is less than average, increased from 42 to 47%. A demographic index of hospital use, with the numbers of bed days per capita in ten age-sex groups in 1963 as weights, indicates that the changing demographic structure had no effect on the overall demand for hospital bed days;[9] the index value changed less than 1% between 1950 and 1968.[10]

[9] The demographic index comparing 1968 and 1950 is defined as

$$\sum_i h_{i,63}\, p_{i,68} \; / \; \sum_i h_{i,63}\, p_{i,50}$$

where $h_{i,63}$ is the average number of hospital days per capita in 1963 for persons in age and sex group i, $p_{i,50}$ is the proportion of the population in that group in 1950, and $p_{i,68}$ is the proportion in 1968. The hospital use rates are reported in National Center for Health Statistics (1966b).

[10] The changing demographic structure could, however, affect the nature of the demand for care per patient day.

Several writers have noted that the changing pattern of disease incidence and the improvements in out-of-hospital care have changed the diagnostic mix of the cases admitted to hospitals. Although there are no general national data for this period, there seems to have been a reduction in the number of patients with infectious and parasitic diseases and an increase in the number with cancer and circulatory system diseases. These diagnoses generally use more hospital days per case. The effect on the cost per patient day is not clear, but it is sometimes stated that the newer cases also use more intensive nursing care.

The sociological literature on hospital use describes a great variation in attitudes toward hospital care among different social groups. The evidence suggests that the increasing educational level and the spread of middle-class norms have stimulated demand both for beds and for higher apparent quality of care. Moreover, because the perceived role of the hospital has changed rather rapidly during the current century, there is also a substantial difference between the attitudes that persons in older age groups had a decade or two ago and the attitudes of persons in the same age groups today. More generally, the growing faith in the power of science, and of curative medicine in particular, accelerates the demand for technologically advanced methods of care.

The impact of hospital bed availability on the demand for care has been a subject of substantial controversy.[11] The observation that the number of hospital beds per 1,000 population differs substantially among areas without any sizable effect on the occupancy rate has led to the proposition that the supply of beds "creates its own demand."[12] This important statement is unfortunately ambiguous. Does it imply that an increase in the number of hospital beds will, all other things being equal, lead to an increase in the quantity demanded *because it depresses the price of hospital care*? If so, this notion of "supply creating demand" is no different from the traditional economic analysis in which a bountiful harvest or a large day's catch of fish would cause the

---

[11] For a review of this discussion, see Klarman (1965, 1969a).

[12] Although the approximate equality of "effective supply" (about 80% of possible total bed days) and bed use could in principle reflect a response of bed supply to the pattern of demand, there is substantial evidence from national experience in Britain (Feldstein, 1964, 1967a, ch. 7) and local area changes in the United States (Roemer, 1961) to show that this is not so. See also the model of bed supply described in Feldstein, 1967b.

price to fall until the quantity demanded was equal to the new quantity supplied. Or does the statement imply that an increase in the number of hospital beds shifts the demand schedule, i.e., increases the number of bed days of care demanded at every price? Such a "pure availability effect" would distinguish the market for hospital services from other markets. This is probably what at least some writers had in mind when they spoke of "demand" being increased by an increase in bed supply.[13] Both interpretations are consistent with the observation that there is little, if any, relation between the percentage occupancy and bed availability, but neither is implied by it; there has in fact been no direct test of the "pure availability effect."[14]

If there is such an effect, how does it operate? A relative scarcity of hospital beds may increase the waiting time for admission for elective procedures, encouraging patients to obtain ambulatory care or to do without treatment. Physicians may change their own criteria of when a condition "requires" hospital care and how long a stay is "appropriate" for each type of case. This may be both a reaction (conscious or unconscious) to their perception of the shortage of hospital beds and a response to pressure from the hospitals themselves.

Of course, the notion that availability directly affects demand does not imply that an independent increase in the bed-to-population ratio would induce sufficient demand to maintain the previous percentage occupancy without a fall in price. Instead, it implies that an increase in the availability of beds would not reduce the price at which demand and supply become equal by as much as the traditional analysis of demand would suggest. The signifi-

[13] See, for example, Roemer and Shain, 1959; Roemer, 1961; and Rosenthal, 1964. In discussing this subject in the context of the British National Health Service, in which there is no price rationing, I referred to the effect of availability on "manifest demand" or "use" (Feldstein, 1967a). At a zero price actual demand may be very much greater than supply; it is possible to observe only the demands that patients are able to effect, not the quantity that they actually demand at the zero price. The same is true for Medicare patients; there are fewer Medicare admissions in states with low bed-to-population ratios, even though these patients face the same "price" (a low deductible and a small copayment after a substantial length of stay) in all states (Feldstein, 1971a).

[14] Such a test would require estimation of a demand function for hospital care in which both price and availability are explanatory variables. This function could not be tested by observing whether prices are lower where there are more beds per capita, since other factors affecting demand also differ across areas.

cance of this implication is that a relatively large increase in the supply of hospital beds would be required to prevent an increase in the demand for hospital bed days due to other factors from causing excess demand; e.g., a 10% increase in the demand for bed days due to higher personal income would not be satisfied by a 10% increase in the number of beds if the greater availability itself induced a further increase in demand. This makes it more likely that price rises were necessary to prevent a growing excess demand during the period since 1950.

3.2 How Hospitals Respond to Increased Demand

Traditional economic theory describes the response of profit-seeking firms to shifts in demand. The conclusion of such analysis is that, in an economy composed of competitive profit-seeking firms, an increase in demand for a product will raise its price because of the higher average cost of producing a larger total quantity. If the firms have some degree of monopoly power, the analysis is more complex. One likely outcome is a higher price, including a greater monopoly profit per unit, even if average cost does not rise. These models of response to changing demand are irrelevant for hospitals in two distinct but related ways. First, hospitals are generally not profit-seeking institutions, and therefore they are not motivated to raise prices in an attempt to increase profits. Second, the traditional models ignore the change in product "quality" as a response to a shift in demand.

If hospitals are not motivated by profit maximization, what does determine their response to changes in demand? The most plausible answer is that subject to the constraint that they break approximately even, hospitals try to maximize the "quantity" of care that they provide. More specifically, when demand increases they try to provide more patient days of care and to raise the "quality" of care.[15] The reason for such behavior need not concern us. It may be that this is the appropriate professional and philanthropic response of institutions dedicated to providing medical care. It may be that administrators and medical staff get

---

[15] This type of assumption has been incorporated in formal models by Feldstein (1967a), Newhouse (1970), and Evans (1970). For some implications of a quite different assumption, that hospitals behave to maximize the personal incomes of the physicians on the staff, see Pauly (1969).

ersonal pleasure and prestige from being part of a larger organization and one that provides more sophisticated care. Or the growth in the hospital budget may be a way of increasing the fees that the medical staff can earn or the salary that administrators receive.[16]

In the short run, hospitals cannot increase the number of bed days of care very much. Percentage occupancy can rise somewhat, but hospitals can expand the number of beds only with substantial delays. Even in the long run, most of the expansion of demand is channeled into higher cost per patient day rather than into more days of care. From 1950 to 1968, the number of days of care per person increased only 29% while the index of inputs per patient day[17] rose 105%. This increase in inputs takes many forms: more staff, more equipment, and more supplies, all of which can be used to increase the sophistication of treatment, to reduce uncertainty, to make patients more comfortable, etc. The relatively greater increase in inputs per patient day than in the number of days per capita reflects both patients' preferences and the choices made by hospital administrators and medical staff. If hospitals had chosen to expand the number of beds even more, patients would not have been willing to pay as large an increase in cost per patient day.

This description of the way hospitals respond to increasing demand should not be misunderstood. The preferences of the hospital administrators and medical staff do not completely determine the final response to changing demand. The structure of the local hospital care market, i.e., the number of hospitals among which the typical patient can choose, has an important influence on the extent to which patients' preferences dominate.[18]

---

[16] This description of behavior applies to voluntary hospitals. Government hospitals are not bound by a break-even constraint and therefore do not respond to demand in the same way. It is likely, however, that they are constrained to keep their cost per patient day at approximately the same level as the voluntary hospitals in their area and that they seek to have similar staffing patterns, equipment, and other technical aspects of the production of care.

[17] This index uses average earnings per employee to measure labor costs and the wholesale price index to measure the price of nonlabor inputs bought by hospitals. See Section 2.3, especially p. 19.

[18] Economists are well aware that, although firms in a competitive market respond to an increase in demand with the aim of increasing their profits, the final effect of a change in demand is to change the quantity produced and the unit cost but not the profits.

It lies beyond the scope of the current discussion to consider what combination of patients' preferences, external labor market pressures, professional standards, and administrative interests determines the actual mix of responses to increasing demand. One aspect of this response, the change in technology, will be discussed in the next chapter. A second aspect, the rise in wages, will be considered in Chapter 5.

In concluding this chapter it is useful to consider what explanations of hospital cost inflation could be developed *without* reference to increasing demand. There are two possible approaches. The first, which might be labeled the "productivity" explanation, is that the prices paid by hospitals for personnel, equipment, and supplies have been rising, while productivity (i.e., output-per-unit-of-input) has not increased as rapidly. This approach cannot explain why the cost per patient day has actually risen faster than input prices. Moreover, the increased number of hospital days per capita is not consistent with increased charges and a constant demand schedule. This suggests the second type of explanation: technical necessity. If the demand for hospital care is completely insensitive to price, hospitals can provide whatever care they consider to be technically appropriate or "necessary" and then charge the resulting cost per patient day. Although experts generally agree that price elasticity of demand is relatively low, both informal observations and specific statistical tests[19] make the complete absence of price sensitivity seem unlikely.

The role of increasing demand for hospital care as the primary cause of the very rapid increase in cost per patient day is not generally understood or widely accepted. It is, however, more than a personal opinion based on casual speculation. The ideas discussed in this chapter have been incorporated into a formal mathematical model with some allowance for changing technology and estimated with a combination of cross-section and time-series state data using annual observations for the period 1958 through 1968. The results (Feldstein, 1971c) support the verbal discussion that has been presented here.

---

[19] See, for example, Rosenthal (1964), Feldstein (1971c).

18. Theories of Hospital Inflation: Some Empirical Evidence

KAREN DAVIS

ABSTRACT

This article examines three alternative hypotheses of hospital inflation: the demand-pull hypothesis, and cost-plus reimbursement hypothesis, and the labor cost-push hypothesis. The theoretical foundation of the cost-reimbursement hypothesis is explored; hospitals desiring to maximize quantity of hospital services or profits will not respond to cost-plus reimbursement by raising costs unless nearly all patients are covered by the plan. Empirical estimation of hospital average costs and average hospital wage rates yield no support for the cost-reimbursement hypothesis. A significant upward shift in hospital costs and hospital wages in the Medicare period, however, was obtained.

With the introduction of the Medicare and Medicaid programs in 1966, average hospital costs per patient day for community hospitals jumped from an annual rate of increase of 6.2 percent in the period from 1962–65 to an annual rate of increase of 13.9 percent in the period from 1967–70.[1] In spite of the plethora of research on hospital costs, little is known about the causes of this dramatic increase in hospital cost inflation.[2] This gap in knowledge is in large part the result of an excessive concern with differences in costs among hospitals at a given point in time rather than with the determinants of hospital

---

The author is a Research Associate at the Brookings Institution.

* The author wishes to thank Herbert E. Klarman, Marian Krzyzaniak, and Stanley Wallack for helpful comments and the Social Security Administration for financial support. The research assistance of Julian Pettengill is gratefully acknowledged. The views expressed here are those of the author and do not necessarily reflect those of the staff, officers, or trustees of the Brookings Institution.

1 [10], Aug 1, 1971, p. 454. Average costs per patient day deflated by the Consumer Price Index for all items other than medical care rose at an annual rate of 5.1 from 1962–65 and 9.1 from 1967–70.

2 Hospital cost studies which have emphasized trends in costs over time include two studies by M. Feldstein [8, 9]; studies of Pennsylvania hospital costs by Lave and Lave [17, 18]; and a study of New York hospitals by Salkever [24]. The Feldstein papers are directed toward a demand-pull type of inflation, while the other papers

cost inflation over time. This paper attempts to remedy this deficiency by reviewing theories of hospital inflation, constructing models of hospital cost determination which permit tests of several hypotheses, and empirically estimating the models.

I. THEORIES OF HOSPITAL INFLATION

To devise appropriate solutions for hospital inflation, it is necessary to have a much clearer understanding of the underlying causes of inflation. If hospital inflation is largely a consequence of increasing demand without increases in supply, an expansion of hospital beds may be warranted. If the inflation is a labor cost-push inflation, attempts to curtail labor costs through wage guidelines or control may be the appropriate policy. If the inflation is induced by certain types of insurance coverage, a restructuring of insurance coverage may be called for. If the inflation is induced by inefficiencies in the hospital market, structural reform of the industry may be a desired course of action. If the inflation is the result of advances in medical technology, inflation may simply be a necessary price of improvement in health.

Three major theories of hospital inflation have been advanced. One views inflation as primarily demand-induced, while two theories view the inflation as originating on the cost side.

1. *Demand-Pull Hypothesis.* M. Feldstein has argued that increases in hospital costs are primarily a response to increase in demand [8, 9]. Essentially, as the price a hospital can charge while maintaining a given level of capacity increases, the hospital raises both prices and costs to the highest level consistent with maintaining a given level of capacity utilization and an equality of prices with average costs. Pressures for costs to rise come partially from patients who, with expanding insurance coverage, demand higher quality care and more amenities such as better food service, more nursing personnel, and more cheerful accommodations. Nonprofit hospitals, legally prevented from distributing profits to owners, are eager to use the potentially higher revenues, generated by increases in demand, to add additional staff, to increase employees' salaries, to introduce more expensive technology, and in general to provide a more expensive "style" of hospital care.

M. Feldstein has estimated this model of hospital inflation using state data for the period from 1958 to 1967 [8]. The focus of the empirical estimation is on the determinants of the demand for hospital care. No attempt is made to test the hypothesis that costs are raised correspondingly in response

concentrate on explaining costs directly. Lave and Lave's study of Pennsylvania hospitals concentrates on determining which types of hospitals have costs rising more rapidly than average, such as teaching hospitals, rural hospitals, and hospitals with initially lower than average costs. Salkever's study of New York hospitals employs essentially a reduced-form approach to estimating hospital costs so that it is impossible to determine whether changes on the demand or on the supply side are the motivating forces influencing costs. He finds that the total effect of cost-reimbursement insurance plans are not more inflationary than charge-reimbursement plans.

to increases in demand. Instead, prices are assumed equal to average costs, and average costs are used to measure price in the demand equation. Recent work, however, has shown that there are substantial variations in hospital profits both among states and over time, and that these variations are systematically related to various supply and demand factors [5]. Judgment on the validity of this theory, therefore, must be postponed until the link between prices and costs is clarified.

   2. *Cost-Reimbursement Inflation.* The second major theory of hospital inflation views the growth of insurance plans which reimburse hospitals on the basis of costs as the principal determinant of rising hospital costs.[3] This theory holds that as hospitals realize that costs can automatically be passed on to third-party payers, they have little incentive to economize on supplies, buy the lowest cost equipment, and keep salaries down. Quantitatively, the potential effect of this source of hospital inflation has increased significantly in recent years with the implementation of Medicare and Medicaid programs.

   An empirical study by Pauly and Drake [23] tested this theory of inflation and found no significant cost-reimbursement effect. Their findings, however, are not conclusive since the study was restricted to hospitals in one geographic area at one point in time and used a very crude measure of cost reimbursement. Since the theoretical basis for this theory has not been developed and since the theory has not been subjected to adequate empirical testing, the following sections will explore in detail this source of hospital inflation. Section II will examine the theoretical basis of the cost-reimbursement theory. Section III will discuss the limitations of the Pauly-Drake study and will develop an empirical model specifically designed to test this theory. Section IV presents some empirical results.

   3. *Labor Cost-Push Inflation.* Since a large proportion of hospital costs are labor costs, this portion of hospital expenses has occasionally been singled out as the principal villain in hospital cost inflation (see, for example, [26]). Rising wage rates are viewed as the principal cause behind rising hospital costs. Increases in wage rates are variously attributed to: (1) a "catching up" of hospital wages with those of comparable occupations, (2) increasing unionization of hospital workers or the threat of unionization, (3) tight labor markets in the mid- and late 1960s, and (4) a change in the composition of hospital employees to more highly skilled personnel.

   To date, no empirical work has systematically investigated the importance of this source of hospital inflation. Therefore, Section V will develop and test a model of hospital wage rate determination.

II. HOSPITAL MOTIVATION AND THE RESPONSE TO COST-REIMBURSEMENT PLANS

Various conjectures concerning the effect of cost-reimbursement schemes on hospital costs have been made. Pauly and Drake, for example, contend that

---

3   For a discussion of this theory of inflation, see Klarman [12, 14, 15].

. . . if hospitals received a fixed percentage of costs as a plus and we assume that they wish to maximize that plus in order to attain maximum growth or to treat the maximum number of patients over the long run, then cost-plus reimbursement leads to a perverse result. Hospitals which are striving to increase funds available for capital investment will try to increase costs, since that will increase the absolute amount of the plus they earn. If, however, payment is based on charges, as in Wisconsin, the long-run growth maximizing hospital has a positive incentive to minimize costs. [23, pp. 302–303]

Klarman, in responding to Pauly and Drake, argues, however, that

. . . a hospital's management is not likely to be influenced by cost reimbursement if only 5 to 10 percent of its income is derived in this manner. It is almost certain to be influenced if the proportion is 90 to 95 percent. [13, p. 317]

In order to determine the likely response of hospital managers to the growth of cost-reimbursement plans, this section will propose several hypotheses of hospital motivation and derive the implications of these hypotheses for response to cost-reimbursement plans.

Initially, it is assumed that hospital managers desire to maximize profits in order to obtain funds for future expansion. Then, an output-maximizing model of hospital behavior will be examined. The relationship of cost-plus reimbursement to the proportion of a hospital's patients covered by the cost plan will be investigated to determine under what circumstances hospital managers will have an incentive to raise costs.

Model 1: Profit Maximization

Let q_n = number of hospital patients not covered by a cost-reimbursement scheme; q_m = number of hospital patients covered by a cost-reimbursement scheme;[4] $p(q_n)$ = price of hospital care facing patients not covered by a cost-reimbursement scheme;[5] $AC(q_n + q_m;\alpha)$ = average cost of providing hospital care, where α is an X-inefficiency[6] shift parameter such that $\partial AC/\partial \alpha > 0$; k = proportion of average cost reimbursed (e.g., $k = 1.05$ if a 5 percent plus is included).

Then, hospital managers are assumed to maximize profits:
$$\pi = p(q_n) \cdot q_n + k \cdot q_m \cdot AC(q_n + q_m;\alpha) - (q_n + q_m) \cdot AC(q_n + q_m;\alpha)$$
= revenue from non-cost-reimbursed patients + revenue from cost-reimbursed patients − total costs.

---

4   Patients covered by a cost-reimbursement scheme are assumed to face a zero net price so that their demand is fixed.

5   Patients not covered by a cost-reimbursement scheme are assumed to have no insurance coverage so that the price paid by the patients is the same as the price charged by the hospital. The demand for hospital care by non-cost-reimbursed patients is then $p(q_n)$. The assumption is not crucial and can be replaced by a relationship between the gross price charged by the hospital and the net price paid by the insured.

6   For a discussion of X-efficiency, see Leibenstein [19].

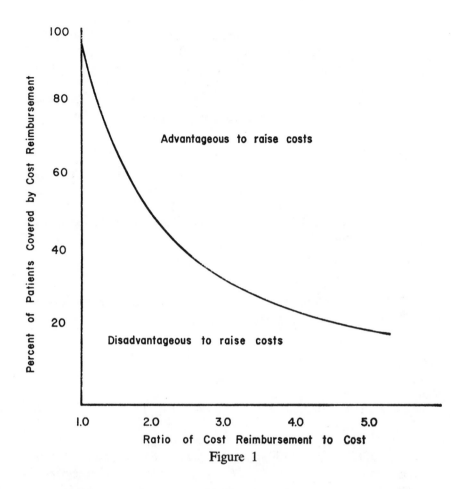

Figure 1

Under what conditions will the hospital gain an increase in profit by increasing X-inefficiency and shifting the average cost curve upward?

$$\partial\pi/\partial\alpha = k \cdot q_m \cdot \partial AC/\partial\alpha - (q_n + q_m) \cdot \partial AC/\partial\alpha$$
$$= \partial AC/\partial\alpha \cdot [kq_m - (q_n + q_m)]$$

Since $\partial AC/\partial\alpha > 0$, profit would increase if

$$k \cdot q_m > q_n + q_m$$
or $$q_m/(q_n + q_m) > 1/k$$

Figure 1 shows various combinations of proportion of total patients covered by cost-reimbursement schemes $[q_m/(q_n + q_m)]$ and various plus factors above which hospital managers would find it desirable to raise costs. As indicated, either the proportion of patients covered by cost-reimbursement schemes would have to be quite high or the plus factor would have to be extremely high before hospital managers would find it desirable to raise costs. For example, if the plus factor were 5 percent so that $k = 1.05$, more than 95 percent of the patients would have to be covered by the cost-plus scheme before a profit-maximizing hospital manager would desire to raise costs. If only 80 percent of the hospital's patients were covered by a cost-plus scheme, the plan would need to reimburse hospitals at a rate greater than one and one-quarter times their cost ($k = 1.25$) before hospital managers would find it advantageous to raise costs. Clearly, these ranges are beyond those found in practice in the United States at the present time.

These results, however, depend upon the assumption of profit maximization which has not found widespread acceptance in the hospital literature.

Model 2: Output Maximization Subject to a Break-Even Constraint

A somewhat more popular model in the hospital literature is the output maximization model.[7] Under this hypothesis, the hospital desires to serve as many patients as possible subject to a break-even constraint.

Since the constraint will always be binding under normal economic conditions, let us examine the constraint:

$$\pi = p(q_n) \cdot q_n + k \cdot AC(q_n + q_m; \alpha) \cdot q_m$$
$$- (q_n + q_m) \cdot AC(q_n + q_m; \alpha) = 0$$

Holding profits equal to zero and allowing output of non-cost-reimbursed patients and the shift parameters to vary,

$$d\pi = 0 = (\partial\pi/\partial q_n)dq_n + (\partial\pi/\partial\alpha)d\alpha$$

or

$$dq_n/d = -(\partial\pi/\partial\alpha)/(\partial\pi/\partial q_n)$$
$$= -[kq_m - (q_n + q_m)]/[MR_{q_n} + k \cdot q_m/(q_n + q_m) \cdot (MC - AC) - MC]$$
$$= [q_n - (k-1)q_m]/[(MR_{q_n} - MC) + k \cdot q_m/(q_n + q_m) \cdot (MC - AC)]$$

Since a quantity-maximizing hospital will increase output beyond that of a profit-maximizing hospital, $(MR - MC)$ can be expected to be negative. If average costs are decreasing or constant over the relevant range, $(MC - AC)$ will be non-positive. Therefore, the denominator in the above expression is negative. If the numerator is also negative, that is, $q_n - (k-1)q_m < 0$, then $dq_n/d\alpha > 0$. If so, a quantity-maximizing hospital will be able to increase the number of patients served by raising costs while continuing to break even. The numerator will be negative provided that

$$q_n - (k-1)q_m < 0 \text{ if and only if } q_n/q_m < k-1$$
$$\text{if and only if } (q_n + q_m)/q_m < k$$
$$\text{if and only if } q_m/(q_n + q_m) > 1/k$$

Therefore, an output-maximizing hospital will find it advantageous to raise costs under exactly the same circumstances as a profit-maximizing hospital— namely, for all points above the combination of cost-plus factors and proportion of patients covered by cost-reimbursement plans drawn in Figure 1. As noted earlier, with 80 percent of a hospital's patients covered by cost reimbursement, the plus factor would have to exceed 25 percent of the hospital's costs before the hospital would find it advantageous to increase costs.

---

7   For an analysis of the output-maximization hypothesis along with other hypotheses of hospital behavior, see Davis [4].

Other models of hospital behavior, however, might lead to different predictions. If the hospital desires to maximize some component of costs, such as nurses' salaries, a cost-reimbursement scheme could be expected to have a more immediate effect on hospital costs even if only a fairly small proportion of patients were covered by the scheme.

The above discussion has been restricted primarily to short-run effects. Although cost-plus schemes may not lead hospitals to raise costs in the short run, hospitals might use the increased funds to make capital acquisitions which would increase costs in the future. This, however, would be true of revenue received from any source—charges, incentive reimbursement, or cost-plus reimbursement.

III. THE MODEL AND ESTIMATION PROCEDURE

Pauly and Drake attempted to assess the effect of cost-reimbursement schemes on hospital costs by analyzing individual hospital data in four states—Illinois, Indiana, Michigan, and Wisconsin— for the year 1966 [23]. They found that hospitals in states in which Blue Cross reimbursed on the basis of costs did not have higher costs than hospitals in states in which Blue Cross reimbursed on the basis of charges.

The empirical model developed here differs from the Pauly-Drake model in several important respects: (1) It presents data before and after the introduction of the Medicare program so that the impact of this important cost-reimbursement scheme can be assessed. (2) A new measure of cost-reimbursement is presented which varies with the extensiveness of coverage. (3) Data are drawn from all areas of the United States rather than from one area. (4) The effect of cost reimbursement is incorporated in a statistical cost model. In addition, hospital wage rates are analyzed to determine if hospital wages are higher when a larger proportion of hospital reimbursement comes from a cost-reimbursement plan.

Estimation is based on state data for 1965, 1967, and 1968. Both single-year, cross-section estimates and pooled cross-section, time-series estimates are obtained.

The model used in the pooled cross-section, time-series estimation is as follows:

$$\log AC = b_0 + b_1 \log Q/B + b_2 \log B + b_3 \log w + b_4 \log MS + b_5 CR$$

$$+ b_6 T_{67} + b_7 T_{68} + \Sigma_{i=1}^{16} d_i F_i + e$$

where AC = average cost of providing hospital care (cost per admission); Q = hospital admissions; B = average bed size; Q/B = case-flow rate (admissions per bed); w = average hospital wage rate; MS = mean length of stay (used as a measure of complexity of case-mix as discussed below); CR = proportion of hospital expenses covered by a cost-reimbursement plan;

T_{67} = time dummy taking a value of 1 in 1967; T_{68} = time dummy taking a value of 1 in 1968; F_i = proportion of hospitals having ith specialized facility.[8]

This functional form (other than for the case-mix, cost-reimbursement, facility, and time dummy variables) can be derived from a short-run, modified, Cobb-Douglas production function relationship.[9] Unlike previous statistical hospital cost analyses, it includes factor costs, complexity of case-mix, and extent of cost reimbursement as explanatory variables.[10] The time dummies are included to pick up time effects including general cost inflation (note that the CPI is a linear combination of the time dummies and the constant term).

The model differs from the Pauly-Drake specification in several respects. It includes wage rates and case-flow rates (Q/B) which are omitted in the Pauly-Drake model. Instead, Pauly and Drake include income and population density in their average cost estimation; both variables are found to be significant. It is very probable that wages paid by hospitals are correlated with income, while population density may be correlated with case-flow rates. If such is the case, income and population density are undoubtedly picking up the significance of the wage rate and case-flow rate variables in the properly specified form.

As presented, this model assumes that cost reimbursement affects cost other than by influencing hospital wages. This assumption is examined in detail in the following section.

A new measure of cost reimbursement is proposed here. Pauly and Drake measured cost reimbursement by a zero-one dummy variable, taking on a value of one for hospitals in states in which Blue Cross reimbursed on the basis of costs and a value of zero in states in which Blue Cross reimbursed hospitals on the basis of charges. Such a measure assumes that the effect on hospital costs is the same whether 5 percent or 95 percent of the hospital's income comes from a cost-reimbursed plan. The measure presented here is the proportion of a hospital's expenses covered by a cost-reimbursement plan. More specifically, it is the sum of Blue Cross reimbursement on the basis of costs plus Medicare reimbursement plus public assistance hospital vendor payments (primarily Medicaid) divided by total hospital expenses. The vari-

---

8   Specialized facilities include: blood bank, pathology laboratory, electroencephalograph, occupational therapy department, physical therapy department, intensive care unit, organized outpatient department, home care program, postoperative recovery room, medical social service department, X-ray therapeutic, radioactive isotope facility, psychiatric inpatient care unit, cobalt and radium therapy, rehabilitation unit.

9   The sum of the coefficients is not constrained to equal one. For derivation of the cost function from the production function, see Nerlove [22]. Also note Lave and Lave [18] for a log linear average cost estimation of hospital costs in Pennsylvania.

10   For reviews of several cross-section cost studies, see Mann and Yett [20] and Lave and Lave [16]. In addition to the combined cross-section, time-series cost studies noted in fn. 2, cross-section cost studies include Berry [1], Carr and P. Feldstein [2], Cohen [3], M. Feldstein [7], and Ingbar and Taylor [11].

able has a value of zero in 1965 for those states in which Blue Cross reimburses on the basis of charges.[11]

One difficulty common to hospital cost estimation is the problem of defining hospital output. Aggregation at the state level obviates some of this difficulty since case-mix variation is less likely to be significant at the aggregated level than at the individual hospital level.[12] Even so, some states may be "healthier" than others because of differences in pollution levels, style of life, etc. The demographic composition of the population may also vary from state to state. To adjust for differences in case-mix and the complexity of cases of a given case type, length of hospital stay and proportion of hospitals possessing various specialized facilities are included. Including length of stay is based on the assumption that length of stay reflects differences in complexity of cases rather than economic factors such as ability to pay. Longer stays are expected to increase the cost per admission. Although estimates are based on hospital admissions, costs per patient day may be derived from the results as follows:

Since $TC/PD = TC/(Adm \cdot MS)$,

$$\log TC/Adm = b_0 + b_1 \log Adm/B + b_2 \log B + b_3 \log w + b_4 \log MS$$
$$+ b_5 CR + b_6 T_{67} + b_7 T_{68} + \sum_{i=1}^{16} d_i F_i + e$$

implies that

$$\log TC/PD = b_0 + b_1 \log Adm/B + b_2 \log B + b_3 \log w + (b_4 - 1)$$
$$\log MS + b_5 CR + b_6 T_{67} + b_7 T_{68} + \sum_{i=1}^{16} d_i F_i + e^{13}$$
$$= b_0 + b_1 \log PD/B + b_2 \log B + b_3 \log w + (b_4 - b_1 - 1)$$
$$\log MS + b_5 CR + b_6 T_{67} + b_7 T_{68} + \sum_{i=1}^{16} d_i F_i + e$$

where TC = total costs; Adm = admissions; and PD = patient days. That is, all coefficients remain unchanged except for that of the mean stay variable. (See the Appendix for detailed definitions of variables and source of data.)

IV. AVERAGE COST REGRESSION RESULTS

Table 1 provides individual year and pooled cross-section, time-series average cost regression estimates for 1965, 1967, and 1968. Overall explanatory power is high with the multiple coefficient of determination adjusted for degrees of freedom ranging from .90 to .95.

The major finding is that the cost-reimbursement variables are insignificant in explaining hospital costs for the individual year results and for the pooled cross-section, time-series results when the time dummy variables are

---

11 An alternative specification, $\log (CR + 1)$, was tried with virtually identical results.
12 See M. Feldstein [7] for a discussion of the importance of adjusting for differences in case-mix.
13 For a demonstration of the econometric equivalence of this formulation and the above formulation, see Vroman [27].

TABLE 1

TOTAL EXPENSES PER ADMISSION, COMMUNITY HOSPITALS, LOG LINEAR RESULTS

	1968 (1)	1967 (2)	1965 (3)	Pooled '65, '67, '68 (4)	Pooled '65, '67, '68 (5)
Constant	−6.60	−4.64	−3.89	−5.99	−3.19
	(3.17)	(1.98)	(1.78)	(5.64)	(3.03)
Admission per bed	− .05	.05	.05	− .03	.04
	(.20)	(1.21)	(.18)	(.17)	(.25)
Average size bed	.26	.32	.28	.32	.30
	(3.76)	(3.15)	(2.52)	(6.08)	(6.40)
Wage rate	1.29	.80	.96	1.21	.86
	(7.98)	(5.29)	(4.75)	(18.63)	(10.64)
Cost reimbursement	.66	.003	.16	.23	.09
	(.62)	(.02)	(1.74)	(4.96)	(1.69)
Mean stay	.49	.51	.22	.35	.25
	(2.09)	(1.52)	(.91)	(2.41)	(1.92)
T_{67}	—	—	—	—	.10
					(5.07)
T_{68}	—	—	—	—	.16
					(6.08)
Facilities	Inc.	Inc.	Inc.	Inc.	Inc.
$\bar{R}^2$	.95	.90	.92	.94	.96
R^2	.97	.95	.95	.95	.96

Note: t-scores in parentheses. Inc. = included.

included. When the time variables are omitted, cost reimbursement is significant in the pooled results. Various interpretations are, therefore, possible. It might be argued that the true explanators of hospital costs are missing variables which are constant across geographic areas but which vary over time, such as the prices of some inputs, interest expenses, the nature of the product provided, and technology. When the time variables are omitted, the cost-reimbursement variable stands as a proxy for these time-series effects. Second, it might also be argued that Medicare had an announcement effect on hospital costs resulting in a shift in average costs with the introduction of Medicare which was independent of the exact proportion of the hospital's patients which were Medicare patients. A third possible interpretation is that the extensiveness of cost-reimbursement plans is the true explanator and the correlation of this variable with the time dummy variables obscured this effect when the time variables are included.

Either of the first two interpretations is consistent with the single year estimations presented in Table 1. The cost-reimbursement variables are insignificant in each of the single year estimations. If the third interpretation were correct, the cost-reimbursement variable should be significant in the single year results as well.

This may be seen somewhat more clearly by examining the percent of hospital expenses covered by cost-reimbursement plans during the period. In 1965, the percent of hospital expenses covered by cost reimbursement varied from zero in states in which Blue Cross reimbursed on the basis of charges to 52.4 percent in Rhode Island. In 1968, the percent of hospital expenses covered by cost reimbursement varied from 18.6 in Louisiana to 87.6 in Rhode Island The single year estimations, then, may be interpreted as finding that as cost reimbursement varied from zero to 52 percent and from 19 to 88 percent, average hospital costs did not change. That is, in 1968 hospitals in states in which cost reimbursement represented 88 percent of costs did not have higher costs, other things equal, than hospitals in states in which cost reimbursement represented only 19 percent of costs. It may be concluded, therefore, that the extensiveness of cost-reimbursement coverage within the ranges observed does not increase hospital costs, but a once-and-for-all shift with the introduction of Medicare cannot be completely ruled out.

As predicted, the length-of-stay variable has a significantly positive coefficient. A 10 percent decrease in mean stay, holding admissions constant, leads to a 3 to 5 percent decrease in cost per admission. To the extent that incentives for reducing mean stay would be desirable depends upon the trade-off between reduced costs and any decline in the quality of care.

The length-of-stay variable has one disadvantage in that it is correlated with the case-flow rate (admissions per bed). The correlation coefficient between the logs of length of stay and the case flow rate is —.83. Including length of stay, therefore, tends to reduce the significance of the case-flow variables. Frequently, the case-flow rate enters with a positive sign rather than the expected negative one. When mean stay is omitted from the estimation, estimated coefficients of the case-flow rate range from —.23 to —.41 and are significantly different from zero.

There is some indication that there are diseconomies of scale. A 10 percent increase in the number of beds per hospital leads to a 2 to 3 percent increase in costs per admission. Average bed size in the sample, however, does not exceed 275 beds so that economies of scale may be evident beyond that range.

The wage variable is positive, as expected, and highly significant. A 10 percent increase in the wage rate leads to an 8 to 9 percent increase in average costs. This is somewhat higher than expected since labor costs account for only 60 percent of hospital expenses. Since other costs of hospital operation, such as food costs, may also vary across geographic areas in the same manner as wage levels, it is possible that the wage rate variable is picking up the influence of other differences in factor costs.

The estimated rate of cost inflation over the period other than that reflected by the increase in wage rates after adjusting for changes in utilization is given by the coefficients of the time dummy variables. In 1967, average costs were 10 percent higher than in 1965; in 1968, average costs were 16 percent higher than in 1965.

Including the proportion of hospitals possessing various specialized facilities increased the coefficient of determination adjusted for degrees of freedom by several points (e.g., from .93 to .96 in the pooled estimation including time variables). Omitting the facilities variables tended to decrease the bed coefficient and increase the wage rate coefficient, suggesting that failure to adjust for specialized facilities may lead to incorrect estimates of the effect of wage rates and size on hospital beds.

TABLE 2

AVERAGE WAGE RATES, COMMUNITY HOSPITALS, LOG LINEAR RESULTS

	1968 (1)	1967 (2)	1965 (3)	Pooled '65, '67, '68 (4)
Constant	6.30	6.24	6.59	4.22
	(5.93)	(4.79)	(8.22)	(6.99)
Manufacturing wages	.24	.25	.19	.46
	(1.81)	(1.59)	(1.96)	(5.93)
Average bed size	−.04	−.08	−.07	−.01
	(.53)	(.84)	(1.07)	(.20)
Hospital density	−.02	−.05	−.02	−.03
	(.95)	(1.80)	(.99)	(2.56)
Cost reimbursement	−.03	.09	.01	.26
	(.31)	(.67)	(.14)	(6.02)
Unionization	−.02	−.02	.01	−.04
	(.43)	(.43)	(.26)	(1.32)
Hospital labor law	.02	.10	.04	.05
	(.62)	(2.23)	(1.27)	(2.12)
T_{67}	—	—	—	—
T_{68}	—	—	—	—
Facilities	Inc.	Inc.	Inc.	Inc.
Regional dummies	—	—	—	—
$\bar{R}^2$	.73	.61	.83	.75
R^2	.86	.79	.91	.79

Note: t-scores in parentheses. Inc. = included.

V. HOSPITAL WAGE RATE DETERMINATION

The previous section assumed that cost-reimbursement schemes affect costs other than by increasing hospital wage rates. This section examines the empirical validity of this assumption. A model of the determination of wage rates in hospitals is developed and the hypothesis that wage rates are higher in states with a larger proportion of hospital revenue stemming from a cost-reimbursement scheme is tested.

The average hospital wage rate is assumed to be a function of a number of factors including: (1) the going wage rate for comparable employment; (2) the monopsony power of hospitals;[14] (3) the skill mix of employees; (4) the threat of unionization; (5) the financial ability of hospitals to pay higher wages; and (6) the extent of cost-reimbursement schemes.

Unfortunately, detailed state data on earnings in comparable occupations are unavailable. The closest proxy for comparable earnings available is average weekly earnings of production workers in manufacturing industries.

Yett has hypothesized that wages for nurses are not competitively determined. He found that

---

14   This hypothesis has been advanced by Yett [29].

TABLE 2
(Continued)

Pooled '65, '67, '68 (5)	1968 (6)	1967 (7)	1965 (8)	Pooled '65, '67, '68 (9)	Pooled '65, '67, '68 (10)
6.33	5.40	5.75	4.99	3.44	5.25
(11.84)	(5.04)	(4.86)	(5.33)	(5.53)	(9.41)
.22	.30	.24	.32	.53	.29
(3.36)	(2.56)	(1.60)	(2.76)	(6.83)	(4.13)
−.07	.12	.15	.12	.10	.13
(1.54)	(3.49)	(3.46)	(3.07)	(3.98)	(6.15)
−.02	.04	.03	.03	.03	.03
(2.35)	(2.35)	(1.27)	(1.54)	(2.39)	(2.98)
−.01	.02	−.05	−.01	.15	−.02
(.20)	(.36)	(−.58)	(.09)	(3.71)	(.42)
−.01	−.02	−.03	−.01	−.06	−.02
(.47)	(.62)	(.74)	(.21)	(2.50)	(.97)
.05	.01	.04	.03	.02	.03
(2.61)	(.49)	(1.04)	(1.25)	(.98)	(1.70)
.10	—	—	—	—	.09
(5.49)					(5.01)
.18	—	—	—	—	.15
(8.46)					(8.12)
Inc.	—	—	—	—	—
—	Inc.	Inc.	Inc.	Inc.	Inc.
.84	.79	.63	.78	.74	.82
.87	.83	.70	.82	.75	.84

> In response to a survey of the 21 largest metropolitan hospital associations, all but one of the 15 that replied reported that they had been successful in establishing and operating a wage standardization program among hospitals in the association. [28, p. 90]

Yett, therefore, feels that hospitals collude to act as monopsonists in the labor market. If the effectiveness of the collusive agreement decreases with the number of hospitals in the area, the monopsony effect will be greater when there are fewer hospitals in the area [25]. To capture the effect, monopsony power is measured by the number of hospitals per square mile in the state. It is expected that wages will be higher in areas of higher hospital density.

The average hospital wage rate is expected to be higher in states in which hospitals hire a higher proportion of skilled personnel. Two measures of the skill composition of employees are used: the average size of hospital and the percentage of the state's hospitals that possess various specialized facilities. Larger hospitals and hospitals with more specialized facilities can be expected to have a higher proportion of skilled personnel and a resulting higher average wage.

In a survey of hospital unionization, Miller and Shortell found that hospitals in areas where they are legally required to bargain have union contracts more frequently than hospitals in other areas and that hospitals in

TABLE 3
AVERAGE WAGE RATES, COMMUNITY HOSPITAL, LINEAR RESULTS

	1968 (1)	1967 (2)	1965 (3)	Pooled '65, '67, '68 (4)
Constant	2423.77	1755.97	2380.53	968.12
	(3.14)	(1.85)	(5.08)	(2.43)
Manufacturing wages	.21	.26	.12	.38
	(2.07)	(2.06)	(1.71)	(6.76)
Average bed size	−2.82	−5.14	−3.94	−2.32
	(1.11)	(1.77)	(1.97)	(1.50)
Hospital density	−7.58	−24.64	−23.00	−12.84
	(.24)	(.70)	(1.11)	(.70)
Net income ratio	−12.32	6.46	−23.95	−.47
	(.33)	(.21)	(1.45)	(.03)
Cost reimbursement	−234.25	163.96	−109.35	959.33
	(.47)	(.27)	(.37)	(5.05)
Unionization	−5.16	−9.72	.72	−9.41
	(.51)	(.89)	(.12)	(1.69)
Hospital labor law	80.82	371.95	128.78	169.85
	(.48)	(1.81)	(1.15)	(1.65)
T_{67}	—	—	—	—
T_{68}	—	—	—	—
Facilities	Inc.	Inc.	Inc.	Inc.
Regional dummies	—	—	—	—
$\bar{R}^2$	.72	.56	.84	.73
R^2	.85	.78	.92	.78

Note: t-scores in parentheses. Inc. = included.

areas that are highly unionized are more likely to have contracts than hospitals in other areas [21]. Two measures of the threat of unionization, therefore, are used: (1) the percent of nonagricultural employment which belongs to a union, and (2) a dummy variable which takes on a value of one in those states with laws requiring nongovernmental, nonprofit hospitals to recognize a collective bargaining unit when a majority of employees of a bargaining unit request recognition.[15]

It is also hypothesized that hospitals with higher profits may be willing to pass along these gains to employees. The ratio of net income to plant assets is used as a measure of ability to pay. The cost-reimbursement variable is the same as described in earlier sections.

In areas in which labor markets are slack or in which hospital employees are relatively more immobile because of a shortage of alternative employment opportunities, hospital wages may lag behind manufacturing wages.

---

15   States with such laws include Connecticut, Hawaii, Kansas, Michigan, Minnesota, Montana, New Jersey, New York, Oregon, and Wisconsin.

TABLE 3
(*Continued*)

Pooled '65, '67, '68 (5)	1968 (6)	1967 (7)	1965 (8)	Pooled '65, '67, '68 (9)	Pooled '65, '67, '68 (10)
1925.34	2672.16	2762.13	2297.08	1391.88	2235.62
(5.75)	(4.56)	(3.93)	(4.21)	(4.24)	(7.31)
.19	.23	.19	.22	.40	.22
(3.68)	(2.23)	(1.50)	(2.18)	(6.49)	(3.75)
−3.31	4.93	4.81	4.34	3.51	4.55
(2.69)	(3.59)	(3.07)	(3.02)	(3.94)	(5.83)
−16.19	15.85	17.76	10.95	11.45	14.41
(1.12)	(.72)	(.72)	(.53)	(.80)	(1.18)
−15.68	27.00	21.30	−14.67	20.90	3.46
(1.28)	(.77)	(.76)	(.73)	(1.37)	(.25)
−192.86	34.44	−256.93	−147.86	586.98	−157.30
(.86)	(.09)	(.55)	(.45)	(3.05)	(.74)
−4.33	.66	−1.41	1.05	−6.11	.33
(.97)	(.08)	(.16)	(.17)	(1.30)	(.08)
188.35	59.27	163.94	145.16	88.71	122.29
(2.31)	(.45)	(1.03)	(1.25)	(1.03)	(1.65)
450.75	—	—	—	—	356.61
(5.41)					(4.20)
766.49	—	—	—	—	641.77
(8.31)					(6.97)
Inc.	—	—	—	—	—
—	Inc.	Inc.	Inc.	Inc.	Inc.
.83	.72	.56	.72	.70	.78
.86	.78	.65	.78	.72	.80

To adjust for any regional differences in labor markets, regional dummy variables are also included.[16]

Multiple regression estimates of hospital wage rates are contained in Tables 2 and 3. Both linear and log functional forms are estimated. About 85 percent of the variation in hospital wage rates is explained by the regressions including time and facilities variables.

Again, the cost-reimbursement variables are insignificant in explaining hospital wages in the individual year results and in the pooled results when the time dummy variables are included, but significant in the pooled results when the time variables are omitted. It may be concluded, therefore, that hospital wage rates do not vary with the extensiveness of cost-reimbursement

---

16 Bureau of the Census region definitions are used: Northeast (Maine, New Hampshire, Vermont, Massachusetts, Rhode Island, Connecticut, New York, New Jersey, Pennsylvania), North Central (Ohio, Indiana, Illinois, Michigan, Wisconsin, Minnesota, Iowa, Missouri, North Dakota, South Dakota, Nebraska, Kansas), South (Delaware, Maryland, Virginia, West Virginia, North Carolina, South Carolina, Georgia, Florida, Kentucky, Tennessee, Alabama, Mississippi, Arkansas, Louisiana, Oklahoma, Texas), and West (Montana, Idaho, Wyoming, Colorado, New Mexico, Arizona, Utah, Nevada, Washington, Oregon, California).

plans, but an important time shift did occur. Several explanations of the time shift may be relevant: the coverage of hospital workers under minimum wage laws in 1967, a gradual adjustment of hospital wages to those of comparable occupations over time, and an announcement effect of Medicare. It is impossible to separate out these influences in the econometric test. There is some evidence, however, to indicate that hospital workers became more militant with the introduction of Medicare and demanded higher wage increases (see, for example, [6]). A shift in hospital wages as a direct consequence of Medicare is therefore plausible.

As expected, average wage rates of hospital employees are positively related to the average earnings of production workers in manufacturing industries and to the measure of skill mix (average bed size and specialized facilities). Part of the increase in hospital wages, therefore, reflects the overall rise in wage rates in all industries.

Evidence on the monopsony hypothesis is mixed. Wages are insignificantly related to hospital density when the facilities variables are included, but excluding specialized facilities leads to a significantly positive relationship. That is, wages are higher in areas with more hospitals, implying that collusive agreements among hospitals either do not exist or break down when there are a large number of hospitals competing for labor. Because of the high correlation between facilities and hospital density, it is difficult to isolate the importance of each issue. Overall explanation is slightly higher when specialized facilities are included.

Little evidence is found to support the contention that the threat of unionization, as measured by the degree of nonagricultural union activity, is significant in raising wages. The unionization variable is insignificant and usually negative. The hospital labor law dummy is somewhat more important in explaining hospital wages. It enters with a positive coefficient which is significant in some of the specifications. This hypothesis, however, can not be conclusively confirmed or rejected without better data on the extent of unionization within the hospital industry.

The ratio of net income to plant assets (or rate of return) was included in the linear estimates. In general, it entered with a negative, insignificant coefficient rather than positive as predicted. The hypothesis that hospitals pass along higher profits to employees, therefore, is not substantiated by these results.

VI. SUMMARY AND CONCLUSIONS

The primary purpose of this paper has been to analyze and test two cost-oriented theories of hospital inflation—the cost-reimbursement theory and the labor cost-push theory. A theoretical examination revealed that under either the profit-maximization or quantity-maximization hypotheses, hospitals will not have an incentive to increase costs unless the percentage of patients covered by the cost-plus reimbursement scheme exceeds about 95 percent (for a 5 percent cost-plus factor). At present, hospitals are unlikely to have cost-reimbursement patients in that range.

The empirical results lead to a rejection of the hypothesis that hospital costs increase with the extensiveness of cost reimbursement within the range observed. Hospitals in states in which cost reimbursement represented 88 percent of costs did not have higher costs, other things equal, than hospitals in states in which cost reimbursement represented 19 percent of costs. However, after adjusting for changes in utilization and rising wage rates, hospital average costs were significantly higher in the Medicare period than in the pre-Medicare period. Time effects such as changes in nonlabor costs, nature of the product provided, and technology may account for the shift in costs over time, but a shift as the direct consequence of the introduction of Medicare cannot be ruled out.

The growth of cost-reimbursement schemes was similarly not important in explaining hospital wage rates. Even though wages did not vary with the extent of cost reimbursement, wages were significantly higher in the Medicare period than in the pre-Medicare period after adjusting for other factors affecting wages. Time effects such as the gradual adjustment of hospital wages to those of comparable occupations or the minimum wage law applied to hospitals may explain the shift. Increased demands of hospital employees as a direct consequence of the introduction of Medicare may also have been a factor.

REFERENCES

1. Ralph E. Berry, Jr. "Product Heterogeneity and Hospital Cost Analysis." *Inquiry* (March 1970): 67–75.
2. W. John Carr and Paul J. Feldstein. "The Relationship of Cost to Hospital Size." *Inquiry* 4 (June 1967): 45–65.
3. Harold A. Cohen. "Variations in Cost Among Hospitals of Different Sizes." *Southern Economic Journal* 33 (Jan. 1967): 355–66.
4. Karen Davis. "Economic Theories of Behavior in Non-profit Private Hospitals." *Economic and Business Bulletin* 24 (Winter 1972).
5. ———. *Net Income of Hospitals: 1961–1969.* Washington: Social Security Administration, 1970.
6. T. L. Ehrich. "Union on the Rise: A Tough Local Presses National Bid to Organize Low-Paid Hospital Help." *Wall Street Journal*, March 3, 1970, p. 1.
7. Martin S. Feldstein. *Economic Analysis for Health Service Efficiency.* Amsterdam: North Holland Publishing Co., 1967.
8. ———. "Hospital Cost: A Study of Nonprofit Price Dynamics." *American Economic Review* 61 (Dec. 1971): 853–72.
9. ———. *The Rising Cost of Hospital Care.* Washington: Information Resources Press, 1971.
10. *Hospitals, Guide Issue* (Aug. 1, year).
11. Mary Lee Ingbar and Lester D. Taylor. *Hospital Costs in Massachusetts.* Cambridge, Mass.: Harvard University Press, 1968.
12. Herbert E. Klarman. "Approaches to Moderating the Increases in Medical Care Costs." *Medical Care* 7:3 (1969): 175–90.
13. ———. "Comment" on Pauly and Drake. In *Empirical Studies in Health Economics,* ed. Herbert E. Klarman. Baltimore: Johns Hopkins Press, 1970.
14. ———. "Policy Alternatives for Controlling Health Services Expenditures." Paper delivered at the annual meeting, American Economic Association, Dec. 28, 1970.

15. ———. "Reimbursing the Hospital: The Difference the Third Party Makes." *Journal of Risk and Insurance* 36 (Dec. 1969).

16. Judith R. Lave and Lester B. Lave. "Economic Analysis for Health Service Efficiency: A Review Article." *Applied Economics* 1 (1970): 293–305.

17. ———. "Estimated Cost Functions for Pennsylvania Hospitals." *Inquiry* 7 (June 1970): 3–14.

18. ———. "Hospital Cost Functions." *American Economic Review* 60 (June 1970): 379–95.

19. Harvey Leibenstein. "Allocative Efficiency vs. X-Efficiency." *American Economic Review* 56 (June 1966): 392–415.

20. Judith Mann and Donald Yett. "The Analysis of Hospital Costs." *Journal of Business* 41 (April 1968): 191–202.

21. J. D. Miller and S. M. Shortell. "Hospital Unionization: A Study of the Trends." *Hospitals* 43 (Aug. 16, 1969): 67–73.

22. Marc Nerlove. *Estimation and Identification of Cobb-Douglas Production Functions.* Chicago: Rand-McNally, 1965.

23. Mark V. Pauly and David F. Drake. "The Effect of Third-Party Methods of Reimbursement on Hospital Performance." In *Empirical Studies in Health Economics,* ed. Herbert E. Klarman. Baltimore: Johns Hopkins Press, 1970.

24. David S. Salkever. "A Micro-Econometric Study of Hospital Cost Inflation." *Journal of Political Economy* 80 (Nov.-Dec. 1972): 1144–66.

25. George Stigler. "A Theory of Oligopoly." *Journal of Political Economy* (Feb. 1964).

26. U.S. Department of Health, Education, and Welfare. *A Report to the President on Medical Care Prices.* Washington: 1967.

27. Wayne Vroman. "Linear Combinations in Regression Analysis." Mimeo, 1971.

28. Donald E. Yett. "Causes and Consequences of Salary Differentials in Nursing." *Inquiry* 7 (March 1970).

29. ———. "The Chronic 'Shortage' of Nurses: A Public Policy Dilemma." In *Empirical Studies in Health Economics,* ed. Herbert E. Klarman. Baltimore: Johns Hopkins Press, 1970.

APPENDIX: DEFINITION OF VARIABLES AND DATA SOURCES

TE/Adm Total expenses per admission in community hospitals. All hospital data for 1965, 1967, and 1968 are taken from [10], Aug. 1, 1966, Aug. 1, 1968, and Aug. 1, 1969.

Adm/B Admissions per bed or case-flow.

B Average bed size of community hospitals in the state.

w Annual earnings of hospital employees divided by number of equivalent full-time personnel.

MS Mean length of stay in community hospitals.

BC Blue Cross–Blue Shield hospital benefit claims expense divided by total expenses for states in which Blue Cross reimburses on the basis of costs; equals zero in states in which Blue Cross reimburses on the basis of charges. In plans in which hospital and medical/surgical claims expenses were combined, the hospital portion was assumed to be the same as in those plans separating the two types of claims expense. It was necessary to make this adjustment in 12 states. Blue Cross–Blue Shield data are taken from Louis S. Reed and Kathleen

Myers, "Enrollment and Finances of Blue Cross and Blue Shield Plans, 1965," *Research and Statistics Note 12* (Oct. 11, 1966), Social Security Administration; Louis S. Reed and Willine Carr, "Enrollment and Finances of Blue Cross and Blue Shield, 1967," *Research and Statistics Note 20*, Social Security Administration; and Louis S. Reed, Willine Carr, and Maureen Dwyer, "Enrollment and Finances of Blue Cross and Blue Shield Plans, 1968," *Research and Statistics Note 22* (Dec. 8, 1969), Social Security Administration. Method of reimbursement is taken from Blue Cross Association, "Hospital Reimbursement Methods of Blue Cross Plans," in *Third-Party Reimbursement for Hospitals* (Bloomington: Indiana University, 1965).

Med   Medicare reimbursement in community hospitals divided by total hospital expenses. Reimbursement data are based on claims approved in calendar year 1967 and 1968 and come from Louise B. Russell, "Hospital Insurance Claims and Reimbursement by Type of Service and by State, 1967 and 1968," *Research and Statistics Note 21* (Oct. 16, 1970), Social Security Administration.

Mcaid   Public assistance and general assistance payments for inpatient hospital care (primarily Medicaid payments) divided by total hospital expenses. Vendor payment data are from *Public Assistance: Vendor Payment for Medical Care by Type of Service, Calendar Year Ended December 31, 1968, and December 31, 1967*, NCSS Report B-2 (CY 68,67), Washington: U.S. Department of Health, Education, and Welfare.

CR $BC + Med + Mcaid$; sum of Blue Cross–Blue Shield hospital claims in states which reimburse on the basis of cost plus Medicare and Medicaid reimbursement divided by hospital expenses.

F_1 to F_{16} Percent of community hospitals with the specialized facilities listed in footnote 8. Data are for all community hospitals which are eligible Medicare providers and come from unpublished records of the Social Security Administration.

w_m Average weekly earnings of production workers in manufacturing industries times 52. Data are from *Statistical Abstract of the United States, 1970*, Table 344.

HD   Hospitals per square mile or hospital density. Area data are drawn from *Statistical Abstract of the United States, 1968*, Table 24.

NI/PA   Net income (revenue minus operating expenses) divided by plant assets in community hospitals.

Union   Percent of nonagricultural employees who are union members. Data for 1968, 1966, and 1964 are from *Statistical Abstract of the United States, 1970*, Table 356, and *Statistical Abstract . . . , 1968*, Table 347.

Labor Law   Dummy variable having a value of one for states with nonprofit hospital labor laws requiring recognition of a collective bargaining unit upon majority request of the employees. Data are from [21].

Region   Dummy variable based on Bureau of the Census region definitions; for definitions, see footnote 16.

T_{67} Time dummy taking on a value of one in 1967

T_{68} Time dummy taking on a value of one in 1968.

19. Inflation and Health Insurance

JOSEPH P. NEWHOUSE

Introduction and Summary

Health insurance and inflation in the medical care sector have long been recognized to be interrelated, although precise measurement of the links between them is not yet available. Since a review article of this area is beyond the scope of this paper, the focus will instead be on certain specific, important issues.

The first issue is the effect of a rise in the relative price of medical care on the demand for health insurance. I believe that the effect of such inflation on demand for insurance is highly uncertain at the present time; there certainly appears to be no compelling empirical evidence that it will be large. Thus, a vicious-circle hypothesis of inflation leading to a higher demand for insurance, which leads in turn to more inflation, can neither be strongly supported nor refuted by the data we now have.

The second issue concerns the effects of medical insurance upon inflation. Additional insurance raises the demand for care; if supply is not perfectly elastic, the relative price will increase. As a result, providers of medical care will be enriched at the expense of the rest of the population. Such enrichment is presumably deemed bad by policy makers; if it were not, there would be much less reason for concern about inflation in this sector.

A third issue relates to a further distributional effect that may occur as insurance approaches full coverage for most of the population. In this case, providers and third-party payers determine the "terms of trade" between the medical care sector and other sectors. In such a situation, the medical care sector may well be able to turn the "terms of trade" in its favor. Recent experience in the United

States hospital sector, as in the Canadian, corroborates this contention. In other words, the medical care sector, if left to its own devices, is likely to expand its control over resources beyond the point that policy makers—ultimately the public—deem desirable. Although, by now, this analysis seems fairly commonplace, present policy with respect to the hospital sector ignores it for the most part. It is also ignored in today's tax policy on insurance premiums.

I want to outline, briefly, three possible policy alternatives for health financing. They are not mutually exclusive, but all hold promise of reducing inflation in medical care. The first two attempt to move back toward the marketplace; the third puts something in its place.

The first alternative is, in essence, maximum liability health insurance. Although variants are possible, essentially there is an annual deductible that is related to income (say 10 percent of annual income or $1,000, whichever is less), and the tax subsidy of insurance premiums is ended. The deductible could be reduced or eliminated for the poor and near poor. Under these arrangements the bulk of the population would choose to self-insure expenditures below the deductible and would not receive insurance benefits for most of their care; thus, the market would essentially regulate the allocation of resources and control inflation.

A second alternative emphasizes the development of health maintenance organizations (HMOs). The consumer is free to choose an HMO and pays the marginal cost for his choice. As a result, the market is retained; providers have incentives to tailor the resource mix to the desires of consumers, to be efficient, and to keep prices down.

A third alternative employs direct controls, such as a fixed budget for medical care. Certificate-of-need legislation and price controls are in the spirit of this alternative. Clearly, direct controls can limit the share of society's resources in medical care.

Pursuing different strategies for different sectors is possible. For example, one might choose to insure hospital services completely and apply direct controls, while retaining the market (by means of a moderate deductible) for ambulatory care.

The preferred alternative depends on answers to very basic questions about which it is difficult to generate scientific evidence. For example, how informed is the consumer relative to the public regulator? What are the consequences of differences in use that arise when the provider is paid by different mechanisms? Knowledgeable persons differ in their answers to these questions. What should be emphasized, however, is that continuing the present trend toward full or nearly full insurance coverage in the context of a nearly unregulated fee-for-service delivery system is likely to produce continued inflation in medical care. Given that such inflation does not appear to be politically acceptable, present institutional arrangements do not appear viable in the long run.

The Effect of Inflation on the Demand for Insurance

Phelps (1973) has derived a theory of demand for insurance. He shows in a simple but plausible model that the amount of insurance demanded may increase or decrease as the relative price of medical services rises. The intuitive reasons for this are that as the price of medical services rises, the consumer bears greater risk and therefore may want more insurance; on the other hand, the insurance is more expensive, and this tends to deter purchase.

Empirical measurement of the relationship between demand for insurance and medical prices has shown mixed results. The strongest support for a positive relationship (that is, quantity demanded increasing with price) has been presented by Feldstein (1973), who used a time series of cross-sectional state data from 1959 to 1965. However, Frech (forthcoming), using data similar to those used by Feldstein, obtained a negative relationship between medical prices and quantity of insurance demanded. Phelps (1973) has investigated the sign of the relationship with both time series and cross-sectional data. In Phelps's time-series data, the sign is positive, but the estimated elasticities range from near zero to near one. In 1963 cross-sectional data (a national probability sample), Phelps found a strong and positive relationship when the variables were entered in linear form; the elasticities ranged from 0.8 to 1.8. When the same variables were entered in logarithmic form, the estimated elasticities were essentially zero.

Whatever one's a priori notions were, a review of this evidence is unlikely to change them a great deal. My own guess is that more insurance will be demanded as medical prices rise, but that the elasticity will be low. In this case, the feedback loop between insurance and price rises and back to insurance is quickly dampened. In any event, a vicious-circle hypothesis that no equilibrium may be possible in the market for insurance short of full coverage (Newhouse and Taylor, 1971; Feldstein, 1971, 1973) is neither strongly supported nor refuted on the basis of existing evidence.

A skeptic may point out that the hospital sector has approached full coverage and that this does appear consistent with the vicious-circle hypothesis. There are other explanations for this phenomenon, however, such as the tax treatment of insurance premiums, discussed below.

The Effect of Insurance on Inflation

The story here is a familiar one, though no less important for its familiarity. Medical insurance can raise prices through two mechanisms. First, subsidizing medical care expenditures raises demand for medical services (Newhouse, Phelps, and Schwartz, 1974). This demand, operating against a less than perfectly elastic supply curve, raises the price of medical care services. As a result of the rise in price, providers' incomes will increase (inframarginal providers will increase their rents).

Second, there may be a "terms of trade" effect. As insurance approaches full or nearly full coverage, the price per unit of service is determined in a transaction between the provider and an intermediary. The intermediary does not have the same incentive as the consumer to substitute away from the good whose price rises and thereby deter the price rise. To the intermediary, increased medical prices reflect themselves in increased premiums (or taxes), but because of risk aversion, the consumer may continue to purchase insurance. In any event, the direct link, found in a usual market, between the quantity of services supplied and the determination of price is broken. In this situation, it may well be that the provider can obtain prices for services that exceed those a consumer would be willing to pay, were he paying them directly (Klarman, 1969, 1974). Thus, once most bills are paid by third parties, there is not only a "one-shot" increase in price stemming from the increase in demand, but there may also be a steady increase in the price of services.

The factors that determine an equilibrium price, given full coverage and a private market, are not clear. One is tempted to invoke the threat of direct price controls through the political process as a deterrent to further price increases, but because the actions of any one institution or provider have only a negligible effect on the overall share of resources in medical care, this explanation is not very convincing. Perhaps the demand for private insurance begins to fall after premiums rise above a certain level. In a public program, there is presumably resistance to higher prices because of the need for tax increases; in this case health becomes no different from education, fire, or police services from the point of view of determining price.

A price rise due to increase in demand will further redistribute income toward providers. (Refer to Table 1.) The assumption is that public policy is seeking to mitigate or eliminate this redistribution when it concerns itself with inflation in medical care. It has been argued that price rises in medical care are "special" and distinct from other price rises, because medical care is a necessity. But analysis shows that whether a good is a luxury or a necessity has little to do with the consequences of a rise in its price for consumer welfare (Newhouse, 1972).

The Medicare-Medicaid legislation is often used as an example (or proof, depending on the biases of the writer) of the effect of insurance on inflation. It is less well appreciated that the change in insurance that this legislation introduced was not large, although the effects were obviously considerable. The change in demand for hospital services (where inflation has been most striking) caused by Medicare-Medicaid was probably on the order of 10 percent. This

TABLE 1   Percentage of Hospital Bills Paid by Third Parties and Expenditure Rate Increases in Selected Years

Year	Percentage of Bill Paid by Third Parties (Fiscal Year)	Percentage Change in Hospital Expense per Adjusted Patient Day	Percentage Change in Hospital Expense per Admission
1960	81.4	7.5[a]	7.5[a]
1965	81.5	7.9	8.7
1966	81.6	7.6	8.6
1967	87.7	13.3	21.2
1968	89.3	12.8	15.2
1969	89.7	15.2	14.4
1970	86.8	14.7	13.1
1971	88.6	13.2	10.6
1972	90.9	13.4	10.4
1973	90.1	9.2[b]	7.4[b]

[a] Data available only for 1963–1965.

[b] The 9.2 and 7.4 values are not strictly comparable to the other figures, because they are based on data in the "Monthly Statistical Report, October 1974," Social Security Administration, Office of Research and Statistics, Division of Health Insurance Studies. This publication contains figures for the 1970–1972 period that are slightly different from those in the *Social Security Bulletin* (1973, p. 37).

Source: Percentage of bill paid by third parties from Cooper et al. (1974), Table 7, and percentage change in hospital expense calculated from Social Security Administration (1973), p. 37.

figure is calculated in a similar way to the 10-to-15 percent estimated increase in demand for ambulatory services that the Medicare-Medicaid programs caused (Newhouse, Phelps, and Schwartz, 1974, Appendix D). Because insurance for hospital services among the aged before Medicare was more common than insurance for ambulatory services, the overall change in demand for hospital services was almost surely less than that for ambulatory services.

Medicare-Medicaid also did not suddenly cause the market for hospital services to become dominated by third parties; this had been true for some time. Table 1 shows the percentage of hospital bills paid by third parties in various years, as well as increases in expenditure per patient day and per admission. The percentage of hospital expenditures not paid by third parties is not the same as the "average" co-insurance rate in the population because elasticity of demand is not zero, so that those with more insurance incur more expenditures. Nevertheless, for our purposes the measure is adequate; it seems unlikely that a "true" average co-insurance rate in the population changed by a much larger amount.

Thus, the introduction of Medicare-Medicaid in (fiscal) 1967 appears to have raised the percentage of expenditures paid by third parties by only 6 percentage points or so. So, in a rough sense, a rise of 10 percent in demand, and a rise from 80 to 90 percent in the portion of the bill paid by third parties, have led to double-digit inflation in United States hospitals for much of the past decade.

Alternative Policy Directions

Three directions for health financing policy are considered which could substantially reduce, if not eliminate, the rise in the relative price of medical services. Comparison of these alternatives will be along several dimensions, including: (1) access to medical care by the poor, or an equity dimension; (2) consumer sovereignty, or an economic efficiency dimension; (3) incentives of providers to produce efficiently, or a technical efficiency dimension. These three dimensions roughly correspond to the three central problems of economic organizations: "For whom? What? How?"

The alternatives to be compared are:

1. Maximum liability health insurance (MLHI), together with elimination of the tax subsidy of private insurance. Families would be given an insurance policy covering all insurance expenditures above 10 percent of their income or $1,000, whichever was less. This deductible could be reduced or eliminated for the poor and near poor. The name is from Elliot Richardson's *Mega Proposal* for the Department of Health, Education and Welfare.

2. Development of health maintenance organizations (HMOs), with several HMOs serving one area. Any remaining legal barriers to HMOs would be removed. So long as the fee-for-service system was large, those electing care in HMOs would receive a voucher equal in value to the amount provided by the national health insurance plan in the fee-for-service system. (Thus, public policy would be neutral toward type of delivery system.) If, ultimately, the delivery system consisted principally of HMOs, the government could give a voucher of sufficient value to purchase care at the average-priced HMO. If the consumer chose an HMO with a less than average price, he would receive the difference in cash. A modification of this arrangement that would make it applicable only to hospitals is also possible (see Newhouse and Taylor, 1971; Kaplan and Lave, 1971). This general thrust has been advocated most predominantly by Paul Ellwood and Walter McClure of InterStudy.

3. Public sector control of resource allocation in medical care, together with full or nearly full insurance coverage. This is the

direction taken by the Health Security Act; in principle, the insurance coverage may be public or private.

The first two alternatives attempt to control inflation by reinstituting the market for the bulk of medical care services. In such an environment, individuals would be motivated to seek efficient providers, and providers would be motivated to provide the style of care that consumers were willing to pay for. The third alternative attempts to eliminate inflation by direct control.

Different strategies could be used for different sectors. For example, the third strategy could be followed with regard to hospitals, while the first could be followed for other sectors of medical care. This would permit a substantial lowering of the health insurance deductible relative to the first alternative, without stimulating demand (from 10 percent of annual income to about $150 per person per year; again the poor could be exempted).

The notion that MLHI would bring into existence a market is challenged by some who believe that most consumers would merely purchase supplementary insurance, so that they would still not face an out-of-pocket price for medical care. Half of the Medicare beneficiaries have supplemented their Medicare insurance. However, supplementation of MLHI should be considerably less frequent than supplementation of Medicare because (a) the tax subsidy could be eliminated and (b) Medicare has upper limits, so that part of the demand for supplementary insurance is for catastrophic insurance.

Supplementary insurance is currently attractive because of tax subsidies. Employer-paid premiums are not taxable income, and half of individually paid premiums are deductible. Feldstein and Allison (1974) estimate that the tax subsidy to health insurance purchases is, on average, greater than the loading charge. If the tax subsidy for supplementary insurance were eliminated, there would be a substantial increase in loading fees (on the order of 15 percentage points) (Mitchell and Phelps, forthcoming). Other data suggest that demand for insurance is considerably reduced by increases in loading charges (Phelps, 1973). Thus tax reform probably would mean that most consumers would not supplement their insurance coverage. It might be that consumers would not supplement their coverage even if there were no change in tax policy, because the true cost of insuring the first dollars of expenditure might not be apparent to them.

The second strategy—HMO development—can also be challenged as not being practical in the short run. But it is important to realize that even gradual expansion of HMOs would increase competition between them and the fee-for-service system, with resulting beneficial effects on inflation. For this reason the MLHI and

HMO strategies are complementary, provided the government pays HMO enrollees the actuarial value of MLHI (plus an administrative allowance), so that HMOs can compete with the fee-for-service system on an equal basis.

Direct controls can clearly control *expenditures,* although whether they can control *inflation* is less obvious. The assumption is that given a fixed budget, supply remains relatively unchanged, so that price per unit of service is also controlled. It could be argued, however, that providers will reduce quality, just as the size of the candy bar may shrink even if its price remains a dime. For now, I will accept the premise that direct controls over expenditure can control inflation, but I will return to this issue in discussing incentives of providers to produce efficiently.

Evaluation of the Alternatives

What are the consequences of these alternatives for equity and efficiency? Access of the poor can be made relatively favorable under any of the three alternatives. If the deductible under MLHI is reduced or eliminated for the poor, their access may be greatest of all under it, because middle and upper classes will pay a substantial amount. Under the HMO alternative, there will be no financial barrier to the average-priced HMO, although there will be to "fancy" HMOs. This raises the specter of several qualities of care, but unless higher income groups are constrained from spending more, such an outcome is inevitable under virtually any institutional arrangement. Clearly there is no financial barrier under the third alternative; thus, the alternatives do not differ very much along this dimension.

By contrast, the alternatives differ substantially in consumer sovereignty. Because the first two alternatives essentially retain a market, a case can be made that consumer preferences dictate the overall amount of resources devoted to medical care, as well as the particular resource mix within medical care. The third alternative starts from the premise that the consumer is uninformed about medical care, and that the physician does not function effectively as his agent. It further assumes that the allocation of resources determined by the regulator better approximates the allocation found in a market of fully informed consumers than does the existing market. Of course, the regulator does not operate independently of consumer preferences because regulation takes place in the context of the political process. Nonetheless, the relationship between the (uninformed) consumer's preferences and resource allocation is clearly greater under the first two alternatives than under the third. Whether this is good or bad cannot be ultimately resolved by scientific evidence, because the standard to which an appeal is made, the outcome in a market of perfectly informed consumers, is essentially unobservable.

Those who wish to argue that the consumer should be permitted to make his own choices could note that insofar as the marginal (or last) unit of medical care produces principally qualitative benefits, such as alleviation of anxiety, consumer choice is probably desirable; the consumer is presumably well informed about his willingness to pay to relieve his anxieties. They could also cite the study by Bunker and Brown (1974), comparing the rates for surgeries performed among other professional groups. Physicians are, by assumption, informed consumers; yet surgery rates for physician-patients were as high or higher than those for other professional groups, contrary to the conventional belief that surgery rates in the United States are inflated by consumer ignorance and the incentives of the fee-for-service system. On the other hand, those who favor central control of resources might deny that the marginal unit of medical care produces principally qualitative benefits.

Insofar as medical care supply generates its own demand, a strong case can be made for suspension of consumer sovereignty. That is, if more hospital beds or more physicians lead to manipulation of the consumer and the creation of artificial demand, the normative significance of consumer demands diminishes sharply. Because of the importance of the "supply-creates-its-own-demand" argument to the issue of centralized resource allocation, further consideration is warranted.

As is well known, the association between the supply of beds and use was first discussed by Roemer and Shain (1959), who postulated that if more beds were built, they would be used. In its simplest form, this empirical association appeared to support the notion that supply created its own demand. Similar associations have been found between use and physician supply (see, for example, Lewis, 1969).

Rosenthal (1964) showed why the association between use and supply could not support the conclusion that supply created its own demand. He observed that because demand for hospital beds was stochastic (that is, some days or seasons are busier than others), supply and use would be positively associated, holding the mean level of demand constant. For example, an area with many beds would have fewer periods in which demand exceeded capacity. Thus, a positive association between beds and use would exist even if supply did *not* create its own demand. Further, there is an identification problem—one cannot tell from the positive association between use and bed supply whether more beds are built where demand is high or conversely. Finally, Rosenthal observed that occupancy rates vary across states, which is not consistent with a simple supply-creates-its-own-demand hypothesis. According to that hypothesis, areas with low occupancy rates ought to have manipulated the demand so that it was kept at a high level. Also, occupancy rates have tended to decrease over time, and one now frequently hears accounts of a hospital bed "surplus," contrary to the "supply-creates-its-own-demand" argument.

The next major contribution to the hospital bed supply-and-demand controversy was that of Feldstein (1968), who analyzed data from the British National Health Service. At the time of Feldstein's study, there had been no beds built in England for about twenty-five years, so he reasonably assumed that current demand was independent of current supply. His data showed approximately a linear relationship between the bed supply and use (across various regions). Feldstein concluded that demand was dependent upon supply and that "Rosenthal's method is inappropriate [because] it seeks to plan supply with reference to an assumed exogenous demand." The writings I have seen since Feldstein's appear to accept his results as conclusive. (See also Evans, 1974, and the comments following his paper by Kehrer.)

In my view Feldstein is drawing the wrong inference from the observation that no beds had been built in twenty-five years. It is probable, with rising income, education, and technological change in medical care, that the demand for hospital services has trended upward over time. In this case, given no new construction of beds, there was likely to have been considerable excess demand for hospital beds in all areas. Accounts of queues for elective surgery support the assumption of general excess demand of the National Health Service (Chant et al., 1972; Todd, 1973). If there was general excess demand, Feldstein's results can tell us nothing about the supply-creates-its-own-demand argument. Rather, his finding shows only that less of the excess demand had to be rationed in areas with greater numbers of beds. Put another way, if there is excess demand, supply "creates" its own use—but not necessarily its own demand.

Because it cannot be established that demand depends on supply, the argument for direct controls and the suspension of consumer sovereignty should not proceed from the basis that supply creates its own demand, but should center on the question of whether the outcomes, when supply responds to the demand of uninformed consumers, are further from or closer to an optimum than when supply responds to the regulator. Unfortunately, there is little evidence to bring to bear on this question.

Before we leave the argument over consumer sovereignty, the effect of HMOs on the consumers' ignorance merits discussion. Some advocates of HMOs believe that the consumer will find it easier to gather information about the capabilities of a few HMOs than about a much larger number of nonaffiliated practitioners. While this argument has a certain plausibility, a more careful analysis leaves it somewhat less than established. The major problem has to do with the consumer's ability to evaluate physicians within the HMO. Even with a *Consumer Reports* type of evaluation of the average quality of the HMO, the consumer is not helped in evaluating a particular physician, unless the evaluation is specific to individual practitioners. And, if the evaluation is that specific, there is no information economy in an HMO. Thus, the argument has to be that information on *average* quality in the HMO is economical to provide, presumably through a sampling from the HMO physician roster, and the consumer will choose his HMO on the basis of average quality. The HMO will, therefore, have incentives to provide appropriate care. A case can be made that all of these assumptions are reasonable, although they are by no means certain.

Considering the incentives of providers to produce efficiently, again, the arguments are well known. Providers paid on a fee-for-service basis have an incentive to deliver more service than providers who are salaried (or paid on a capitation basis); in fact, fee-for-service providers actually do deliver more hospital services. As a result, under MLHI and a fee-for-service system (the first alternative), one might expect more hospital services delivered than if HMOs were developed (the second alternative). Whether this difference is good or bad is open to question. Except for arguments based on consumer ignorance, whether or not the consumer is permitted a nonsubsidized choice of either delivery system has no important policy significance, because the consumer who chose the fee-for-service system would pay more.

The implications for services supplied under the third alternative, direct controls, is unclear. There is no tradition in the United States of strongly enforced controls that are expected to last for an indefinite time. (Phase IV was not expected to last very long.) The closest analogue of direct controls appears to be certificate-of-need legislation, but there has been no evaluation of this legislation.

What might one expect? On a theoretical basis, there is a question as to whether price can be lowered without affecting supply (that is, whether controls are keeping down provider rents or whether providers are simply being shifted down a supply curve). There is a further question of whether the entire control process is ineffective and nothing is affected. If one believes that prices are artificially high (namely, that substantial rents exist because of lack of competition or entry restriction), price controls need not affect provider behavior. (They will not so long as the rent is never more than that appropriated by direct price controls. If the rent is taken in the form of inflated input costs, controls over inputs or total costs are necessary as well.) The judgment must be made that controls are preferable to changing the institutions that are generating the artificially high prices (rents), taking into account the costs of generating the information and the possibility of error.

If the controls go far enough (that is, do more than appropriate rents), providers will presumably shift down their supply curves and fewer services will be supplied. If one believes that too many of the "wrong" kind of services are being supplied, this is a good thing, but this leads us back to the consumer-sovereignty set of arguments.

In the case of physicians, it is possible that a backward-bending supply curve of hours exists. Even if this is the case (and the empirical evidence is far from conclusive), it seems probable that the supply curve of ambulatory medical services is positively sloped (through introduction of paramedical personnel, expansion of emergency rooms, expansion of the physician stock, and so forth, as prices rise).

A case can be made that controls (given the present delivery system) will ultimately be ineffective or perverse. There are large numbers of providers (both hospitals and physicians) in the health care sector producing certain intangible services. As a result it is difficult for the regulator to obtain information. In the short run, providers may be able to circumvent the intent of the regulations by billing for services that were not previously billed for or by creating new services. In the long run, there are serious questions about whether the providers will "capture" the regulators and whether regulation will retard innovation and technological change. Experience with price regulation in other sectors is not encouraging. In natural monopolies, such as electric power, regulation appears to have little effect; in oligopolistic or competitive industries, such as airline services, regulation appears to have raised prices (Jordan, 1972; Noll, 1974). Exactly where medical care falls on this spectrum is not clear, but in either case the outlook is not favorable. The Canadian medical care experience is that government-negotiated fee schedules for physicians and approval of budgets for hospitals do not preclude inflation (Evans, forthcoming); indeed, the Canadian experience in medical care inflation is quite similar to ours.

Fixing an annual budget, as in the United Kingdom, can be effective in controlling expenditure, but what will happen to supply if this were done in the United States is open to question, as pointed out above.

Conclusions

All three of the policy alternatives hold some promise of reducing inflation, but none can be guaranteed to accomplish it. Under the first alternative, consumers may purchase supplementary insurance, so that the market will not exist. The second alternative, on a large enough scale, simply may not be feasible in the short run, because HMO development may not be that rapid. And direct controls may not be very effective, or may produce undesirable side effects, because of the difficulty of obtaining information.

In spite of the uncertainties, the possibilities for reducing inflation afforded by these three alternatives should be compared with those of the present trend toward full insurance coverage in the context of an essentially unregulated fee-for-service system. Public policy has played a significant role in encouraging this trend through its tax subsidy of insurance premiums, while at the same time attempting to minimize direct intervention in the delivery system. It seems that the probability of substantial, continuing inflation is higher under present policies than under any of the three alternatives.

20. Changes in the Costs of Treatment of Selected Illnesses

ANNE SCITOVSKY AND NELDA McCALL

Reprinted from *NCHSR Research Digest* DHEW Publication No. (HRA) 77-3161, 1-36.

INTRODUCTION

BACKGROUND AND PURPOSE OF THE STUDY

In the mid-1960's, we conducted a study of changes in the costs of treatment of selected illnesses between 1951 and 1964.[1] The purpose of the study was twofold. First, we wanted to explore the feasibility of a new way of constructing a medical care price index, proposed by Anne Scitovsky in an earlier paper.[2] The proposed index would be based on costs of treatment of specific illnesses rather than on the prices of the various medical care services which the Bureau of Labor Statistics (BLS) uses in constructing the medical care component of the Consumer Price Index (CPI). Second, if the method was feasible, we wanted to compare our data on changes in medical care costs with those compiled by the medical care component of the CPI during this 13-year period.

To summarize briefly the results of this earlier study,[3] we found that, by and large, the cost-of-illness approach was feasible. This method of constructing a medical care price index, however, is much more costly than the method used by the BLS. We therefore recommended it not as a substitute for the present index but as additional index to be prepared every few years for comparison with and evaluation of the present index. The BLS has at various times expressed an interest in constructing an additional index of this kind but so far has not implemented it, concentrating instead on improving the present medical care component of the GPI.

In addition, we found that for the period 1951-1964, the medical care component of the CPI probably understates the rise in medical care costs. One of the principal reasons for this understatement was that the BLS measures changes in the customary fee for physician office visits. We found that in 1951, the *average* office fee was considerably below the customary fee, whereas by 1964 the gap between customary and average fees had narrowed considerably, with the average fee being only about 10% below the custom-

383

ary fee. Another reason for concluding that the BLS index probably understated the rise in medical care costs was the assumption by the BLS that fees for services that it did not price separately during this period (mainly fees for laboratory tests and x-rays in and out of the hospital, operating room charges, and anesthetists' fees) had risen by the average percent of all medical care items it priced. Our figures indicated that the fees for these services had risen at a considerably greater rate than the medical care price index for all services.

Finally, more or less as a by-product of the study, we gained some insight into the effects of changes in treatment on costs. The term "changes in treatment" is used to denote all changes in inputs of different medical services for a given diagnosis. These changes include the use of new techniques or new drugs, the substitution of specialists for non-specialists, increases or decreases in the use of specific services such as laboratory tests or days of hospital stay, the substitution of inpatient for outpatient treatment, or changes in the "mix" of services. Pricing 1951 treatment in 1964 prices, we found that in five of the eight conditions studied, costs rose more (some of them substantially more) than they would have risen if treatments had remained unchanged. In other words, the net effects of changes in treatment during the period 1951-1964 were largely cost-raising.

This paper discusses a follow-up of the earlier study, and compares the 1964 data with new data for 1971[4] for the same conditions covered by the original study. These are otitis media (middle ear infection) in children, acute appendicitis (subdivided in simple appendicitis and perforated appendicitis), maternity care, cancer of the breast, and forearm fractures in children (subdivided into cases requiring a cast only, cases requiring a closed reduction without a general anesthetic, and cases requiring a closed reduction with a general or regional anesthetic). In addition, the new study also includes pneumonia, duodenal ulcer, and myocardial infarction for the years 1964 and 1971.[5] For these latter conditions, data from the 1964 study could not be used at that time because no data from 1951 were available for comparison.[6]

The purpose of the present study is again twofold. First, to explore what light, if any, the data might shed on the BLS medical care price index for the period 1964-1971; and, second, to analyze in more detail the effects of changes in treatment on costs. Little information is available on this subject. With the constant rise in medical care costs in the past 20 years, this problem deserves more attention than it has received. Moreover, the subject is of particular importance at the present time because Professional Standards Review Organizations (PSROs) are being organized throughout the United States.

This paper will therefore be divided into two parts. Because of its timeliness, we begin with an analysis of our findings regarding the effects of changes in treatment on costs for both the 1951-1964 and the 1964-1971 periods (Part I). In Part I, we also discuss briefly the problem of quality change in the medical care sector. Part II consists of comments on the BLS medical care price index based on the findings of our 1964-1971 study.

With regard to data sources and methodology, in both studies the study population consisted of patients treated by physicians at the Palo Alto Medical Clinic (PAMC), a multi-specialty, largely fee-for-service group practice of about 140 physicians in Palo Alto, California.[7] The PAMC has its own laboratory, radiology, physiotherapy, and EKG departments. It does not operate its own hospital. Patients needing hospitalization are in almost all cases treated at the Stanford University Hospital. Accordingly, we obtained almost all the data on medical care inputs and costs from the medical and financial records of the PAMC and the Stanford Hospital. For data on disease-related medical care goods and services not rendered (and hence not billed) by either the PAMC or the Stanford University Hospital, the patients were contacted directly. Such information primarily covered expenses for drugs and prescriptions but also included some expenses for private nursing services, ambulance services, and medical supplies.

In our earlier study, we devised our own system for coding the various medical services used by PAMC physicians in the treatment of the conditions studied. While the PAMC had fee schedules in both periods (a rather short one in 1951, a more detailed one in 1964), it did not adopt the 1964 California Relative Value Studies (CRVS)[8] coding system until some time in 1965. At that time, the data collection for 1951 and 1964 was practically completed. In the new study, we used the 1969 edition of the CRVS coding system, which the PAMC began using in the latter part of 1970. To make the 1964 and 1971 data comparable, all 1964 data was recoded in terms of the 1969 CRVS system. Because of budgetary constraints, the 1951 data were not recorded.

PAMC fee schedules are not binding on PAMC physicians, who can and do depart from them, mainly by giving discounts or making adjustments in special cases. Judging by our data over the 20-year period, they did so considerably more frequently in 1951 than in 1964, and somewhat more frequently in 1964 than in 1971. For hospital services, as well as for drugs and prescriptions and other services not provided by either the PAMC or the Stanford Hospital, we used our own coding system in all three periods since the CRVS does not include such services.

For purposes of pricing, episodes of illness were defined as follows:

Otitis media and forearm fractures: from date of diagnosis until there were no further entries in the patient's medical record for the episode.
Appendicitis: from date patient first sought medical care for abdominal pain until there were no further entries in the patient's medical record for the episode.
Maternity care: from date patient first consulted a physician for possible pregnancy through the last post-partum visit. We included only normal pregnancies and excluded cases requiring a Caesarian section.
Cancer of the breast: from date patient first consulted a physician for a lump in her breast until six months after the mastectomy.
Pneumonia: up to three months, beginning with date of diagnosis.
Duodenal ulcer: six months beginning with date of diagnosis.
Myocardial infarction: three months, beginning with date of diagnosis. Patients who died before the end of the three-month period were excluded.

PART I

EFFECTS OF CHANGES
IN TREATMENT ON COSTS,
1951-1964 AND 1964-1971

Introduction

One of the factors that is considered to have contributed to the rapid rise in medical care expenditures over the past 20 or 25 years is a change in inputs of medical goods and services. Such a change in inputs may occur as a result of technological innovations such as new drugs, or new procedures such as renal dialysis, heart by-pass surgery and organ transplants. Alternatively, it may occur because there is a change in the use or in the "mix" of existing medical services. Examples of this latter type of change are the substitution of physician office visits for home visits, or of inpatient care for outpatient care, or of specialists for general practitioners, or a change in the number and/or type of diagnostic tests.

A number of economists have estimated the quantitative importance of various factors, including changes in inputs, that have resulted in the steep rise in medical care costs in recent decades. The most notable of these studies are by: Klarman and Rice on the increase in expenditures for dentists, physicians, and hospital services in the period 1929-1969;[1] Martin Feldstein on the rising cost of hospital care in the period 1950-1968;[2] and Fuchs and Kramer on the increase in expenditures for physicians' services in the period 1948-1968.[3]

All the above studies are based on national data. The present studies, based on changes in the costs of treatment of selected illnesses, are more specific but also more limited. They are more specific because, for the illnesses covered, it is possible to identify and quantify the exact changes in inputs of medical services that have occurred, such as the use of new techniques or changes in the number and type of diagnostic tests, the number of physician visits and the average length of hospital stay. Such a detailed analysis is not possible on the basis of currently available national data. The present studies are more limited, however, because they cover only a few illnesses and are based on data for patients of a single group of providers. In most instances they are also based on small numbers of cases. The findings should therefore be regarded as suggestive rather than conclusive. Nevertheless, the trends revealed in the findings appear to reflect general trends since, taken together, the various types of illnesses showed much the same changes.

Effects of Changes in Treatment on Costs, 1951-1964

Some of the effects of changes in treatment on costs for the conditions covered by our 1951-1964 study were discussed in a previous publication.[4] These are investigated in more detail here, mainly to show the continuity of major trends in the periods 1951-1964 and 1964-1971 for appendicitis (subdivided in simple and perforated cases),[5] and maternity care. The conditions covered by this earlier study, as mentioned above, are otitis media (children), cancer of the breast,[6] and forearm fractures in children (subdivided into cases requiring a cast only, cases requiring a closed reduction without a general anesthetic, and cases requiring a closed reduction with a general or regional anesthetic).

TABLE 1
Average costs of treatment of selected illnesses, 1951 and 1964;
and 1951 treatment in 1964 prices

	1951		1964		1951 treatment in 1964
	$	N	$	N	prices
Otitis media (children)	$ 10.83	96	$ 18.34	156	$ 22.31
Appendicitis					
Simple	341.13	99	591.51	89	571.21
Perforated	516.36	6	958.72	17	888.18
Maternity care[1]	291.13	52	502.92	100	505.80
Cancer of the breast[2]	739.39	21	1503.93	30	1295.06
Forearm fractures (children)					
Cast only	54.36	7	82.89	37	82.89
Closed reduction, no general anesthetic	65.67	3	121.76	25	89.30
Closed reduction, general or regional anesthetic[3]	80.35	5	365.33	23	167.93

[1] Exclusive of costs of outpatient drugs and prescriptions.

[2] Exclusive of costs of surgery performed as a procedure independent from the mastectomy, and of miscellaneous minor outpatient medical goods and services.

[3] The actual average cost obtained on the basis of the 1964 data was $331.85. However, when recoding 1964 data, we found that through a billing mistake on the part of the Stanford Hospital, most patients were not charged for the use of the operating room, although the reduction had clearly been performed there. The 1964 figure has been adjusted upward for this omission by using the 1964 operating room charge for the patients who were billed.

Table 1 and 2 summarize the findings of the earlier study. Table 1 shows average costs of treatment for the eight conditions in 1951 and 1964, and the average costs of 1951 treatment in 1964 prices. Table 2 shows the percentage increase in actual average costs, and the percentage increases due to pure price changes and due to *net* changes in inputs,[7] both for the whole 13-year period and as annual rates of change. The emphasis is on "net." In almost every instance, there were cost-raising and cost-saving changes in treatment. Thus the figures of 1951 treatment in 1964 prices, as well as the figures of "pure" changes in inputs, reflect the net effect of both types of changes.

As these tables indicate, most of the changes in treatment during the period 1951-1964 were, on balance, cost-raising. The one exception was

TABLE 2

Percentage change in average costs of treatment of selected
illnesses, 1951-64: Total change, change due to price
changes, and change due to net changes in inputs of
medical services

	Percentage change, 1951-1964			Annual rate of change		
	Total	Price	Inputs	Total	Price	Inputs
Otitis media (children)	69	106	(18)	4.1	5.7	(1.5)
Appendicitis						
Simple	73	67	4	4.3	4.0	0.3
Perforated	86	72	8	4.9	4.3	0.6
Maternity care[1]	73	74	(1)	4.3	4.4	(0.1)
Cancer of the breast[2]	103	75	16	5.6	4.4	1.2
Forearm fractures (children)						
Cast only	53	53	–	3.3	3.3	–
Closed reduction, no						
general anesthetic	85	36	36	4.8	2.4	2.4
Closed reduction, general						
or regional anesthetic[3]	355	109	117	12.4	5.8	6.1

[1] Exclusive of costs of outpatient drugs and prescriptions.

[2] Exclusive of costs of surgery performed as a procedure independent from the mastectomy, and of miscellaneous minor outpatient medical goods and services.

[3] The actual average cost obtained on the basis of the 1964 data was $331.85. However, when recoding 1964 data, we found that through a billing mistake on the part of the Stanford Hospital, most patients were not charged for the use of the operating room, although the reduction had clearly been performed there. The 1964 figure has been adjusted upward for this omission by using the 1964 operating room charge for the patients who were billed.

otitis media in children. The main explanation in this case was the shift from home visits to office visits. In 1951, one-third of all physician visits for this condition were home visits; by 1964, only three percent were home visits. Another, though minor, cost-saving factor was the change from parenterally administered drugs (penicillin injections) to orally administered antibiotics, which began to come on the market in the early 1950s.

In the case of one other condition, maternity care, changes in treatment were more or less neutral, cost-raising changes more or less offsetting cost-saving changes. Despite a decrease in the average length of hospitalization by almost one day (from 4.6 days in 1951 to 3.8 days in 1964), and despite an increase in the percentage of women delivered without a general anesthetic (from two percent in 1951 to 12 percent in 1964), the increase in the average number of laboratory tests per case (from 4.8 in 1951 to 11.5 in 1964) just about offset the cost-saving changes.

For conditions where changes in treatment were, on balance, cost-raising, the main factors that raised costs for both types of appendicitis were: increase in the number of laboratory tests per case (from 4.7 to 7.3 for simple appendicitis, from 5.3 to 14.5 for perforated appendicitis); an increase in the average number of postoperative intravenous solutions (from 0.1 to 2.4 for simple appendicitis, from 6.7 to 12.7 for perforated appendicitis); and the use of postoperative room, which was not available in 1951. The only cost-saving change, a minor one, was a shift in the hospital accommodation pattern from private and semi-private rooms to ward beds.

In the case of cancer of the breast,[8] the principal change in treatment that raised costs was the greatly increased use of radiotherapy. This increase took two forms: more patients received radiotherapy in 1964 (37 percent as against 13 percent in 1951); and patients receiving this type of treatment received almost twice as many treatments in 1964 as in 1951 (28.9 per case in 1964 as against 13.3 in 1951). As a result, the average number of radiotherapy treatments per case rose from 1.7 in 1951 to 11.0 in 1964. Additional factors that raised costs were an increase in the number of diagnostic x-rays per case (from 0.7 to 2.0); an increase in the average number of laboratory tests per case (from 5.9 to 14.8); and as in the case of appendicitis, the use of a postoperative room. The combined costs of these additional services outweighed considerably the substantial reduction in the average length of hospitalization by 2.5 days (from 12.7 days to 10.2 days).

This brings us to changes in the treatment of forearm fractures in children. In 1966, when analyzing the data of our 1951-1964 cost of illness study, we planned not to present the data on forearm fractures because of the very small number of cases available for 1951. However, a discussion with five PAMC orthopedists (three of whom were at the PAMC in 1951) changed our minds. They expressed the opinion that, despite the limitations of the data, the average cost figures for the three types of fractures were fairly good approximations of actual average costs. They also felt that the increases in average costs which we found seemed reasonable, considering the changes in treatment that had occurred. Accordingly, the findings were included in our report and are presented here again, with the reservation that they are to be regarded as rough estimates.

Two changes in treatment considerably raised the average costs of forearm fractures requiring a closed reduction.[9] One was the substitution of orthopedic surgeons for general surgeons. In 1951, over half of the cases studied were treated by general surgeons. By 1964, all cases were treated by orthopedic surgeons. The 1951 data showed that the average fee of an orthopedic surgeon was about 75 percent higher than that of a general surgeon for the same procedure. On the basis of this differential in fees, we estimated that about half the actual increase in the costs of treating forearm fractures requiring a closed reduction without a general anesthetic was due to the shift to orthopedic surgeons. In the case of forearm fractures requiring a closed reduction *with* a general anesthetic, there was an additional cost-raising change. While in 1951 some of these cases were still treated in the physician's office, in 1964 all such cases were treated in the hospital and required at least an overnight stay. This raised costs not only because of the additional hospital charges but also because, as seen in the 1951 figures, surgeons (general surgeons and orthopedists) and anesthetists charged more for services performed in the hospital than in the office. We estimated that over half of the increase in the cost of treatment of these cases was due to the combined effect of the increased use of orthopedic surgeons and of hospital care instead of office care.

In summary, we found that for the conditions covered, the period 1951-1964 was characterized predominantly by cost-raising changes, primarily increases in the number of diagnostic tests and therapeutic procedures per case. There was an increase in the use of specialists and a shift from outpatient to inpatient treatment. In almost all instances, these changes outweighed the main cost-saving change, which was the reduction in the average length of hospital.stay.

TABLE 3

Average costs of treatment of selected illnesses, 1964 and 1971,
and 1964 treatment in 1971 prices

	1964		1971		1964 treatment in 1971 prices
	$	N	$	N	$
Otitis media (children)	$ 18.34	156	$ 25.13	257	$ 24.18
Appendicitis					
Simple	591.51	89	1062.58	41	1040.02
Perforated	958.72	17	2062.17	11	1811.53
Maternity care[1]	502.92 [527.47]	100	786.32 [807.08]	154	852.87 [880.53]
Cancer of the breast[2]	1503.93 [1558.57]	30	2356.71 [2557.35]	35	2491.52 [2582.40]
Forearm fractures (children)					
Cast only	82.89	37	97.01	48	94.04
Closed reduction, no general anesthetic	121.76	25	245.79	20	199.32
Closed reduction, general or regional anesthetic[3]	365.33	23	521.92	18	573.61
Myocardial infarction	1448.98	28	3279.87	48	2461.08
Pneumonia (non-hospitalized)	75.04	71	84.98	183	98.88
Duodenal ulcer (non-hospitalized)	159.49	35	186.90	27	211.63

[1] The figures in brackets include costs of outpatient drugs and prescriptions, the others exclude such costs.

[2] The figures in brackets include the costs of surgery done as a procedure independent from the mastectomy, and of miscellaneous minor medical goods and services.

[3] The 1964 figure is the adjusted figure shown in Table 1 that made amendment for the missing operating room charges. 1964 operating room charges in 1971 prices were estimated by using the average operating room charge of those patients who were billed for use of the operating room. Again, through a billing mistake, three of the 14 patients who were treated in the operating room in 1971 were not billed for its use.

Effects of Changes in Treatment on Costs, 1964-1971

Tables 3 and 4 are the 1964-1971 counterparts of Tables 1 and 2. Table 3 shows actual average costs of treatment for the 11 conditions for which we have data in 1964 and in 1971, and the average cost of 1964 treatment in 1971 prices. Table 4 shows the percentage increase in actual average costs, and the percentage increases due to pure price changes and due to net changes in the input of medical services, again for the whole period and in terms of annual rates of change. It is interesting, though not surprising to anyone familiar with the changes in the different components of the BLS medical care price index during this period, to discover that costs of treatment of conditions requiring hospitalization rose at a considerably faster rate than those of conditions treated on an ambulatory basis. Detailed tables for each condition are given in Appendix A. They break down total costs of treatment of each condition into costs of the major inputs of medical serv-

TABLE 4

Percentage change in average costs of treatment of selected
illnesses, 1964-1971: Total change, change due to price
changes, and change due to net changes in inputs of
medical services

	Percentage change, 1964-1971			Annual rate of change		
	Total	Price	Inputs	Total	Price	Inputs
Otitis media (children)	37	32	4	4.6	4.0	0.6
Appendicitis						
Simple	80	76	2	8.8	8.4	0.3
Perforated	115	89	14	11.6	9.5	1.9
Maternity care[1]	56	70	(8)	6.6	7.9	(1.2)
	[53]	[67]	[(8)]	[6.3]	[7.6]	[(1.2)]
Cancer of the breast[2]	57	66	(5)	6.7	7.4	(0.7)
	[64]	[66]	[(1)]	[7.3]	[7.5]	[(0.1)]
Forearm fractures (children)						
Cast only	17	14	3	2.3	1.9	0.4
Closed reduction, no general						
anesthetic	102	64	23	10.6	7.3	3.0
Closed reduction, general						
or regional anesthetic[3]	43	57	(9)	5.2	6.7	(1.3)
Myocardial infarction	126	70	33	12.4	7.9	4.2
Pneumonia (non-hospitalized)	13	32	(14)	1.8	4.0	(2.1)
Duodenal ulcer (non-hospitalized)	17	33	(12)	2.3	4.2	(1.8)

[1] The figures in brackets include costs of outpatient drugs and prescriptions, the others exclude such costs.

[2] The figures in brackets include the costs of surgery done as a procedure independent from the mastectomy, and of miscellaneous minor medical goods and services.

[3] The 1964 figure is the adjusted figure shown in Table 1 that made amendment for the missing operating room charges. 1964 operating room charges in 1971 prices were estimated by using the average operating room charge of those patients who were billed for use of the operating room. Again, through a billing mistake, three of the 14 patients who were treated in the operating room in 1971 were not billed for its use.

ices in 1964 and 1971 and also show the costs of the major 1964 inputs of services in 1971 prices. Thus, one can see not only which specific changes in inputs were cost-saving and which were cost-raising, but also their magnitude in 1971 prices. Again, what stands out for all conditions requiring hospitalization is the increase in hospital costs as a percentage of total costs over the period 1961-1971. Appendix B shows the results of a number of tests of significance.

Although an analysis of the 1964-1971 data showed a continuation of most of the trends observed in the earlier period, it also revealed more conditions where changes in treatment were, on balance, cost-saving. Of the eight conditions for which data are available for both periods, net changes in inputs of medical services were cost-saving in the cases of three: maternity care, breast cancer, and forearm fractures requiring a closed reduction with a general or regional anesthetic. Net changes in inputs were also cost-saving for two of three conditions, pneumonia and duodenal ulcer,[11] where data exist for 1964 and 1971 only.

In the following analyses, we discuss first the conditions where changes in treatment were, on balance, cost-saving. The maternity care data show two changes which stemmed the rise in costs. The principal cost-saving change was the further reduction in the average length of hospital stay by one day (from 3.8 days per case in 1964 to 2.8 days in 1971). The other was the continued increase in the percentage of women delivered without a general anesthetic (from 12 percent in 1964 to 24 percent in 1971). These changes more than offset the continued increase in laboratory tests (from 11.5 per case in 1964 to 13.5 in 1971) and the increased use of in-hospital drugs and miscellaneous hospital supplies.

As in the case of maternity care, the main cost-saving change in cancer of the breast was the further decline in the average length of hospital stay by 1.3 days (from 10.2 days in 1964 to 8.9 days in 1971). An additional cost-saving change was the partial substitution of modified radical mastectomies for radical mastectomies. In 1964, all the patients in the study had radical mastectomies, while in 1971, only 26 percent had radical mastectomies, the rest having modified radicals, the fee for which is somewhat lower. Minor cost-saving changes were the reduction in the average operating room time (presumably attributable to the somewhat simpler surgical procedure), the resulting reduction in anesthetist time, and slight reduction in the average number of radiotherapy treatments. Cost-raising changes were minor and were due largely to the use of somewhat more expensive inpatient drugs. Although the number of laboratory tests (inpatient and out-patient) per case increased (from 14.8 per patient in 1964 to 27.4 in 1971), this had little effect on costs. There seems to have been a shift to lower-priced tests because the actual 1971 average cost of laboratory tests per patient was just about the same as the average costs of 1964 tests in 1971 prices.

In the case of pneumonia, there was a slight reduction in the number of physician visits per case (from 3.0 in 1964 to 2.6 in 1971) and, as will be shown in Part II, a shift to lower-priced visits; a reduction in the average number of laboratory tests per case (from 3.0 to 2.3); and a very slight reduction in the number of x-rays (from 2.0 to 1.8). These cost-saving changes more than offset the use of slightly more expensive drugs and the increase in miscellaneous outpatient services, such as nursing care.

Much the same changes took place in the treatment of duodenal ulcer: a decline of almost one physician visit per case (from 4.7 visits in 1964 to 3.8 in 1971) and, as in the case of pneumonia, a shift to less expensive visits; a slight decline in the number of x-rays per case (from 2.4 to 2.2); and a minor shift to somewhat less expensive laboratory tests. Again, these cost-saving changes out-weighed the increased cost due to the use of somewhat more expensive drugs.

It is possible that, in both instances, there were less serious cases in the 1971 study population than in the 1964 groups. This is doubtful, however, especially in the case of pneumonia. Of the total study population (hospitalized and non-hospitalized cases), eight percent were hospitalized in 1964 compared to three percent in 1971. Furthermore, the hospitalized cases had an average length of stay of 5.0 days in 1964 and of 6.6 days in 1971. The two figures together indicate that, if anything, the patients hospitalized in 1971 were more serious cases than those hospitalized in 1964, and hence that there was a higher proportion of more serious cases in the non-hospitalized group in 1971 than in 1964.

Forearm fractures in children have been left to the last so that both types of closed reductions can be discussed together.[12] As Tables 3 and 4 show, the net effects of changes in treatment of fractures requiring a closed reduction without a general anesthetic were cost-raising, while the net effects of changes in treatment of fractures requiring a general or regional anesthetic were cost-saving. It is possible, however, that the figures on fractures requiring no general anesthetic are misleading.

There was an important change in the use of hospital care in forearm fractures requiring a closed reduction with a general or regional anesthetic.[13] As mentioned earlier, all the 1964 cases were treated in the hospital and remained there at least one night. By contrast, of the 1971 cases, four (22 percent) were treated in the orthopedist's office, with the orthopedist administering a regional anesthetic. Of the remaining cases, half were treated in the hospital but discharged on the same day, while the other half were treated in the hospital, staying at least one night. What this change implies in terms of costs is shown below:

Place of treatment	Average cost per case
Physician's office	$269
Hospital, in-out in one day	532[14]
Hospital, inpatient	639

This change in the hospitalization pattern, combined with the resulting reduction in operating room charges and anesthetists' fees, more than offset the increase in the number of x-rays (from 5.4 per case in 1964 to 6.4 in 1971) and the very minor increase in the number of physician visits per case.

In the case of forearm fractures requiring a closed reduction without an anesthetic or with a local anesthetic only, there was an increase in the number of physicians visits per case (from 6.1 in 1964 to 7.0 in 1971), as well as in the number of x-rays per case (from 2.7 in 1964 to 3.9 in 1971). It is possible, however, that in 1971, orthopedists treated a greater percentage of forearm fractures in the office with a local anesthetic, and that some of the patients in this group might have been treated in the hospital in 1964. This would explain the increase in visits and x-rays per case in this group. It would also explain the increase in the per capita number of x-rays for patients given a general or regional anesthetic in 1971 since it would mean that in 1971 this type of treatment was only given in the most serious cases. If such a change in the mix of these two types of cases occurred, our figures for fractures treated without a general or regional anesthetic would show a cost-raising change when in reality the change was cost-saving. The figures do not bear out this hypothesis since, in both years, about the same percentage of closed reductions were treated with a local or no anesthetic (52.1 percent in 1964, 52.6 percent in 1971).

We can only hypothesize, however, because we are dealing with small numbers. Because of the considerable difference between the cost of cases treated on an ambulatory rather than an inpatient basis, we hope that others will be stimulated to do a more comprehensive study of the treatment of common fractures.

Conditions where changes in treatment were, on balance, cost-raising include otitis media, appendicitis and myocardial infarction. Only minor changes were seen in the case of otitis media. The main shift was to more expensive drugs. Changes in treatment of simple appendicitis also were minor. The main cost-raising factors were an increase in the number of laboratory tests per case (from 7.3 in 1964 to 9.3 in 1971), an increase in the number of postoperative intravenous solutions, the use of more expensive drugs, and an increase in operating room time. A surgeon explained the latter puzzling statistic. In recent years such surgery has frequently been done by residents of Stanford University Hospital under the supervision of the surgeon. Residents, being less experienced, tend to take more time. It is a good example (and the only one we know of to which a dollar figure can be attached) of the way in which patients subsidize the teaching of medicine. The above changes, taken together, slightly more than offset the cost-saving reduction in the average length of hospital stay (from 4.2 in 1964 to 3.8 days in 1971).

In the case of perforated appendicitis, a number of cost-raising changes far outweighed the reduction in the average length of hospital stay of over half a day (from 10.7 days in 1964 to 10.1 days in 1971). The most important of these was the continued increase in the number of laboratory tests per patient (from 14.5 in 1964 to 31.0 in 1971). In terms of 1971 dollars, these additional tests alone cost over twice the saving brought about by the reduction in the average length of hospital stay. Other changes that raised costs were the use of more drugs—and more expensive ones; an increase in the number of postoperative intravenous solutions per patient; and an increase in a number of miscellaneous inpatient and out patient services (e.g., in the number of physician visits per case, in operating room time, and in hospital supplies).

Of the conditions covered by the 1964-1971 study, the changes in treatment in myocardial infarction had their most drastic effect on costs. This was due principally to the increased use of intensive care units. In 1964, the Stanford Hospital had a relatively small Intensive Care Unit (ICU). It was used by only three of the 1964 coronary cases whose average stay was 7.3 days (or 0.8 days for all 1964 cases). By 1971, the hospital had not only an ICU but also a Coronary Care Unit (CCU) and an intermediate CCU. Of the 1971 cases, only one did not receive at least some care in either the CCU or the intermediate CCU. The majority (85 percent) were admitted directly to the CCU, where they spent an average of 4.4 days; after their stay in the CCU, most of these patients (83 percent) proceeded to the intermediate CCU, where they spent an additional 4.6 days on the average. The rest of the cases (13 percent) were admitted to the intermediate CCU, where they stayed an average of 8.5 days. Taking into account the saving due to the reduction in the average length of hospital stay of the coronary cases by about one day (from 19.7 days in 1964 to 18.8 days in 1971), our estimates show that the net additional cost of the substitution of care in the CCU and intermediate CCU for the 1964 type of care in regular hospital beds (and minimal use of the ICU) amounted to about $385 per case in 1971 dollars.

The above figure is only the net additional cost of the intensive care unit days.[15] Along with the increased use of intensive care units went increases in the inputs of other services. The average number of laboratory tests increased (from 37.9 in 1964 to 48.5 in 1971). So did the number of electrocardiograms (from 5.4 per patient in 1964 to 9.0 in 1971); the number of intravenous solutions (from 1.6 to 10.6); the number of x-rays (from 1.3 to 6.3); and the number of inhalation therapy treatments (from 12.8 to 37.5). There was also an increase in the use of drugs in the hospital. The increased costs resulting from all these additional services (CCU care and other services) were only partially offset by the reduction in the average length of hospital stay (already taken into account above), a decrease in the average number of physician visits (from 27.6 in 1964 to 26.0 in 1971), and a decline in miscellaneous outpatient services such as nursing care.

Overview 1951-1964-1971

To give an overview of the major trends in inputs of medical services shown by our studies for the period 1951-1971, Tables 5 and 6 show data on the per capita number of the more important medical services for the diagnoses covered by the studies. Table 5 shows the average number of various diagnostic tests and some therapeutic procedures (intravenous solutions and inhalation therapy) by diagnosis for the years for which we have data. Table 6 shows the average number of physician visits and average length of hospital stay by diagnosis.

Table 5 shows striking changes. With minor exceptions, there was a steady and consistent increase in the average number of diagnostic tests per diagnosis over the 20-year period. There was also a steady increase in the two therapeutic procedures for which there is data. To take just a few examples, the average number of laboratory tests for perforated appendicitis increased from 5.3 per case in 1951 to 14.5 in 1964, to 31.0 in 1971. For maternity care, the number rose from 4.8 per case in 1951, to 11.5 in 1964, to 13.5 in 1971. Similarly, the number of x-rays per case of forearm fracture requiring a closed reduction with a general or regional anesthetic increased from 2.0 in 1951, to 5.4 in 1964, to 6.4 in 1971. The average number of electrocardiograms for myocardial infarction rose from 5.4 in 1964 to 9.0 in 1971. Much the same picture emerges for most of the other conditions.

The average number of physician visits per diagnosis, shown in Table 6, did not exhibit any consistent trend. The number rose slightly for some conditions, declined slightly for others, and remained more or less stable for others. For all conditions taken together, those for which there are data for all three years showed a rise in the average number of physician visits in both periods 1951-1964 and 1964-1971. For the three conditions for which there are data only for 1964 and 1971, the average number of physician visits for all conditions taken together stayed almost unchanged in the period 1964-1971. By and large, the data did not show any major change in inputs of physician services.

TABLE 5

**Number of diagnostic and other services per case, selected
illnesses, 1951, 1964, and 1971**

Type of service and illness	1951	1964	1971
Laboratory tests			
Appendicitis			
Simple	4.7	7.3	9.3
Perforated	5.3	14.5	31.0
Maternity care	4.8	11.5	13.5
Cancer of the breast	5.9	14.8	27.4
Myocardial infarction	NA	37.9	48.5
Pneumonia	NA	3.0	2.3
Duodenal ulcer	NA	5.4	5.4
X-Rays			
Cancer of the breast			
Diagnostic	0.7	2.0	2.3
Radiotherapy	1.7	11.0	10.6
Forearm fracture			
Cast only	2.3	2.3	2.2
Closed reduction, no			
general anesthetic	3.7	2.7	3.9
Closed reduction, general			
or regional anesthetic	2.0	5.4	6.4
Myocardial infarction	NA	1.3	6.3
Pneumonia	NA	2.0	1.8
Duodenal ulcer	NA	2.4	2.2
Intravenous solutions			
Appendicitis			
Simple	0.1	2.4	4.6
Perforated	6.7	12.7	14.2
Cancer of the breast	1.0	1.7	1.7
Myocardial infarction	NA	1.6	10.6
Electrocardiograms			
Myocardial infarction	NA	5.4	9.0
Inhalation therapy			
Myocardial infarction	NA	12.8	37.5

By contrast, the data showed a consistent downward trend in the average length of hospital stay over the 20-year period 1951-1971. This is true especially of maternity care, where the average length of hospital stay declined from 4.6 days in 1951 to 2.8 days in 1971, and of cancer of the breast, where it declined 12.7 days in 1951 to 8.9 days in 1971.

TABLE 6

Average number of physician visits and average of length of
hospital stay per case, 1951, 1964 and 1971

Type of service and illness	1951	1964	1971
Average number of physician visits			
Otitis media	1.8	1.7	1.9
Appendicitis			
Simple	2.9	5.6	5.5
Perforated	6.8	9.1	11.8
Maternity care (obstetrician)	12.7	14.5	14.9
Cancer of the breast			
Surgeons	12.6	13.7	12.0
Other MDs	1.3	3.1	1.9
Forearm fractures			
Cast only	5.3	4.5	4.4
Closed reduction, no general			
anesthetic	6.7	6.1	7.0
Closed reduction, general			
or regional anesthetic	5.8	7.9	8.1
Myocardial infarction	NA	27.6	26.0
Pneumonia	NA	3.0	2.6
Duodenal ulcer	NA	4.7	3.8
Average length of hospital stay			
Appendicitis			
Simple	4.3	4.2	3.8
Perforated	10.8	10.7	10.1
Maternity care	4.6	3.8	2.8
Cancer of the breast	12.7	10.2	8.9
Forearm fractures			
Closed reduction, general			
or regional anesthetic (all cases)	0.4	1.2	0.6
Closed reduction, general			
or regional anesthetic, (hospitalized			
cases)	1.0	1.2	1.4
Myocardial infarction	NA	19.7	18.8

The decline in the average length of hospital stay was the major cost-saving factor found. Without it, the net effects of changes in inputs for the conditions requiring hospitalization would have been even greater in cases where they were cost-raising. In the case of maternity care and cancer of the breast in 1964-1971, they would have been more or less neutral rather than cost-saving. It is doubtful that the increased input of other medical services, mainly diagnostic tests, had anything to do with the decline in the average length of hospitalization.

Medical Care Costs and Changes in the Use of "Mix" of Existing Services

There is general concern on the part of government, the general public, and some of the medical profession over the increase in medical care costs resulting from technological innovations such as renal dialysis, open-heart surgery and organ transplants. What has received little, if any, attention is the effect on medical care costs of changes in the use or "mix" of existing services, such as most of those decribed in this study. While, as Tables 2 and 4 show, the effects on costs of "pure" changes in inputs (i.e., in constant dollars) have been small compared to the effects of pure price changes, they have not been small compared to the effects of pure price changes, they have not been negligible in terms of current dollars. On the basis of our data, we have made rough estimates of the costs of the net additional inputs in current dollars on a national basis for conditions for which data on total number of cases were readily available. We have also made rough estimates of the savings in current dollars on a national basis for conditions where data on total number of cases were available.

For 1964, we estimated that the net additional inputs compared to 1951 inputs for appendicitis cost about $8.7 million in current dollars and those for cancer of the breast about $21.7 million.[16] These costs, taken together amount to only about 0.1 percent of total personal health care expenditures in 1964. But when they are multiplied by the total number of other conditions whose treatment probably changed in much the same way, it is clear that they are not negligible.

For 1971,[17] we estimated that the net additional inputs (compared to 1964 inputs) for appendicitis cost about $18.7 million in current dollars. Those for myocardial infarction cost about $275.2 million. Together, these costs are about 0.4 percent of total personal health care expenditures in 1971. Considering that treatment in other conditions is likely to have changed in a similar way, the costs begin to mount.

For pneumonia and maternity care, where changes in net inputs were found to have been cost-saving in the period 1964-1971, the savings for pneumonia were estimated at about $14.2 million. Those for maternity care were estimated at about $185.6 million. Although our study covers too few illnesses to draw a definite conclusion, we suspect that, in terms of numbers of cases and costs, conditions where changes in inputs were cost-raising probably outweighed those where they were cost-saving.

The above estimates are rough. While we believe that the directions shown by our data are probably accurate (i.e., whether changes in treatment were, on balance, cost-raising or cost-saving), the actual dollar figures will vary considerably according to geographic area, and by provider and patient characteristics. We therefore present the data mainly to show the need for greater attention to changes in the treatment of the common, everyday conditions that make up the bulk of medical practice. While the increase in medical care costs due to to the increase in net inputs may be relatively small for each individual diagnosis, taken together (even when allowance is made for net cost-saving changes) they may well approach, or possibly exceed, the additional costs resulting from technological innovation.

Accordingly, we recommend that additonal studies of changes in costs of treatment be carried out periodically in different areas of the United States, on a larger scale than ours and covering more diagnoses. The time is right. PSROs are in the process of being organized throughout the country. While their present scope of reveiw is limited, there is every reason to believe that it will expand. Now is the time, therefore, for the medical profession to examine in detail current patterns of treatment, especially of the more common diseases, with a view to evaluating them carefully in terms of both outcomes and costs. If this is not done now, there is a danger that current standards of treatment may simply be "frozen," regardless of their effective-ness and cost. We realize it is easier to curb the increase in medical care costs by limiting the implementation of new technology (e.g., the construction of additional renal dialysis facilities or intensive care units) than by influencing physicians to modify accepted forms of treatment. But if the rise in medical care costs is to be brought under control, it is necessary to evaluate both technological innovations and currently accepted forms of treatment. To do the latter, additional detailed and more comprehensive studies are essential.

Medical Care Costs and Changes in Quality

We want to touch briefly on the problem of quality change in the medical care sector. It is clear that members of the medical profession regard in-creases in inputs as an improvement in the quality of care. But it is some-what surprising that many economists also assume that more care, or more expensive care, is better care. In constructing the CPI and its components, the BLS has always assumed, when "linking in" a new and more expensive product or service, that the entire price difference between the new and the old product reflects improved quality. This method has often been criticized, but no better method has yet been developed. Other economists also have tended to equate more medical care inputs with higher quality care, as did one of the authors of this paper an earlier publication.[18].

A more recent example of the "more care is better care" school of thought is Karen Davis in a study of Medicare and Medicaid benefits for the elderly.[19] She constructs a measure of "real hospital care received by the elderly which includes both additional quantity and higher quality of care" by deflating hospital expenses of the elderly by a constant quality index of hospital expenses per adjusted patient day. This index takes account of the increased amounts of labor and non-labor inputs used to provide a day of hospital care. She estimates that if hospitals had continued to use the same inputs to provide a day of hospital care over the period 1966-1973, hospital costs would have risen by 62 percent, rather than 133 percent as shown by the index of the cost per adjusted patient day.

Looking over the data from our cost of illness studies, it is hard to know how much the net increase in inputs of all kinds has really improved the quality of care. For example, is a patient with perforated appendicitis really better off when he gets almost six times as many laboratory tests as he did in 1951? How much better off is a child with a broken forearm who has it reduced by an orthopedist instead of by a general surgeon? Even if we assume that the child does get better treatment from an orthopedic surgeon than from a general surgeon, is the improvement really as great as the full difference in the fees of the two types of physicians (which is what the BLS would assume)?

To use two other examples, how much has increased radiotherapy improved the outcome of breast cancer? How much has the increased use of coronary units improved the outcome of myocardial infarction? A look at the age-adjusted mortality rate from breast cancer in women in the United States is somewhat discouraging: it actually rose slightly from 22.3 per 100,000 women in 1960 to 22.8 in 1971.[20] In myocardial infarction, there was a decline in the age-adjusted mortality rate from 141.1 per 100,000 population in 1968 (the earliest year for which the National Center for Health Statistics has data) to 127.8 in 1971. Yet, according to some clinical studies reported in medical journals, there seems considerable doubt about the effectiveness of coronary care units.[21] One study even found no difference in mortality rates between coronary patients treated in the hospital and those treated at home.[22]

None of these studies can be regarded as conclusive. But they do suggest that we do not yet have the last word on the effectiveness of coronary care units. On the basis of currently available data, we would regard it as an understatement of the "pure" price increase (and implied overestimate of the quality increase) if the BLS were to "link in" the daily rate of a bed in a coronary care unit on the assumption that the entire difference in price between the rate for semi-private room and the rate for a coronary care unit bed represented an increase in quality.

We are aware of the difficulties of devising a better medical care price index than the BLS index. Although we still believe that it would be worthwhile to construct a medical care price index based on costs of treatment of selected illnesses every few years, it is not thought of as a replacement of the BLS index. For the time being, we shall have to continue using the BLS index to deflate medical care expenditures, though we should keep in mind its shortcomings.

Some thought might be given, however, to the construction of an index of the quality of medical care with which to deflate a medical care price index that does not attempt to adjust for quality changes. Such a quality index might include specific mortality rates and data on disability days, as well as data on adverse effects of medical care such as number of hospital days and/or number of disability days for iatrogenic diseases. In selecting items to be included in such a quality of care index, it would be essential to make sure that it is an index of the quality of medical care, not a health status. For example, mortality rates for diseases where other factors (such as environmental factors, the quality of housing and nutrition, occupation, and similar factors) play no role, or at least only a limited role, should be selected rather than the overall mortality rate. Disability days would have to be treated in the same way, i.e., they would have to relate to conditions where factors other than medical care have little influence. It is beyond the scope of this paper to attempt to work out the details of such an index. We have no illusion that it will be easy to construct but suggest that it is a possibility worth exploring.

PART II

COMMENTS ON THE BLS MEDICAL CARE PRICE INDEX

In 1964, the CPI underwent a major revision which undoubtedly improved the BLS medical care price index as a measure of changes in medical care prices. Nevertheless, on the basis of our findings, we have a few brief comments on two issues: the measurement of changes in physicians' fees for office visits, and the problem of selecting representative medical services for inclusion in the index.[1]

Physicians' Fees for Office Visits

One of the services which the BLS prices to measure changes in physician fees is the customary fee for a routine office visit. In our 1951-1964 cost-of-illness study, we found that the customary fee for such a visit had risen less than the average fee. This was because in 1951 the average fee was considerably below that of the customary fee, while by 1964, the gap between them had narrowed. We concluded that if this was a nationwide phenomenon and there were reasons to believe that it was the BLS index understated the increase in the fee for a routine physician office visit for the period 1951-1964.[2] In our 1964-1971 study, we found that the gap between average and customary fees had narrowed still further. If in the United States as a whole, there was similar continued shrinking of the gap between average and customary fees, the BLS index for a routine office visit still understated the rise in this type of fee during the period 1964-1971. However, the understatement was very much less than for the period 1951-1964 because in 1964 the average fee was already only between 5 percent and 17 percent below the customary fee, decreasing to between 2 percent and 7 percent in 1971.

The BLS uses the fee for a routine office visit to represent changes in the fees for all physician office visits. It may be of interest to note that our data on office visit fees of internists and pediatricians (for pneumonia, myocardial infarction, duodenal ulcer, and otitis media) with one exception showed that the average fee for all offices visits rose less than that for a routine office visit. The explanation lies in a shift from more expensive to less expensive visits. For example, in 1964, 17 percent of all office visits for myocardial infarction had fees above that for a routine office visit, as against only 5 percent in 1971. This decline was accompanied by a slight increase in visits at the scheduled fee for a routine office visit (from 78 percent in 1964 to 84 percent in 1971) and a considerable increase (from 5 percent in 1964 to 10 percent in 1971) of visits at fees below that for a routine office visit. Our data for the other conditions show much the same picture.

If this shift from higher priced to lower priced physician office visits were true on a nationwide basis, the fee for a routine office visit would overstate the increase in physician office visit fees. We doubt, however, that such a shift did not occur on a nationwide basis. Data from a later study in which we compared the distributions of all office visits for primary care physicians at the PAMC between 1969 and 1971 showed no change; by contrast, a Social Security Administration study showed a shift to more expensive office visits for California Medicare patients during this same period.[3] What all these data suggest is that there is a need for periodic studies of the "mix" of physician office visits and the changes in their fees, in order to evaluate whether the fee for a routine office visit can really represent changes in the fees for all office visits. The need for such periodic reviews increases as increasingly complex and fractionated coding and terminology systems are developed for processing claims under public and private health insurance plans.

Selection of Medical Services for a Medical Care Price Index

There was some evidence in our study that the fees for the more common and less expensive medical care services rose more than those for the more expensive ones. For example, the fee for an appendectomy rose 46 percent between 1964 and 1971, while the fee for the more complex and expensive radical mastectomy rose only 36 percent. There was similar difference in the increase in charges for x-rays. Charges for the relatively inexpensive x-rays performed in connection with pneumonia and fractured forearms (such as chest, single view; chest, two views; wrist, two views, forearm, including one joint) rose between 30 percent and 50 percent, while the charge for the more expensive upper G.I. series x-rays rose only 24 percent. If this difference between the rate of increase in the fees for the more common and less expensive services and the fees for the less common and more expensive services should be found to be general, this would become an important consideration in the selection of items to be included in a medical care price index. If the index priced mainly the cheaper procedures, it would tend to overstate the increase in medical care prices. Conversely, if the index included too many expensive procedures, or selected a relatively expensive procedure to represent a group of services, it would tend to understate the price increase.

An attempt was made to determine if there was evidence to support our tentative hypothesis that fees for cheaper procedures rose more than those for more expensive ones. Because the subject was beyond the scope of our study, we were able to do only a cursory exploration, based on the PAMC fee schedules for 1966 and 1971.[4] We found that the hypothesis was not borne out by fees for physician office visits, although there was some evidence that it held in the case of fees for physician hospital visits. There was also some confirmation of it in the case of fees for surgical procedures. We next looked at the fees for 22 common diagnostic x-rays and found some support for our hypothesis, although it was not overwhelming. The same was true of laboratory tests. None of our findings gave conclusive proof of our hypothesis, and it must also be borne in mind that our data are based on a small sample of procedures and only one group of providers. However, they are suggestive enough to deserve further exploration, especially since some physicians with whom we discussed our hypothesis said they would not be surprised if it proved to be correct.

They offered two explanations. According to the first, if a physician, or a laboratory, or a radiology department wants to increase their revenue, they can do it most effectively by raising the fees for the common, "bread and butter" procedures. The second explanation has a "Robing Hood" promise. The medical profession, according to this reasoning, is reluctant to charge a very sick patient, or a patient requiring very costly procedures, the full cost of treatment. Instead, providers spread some of this cost over patients requiring less costly care by raising the fees for the more common and less expensive services and procedures. An additional explanation, which would apply to surgeons' fees, is that surgeons prefer more interesting procedures to common, everyday procedures. Any or all of these explanations have some validity. We hope that this question will be investiaged more fully.

NOTE: The numbers of hospital and non-hospital laboratory tests shown in these tables do not add up to the total figures for laboratory tests shown in the text and text tables. In these tables, the number of hospital laboratory tests shown is the number of tests billed, while the number of non-hospital tests is the actual number of tests performed. Thus, a hospital laboratory procedure consisting of several tests (such as a complete blood count) was counted as one test in these tables. In the text and text tables, we have adjusted the hospital laboratory test figures to reflect the actual number of tests.

APPENDICES

Appendix A

TABLE 1

Otitis Media: Average cost and average inputs
of services by type of service, 1964 (N=156),
1971 (N=256), and 1964 treatment in 1971 prices

	Actual 1964 $	Actual 1964 #	Actual 1971 $	Actual 1971 #	1964 treatment 1971 prices	% increase actual	% increase pure price
Total cost	18.34	–	25.13	–	24.18	37	32
Physician	11.72	1.7	17.02	1.9	16.91	45	44
Drugs	6.44	2.4	7.70	2.4	7.05	20	9
Prescriptions	4.53	1.3	6.58	1.5	4.40	45	–3
Injections	1.23	0.4	0.44	0.1	1.85	–64	50
Over-the-counter items	0.67	0.7	0.68	0.8	0.80	2	19
Miscellaneous[1]	0.18	–	0.42	–	0.23	133	28

[1]   Includes outpatient laboratory tests in both years and outpatient medical supplies in 1971

TABLE 2

Simple Appendicitis: Average cost and average inputs of
services by type of service, 1964 (N=89), 1971 (N=41), and 1964
treatment in 1971 prices

	Actual 1964 $	Actual 1964 #	Actual 1971 $	Actual 1971 #	1964 treatment 1971 prices	% increase actual	% increase pure price
Total cost	591.51	–	1062.58	–	1040.02	80	77
Non-hospital	318.25	–	468.79	–	482.13	47	51
Physician	312.08	5.6	461.45	5.5	473.80	48	52
Surgeon	253.03	3.6	366.60	3.7	373.40	45	48
Anesthetist	48.53	1.0	80.10	1.0	81.00	65	67
Other physician	10.51	1.0	14.75	.8	19.40	40	85
Laboratory tests	4.59	1.9	6.05	2.3	5.29	32	15
Miscellaneous[1]	1.58	–	1.29	–	3.04	–18	92
Hospital	273.25	–	593.80	–	557.90	117	104
Room and board	131.44	4.2	305.22	3.8	334.90	132	155
Operating room, post-operating room	79.23	1.8	139.76	2.0	120.29	76	52
Laboratory tests	25.98	3.9	55.07	4.2	45.98	112	77
Drugs	33.00	–	76.20	–	50.81	131	54
Anesthesia	18.68	1.0	23.88	0.9	22.43	28	20
Intravenous solutions	6.74	2.4	36.32	4.6	17.89	439	165
Other drugs	7.58	2.3	16.00	6.7	10.49	111	38
Miscellaneous[2]	3.61	–	17.56	–	5.91	386	64

[1]   Includes outpatient X-rays, miscellaneous services, drugs and ambulance services in 1964. In 1971, it includes outpatient X-rays, miscellaneous services, drugs and medical supplies.

[2]   Includes emergency room charges, electrocardiograms, X-rays, supplies and inhalation therapy in 1964. In 1971, it includes emergency room charges, electrocardiograms, X-rays and supplies.

TABLE 3

Perforated Appendicitis: Average cost and average inputs of
services by type of service, 1964 (N=17), 1971 (N=11), and 1964
treatment in 1971 prices

	Actual 1964 $	#	Actual 1971 $	#	1964 treatment 1971 prices	% increase actual	pure price
Total cost	958.72	–	2062.17	–	1811.53	115	89
Non-hospital	359.64	–	602.27	–	538.81	167	50
Physician	342.53	9.1	571.07	11.8	517.65	67	51
Surgeon	265.15	5.5	403.89	5.8	390.20	52	47
Anesthetist	55.29	1.1	88.27	1.1	86.45	60	57
Other physician	22.09	2.5	78.91	4.9	41.00	257	86
Laboratory tests	7.03	2.7	17.86	6.8	7.99	154	14
Miscellaneous[1]	10.08	–	13.34	–	13.17	32	31
Hospital	599.07	–	1459.91	–	1272.72	144	112
Room and board	323.15	10.7	807.50	10.0	853.72	150	164
Operating room, post-operating room	85.59	2.0	142.57	2.2	131.90	67	54
Laboratory tests	62.32	9.1	174.27	16.0	77.09	180	24
Drugs	96.11	–	280.50	–	167.05	192	174
Anesthesia	19.65	1.1	25.08	1.1	23.71	28	21
Intravenous solutions	33.19	12.7	112.04	14.2	88.51	238	167
Other drugs	43.28	12.1	143.39	21.3	54.84	231	27
Miscellaneous[2]	31.90	–	55.06	–	42.94	73	35

[1] In both years, it includes outpatient X-rays, drugs and medical supplies.

[2] Includes emergency room charges, electrocardiograms, X-rays, blood, supplies and inhalation therapy in 1964. In 1971, it includes emergency room charges, electrocardiograms, X-rays and supplies.

TABLE 4

Maternity Care: Average cost and average inputs of
services by type of service, 1964 (N=100), 1971 (N=154), and 1964
treatment in 1971 prices

	Actual 1964 $	#	Actual 1971 $	#	1964 treatment 1971 prices	% increase actual	pure price
Total cost	527.47	–	807.08	–	880.53	53	67
Non-hospital	315.85	–	445.56	–	461.98	41	46
Physician	264.98	15.6	385.86	15.8	395.06	46	49
Obstetrician	236.96	14.5	344.91	14.9	347.17	46	47
Anesthetist	26.41	0.9	39.17	0.8	45.13	48	71
Other physician	1.61	0.2	1.79	0.2	2.76	11	71
Laboratory tests	19.00	9.5	36.36	11.9	29.14	91	53
Drugs	24.55	6.3	20.76	5.2	27.66	–15	13
Miscellaneous[1]	7.32	–	2.58	–	10.12	–65	38
Hospital	211.61	–	361.52	–	418.55	71	98
Room and board	124.05	3.8	196.44	2.8	264.98	58	114
Delivery room	54.75	1.0	100.51	1.0	101.17	84	85
Laboratory tests	9.01	2.0	8.59	1.5	9.38	–5	4
Drugs	20.77	–	44.54	–	39.11	114	88
Anesthesia	10.38	0.9	19.51	0.7	23.13	88	123
Other drugs	10.40	4.6	25.03	9.0	15.98	141	54
Miscellaneous[2]	3.04	–	11.44	–	3.92	276	29

[1] Includes outpatient X-rays, medical supplies, special nurses and dressings in 1964. In 1971, it includes outpatient X-rays, miscellaneous services, and dressings.

[2] Includes emergency room charges, blood transfer issue fees, X-rays, blood and supplies in 1964. In 1971, it includes electrocardiograms, X-rays, blood and supplies.

TABLE 5

Cancer of the Breast: **Average cost and average inputs of services by type of service, 1964 (N=30), 1971 (N=35), and 1964 treatment in 1971 prices**

	Actual 1964 $	#	Actual 1971 $	#	1964 treatment 1971 prices	% increase actual	pure price
Total cost	1503.93	–	2356.71	–	2491.52	57	66
Non-hospital	879.51	–	1215.63	–	1238.11	38	41
Physician	609.43	17.8	786.06	14.9	847.02	29	39
Surgeon	505.33	13.7	650.90	12.0	690.80	29	37
Anesthetist	79.40	1.0	109.14	1.0	111.11	38	40
Other physician	24.71	3.1	26.02	1.9	45.12	5	83
Laboratory tests	14.73	4.3	32.15	16.9	14.38	118	–2
X-rays	235.55	13.1	379.49	12.9	357.07	61	52
Diagnostic	31.82	2.0	84.72	2.3	49.65	166	56
Therapeutic	203.73	11.0	294.77	10.6	307.42	45	51
Miscellaneous[1]	19.79	–	17.93	–	19.64	–9	–1
Hospital	624.42	–	1141.08	–	1253.41	83	101
Room and board	361.15	10.2	732.04	8.9	835.20	103	131
Operating room, post-operating room	127.09	2.0	189.48	2.1	190.74	49	50
Laboratory tests	56.18	7.3	108.61	5.2	124.22	93	121
Drugs	50.54	–	72.01	–	57.03	43	13
Anesthesia	33.17	1.0	35.38	1.0	36.17	7	9
Intravenous solutions	4.84	1.7	13.29	1.7	13.54	175	180
Other drugs	12.53	4.1	23.34	13.5	7.32	86	–42
Miscellaneous[2]	29.46	–	38.94	–	46.22	32	57

[1] In both years, it includes miscellaneous outpatient services and drugs.

[2] Includes emergency room charges, electrocardiograms, blood transfer issue fees, X-rays, blood, supplies and inhalation therapy in 1964. In 1971, it includes electrocardiograms, blood transfer issue fees, X-rays, blood, supplies and inhalation therapy.

TABLE 6

Fractured Forearms, cast only: **Average costs and average inputs of services by type of service, 1964 (N=37), 1971 (N=48), and 1964 treatment in 1971 prices**

	Actual 1964 $	#	Actual 1971 $	#	1964 treatment 1971 prices	% increase actual	pure price
Total cost	82.89	–	97.01	–	94.04	17	13
Physician	51.96	4.5	55.19	4.4	53.29	6	3
Orthopedic surgeon	48.88	3.7	45.09	3.6	45.94	–8	–6
Other physician	3.08	0.8	10.10	0.8	7.35	228	139
X-Rays	29.16	2.3	30.98	2.2	32.96	6	13
Miscellaneous[1]	1.77	–	10.83	–	7.79	512	340

[1] Includes miscellaneous services, drugs and supplies in 1964. In 1971, it includes miscellaneous services, hospital emergency room charges and drugs.

TABLE 7

Fractured Forearms, closed reduction, no general anesthetic: Average costs and average inputs of
services,1964 (N=25), 1971 (N=20), and
1964 treatment in 1971 prices

	Actual 1964 $	#	Actual 1971 $	#	1964 treatment 1971 prices	% increase actual	pure price
Total cost	121.76	–	245.79	–	199.32	102	64
Physician	88.04	6.1	176.03	7.0	152.28	100	73
Orthopedic surgeon	85.84	5.5	171.13	6.5	145.77	99	70
Other physician	2.20	0.6	4.90	0.6	6.51	122	196
X-Rays	32.09	2.7	53.05	3.9	40.37	65	26
Miscellaneous[1]	1.64	–	16.71	–	6.66	919	306

[1] Includes miscellaneous services and drugs in 1964. In 1971, it includes miscellaneous services, hospital emergency room charges and drugs.

TABLE 8

Fractured Forearms, closed reduction with general or regional anesthetic:
Average cost and average inputs of services, 1964 (N=23), and 1971 (N=18), and 1964 treatment
in 1971 prices

	Actual 1964 $	#	Actual 1971 $	#	1964 treatment 1971 prices	% increase actual	pure price
Total cost	331.85	–	521.92	–	476.28	57	44
Non-hospital	232.90	–	339.91	–	285.05	46	22
Physician	200.67	7.9	270.42	8.1	242.15	35	21
Orthopedic surgeon	165.35	6.4	226.86	7.0	183.68	37	11
Anesthetist	33.17	1.0	39.72	0.7	51.50	20	55
Other physician	2.15	0.5	3.83	0.4	6.98	78	225
X-rays	31.14	2.7	56.78	4.1	37.64	82	21
Miscellaneous[1]	1.09	–	12.71	–	5.25	1066	382
Hospital	98.95	–	182.02	–	191.23	84	93
Room and board	36.74	1.2	48.89	0.6	108.81	33	196
Operating room, post-operating room	5.54	0.5	71.01	0.9	9.93	1182	79
Laboratory tests	10.70	2.0	6.84	1.4	9.67	−36	−10
X-rays	22.28	2.7	23.19	2.3	29.39	4	32
Drugs	13.12	–	15.23	–	16.98	16	29
Anesthesia	12.48	1.0	12.26	0.7	16.56	−2	33
Other drugs	0.65	0.3	2.96	1.6	0.42	355	−35
Miscellaneous[2]	10.56	–	16.85	–	16.45	60	56

1   In both years, it includes outpatient miscellaneous services and drugs.

2   In both years, it includes emergency room charges and supplies.

Note: See p. 35, Table 4, footnote 3 for reason for differences in cost figures for 1964 and for 1964 treatment in 1971 prices.

TABLE 9

Myocardial Infarction: **Average cost and average inputs of services by type of service, 1964 (N=28), 1971 (N=48), and 1964 treatment in 1971 prices**

	Actual 1964 $	#	Actual 1971 $	#	1964 treatment 1971 prices	% increase actual	pure price
Total cost	1448.98	–	3279.87	–	2461.08	126	70
Non-hospital	406.88	–	511.44	–	616.00	26	51
Physician	257.49	27.6	405.27	26.0	436.32	57	69
Office	28.59	3.5	54.54	4.3	50.28	91	76
Hospital	187.83	20.8	341.20	21.1	326.15	82	74
Home	41.07	3.3	9.53	0.6	59.89	–77	46
Laboratory tests	22.57	5.5	11.40	3.3	23.23	–50	3
Electrocardiograms	21.43	1.4	31.13	1.7	25.04	45	17
Drugs	28.55	5.5	25.56	4.6	26.42	–11	–8
Miscellaneous[1]	76.84	–	38.08	–	104.99	–50	37
Hospital	1042.09	–	2768.44	–	1845.08	166	77
Room and board	688.86	19.7	1864.66	18.8	1479.91	171	115
Intensive care units [2]	49.29	0.8	710.18	4.0	104.99	1341	113
Intermediate coronary care units	–	–	372.75	4.1	–	–	–
Ward, semi-private, private	639.57	18.9	781.72	10.7	1374.92	22	115
Laboratory tests	174.80	27.4	389.05	37.7	162.99	123	–7
Electrocardiograms	58.84	4.0	138.64	7.3	76.09	136	29
X-rays	18.21	1.2	79.06	5.9	26.12	334	43
Drugs	60.39	–	123.58	–	55.84	105	–8
Intravenous solutions	4.62	1.6	47.48	10.6	10.45	927	126
Other drugs	55.78	16.1	76.10	32.1	45.39	36	–19
Inhalation therapy	34.46	12.8	50.22	37.5	35.95	46	4
Miscellaneous[3]	6.52	–	123.25	–	8.17	1790	25

[1] Includes outpatient X-rays, miscellaneous services, ambulance services, medical supplies and nursing services in both years.

[2] Includes Intensive Care Units and Coronary Care Units.

[3] Includes emergency room charges and supplies in 1964. In 1971, it includes operating and emergency room charges, blood transfer issue fees, blood, supplies, nuclear medicine, physical and occupational therapy.

TABLE 10

Pneumonia, non-hospitalized: Average cost and average inputs of
services by type of service, 1964 (N=71), 1971 (N=183), and
1964 treatment in 1971 prices

	Actual 1964 $	#	Actual 1971 $	#	1964 treatment 1971 prices	% increase actual	pure price
Total cost	75.04	–	84.98	–	98.88	13	32
Physician	21.68	3.0	28.59	2.6	40.70	32	88
Laboratory tests	8.65	3.0	6.89	2.3	9.77	−20	13
X-Rays	30.50	2.0	31.67	1.8	36.13	4	19
Drugs	13.97	3.1	13.74	3.7	12.09	−2	−14
Prescriptions	11.71	2.1	11.32	2.4	9.17	−3	−22
Injections	0.87	0.3	0.78	0.2	1.21	−10	39
Over-the-counter items	1.39	0.7	1.64	1.1	1.71	18	23
Miscellaneous[1]	0.24	–	4.09	–	0.19	1604	−21

[1] Includes miscellaneous outpatient services and medical supplies in both years, and nursing services in 1971.

TABLE 11

Duodenal Ulcer, non-hospitalized: Average cost and average inputs of
services by type of service, 1964 (N=35), 1971 (N=27), and
1964 treatment in 1971 prices

	Actual 1964 $	#	Actual 1971 $	#	1964 treatment 1971 prices	% increase actual	pure price
Total cost	159.49	–	186.90	–	211.63	17	33
Physician	44.17	4.7	54.94	3.8	72.42	24	64
Laboratory tests	15.19	5.4	12.59	5.4	17.11	−17	13
X-Rays	60.60	2.4	72.30	2.2	78.59	19	30
Drugs	35.49	13.3	40.40	15.2	38.17	14	8
Prescriptions	19.15	3.8	17.30	4.0	21.30	−10	11
Injections	0.29	0.1	–	–	0.30	–	3
Over-the-counter items	16.06	9.4	23.10	11.2	16.57	44	−59
Miscellaneous[1]	4.04	0.4	6.67	0.2	5.36	65	33

[1] Includes miscellaneous outpatient services.

Appendix B

TABLE 1

Average costs of treatment of selected illnesses, 1964 and 1971

	Actual 1964		Actual 1971		Significant at 5%
	Mean	Standard Deviation	Mean	Standard Deviation	
Otitis media (children)	18.34	(7.77)	25.13	(10.70)	yes
Appendicitis					
Simple	591.50	(87.19)	1062.58	(135.43)	yes
Perforated	958.72	(407.69)	2062.17	(1737.59)	yes
Maternity care[1]	527.47	(81.16)	807.08	(115.90)	yes
Cancer of the breast[2]	1558.57	(476.91)	2557.35	(636.58)	yes
Forearm fractures (children)					
Cast only	82.89	(16.02)	97.01	(36.52)	yes
Closed reduction, no general anesthetic	121.76	(20.89)	245.79	(84.13)	yes
Closed reduction, general or regional anesthetic[3]	331.85	(58.07)	521.92	(168.27)	yes
Myocardial infarction	1448.98	(747.98)	3279.87	(1682.19)	yes
Pneumonia (non-hospitalized)	75.04	(50.18)	84.98	(56.27)	no
Duodenal ulcer (non-hospitalized)	159.49	(65.63)	186.90	(100.43)	no

[1] Includes drugs.

[2] Includes costs of surgery performed as a procedure independent of the mastectomy and miscellaneous medical goods and services.

[3] This is the actual figure unadjusted for missing operating room charges.

TABLE 2

Average costs of treatment of selected illnesses, treatment unchanged

	Actual 1964		1964 Treatment 1971 Prices		Significant at 5%
	Mean	Standard Deviation	Mean	Standard Deviation	
Otitis media (children)	18.34	(7.77)	24.18	(11.14)	yes
Appendicitis					
Simple	591.50	(87.19)	1040.02	(162.82)	yes
Perforated	958.72	(407.69)	1811.53	(718.21)	yes
Maternity care[1]	527.47	(81.16)	880.53	(115.01)	yes
Cancer of the breast[2]	1558.57	(476.91)	2582.40	(699.94)	yes
Forearm fractures (children)					
Cast only	82.89	(16.02)	94.04	(13.73)	yes
Closed reduction, no general anesthetic	121.76	(20.89)	199.32	(14.34)	yes
Closed reduction, general or regional anesthetic[3]	331.85	(58.07)	476.28	(76.32)	yes
Myocardial infarction	1448.98	(747.98)	2461.07	(1200.01)	yes
Pneumonia (non-hospitalized)	75.04	(50.18)	98.88	(72.80)	yes
Duodenal ulcer (non-hospitalized)	159.49	(65.63)	211.63	(92.38)	yes

[1] Includes drugs.

[2] Includes costs of surgery performed as a procedure independent of the mastectomy and miscellaneous medical goods and services.

[3] This is the actual figure unadjusted for missing operating room charges.

TABLE 3

Average costs of treatment of selected illnesses, 1971 prices

	1964 Treatment 1971 Prices		Actual 1971		Significant at 5%
	Mean	Standard Deviation	Mean	Standard Deviation	
Otitis media (children)	24.18	(11.14)	25.13	(10.70)	no
Appendicitis					
Simple	1040.02	(162.82)	1062.58	(135.43)	no
Perforated	1811.53	(718.21)	2062.17	(1737.59)	no
Maternity care[1]	880.53	(115.01)	807.08	(115.90)	yes
Cancer of the breast[2]	2582.40	(699.94)	2557.35	(636.58)	no
Forearm fractures (children)					
Cast only	94.04	(13.73)	97.01	(36.52)	no
Closed reduction, no general anesthetic	199.32	(14.34)	245.79	(84.13)	yes
Closed reduction, general or regional anesthetic[3]	476.28	(76.32)	521.92	(168.27)	no
Myocardial infarction	2461.07	(1200.01)	3279.87	(1682.19)	yes
Pneumonia (non-hospitalized)	98.88	(72.80)	84.98	(56.27)	no
Duodenal ulcer (non-hospitalized)	211.63	(92.38)	186.90	(100.43)	no

[1] Includes drugs.

[2] Includes costs of surgery performed as a procedure independent of the mastectomy and miscellaneous medical goods and services.

[3] This is the actual figure unadjusted for missing operating room charges.

REFERENCES

Introduction

1. The periods covered by our study were the 18-month periods January 1951 through June 1952, and January 1964 through June 1965. These periods are referred to as 1951 to 1964. In the article on this study, these periods were referred to as 1951 and 1965.

2. Scitovsky, Anne., "An Index of the Cost of Medical Care—A Proposed New Approach," *The Economics of Health and Medical Care*, Proceedings of the Conference on the Economics of Health and Medical Care (May 10-12, 1962). Ann Arbor: University of Michigan, 1964, pp. 128-142.

3. For a more detailed discussion, see Scitovsky, Anne A., "Changes in the Costs of Treatment of Selected Illnesses, 1951-65," *American Economic Review*, December 1967, vol. LVII, pp. 1182-1195. See also Barzel, Yoram, "Costs of Medical Treatment: Comment," and Scitovsky, Anne A., "Costs of Medical Treatment: Reply, "*American Economic Review*, September 1968, vol. LVIII, pp. 936-940. The detailed unpublished report on the study is available from University Micro-films, 300 North Leek Road, Ann Arbor, Michigan 48106 (Film reel #387).

4. Our study again covered an 18-month period, January 1971 through June 1972. This period is referred to as 1971.

5. For pneumonia and duodenal ulcer, we shall present data only for patients treated on an ambulatory basis since there were too few hospitalized cases in the study.

6. For a description of the selection, and the reasons for the selection, of the particular conditions covered by the studies, see the papers cited in footnote 3.

7. The PAMC offers a few prepaid plans. However, these account for only about 15% of its total revenue.

8. The California Relative Value Studies, prepared and revised periodically by the California Medical Association, is:

> . . .a reflection of the practice of medicine in California. It is a coded listing of physician services with unit values to indicate the relativity within each individual section of median charges by physicians for these services. . .

> The primary purpose of the RVS is to precisely describe and code the services provided by physicians. The general acceptance of the RVS by insurance carriers and government agencies assures the physician who uses its coding and terminology that the services and procedures he performs are identifiable. With appropriate consideration to individual and local variations in practice, the RVS may also be used:

> 1. as a guide to physicians in establishing fees;

> 2. as a guide for insurance carriers and government agencies in determining their commitment;

> 3. and as a guide in evaluating individual claims."

The CRVS consists of five independent sections: (1) Medicine; (2) Anesthesia; (3) Surgery; (4) Radiology; and (5) Pathology (formerly Laboratory). The unit values of one section bear no relation to those of any other. Thus, if a physician wants to use the CRVS as a guide to establishing his fees, he would use one particular dollar conversion factor for, say, an office visit (Medicine) and an entirely different one for a surgical procedure (Surgery). For details, see *1969 California Relative Value Studies*, 5th ed., California Medical Association, 693 Sutter Street, San Francisco, California 94102.

Part I

1. Klarman, Herbert E., Dorothy P. Rice, Barbara S. Cooper, and H. Louis Stattler III, *Sources of Increase in Selected Medical Care Expenditures, 1929-1969*. Department of Health, Education, and Welfare, Social Security Administration, Office of Research and Statistics, Staff Paper No. 4, April 1970.

2. Feldstein, Martin S., *The Rising Cost of Hospital Care*. Information Resources Press, Washington, D.C., 1971.

3. Fuchs, Victor R. and Marcia J. Kramer, *Determinants of Expenditures for Physicians' Services in the United States, 1948-68*. Department of Health, Education, and Welfare, National Center for Health Services Research and Development, DHEW Publication No. (HSM) 73-3013, December 1972.

4. Scitovsky, Anne A., "Changes in the Costs of Treatment of Selected Illnesses, 1951-1965, "*American Economic Review*, December 1967, vol. LVII.

5. We are omitting our data on gangrenous cases which, in terms of severity and costs, are somewhere between simple and perforated cases of appendicitis. There were few cases and their costs varied much more widely than those of simple and perforated cases.

6. Cases treated by radical mastectomy only. Cases treated by simple mastectomy were excluded because of their small number.

7. To calculate theses percentages, we used the usual formula:

$$\frac{Q_i P_i}{Q_o P_o} = \frac{Q_o P_i}{Q_o P_o} \times \frac{Q_i P_i}{Q_o P_i}$$

where Q_o and P_o are quantities and prices, respectively, in the base year and Q_i and P_i quantities and prices, respectively, in the later year. Thus, the first term in the equation expresses the total change in costs (the ratio of actual average costs in the later year to those in the base year). The second expresses the pure price change (the ratio of quantities in the base year in prices of the later year to actual average costs in the base year). The third term expresses the net effect of changes in inputs (the ratio of actual average costs in the later year to quantities in the base year in prices of the later year). In cases where the net effects of changes in treatment were cost—saving, the "pure" price increase is greater than the actual increase in average costs and shows the increase that would have occurred if only prices had changed and treatment had remained constant.

To illustrate the method, it may help to use some actual dollar figures from Table 1, e.g., those for cancer of the breast. The formula is:

$$\frac{\$1503.93\ (Q_i P_i)}{\$739.39\ (Q_o P_o)} = \frac{\$1295.06\ (Q_o P_i)}{\$739.39\ (Q_o P_o)} \times \frac{\$1503.93\ (Q_i P_i)}{\$1295.06\ (Q_o P_i)}$$

This gives us the following index numbers:

203 (actual changes in average costs) = 175 (pure price change) x 116 (pure change in inputs)

or the following percentage changes:

103% increase in actual average costs, 75% pure price increase, and 16% pure input increase.

8. Cases treated by simple mastectomy were excluded because of their small number.

9. There were no changes in the treatment of cases requiring a cast only.

10. We did not reproduce the detailed 1951-1964 tables because they can be found in the unpublished complete report on our earlier study (see footnote 4 above).

11. Data on hospitalized cases of both conditions are excluded because of the small number of cases.

12. Cases requiring a cast only are omitted from the discussion because treatment stayed practically unchanged.

13. One of the PAMC orthopedists advised us which of the regional anesthetics were given in place of a general or a local anesthetic and should therefore be included in this group. In our comparable 1964 group, only three cases had such regional anesthetics, the rest a general anesthetic; and all cases were treated in the hospital on an inpatient basis.

14. Omitted from this calculation was one patient who had the same fracture reduced twice, involving two separate hospital episodes.

15. i.e., days in the ICU, CCU and intermediate CCU.

16. In the absence of readily available data on total number of cases in 1964, data for 1965 was used. In addition, since for 1965 no separate data on the number of radical mastectomies were available, we applied in 1971 ratio of mastectomies to all other breast surgery to the 1965 data for breast surgery. Source: National Center for Health Statistics, *Surgical Operations in Short-Stay Hospitals for Discharged Patients, United States—1965*, Vital and Health Statistics, Series 13, No. 7.

17. Data on the total number of appendectomies in 1971 from *Surgical Operations in Short—Stay Hospitals, United States—1971*, National Center for Health Statistics, Vital and Health Statistics, Series 13, No. 18. The data for total number of myocardial infarctions are from *Inpatient Utilization of Short—Stay Hospitals by Diagnosis, United States—1971*, National Center for Health Statistics, Vital and Health Statistics, Series 13, No. 16. Our estimates of the costs of the net additional inputs for myocardial infarction are probably on the high side since we excluded in our study cases who died within three months of the onset of their coronary attack.

18. Scitovsky, Anne A., *op. cit.*

19. Davis, Karen, "The Distribution of Medicare and Medicaid Benefits Among the Elderly," paper presented at the American Economic Association, San Francisco, December 30, 1974. See especially pp. 14-21.

20. Data from National Center for Health Statistics. We were unable to get data going back to 1951.

21. See Martin, Samuel P., *et al.*, "Inputs into Coronary Care During 30 Years—A Cost Effective Study, *"Annals of Internal Medicine*, September 1974, Vol. 81, No. 3. Astvad, K., *et al.*, "Mortality from Acute Myocardial Infarction Before and After Establishment of a Coronary Care Unit," *British Medical Journal*, March 23, 1974. Bloom, Bernard S. and Osler L. Peterson, "End Results, Cost and Productivity of Coronary Care Units," *The New England Journal of Medicine*, January 11, 1973, Vol. 288, No. 2.

22. Mather, H.G., *et al.*, "Acute Myocardial Infarction: Home and Hospital Treatment," *British Medical Journal*, August 7, 1971.

Part II

1. See also our brief discussion of quality change in Part I, pp. 33-36 above.

2. For details, see Scitovsky, Anne A., "Changes in the Costs of Treatment of Selected Illnesses, 1951-1965," *American Economic Review*, December 1967, vol. LVII.

3. Sobaski, William J., Anne A. Scitovsky and Nelda McCall, *The 1969 California Relative Value Studies and Costs of Physician Office Visits: Two Studies*. Health Policy Program, School of Medicine, University of California, San Francisco, Calif., September 1975. See also Social Security Administration, Office of Research and Statistics, *Effects of the 1969 California Relative Value Studies on Costs of Physician Services Under SMI*. DHEW Pub. No. (SSA)75-11702 (June 20, 1975). SMI—Supplementary Medical Insurance—is a voluntary program covering a large part of the cost of physician services and some other services not covered under the basic Medicare plan. This is the complete Social Security Administration study and also shows that fees for physician hospital visits showed much the same pattern as those for office visits.

4. We have used the 1966 fee schedule since we did not have a complete 1964 fee schedule.

SECTION V

HUMAN CAPITAL

21. The Production of Health: An Exploratory Study

RICHARD AUSTER, IRVING LEVESON, AND DEBORAH SARACHEK

ABSTRACT

The relationship of mortality of whites to both medical care and environmental variables is examined in a regression analysis across states in 1960. Medical care is alternatively measured by expenditures and by the output of a Cobb-Douglas production function combining the services of physicians, paramedical personnel, capital, and drugs. Simultaneous equation bias resulting from the influence of factor supply curves and demand for medical care is dealt with by estimating a more complete model. Both two-stage least squares and ordinary least squares estimates are presented.

The elasticity of the age-adjusted death rate with respect to medical services is about −0.1. Environmental variables are far more important than medical care. High education is associated with relatively low death rates. High income, however, is associated with high mortality when

Richard Auster is an Assistant Professor, City College of the City University of New York. Irving Leveson is Chief Research Specialist, Office of Comprehensive Planning, New York City Department of City Planning. Deborah Sarachek is testing her local postnatal care facilities.

* The research was done under the auspices of the National Bureau of Economic Research "Productivity in the Service Industries" project, financed by a grant from the Ford Foundation; the "Health" project, financed by a grant from the Commonwealth Fund; with a grant of computer time from IBM Corporation. The authors wish to express thanks to Victor R. Fuchs for his encouragement and support as well as for his extensive comments and suggestions. Without his pioneering work, this study would not have been possible. Also appreciated is the assistance rendered in the form of comments and criticisms by Gary Becker, Philip Enterline, Michael Grossman, Reuben Gronau, Herbert Klarman, Sidney Leveson, John Meyer, Robert Michael, Jacob Mincer, David O'Neill, Melvin Reder, and Morris Silver. Finally, thanks are due to Robin Ringler, Ira Silver, Lorraine Wolch, and especially Henrietta Lichtenbaum for research assistance.

All appendixes referred to and additional tables are available from the authors upon request.

medical care and education are controlled for. This may reflect unfavorable diets, lack of exercise, psychological tensions, etc. The positive association of mortality with income may explain the failure of death rates to decline rapidly in recent years. Adverse factors associated with the growth of income may be nullifying beneficial effects of increases in the quantity and quality of care. If so, the view that we have reached a biological limit to the death rate is not valid.

INTRODUCTION

The Problem

The medical industry is one of the more important industries in the U.S. and one of the fastest growing. Moreover, it is an industry in which government plays a large and increasing role.[1] Government activities now encompass the sponsorship or undertaking of most medical research, the financing of medical care and hospital construction, the regulation of the supply of personnel and the practice of medicine, and the financing of medical education. Government decisions affect the way in which resources are allocated between health and other goals, between medical services and other determinants of health, and among the various types of medical services. (The term "medical" services is used here to include public health activities.) If such allocation decisions are to be optimal, it is necessary to know both the costs of and returns to each possible use. While in similar fields, such as education, information on returns has become increasingly available, in the health field, work has largely centered on costs alone.

Recently some attempts have been made to evaluate the economic benefits of improvements in health.[2] However, as yet no one has answered in a satisfactory way the very basic question: "What is the contribution of medical services as opposed to environmental factors and to changes in the health of the population?" (The term "environmental factors" is used here simply to refer to all factors other than medical and health services.) Certainly more studies of the effects of specific therapeutic techniques on

---

1   In recent years almost one-third of national health expenditure has been made by government. Total medical care spending is now running at an annual rate in excess of $50 billion. While employment in the U.S. has grown at a rate of 1.2 percent per year since 1929, employment in the health industry has grown at 3.5 percent.

2   For example, see Selma J. Muskin, "Health as an Investment," *Journal of Political Economy*, 70:5, Pt. 2, Supp. (October 1962), pp. 129–57; Burton A. Weisbrod, *Economics of Public Health* (Philadelphia: University of Pennsylvania Press, 1961); Victor R. Fuchs, "Some Economic Aspects of Mortality in the United States," unpublished ms., National Bureau of Economic Research, July 1965; Mary Lou Larmore, "An Inquiry into an Econometric Production Function for Health in the United States" (Ph.D. diss., Northwestern University, August 1967).

health and of the role of the factors of production in individual health programs are needed.[3] However, for broad policy questions, there is also a
need for the measurement of the over-all effect of "medical services" on
health and of the contribution of each of the factors of production which
combine to produce "medical services."

Past studies of the factors influencing health have commonly dealt
with a few variables at a time. Information on the effectiveness of medical
services in improving health has typically been derived from the relatively
few deliberate or "natural" experiments whose results were such as to make
the impact of medical care easily discernible. The situations that were the
subject of these experiments have been limited to a relatively small part of
the health spectrum; most of them were in areas where medical accomplishments have been atypically great. Moreover, for a growing range of problems the importance of environmental conditions makes it impossible to
determine adequately the impact of medical services on health solely in
experimental circumstances. For these problems, a broad attempt to separate environmental effects from the impact of medical care on health is
desirable, both as a policy guide and as an indicator of directions for further study. The influence of socioeconomic factors on health has frequently
been considered apart from studies of the impact of medical care. In order
to properly determine the role of medical care and other forces, both are
best considered together.

The following sections describe variants of an econometric model
designed to determine the causes of geographic variation in health, estimate
the coefficients of the model, and consider some of their implications.

The Model

Some of the most difficult problems in medical economics revolve around
the definition and measurement of the output of the medical and health
services industry. If we define output according to the services provided,
our definition would imply such measures as physicians' visits and patient
days in hospitals. Under such a definition, productivity analysis would be
concerned with the production of medical services themselves. If, however,
the production process is viewed as one that changes the health status of
the population, medical services must be considered as an intermediate
product in the "production" of health.[4] Because of our concern with the
impact of medical services on health, we take the latter approach. This
deviates from the usual practice of defining output as a good or service.
We define output as the result derived from the use of that good or service,

3   For a summary of some of these studies, see Victor R. Fuchs, "The Contribu-
    tion of Health Services to the American Economy," *Milbank Memorial Fund
    Quarterly*, 44:4 (October 1966), pp. 65–101.
4   See Victor R. Fuchs, "The Contribution of Health Services . . . ," pp. 66–70,
    and Kenneth E. Boulding, "The Concept of Need for Health Services," *Milbank
    Memorial Fund Quarterly*, 44:4 (October 1966), pp. 202–21.

because we are primarily interested in finding ways to improve health.[5] Moreover, because of consumer ignorance about the impact of medical services on health, the possibility that medical services are not competitively priced, and a possible divergence between private and social benefits, we are not willing to assume that the optimum quantity of medical care is already being provided. Instead, we would like to determine the benefits of medical care and compare them with costs, to arrive at judgments as to whether additional expenditures are warranted.

Given the amount of medical services that a group of individuals consumes and socioeconomic variables, it should be possible to predict what the health of the group will be. We assume that genetic factors either are reasonably constant across states, or do not vary systematically with our independent variables, so that the other variables are assumed not to be influenced by genetic effects on health. Thus we hypothesize that health will be a function of the amount of medical services (M) consumed in that state and certain environmental variables.[6]

Percent nonwhite (X_0). At a given level of income, education, etc., nonwhites may have poorer sanitation, housing, etc., as a result of discrimination.

Income (X_1). It has been observed that higher income people tend to consume higher quality goods, better housing, etc., which may favorably affect their health. On the other hand, high incomes may permit a general style of life that is not conducive to health, particularly because the individual may be able to compensate for the adverse effects of his consumption pattern by simultaneously consuming more medical care. In addition, an increase in income may require entering those occupations which involve less exercise and/or more tension. This variable acts as a proxy for a host of factors for which we would prefer specific measures.

Education (X_2). Higher levels of education may be associated with relatively more medical care at preventive stages. In addition, the better educated may provide more care for themselves or members of their families, or simply be more willing to take the doctor's advice.

Standard Metropolitan Statistical Areas (SMSA's), percent of population inside SMSA's (X_3). Urbanization may have adverse effects on health because of such factors as air and water pollution, congestion, etc.

Percent employed in manufacturing (X_4). This index of industrialization was found to be significant by Fuchs. It may reflect patterns of work or simply general air pollution.

Alcohol consumption per capita (X_5) *and cigarette consumption per capita* (X_6). These two consumption items are included explicitly because of their special interest and our ability to measure them.

---

5 Defining the output of the medical industry by medical outcomes is similar to Lancaster's focus on attributes of goods and services and Becker's on characteristics. See Kelvin Lancaster, "A New Approach to Consumer Theory," *Journal of Political Economy*, 74 (April 1966), and Gary S. Becker, "A Theory of the Allocation of Time," *Economic Journal*, 75 (September 1965).

6 The sources and methods used are contained in Appendix A.

Percent in white-collar occupations (X_7). This is a proxy variable for factors like stress and exercise.

Females not in the labor force (percent of females not in the labor force, married, with husband present) (X_8). If labor force activity is more adverse to health than household activity, this variable will be positively related to health. In addition, women out of the labor force provide medical services to other members of their families. It may not be highly skilled care, but it is personal and in the right place at the right time. If there is important variation in such home production, the variable will also tend to have a positive relation to health.

We also add a variable indicating the effectiveness of medical care:

Medical school (a dummy variable coded 1 for states with medical schools and 0 for those without) (X_9). It is hypothesized that the quality of medical care will be higher and the technology more advanced in hospitals associated with medical schools than in others. Also, it is assumed that medical schools disseminate information and provide continuous training to physicians in the community.

Specifically, we write the following production function for health:[7]

$$(1) \qquad H = A_1 M^{\sigma_0} \prod_{i=1}^{9} X_i^{\sigma_i} e^{\epsilon_1}$$

where ϵ_1 is a random disturbance term which is assumed to be normally distributed. We intend in this formulation (Model I) to measure M by expenditures on medical care per capita (E). The price elasticity of demand for medical services appears to be very close to zero. Price variation may therefore act similarly to measurement error in an independent variable which, if uncorrelated with the dependent variable, would bias the regression coefficient of expenditures downward. An alternative formulation will be considered later.

The primary purpose of this paper is to estimate σ_0, the elasticity of health with respect to medical services. This could be done directly by estimating equation (1) by ordinary least squares. However, to do so would result in biased estimates owing to the simultaneous nature of the problem. This can be illustrated by considering the meaning of the coefficient of physicians in an equation relating it and other variables to health.

---

7 The writing of this equation involves two further assumptions: first, that the amount of medical services produced in an area equals the amount consumed there; second, that health is a function of this year's medical services only, e.g., that the state of the group's health is not affected by the amount of medical services or environmental factors prevailing over the lifetimes of members of the group. Correlations for the various variables by state between the years 1940, 1950, and 1960 are very high, indicating that relative conditions in each state have not changed greatly over time. As a test of whether this is a source of serious bias, a migration variable was introduced into the production equation. The results (not shown) were not materially affected. Inclusion of variables for the years in question would introduce a high degree of multicollinearity into our estimates. The adverse effects of this would most likely

One is tempted to interpret this coefficient as a measure of the effect of doctors on health. Consider, however, that where health is poor, *ceteris parabis,* the demand for doctors will tend to be high. If doctors move around the country in such a way as to equalize returns to medical practice, then areas with poor health will tend to attract a greater than average number of doctors per capita. Or, to put the matter more precisely, not only does the coefficient in question measure the elasticity of health with respect to doctors, but also the elasticity of doctors with respect to health. In order to deal with the simultaneity, estimates are obtained by using two-stage least squares. This technique involves the replacement of each independent endogenous variable in equation (1) by predicted values obtained by regressing that variable on all of the exogenous variables in the model.[8] Equations for the demand for medical services, and the supplies of physicians, paramedical personnel,[9] and hospital capital[10] were specified. These equations, together with equation (1) give us the following set of exogenous variables:

X_0 Percent white.
X_1 Income.
X_2 Education.
X_3 Percent of population inside SMSA's.
X_4 Percent employed in manufacturing.
X_5 Alcohol consumption per capita.
X_6 Cigarette consumption per capita.
X_7 Percent in white-collar occupations.
X_8 Married women out of the labor force.
X_9 Medical school.
X_{10} Percent of population more than 60 years old.
X_{11} Birth rate.
X_{12} Percent foreign born.
X_{13} Percent of health expenditures financed by health insurance.
X_{14} Percent of health expenditures in state and local governmental short-term hospitals.
X_{15} Percent of population rural.
X_{16} Percent of population in SMSA's of 1 million or more.
X_{17} Ratio of 1960 to 1950 population.
X_{18} Total property income.
X_{19} Labor force participation rate of females.

The classification of variables as endogenous or exogenous is necessarily somewhat arbitrary and is dictated in part by the completeness of our

---

outweigh the benefits from improved specification. The related problem of selective migration was examined by comparing the difference between deaths by state of residence and deaths by state of occurrence with residuals from early runs and found unimportant.

8 See J. Johnston, *Econometric Methods* (New York: McGraw-Hill Book Co., 1963), ch. 9.

9 All persons employed in the industry "medical and other health services," with the exception of physicians and surgeons.

10 The derivation and estimation of these equations is contained in Appendixes C and D and the basic data in Appendixes F and G.

model. Consideration of classifications implied by other models is beyond the scope of this article.

As an alternative to measuring medical services by expenditures, we can specify a production function for medical services. Specifically, we can write

(2) $$M = A_1 D^{a_1} N^{a_2} K^{a_3} R^{a_4} G^{a_5} X_9^{a_6} e^{\epsilon_2}$$

where

D = number of physicians per capita.
N = number of paramedical personnel per capita.
K = medical capital per capita.
R = prescription drug expenditures per capita.
G = percent of practicing physicians in group practice.
X_9 = medical school.

Note that in addition to the four input measures, two efficiency variables, group practice and medical school, are included.

Group practice (G). Many people believe that medical care produced in group practice tends to have a more favorable end result because the care is more continuous and there is better exchange of information between the physicians. We expect a positive coefficient for this variable in equation (2) and a negative coefficient in equation (3) below. Substituting equation (2) into equation (1) yields

$$H = (A_1 A_2^{\sigma_0}) (D^{a_1} N^{a_2} K^{a_3} R^{a_4} G^{a_5} X_9^{a_6})^{\sigma_0} \prod_{i=1}^{9} X_i^{\sigma_i} e^{\epsilon_1 + \epsilon_2}$$

If we then impose the restriction that $\sum_{i=1}^{4} a_i = 1$, that is, that the production function of medical services exhibits constant returns to scale, we can obtain an estimate of σ_0 by summing the coefficients of D, N, K, and R; that is,

(3) $$\sigma_0 a_1 + \sigma_0 a_2 + \sigma_0 a_3 + \sigma_0 a_4 = \sigma_0 \sum_{i=1}^{4} a_i = \sigma_0$$

Equation (3) together with the exogenous variables listed for Model I will be referred to as Model II; Models I and II will enable us to investigate the impact of medical services and environmental factors on health. This will be done by an analysis of interstate differences in health in 1960.[11]

---

11 The use of individuals rather than states as the unit of observation would present many problems because of transitory influences. For example, high income individuals might have better health because those with poor health can work less frequently or earn lower wages. The use of states requires attention to the

Measurement of Health

The growing awareness that as the incomes of nations grow, medical services are devoted to an increasing number of problems—disability, mental
illness, problems of aging, etc.—has caused researchers to devise an ever
increasing number and variety of measures to supplement the use of death
rates. Among these are measures of the prevalence of chronic conditions
and activity limitations, and measures of work loss and bed disability.

Measures of mortality possess a number of properties which make
them suitable for health research. They are objectively measured, reasonably accurate, readily available, and universally understood. Their use in
any new study has the feature of comparability with earlier work.[12] However, even within the class of mortality measures, many indices have been
used in the past. These indices differ according to whether they are crude
death rates or rates standardized to a common age distribution, or whether
they are death rates for specific age groups or for all age groups combined.
In some cases life expectancy has been used.[13]

Age and sex specific death rates are preferred in principle, but not
enough information was available to derive measures of the amount of
medical care each age or sex group receives. It did not seem reasonable to

---

distribution of characteristics and resources among individuals because relationships among aggregates may depend on them. However, it reduces the importance of transitory factors. One reason for this is that health is likely to vary
much less relative to variation in income across states than across individuals.
Another advantage of using states is that medical knowledge probably varies
less across them than over time or across countries, at least for recent years
when the death rate has changed little. Finally, with states, variations in reporting practices and in the accuracy of information, which may be serious at the
individual level, tend to average out.

12　Fuchs points out that the ranks across geographic divisions of measures of
mortality and morbidity tend to be correlated in spite of inadequacies in the
morbidity measures. The lowest correlations are with measures indicating the
presence of chronic conditions. For example, the rank correlation of age-
adjusted death rates with age-adjusted average work loss days per person 17
years and older is .65, while it is only 0.08 with the age-adjusted percentage
of persons with one or more chronic conditions and some activity limitation.
See "Some Economic Aspects of Mortality . . . ," Table 2.

13　Different patterns of age-specific death rates can result in the same average age
at death; even when they do, people may prefer one pattern over another.
Average life expectancy is in principle superior to age-adjusted death rates since
it takes into account not only variation in the average age at death, but also
differences in patterns of age-specific death rates. Once the importance of the
entire distribution of age-specific death rates is recognized, a number of other
measures of aspects of health are immediately suggested. For any given average
age at death, a greater or lesser dispersion of the average age at death across
individuals, or other characteristics of the distribution, may be considered
desirable. Persons who weigh more immediate improvements more heavily than
later ones may at any given age feel better off from a reduction in age-specific
death rates in age groups which they are immediately approaching than from
an even larger reduction in the future, even though that larger reduction has a
greater effect on average life expectancy. This suggests still another measure: a
"discounted life expectancy" that gives greater weight to more immediate
gains.

TABLE 1

PRODUCTION OF HEALTH, TOTAL POPULATION, MODEL I,
ORDINARY LEAST SQUARES

		Linear		Log	
		Regression Coefficient	Standard Error	Regression Coefficient	Standard Error
Intercept		6.776	.783	.860	.164
Percent nonwhite	(X_0)	.054	.008	.048	.009
Income	(X_1)	.057	.029	.023	.084
Education	(X_2)	—.152	.086	—.153	.138
Percent in SMSA's	(X_3)	—.002	.003	—.012	.006
Percent in manufacturing	(X_4)	.008	.007	.049	.020
Alcohol consumption per capita	(X_5)	.060	.197	.031	.046
Cigarette consumption per capita	(X_6)	—.019	.011	.141	.063
Health expenditures per capita	(E)	—.084	.007	—.084	.081
Medical school	(X_9)	—.020	.158	—.020	.011
R^2		.761		.674	

assume that the relative use of medical services per capita in each age group was the same in every state, in spite of variations in relative income, education, etc. The decision was made to examine age-sex-adjusted death rates.

The use of age-adjusted death rates as the measure of health for the purpose of determining the impact of medical services presumes that a constant proportion of medical services is devoted to prolonging life as opposed to reducing pain or other health-related goals. The use of an insufficiently comprehensive measure of health can lead to biased measurement of the impact of medical services on health. For example, we might understate the effect of medical care on mortality if a relatively large proportion of medical services tended to be used for goals other than to prolong life in states using large amounts of medical care per capita. This problem is considered further in discussing the results.

The difference in geographic patterns between life expectancy and age-adjusted death rates (adjusted to the U.S. age distribution by the indirect method) is small in the U.S. at the present time. The correlation coefficient between the two measures across states in 1960 is 0.96. The life expectancy data were supplied by Harley B. Messenger.

A number of readers have mentioned the possibility of omitting violent deaths. These are intended to be influenced by medical care, as are "natural" deaths. In any event, they are a small part of the total and their exclusion would have little effect.

TABLE 2

CORRELATION COEFFICIENTS, WHITE POPULATION, LOGARITHMS

	Income (X_1')	Education (X_2')	Percent in SMSA's (X_3')	Percent in Manufacturing (X_4')	Alcohol Consumption per Capita (X_5')	Cigarette Consumption Per Capita (X_6')	Health Expenditures per Capita (E)	Medical School (X_9')
Age-sex adjusted death rate (H')	.447	−.044	.112	.381	.378	.478	.166	−.100
Income (X_1')		.551	.265	.278	.671	.463	.680	.085
Education (X_2')			−.112	−.195	.330	.224	.467	−.161
Percent in SMSA's (X_3')				.273	.172	.050	.230	.352
Percent in manufacturing (X_4')					.021	.116	.061	.611

THE RESULTS

Determinants of Death Rates—Model I

Initially, we attempted to determine the production relationship for whites and nonwhites combined. Table 1 presents Model I results for this specification, estimated by ordinary least squares. The large positive coefficient of color would imply that nonwhites experience higher death rates than whites, holding constant both the levels of socioeconomic variables and the quantity of medical care. Percentage nonwhite is correlated with many of the other variables, making it difficult to separate their effects from variation associated with color and introducing some doubt as to the accuracy of the estimated effect of the color variable itself. For example, the partial correlation between color and education, given income, is .44. Because differences between whites and nonwhites are great for many of the other independent variables, treating whites and nonwhites together raises the intercorrelation among these variables. Because color may interact with other variables, there is also a possibility of specification error. When whites are considered alone, correlation between education and income falls from .73 to .55 (see Table 2) and between education and medical care from .67 to .47. On the basis of the above considerations, it was decided to restrict the analysis to whites.

Table 3 presents Model I estimates by ordinary least squares for whites, in both linear and logarithmic forms. In the logarithmic form, the

TABLE 3

PRODUCTION OF HEALTH, WHITE POPULATION, MODEL I,
ORDINARY LEAST SQUARES

		Linear		Log	
		Regression Coefficient	Standard Error	Regression Coefficient	Standard Error
Intercept		.957	.099	—.196	.152
Income	(X_1')	.003	.002	.204	.076
Education	(X_2')	—.016	.011	—.218	.112
Percent in SMSA's	(X_3')	—.000	.000	—.000	.005
Percent in manufacturing	(X_4')	.002	.001	.040	.018
Alcohol consumption per capita	(X_5)	.013	.027	—.002	.038
Cigarette consumption per capita	(X_6)	.002	.002	.102	.056
Health expenditures per capita	(E)	—.001	.001	—.065	.065
Medical school	(X_9)	—.042	.021	—.023	.010
R^2		.517		.539	

regression coefficients are elasticities. Variables for whites were used where possible. These are indicated by a "prime" over the variable number. It was necessary to assume that the per capita usage of medical services by whites in a state is the same as for the entire population. Fuchs experimented with the assumption that the share of medical services received by whites is the same as their share of income, and found that the regression coefficients of the modified measures of medical services differed little from the original ones. This was found for our study also.

More than 50 percent of the variation among states in age-sex-adjusted death rates is associated with the combination of medical and environmental variables. The sign of health expenditures is negative, contrary to the positive zero order correlation. A 10 percent increase reduces mortality by two-thirds of a percent in the logarithmic form. Income is positively related to the death rate, while education has a negative association. This finding is not the result of intercorrelation between the two variables. The coefficient for income remains positive after the education variable is omitted. The same signs appear even in the simple correlations. Also, the use of the age-adjusted income and education measures does not change the results. Urbanization does not appear to be important when other factors are held constant, either in the form shown or when alternative measures are used. However, the index of industrialization—percentage of employment in manufacturing—is positively related to mortality. Cigarette

TABLE 4

PRODUCTION OF HEALTH, WHITE POPULATION, MODEL I,
TWO-STAGE LEAST SQUARES, LOGARITHMS

		Regression Coefficient	Standard Error
Intercept		—.135	.162
Income	(X_1')	.212	.075
Education	(X_2')	—.194	.114
Percent in SMSA's	(X_3')	—.000	.005
Percent in manufacturing	(X_4')	.039	.018
Alcohol consumption per capita	(X_5)	.014	.041
Cigarette consumption per capita	(X_6)	.099	.056
Health expenditure per capita[a]	(E)	—.116	.082
Medical school	(X_9)	—.021	.010
R^2		.551	

[a] Endogenous.

consumption per capita exhibits a positive association with mortality, but alcohol consumption does not have a consistently positive sign.[14] The effect of per capita medical services appears to be small, but, as was indicated in the previous section, estimates of the effect of medical services on the death rate by ordinary least squares are subject to simultaneous equations bias. States with medical schools tend to have lower mortality rates than those without them. A coefficient of —.02 in the logarithmic form implies that states with medical schools, all other things being equal, have lower death rates by 4.5 percent than states without medical schools.[15] A related variable—percentage of physicians in active practice under age 35 (excluding interns and residents)—was also tested. It was intended to measure the vintage of the available technology. The effects of the variable, however, disappeared when the medical school variable was introduced. Another efficiency parameter considered was hospital size, which was thought a possible reflection of quality of care. However, it did not show the expected sign, while it increased problems of multicollinearity.

Table 4 presents estimates for Model I using two-stage least squares (2SLS). The standard errors cannot be clearly interpreted, since when 2SLS is used, the underlying distributions are not known. They may nevertheless serve as a guide. As expected, the coefficient of per capita medical expenditures was increased (to —.116 with a standard error of .082).[16] The other coefficients were essentially unchanged.

In Table 5, two variables are added to the two-stage least squares equation. At this point, it should be emphasized that with the nature of the data available, improved specification often comes at the price of a radical increase in multicollinearity. While the increase in multicollinearity from the addition of the white-collar and labor force variables is not very destructive in this case, it would be if they were included in Model II. The proportion of workers in white-collar occupations is positively associated with death rates, while the proportion of married females with

---

14 Alternative estimates of the coefficients of alcohol, cigarettes, and percentage in manufacturing were derived from the demand estimating equation in Appendix C. These are .006, .200, and .029, respectively; all three are very similar to those presented in this section. In the case of alcohol, some measure of the distribution of its use might be helpful. While we have hypothesized a positive coefficient for urbanization, it should be noted that the single most important variable explaining interstate differences in motor vehicle accident death rates is population density—with a negative sign. See Victor R. Fuchs and Irving Leveson, "Motor Accident Mortality and Compulsory Inspection of Vehicles," *Journal of the American Medical Association,* 201 (August 28, 1967), pp. 657–61. Since we include accidental deaths and since population density is positively related to urbanization, urbanization may be measuring two things with opposite effects on "health," i.e., pollution and speed of cars.

15 A continuous form of this variable performed less satisfactorily. The dummy variable is still coded zero and one in logarithmic equations but is interpreted as the log of a variable coded one and ten.

16 This probably results not only from the removal of simultaneous equation bias, but also in part from the elimination of measurement error in medical expenditures variable by the use of the instruments in the first stage.

TABLE 5

PRODUCTION OF HEALTH, WHITE POPULATION, TWO-STAGE LEAST SQUARES, LOGARITHMS

		White-Collar Workers		Females Not in Labor Force		White-Collar Workers and Females Not in Labor Force	
		Regression Coefficient	Standard Error	Regression Coefficient	Standard Error	Regression Coefficient	Standard Error
Intercept		−.287	.175	.232	.251	.126	.240
Income	(X_1')	.168	.076	.226	.074	.177	.072
Education	(X_2')	−.243	.113	−.244	.113	−.312	.110
Percent in SMSA's	(X_3')	−.002	.005	.000	.005	−.003	.004
Percent in manufacturing	(X_4')	.048	.018	.025	.019	.034	.018
Alcohol consumption per capita	(X_5)	.014	.040	.006	.040	.004	.038
Cigarette consumption per capita	(X_6)	.099	.054	.084	.054	.080	.051
White-collar workers	(X_7')	.145	.075			.173	.072
Females not in labor force	(X_8')			−.233	.124	−.281	.119
Health expenditures per capita[a]	(E)	−.096	.080	−.090	.081	−.061	.077
Medical school	(X_9)	−.028	.010	−.016	.010	−.023	.010
R^2		.591		.589		.645	

[a] Endogenous in two-stage least squares runs.

husband present and out of the labor force is negatively associated with mortality. The inclusion of these two variables appreciably increases the coefficient of determination at the same time as it reduces the estimated effect of medical care on mortality.[17]

Determinants of Death Rates—Model II

Model II disaggregates medical services into four components. It is expected that this disaggregation will raise the estimate of the effect of medical services on the death rate. In the form "medical expenditures," part of the variation results from variations in price as distinguished from quantity, the former having no relevance for the death rate. To the extent that price variation operates as a kind of random measurement error, variation in expenditures will tend to overstate the true variation in quantity and result in an understatement of the regression coefficient.[18] All Model II equations are in logarithmic form. Table 6 presents estimates of Model II by ordinary least squares and instrumental variables. Capital is measured by the value of plant assets. (The problem of capital measurement is discussed in Appendix B.) As was to be expected, the instrumental variables estimation yields a higher estimate of σ_o than ordinary least squares; higher values for σ_o are also obtained vis-à-vis Model I. The coefficients of the environmental variables differ little between the two models. While σ_o, the sum of the coefficients of the factors of production, is fairly constant between alternative formulations, determination of the effects of individual factors of production is hampered by the high intercorrelations among these factors. The highest degree of correlation is between paramedical personnel and capital. In an attempt to eliminate this, the two variables were combined by linearly regressing the total number of paramedical personnel on capital and combining the factors according to the estimated conversion.[19] Estimates using this "composite" are shown in Table 7.

---

17 Two hypotheses can be advanced to explain the effect of the female labor force variable. Labor market activity may be less favorable to health than nonmarket activity. Also, females at home may provide unmeasured medical services. The former would suggest that the relationship would hold for females; the latter that it would hold for males. In fact, the coefficient is very close to zero in regressions against the white male age-adjusted death rate but is quite large for females. However, this cannot be clearly interpreted as support for the market activity hypothesis. In states where the death rate of males relative to females is high, relatively more females will be widowed and/or working. The female labor force variable, therefore, is in part a proxy for the ratio of the male to the female death rate which is correlated with the sex-specific death rates in such a way as tend to produce the observed result. On the other hand, relatively more women will be out of the labor force where the health of women is poor. The net effect of these two biases is not known.

18 Even if price did not vary, the expenditure variable, which as measured here is essentially total cost, would only be an error-free measure or the quantity of medical services, if the production function were homogeneous of degree one and factors of production were being combined in a cost-minimizing way. The latter in particular is not necessarily true in a nonprofit industry.

19 The relationship indicated fixed proportions.

TABLE 6

PRODUCTION OF HEALTH, MODEL II, WITHOUT COMPOSITES

		Ordinary Least Squares		Two-Stage Least Squares	
		Regression Coefficient	Standard Error	Regression Coefficient	Standard Error
Intercept		−.065	.157	.037	.251
Income	(X_1')	.105	.079	.183	.116
Education	(X_2')	−.161	.121	−.288	.216
Percent in SMSA's	(X_3')	−.001	.005	−.001	.005
Percent in manufacturing	(X_4')	.051	.023	.042	.040
Alcohol consumption per capita	(X_5)	−.002	.037	.013	.044
Cigarette consumption per capita	(X_6)	.094	.053	.097	.058
Drug expenditures per capita[a]	(R)	−.070	.040	−.076	.066
Physicians per capita[a]	(D)	.143	.064	.044	.111
Paramedical per capita[a]	(N)	−.190	.076	−.031	.195
Capital per capita[a] (plant assets)	(K)	−.004	.048	−.109	.141
Group practice[a]	(G)	.007	.012	.007	.021
Medical school	(X_9)	−.034	.012	−.024	.019
R^2		.639		.586	
Elasticity of the death rate with respect to medical services (σ_o)		−.121		−.172	

[a] Endogenous in two-stage least squares runs.

TABLE 7

PRODUCTION OF HEALTH, MODEL II, COMPOSITE OF CAPITAL AND PARAMEDICAL

		Ordinary Least Squares		Two-Stage Least Squares	
		Regression Coefficient	Standard Error	Regression Coefficient	Standard Error
Intercept		.018	.181	−.044	.213
Income	(X_1')	.165	.075	.183	.080
Education	(X_2')	−.263	.108	−.231	.116
Percent in SMSA's	(X_3')	−.002	.005	.000	.006
Percent in manufacturing	(X_4')	.035	.023	.039	.029
Alcohol consumption per capita	(X_5)	−.014	.038	.008	.044
Cigarette consumption per capita	(X_6)	.108	.055	.098	.059
Drug expenditures per capita[a]	(R)	−.062	.042	−.051	.064
Physicians per capita[a]	(D)	.089	.061	.003	.090
Composite of capital and paramedical per capita[a] (plant assets)	$(K+N)$	−.124	.061	−.086	.072
Group practice[a]	(G)	.001	.012	.001	.017
Medical school	(X_9)	−.028	.012	−.022	.015
R^2		.595		.557	
Elasticity of the death rate with respect to medical services (σ_o)		−.097		−.134	

[a] Endogenous in two-stage least squares runs.

The elasticity of the death rate with respect to medical services is —.134 in the two-stage least squares run, and the positive coefficient of physicians is reduced to zero. The environmental coefficients are essentially unchanged.[20] In such gross comparisons, no impact of group practice on mortality is discernible.

An attempt was made to deal more adequately with variations in the quality of physicians, in particular between general practitioners and specialists. A fixed weight composite of G.P.'s and specialists based on the national difference in their earnings was used. In addition, composites of paramedical and alternative measures of capital input were considered. The use of the physicians' composite had no effect on the results. All coefficients remain basically unchanged. Use of alternative measures of capital had a relatively negligible effect on the estimate of σ_o. However, the estimates of the individual effects of the various medical inputs did appear to be quite sensitive to alternative measures of capital. Clearly, further research is called for before the productivity of individual factors of production can be ascertained.

Attempts were made at various points in the investigation to add distribution parameters such as variables for low income and low education. It was found that in the cases considered, the explanatory power of the measures of the variables could not be improved upon by replacing them with the distribution parameters, and serious multicollinearity resulted when both forms were introduced simultaneously.

Discussion

Both models indicate that a 1 percent increase in the quantity of medical services is associated with a reduction in mortality of about 0.1 percent. Environmental conditions are a more important determinant of interstate variation in death rates. Among these, income and education play the greatest role. The effect of income on mortality is positive while that of education is negative. Urbanization is not important, but a number of labor force variables are. There is also some indication of harmful effects from cigarette smoking.

The positive coefficient of income is particularly interesting since it is contrary to gross relationships in most data. It should be borne in mind that the analysis holds constant the effects of medical care and education, variables that increase with income. Also, use of state averages, unlike use of individual observations or data grouped by income, greatly reduces the extent to which observed patterns are influenced by the tendency for some persons to have low income because their health is poor. Abstracting from these considerations, there are many reasons why income and mortality might be positively related.

---

20   In an attempt to treat incomes as an endogenous variable, the endogenous form was more highly correlated with other variables and its coefficient increased.

We view persons as simultaneously determining consumption patterns, occupation, and life styles. As incomes rise, they might choose more adverse diets, faster cars, less exercise, etc. Also, occupations with less exercise, more strain, high risk of accident, etc., might be selected in order to obtain higher income. The results of this study suggest that both occupation- and consumption-related factors may be important.

The education variable may also represent quite complex forces. We do not know if we have isolated effects of the educational process or simply greater ability or willingness to learn. Even if what we have found does represent the effects of education, it is not clear whether general education or specific health training, such as in hygiene classes and exposure to school health programs, is relevant. There are many unanswered questions as to the patterns of care to which learning leads. The more educated may seek more preventive care, obtain medical care at earlier stages of an illness, have a better follow-up on drugs prescribed and referrals, or receive more continuous care. The last factor may be related to differences in the year-to-year variability of income between the more and less educated.

In comparisons among both developed and underdeveloped countries, Irma Adelman estimated the elasticity of the death rate with respect to the number of physicians per capita for specific age groups.[21] Her estimates of the impact of medical services on health are remarkably close to those in our study. Income, the rate of growth of income, and the proportion of the labor force employed outside agriculture were held constant. It seems likely that in international comparisons the number of physicians per capita is a good index of the total quantity of death-related medical services. Furthermore, since there is limited international factor mobility, it is probable that her estimates are relatively unbiased by her use of a single equation procedure. Her negative coefficient for income may reflect such factors as education, public health, and sanitation. Also, the effect of income may not be the same at all levels. She reports no significant difference between the coefficients for underdeveloped and developed countries, which may not hold true when education is added. Education has a positive sign in the Adelman study. Across countries, it may be associated with many of the factors with which income is associated across states. The income results with education included are not reported.

IMPLICATIONS AND CONCLUSIONS

One application of our results is to provide a possible explanation of recent trends in mortality in the U.S. The age-adjusted death rate has not declined appreciably between about 1955 and 1965 (see Table 8), in spite of a substantial increase in the quantity of medical services produced per capita and probably some technological change as well. If we deflate

---

21 See "An Econometric Analysis of Population Growth," *American Economic Review*, 52 (June 1963), pp. 314–39.

TABLE 8

CONTRIBUTION OF SELECTED MEDICAL SERVICES AND
ENVIRONMENTAL FACTORS TO CHANGES IN THE
AGE-ADJUSTED DEATH RATE, 1955–65

	Percentage Change in Variable	Percentage Change in Mortality per Percentage Change in Variable	Percentage Change in Mortality
Actual change in U.S. death rate			—3.9%
National health expenditures per capita deflated by CPI for medical care	+35%	—.1%	—3.5%
Median family income deflated by CPI for all items	+32%	.2%	+6.4%
Education	+17%	—.2%	—3.4%
Cigarette consumption per capita	+18%	.1%	+1.8%

Source: U.S. Bureau of the Census, Statistical Abstract of the United States, 1967, various tables.

national health expenditures by the Consumer Price Index for medical care, we find an increase in real expenditures per capita of 35 percent between 1955 and 1965. This alone would lead us to expect a decline in the death rate of about 4 percent. The effect of the medical school variable over time cannot be similarly derived, because its effects will be spread out and depend more on the past rather than on the present growth of the schools. What, then, has offset the expected decline? The answer is provided by the environmental factors, although a literal application of the estimated coefficients to time series may not be fully justified. The growth of education would have led to a decline of about 3 percent. On the other hand, changes in real family income would have increased mortality. With a literal application of the estimates, the effect of income is 6 percent. However, occupation will tend to vary less with income over time than in cross sections, because technological change also contributes to changes in income. This suggests that a smaller estimate of the effects of income on changes in mortality is appropriate. Changes in cigarette consumption per capita would have led to a further increase of 2 percent, although this is a case for which changes over a longer period are clearly more appropriate. Our results, then, would imply that adverse environmental factors have been offsetting the advantages of increases in the quantity and quality of medical care. We can estimate the effects of improvements in the effectiveness of medical services as all changes not attributable to either changes in the quantity of medical care or environment. Literal predictions based on the variables in Table 8 would imply that in the period 1955–65 technological change reduced mortality by —3.9 minus 1.3 percent, or a total of 5.2 percent. Converted to an annual rate, this change is a change in mortality due to technology of 0.5 percent per year. Allowing for the effects of medical schools and modifying the coefficient of income would produce an even smaller estimate of the contribution of technology change in the 1955–65 period. What may be an appropriate explanation since 1955 is not likely to be for a longer period of time since in prior years the death rate fell precipitously. Unless the marginal effectiveness of medical care is substantially lower than in the past, one would have to infer that a slowdown in technological advance occurred.

It is also interesting to examine the implications of our results for white-nonwhite mortality differentials. In 1960, the white death rate was only 69 percent of the nonwhite death rate when both are adjusted to the U.S. age distribution. Medical care spending and education would account for a large part of the difference with small offsets from cigarette and possibly alcohol consumption. The application of the results on income to this problem seems highly questionable, since income may represent different variables at different ends of the income distribution. The color differential in mortality could be "explained" by our equations only if the predicted effect of income were omitted.

Some useful cost-benefit implications can be derived from the results. Dorothy P. Rice has estimated the economic cost of mortality using the present discounted value of future earnings as a measure of the loss of production to the economy. For 1963, she estimates these costs alternatively as $49.9 billion and $40.6 billion, depending on whether a 4 percent or a 6 percent rate of discount is used.[22] If the effect of a 1 percent increase in medical expenditures is to reduce death rates by 0.1 percent, as our estimates suggest, the benefit in increased production would be $40–50 million. Adding an equal percentage reduction in the loss from morbidity would bring the benefits to about $60–70 million. In 1963, however, national health expenditures were $32.9 billion, so that the costs of a 1 percent increase in medical services would have been $329 million. While this comparison implies that costs exceed benefits, it should be noted that we have only considered economic losses due to the loss of productive time. No allowance has been made either for the loss of productivity due to illness or for the large psychic costs resulting from poor health. Also, the percentage effect of an across-the-board increase in the quantity of medical care may reduce morbidity losses by a very different percentage than mortality losses. We have examined the impact of variation in medical care generally. This type of cost-benefit comparison is relevant to a general increase in the quantity of medical care such as results from increased health insurance coverage. Specific programs may be able to select problems and areas with higher returns.

---

22 Dorothy P. Rice, *Estimating the Cost of Illness,* U.S. Public Health Service Publication No. 947-6 (May 1966), Tables 31 and 32.

Statements regarding the merits of increments to educational spending *relative* to medical care can be made with less concern about the problems of benefit measurement. The effects on mortality of education are about double those of medical care, according to our estimates. Increases in education would presumably save medical resources as well. Yet a 1 percent increase in the quantity of education involves only about one and one-half times the additional dollars. This would suggest that the trade-off favors education, although again we need to know the relative effects on morbidity.[23, 24] In view of the many other benefits of education, however, this result strongly suggests that the return to expenditures on additional education are far greater than to additional expenditures on medical care.

It is possible to integrate a great many of our findings, and in particular the observed effect of income on health, into a coherent, although somewhat conjectural, framework. Let us begin with the empirical observation that the gross relationship between health and income has the form H_T in Figure 1, increasing at a decreasing rate until it becomes approximately level over a wide range. This has been found to be the case for a large number of health measures, e.g., 365 minus the number of the disability days per person per year.[25] The beneficial effects of medical care and education on health, both of which rise with income, are represented by H_{M+E}, which is monotonically increasing at perhaps a decreasing rate. H_T can be considered as resulting from H_{M+E} and the effects of factors other than medical care and education which are associated with income, H_Y. Alternatively, H_Y can be derived as a residual by subtracting H_{M+E} from H_T. In effect, we can consider H_Y to represent approximately the same factors as the income variable in our regressions. H_Y rises steadily and reaches a maximum at relatively low levels of income, declining continuously thereafter. The rising portion represents the effects of factors such as basic nutrition, sanitation, and housing, while the declining portion represents such factors as diet, exercise, and stress.[26]

This model is consistent with our finding of an adverse effect of income and also with the findings of Irma Adelman across countries, because of the unique income level of the U.S. More generally, the model tends

---

23 The value of the effect on education of improvement in health attributable to an increase in medical care is likely to be much smaller than the saving in medical care due to an increase in education. See Irving Leveson, Doris Ullman, and Gregory Wassall, "The Effects of Improved Health on Productivity Through Education," *Inquiry*, forthcoming.

24 This comparison might overstate the merits of increasing education because forgone earnings of students may be greater than forgone earnings of medical patients. Also, to some extent, interstate differences in education may reflect interstate differences in native ability which would not be increased when education is increased over time.

25 For example, see U.S. Public Health Service, *Medical Care, Health Status, and Family Income, United States,* National Center Health Statistics Report, Series 10, No. 9 (Washington: U.S. Government Printing Office, May 1964).

26 If this is correct, then by fitting a monotonic relationship to H_Y one tends to underestimate the adverse effects of factors associated with income on health.

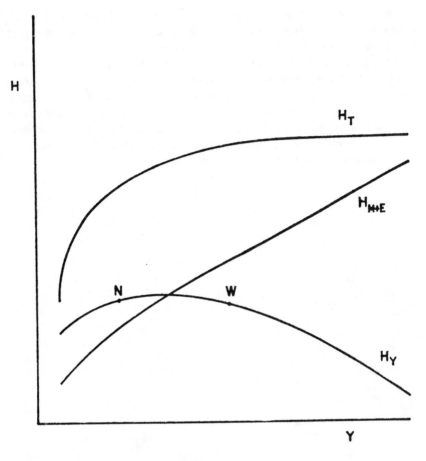

FIGURE 1

to explain the difference between our results and those of other studies concentrating on low income groups. It should also be noted that replacing the mean-income variable by the percentage of persons with low income would give a greater weight to the rising portion of the curve. When this was done, a smaller adverse effect of income was found.

Now consider the attempt to explain the white-nonwhite differential. We noted that a reconciliation could be made only if the predicted effects of income were not included. Suppose, however, that the average income of whites was at a point on H_Y such as W and those of nonwhites at N. Factors associated with income would then have both positive and negative effects on the differential. If these cancelled, the reconciliation of the color difference would be successful. If the income effect were not important in explaining the color differential, however, the fact that the death rate for whites and nonwhites combined is strongly influenced by color would mean that effect of income on the total death rate ought to be much less than on white mortality. This view is supported by the results in Table 1.

At this point we are tempted to speculate that those factors which account for the declining portion of H_Y are also responsible for the higher death rates in the United States than in many European countries. Perhaps in that comparison, differences in the way people make a living, spend money, and allocate their time more than outweigh the effects of medical care and education. We might also expect that adverse effects of stress, exercise, and diet associated with income will not apply to infants. This model would therefore predict the negative association between income and infant mortality which has commonly been found. Again, the speculative nature of these remarks needs emphasis.

22. The Relation of "Human Capital" Preservation to Health Costs

JOHN S. SPRATT, JR.

Reprinted with permission from *American Journal of Economics and Sociology* 34. Copyright © 1975, American Journal of Economics and Sociology, Inc., 295-307.

ABSTRACT. The concept of *'human capital'* has evolved in economics as a way of measuring the value society places on an individual. This value, it is argued, constitutes a real but seldom discussed limit on how much money either an individual or society will pay for the *health costs* of an individual. Conversely, it can be argued that the capacity of the health system to preserve 'human capital', as created by nature and nurture and by 'investments' in education and training, is an economic justification for health costs, just as military costs are justified for the defense of the population. In the latter instance, the greatest *public health benefit* for the dollar would be obtained by *Pareto optimal expenditures*. Similarly a microeconomic model for the *clinical process* involved in diagnosing, treating and rehabilitating the diseased individual is suggested that relates the time consumed by the elements of the clinical process to the probabilities of maximizing the preservation of the greatest number of functional man-days obtainable for an aging individual's cohort. For the model to work there would have to be an economic incentive for the *health provider* to engage in objective-oriented, interdisciplinary, cost-effective actions in the clinical process that would minimize the diseased individual's *downtime* and maximize his *functional longevity* in an *operations research* framework.

THE PURPOSES of this paper are to define the nature of 'human capital'—what the classical economists defined as the productive power of labor—to review the background of the concept of 'human capital' and the relation of this 'asset' to the economic strength of a society and to consider the relation of 'human capital' to health costs. In this view, every individual has both a current capital value based on his net worth at the moment and a potential capital value based on his future earnings. Both society and the individual have an 'investment' in this potential 'capital value' through the contribution of human time and money for nurturing,

* This investigation was supported in part by USPHS Grant No. CA 08023.

445

housing, protecting, educating and training the individual. This potential capital value is not known absolutely in any specific case, but the general parameters are known from current economic and demographic statistics. A recent study by the present writer entitled "The Measurement of the Value of the Clinical Process to Individuals by Age and Income" (1) attempts to utilize these data sources. The observation is made in that study that the forces of a market economy are a dominant determinant of the potential capital value of each individual and that this value is measurable in terms of dollar earnings. Though an individual may have varying intelligence, talents, drive and opportunity, his dollar value is still very strongly influenced by market value exterior to himself. The individual's inherited or developed relation to the oligarchy and the value the market places on different levels and types of education and work capability are fundamental determinations of the 'capital value' of a human being.

I

Since the dollar value of individual productivity is also a function of time, the potential 'capital worth' of an individual is a function of his residual longevity and functional capacity during this period. Thus, through no fault of the health care system, the same clinical process which may be enormously valuable to one individual in terms of dollars, may be of no value to another. The mean limits placed on the potential capital value of various clinical processes are given in Figures 1, 2 and 3. The frequency distributions of wealth and income are usually lognormal giving a wide distributional skew (2). Such a skew is apparently the natural consequence of the Pareto optimal equilibrium condition of wealth distribution that develops in a society managed largely by market competition (3). The disparity of a value is so great that with a uniform fee system persons with high potential incomes pay health fees that are a pittance of the potential human capital value of health services, while the very poor, paying the same fees, may pay a price far in excess of the potential capital value preserved by identical clinical procedures. Thus, a paradox can exist whereby the working poor subsidize the health care of the rich. In fact, these data support the obvious conclusion that any reimbursement system for health services based on uniform fees not subsidized by a levelling form of taxation or paid for by a uniform premium to a non-tax subsidized third-party would constitute the most pernicious form of regressive taxation. Uniform premiums and fees are equivalent to a per capita head tax that must be paid to give one a chance to survive major illness. Though the head tax is uniform, the economic value of surviving is highly variable and there is often an inverse relation between the amount of the head tax and the real dollar value of survivorship.

The peculiar disparities that exist between the perceived value of people as opposed to property were pointed out in 1875 by Johann H. von Thünen who noted that a hundred men might be expended in battle to save one cannon (4). He observed that the value of the cannon was explicit in terms of public funds, whereas the public accounting system

Table 1
Individual Downtime Factors in the Clinical Process Accruing to the Advantage of the
   Individual (a)

Time spent in diagnostic effort leading to discovery and effective treatment of diseases
   that could reduce life span or function.
Time spent in beneficial treatment (b).
Time spent in beneficial rehabilitation.
Time spent in educating and motivating people to remain well.
Time spent in educating and motivating people to make logical requests for health ser-
   vices that will accrue to their benefit.
Time spent in educating and motivating people to participate effectively in their own
   care and rehabilitation when they do become sick.

(a) Reprinted from J. S. Spratt Jr. and F. R. Watson, "The Decision Making Process
   in Cancer Patient Care," *Ca-A Cancer Journal for Clinicians*, 23 (1973), p. 155.
(b) Beneficial treatment is defined as treatment that will alleviate symptoms, preserve
   a functional attitude and motivation, restore function or preserve longevity at a
   tolerable cost.

Table 2
Individual Downtime Factors in the Clinical Process Accruing to the Disadvantage of
   the Individual (a)

Time lost for diagnostic effort not leading to beneficial treatment (b).
Treatment not restoring or preserving function.
Treatment not preserving maximum longevity.
Cost in excess of ultimate value.
Time consumed in the coordination of interdisciplinary consultation and treatment that
   does not lead to added patient benefit.
Time wasted in travel and waiting.
Time wasted by avoidable morbidity.
Avoidable mortality from elements of the clinical process.
Time spent in treatment not preserving longevity or function.
Time lost from delay in rehabilitation.

(a) Reprinted from Spratt and Watson, *op. cit.*
(b) Beneficial treatment is defined as treatment that will alleviate symptoms, restore
   function or preserve longevity at a tolerable cost.

gave human beings no explicit value. By conscription, they could be obtained for nothing. Von Thünen noted that people protested against
the uncompensated confiscation of property, but not of men. The uncompensated loss of human capital during a war has been estimated to
be of enormous proportions. Such losses deplete the wealth or potential
wealth of individuals, families and the nation as a whole.

The field of modern economics may be said to have begun with William Petty's "Essay in Political Arithmetick" of 1682 (5). The evolution
of the economic concept of 'human capital' has been well reviewed by
B. F. Kiker (6), whose work contains an excellent bibliography.

The preservation of 'human capital' is divisible into two categories of
effort. First is the effort associated with the avoidance of disease through
health-preserving individual and social practices guided by the insights
of preventive medicine. Second is the effort expended in clinical medicine for the diagnosis, treatment and rehabilitation of extant disease. In
both instances, the ability to preserve 'human capital' is confronted by an

ever closer and greater time and risk of dying created by the progressive and irreversible process of aging. This process can be slowed but never stopped. How to maximize the preservation of functional longevity while minimizing the downtime of the individual from clinical effort or disease morbidity is an operations research problem. Operations research seeks to maximize the chance of achieving specific objectives in a systematic and cost-effective way.

Reorientation of clinical decision-making to cost-effective considerations certainly requires an operations research approach. Consistent acquisition of an oversized data base, for example, can result in a chronic oversell of diagnostic laboratory and roentgen studies. Note, for example, the cost-effective consideration of the clinical actions listed in Tables 1 and 2.

Maximizing the potential 'capital value' of every individual in the society is an even more complicated operations research problem into the total cultural, social and economic fabric of the country that would set plans and priorities for the cost-effective expenditure of the entire social overhead. The social overhead is defined for present purposes as that portion of the gross national product which a society spends on health, education, welfare and the protection of its population.

Von Thünen recognized the importance of education in enhancing the value of 'human capital.' However, he did not pursue the value of maximizing the worth of the educational 'investment' through preserving longevity and function. More recent economists have tended to accept that health is a marketable commodity and that the consumer will decide what he is willing to pay to remain healthy. E. J. Mishan would have us search for Pareto improvement as a basis for public health expenditures (7). A Pareto improvement occurs when at least one person is made better off and no one is made worse off through social expenditures. The measured extent of this benefit can be related to cost and thereby become the basis of public health cost/benefit analysis. However, no sum of money is adequate to compensate an individual for his life, and here market forces play an important role by leaving the individual consumer some choice in what he will pay for health. Thus, the value of health will always remain partially a function of what the individual, on one hand, and society, on the other, will pay for health services.

What the economists dismiss rather lightly is the adverse effect that market forces may have on 'human capital' preservation. The unrestrained market can make products attractive to the consumer, motivating him to

Table 3

Life Time and Mean Income of Males 25 Years Old and Over by Years of School Completed (a)

	Elementary		High School		College	
	0–7 Yrs.	8 Yrs.	1–3 Yrs.	4 Yrs.	1–3 Yrs.	4 Yrs/More
Life Time Income ($1,000s) (b)	196	258	294	350	411	586
Annual Mean Income	3,981	5,467	6,769	8,148	9,397	12,938

(a) Adapted from U.S. Bureau of the Census *Statistical Abstract of the United States, 1972* (Washington, D.C.: U.S. Government Printing Office, 1972).

(b) Computed from ungrouped data, 1968.

buy and use things that are detrimental to his own well-being. He may do this in ignorance or in faith that the market has some rationality in its selling practices. The market, for example, does not offer a complete, economical, nutritional diet system; it offers a discordant selection of food products that through consumer selection can lead to malnutrition. The consumer must have the motivation and knowledge requisite to select a nutritional disease-preventing diet from among these discordant products. His inability to select a nutritious diet can be verified by the excess consumption of just a single non-nutritional commodity—sucrose (refined sugar)—which is a major contributor to obesity and the premature appearance of various chronic diseases (8). Such indiscretions created by the market reduce the 'human capital value' of the population through shortened life span and down time from illness. Also, the costs of health care increase.

Market economists have a very convenient escape from such unpleasant truisms by attributing to the consumer the capacity to determine priorities. However, this is less and less true as new industries, in collaboration with the motivational methods of the advertising industry, have consistently shown that consumer tastes can be directed. The political system has a certain rationality in setting consumer priorities through political action, but the process is slow and constantly behind the more versatile and aggressive promoters and advertisers.

With the assumption that all extant factors contributing to the destruction of 'human capital' are eliminated, the limits imposed on the preservation of 'human capital' are presently determined by the aging process which is progressive and irreversible (9). Strehler and Mildvan provide a stochastic model of the aging process based on a progressive loss of physiological reserve in various systems (10). Bjorksten estimates that without control over or restraint of the aging process, few would live longer than 105 years (11). Potential 'human capital value' would terminate at an even earlier age, leaving the individual dependent upon his current assets and deferred earnings (annuities).

II

KIKER AND BIRKELI have recently published a theoretical model for ascertaining the value of 'human capital' that could be advantageous in justifying or evaluating health system costs (12). These economists were concerned primarily with 'human capital' losses from war. However, if we substitute 'illness' for 'casualty' their model is adaptable to a consideration of the economics of health.

They postulated that certain variables such as education, skills, health and availability in time and space are related to the individual's capacity to earn. However, education, as measured by time spent in school, has not been well correlated with economic value of effort to the rest of society, though it is correlated with individual earnings. In fact, education not leading to the preservation or creation of products with capital value may be inflationary; *i.e.,* it depletes the value of a society's money by the wasteful expenditure of human energy often with conspicuous overconsumption by the population. As an example, witness the enormous waste of human energy and the overconsumption that occurs on a collegiate Saturday football afternoon, all occurring in the name of education and sponsored by an academic department with full backing from the academic bureaucracy that may be supported in whole or in part from the earnings of such exhibitions.

The Kiker and Birkeli model considers lost earnings based on age and educational level. Substituting clinical terms in their model, the jth patient's 'capital value' (K_j) can be estimated with the following equation:

$$K_j = \sum_{t=1}^{h-1} d_j P^*_{jt} W^e_{jt} (1+v)^{t-1} / (1+r)^{-t} \tag{1}$$

where

$$P^*_{jt} = \prod_{s=1.}^{t+1-1} \{1 - P(s)\}$$

The symbols have the following meanings:

P^*_{jt} = the probability of the jth individual's being alive at the end of the tth period after becoming ill.

W^e_{jt} = earnings of the jth individual in the tth period by preillness educational level, e.

d_j = degree of disability of the jth individual $(0 \leq d \leq 1)$.

v = rate of increase in labor productivity.

r = an 'appropriate' discount rate.

l = age of patient.

h = upper extreme of the age range (retirement age) for the jth individual $(h-1$ = number of potential earning periods).

$P(s)$ = probability of dying in periods, conditional upon being alive at the end of period $s-1$.

The total human capital loss (K) can be calculated as a per annum rate by using annual data instead of war specific data as did Kiker and Birkeli. Thus,

$$K = \sum_{j=1}^{n} K_j, \tag{2}$$

where: n denotes the total patients per annum.

Kiker does not consider that an individual retains future value to the end of his life. He simplifies the concept by retiring everyone at age 65 (13). This is an unacceptable simplification in medicine and in economics for, in fact, many persons continue productive work past age 65, maintaining their earning stream through productive work and through various types of deferred earning accounts—annuities, pensions, social security, etc. By remaining functional, they also avoid placing non-productive costs on family, friends and nursing home staffs. The consumer incomes of those past age 65 is a documented value (14).

The model in equation 1) makes certain economic assumptions. It assumes that an individual's productivity is subject to a constant positive rate of growth. The authors avoid the complexity of considering a

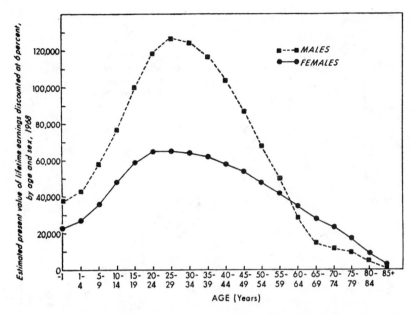

Figure 1. The average age and sex specific residual earning capacity is expressed in dollars. (These statistics are taken from Table V in D. P. Rice, B. S. Cooper and N. L. Worthington, "The Economic Cost of Digestive Diseases," presented by Rice at the Second Conference on Digestive Disease as National Problem, Bethesda, Maryland, May 8, 1973.)

variable rate of growth, but such variation does, in fact, exist and few human situations can have as adverse an effect on the rate of economic growth as can certain acute and chronic illnesses. The model provides for an adjustment based on 'normal' mortality, a value also subject to change with the more effective utilization of medical and other knowledge. The model also assumes an equilibrium state between rates of human loss and the needs of the work force. Kiker and Birkeli used common data sources on consumer income, educational data and vital statistics of the United States (15). They estimated that the human capital loss to the United States from the Vietnam War as of early 1970 was between 5.8 and 11.6 billion dollars. In the case of this war, still another source of unquantified capital loss exists. The human capital loss created in the population of the U.S. from the narcotics epidemic aggravated by this war and the security costs created by trying to control the illicit narcotic traffic are not known. The model previously published in reference 1 provides a framework for considering the significance of human capital preservation in a single individual based on the average residual earnings of his cohort of the same age and sex.

The data in Figures 1 and 2 were used in a simple way to ascertain the limiting value (L_T) of any clinical process (CP) in functional man-days (T):

as f (functional capacity of the individual) → 0, and

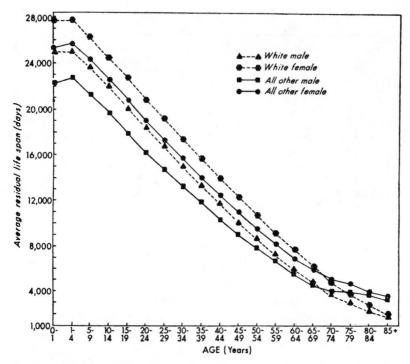

Figure 2. The average age specific residual life span in days. (This information is computed from *Vital Statistics of the United States, 1971* (Washington, D.C.: U.S. Government Printing Office, 1971), Vol. II, sect. v., "Life Tables," DHEW publication No. (HRA) 74–1147.

as T_R (age specific average number of residual man-days) $\rightarrow 0$,

$$L_T \rightarrow T_R - T_{CP} - T_r - T_W - T_M. \qquad 3)$$

Other symbols in the equation follow:

T_{CP} = Man-days consumed by activities in the clinical process.

T_r = Man-days consumed by reduced function from disease or its treatment ($r = 1 - f$).

T_W = Man-days consumed by travel, waiting, redundancies and other inefficiencies.

T_M = Man-days not salvageable by treatment.

In the complete model, the physician must decide on the course of action having the highest probability (P) for maximizing functional longevity, while minimizing patient downtime, mortality and cost. The course of action must then be negotiated as a 'trade-off' of options between the physician and the patient—commonly referred to as 'informed consent.' These options often have an estimated probability of dying (p) usually based on past experience with similar problems. The model by which the clinical process is negotiated is as follows:

$$P_p = \frac{T_R - T_{CP} - T_r - T_W - T_M}{T_R}$$

This is read that the probability (P) of preserving the optimum number of functional residual man-days of life (T_R) with a given clinical

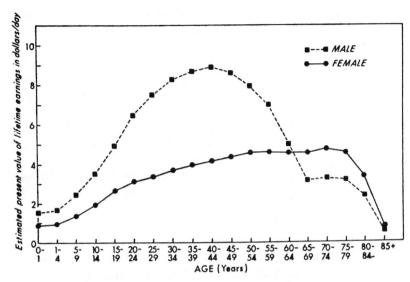

Figure 3. The average age specific number of dollars that an individual can earn per day. (These data are determined by dividing the average age specific residual income in Figure 1 by the average age specific number of man-days in Figure 2. The quotient is designated the dollar value of one functional man-day (Tarp). This is a very crude statistic derived from a series of estimates but serves the purpose of indicating an order of magnitude for the average daily dollar value of human existence in the United States, as measured by the material (and not necessarily economic) standard. Obviously public expenditures, third party disbursements, must provide cost/benefit parameters to health expenditures to avoid undue economic morbidity from illness. All health costs produce a real overhead for the provider (preparation and training, fees, contractual expenses, salaries, equipment, supplies, etc.). Presently there is no economic incentive to the provider for practicing cost-effective medicine in a market economy that is driven by the profit incentive.)

process (CP) is equal to the expected T_R for the specific age and sex less the time consumed by the clinical process (T_{CP}) (diagnostic, therapeutic and rehabilitative for his illness), time consumed from reduced function (T_r), time consumed from waste and inefficiences (T_W) and time not salvageable as a result of limitation imposed by the disease itself or the technological inability of the clinical process to measurably alter the course of the disease (T_M). The subscript (p) for P denotes the probability that the patient will die from the risks of the contemplated clinical process (CP). P_p is increasingly known from various reports on end results and risks of treatment available in the clinical literature.

Reverting to Kiker's battle casualty considerations, the health care system wages a war continuously against 'human capital' losses. Common losses secondary to illness result from 'educational' interruptions or delays, loss of existing skills or knowledge, impairment of health through drug use and decreased 'investment' by both the government, patients and the families of patients in 'industries' that normally produce 'human capital,' such as schools. The health care system can preserve 'human capital' as its economic contribution to society, and it can enhance the 'human capital value' of the society through the training, efficiency and productivity of its manpower and resources. The largest single low-cost health manpower resource is the people themselves. They can contribute to the preservation of their own potential 'capital value' and the potential 'human capital value' of their society through knowledgeable self-protective behavior. This requires consumer education against market exploitation just as Thomas Jefferson originally advocated (16). Maximizing the functional longevity of each individual in the most cost-effective way is an operations research problem within the social system of the United States and no perfect model to obtain such an ideal objective exists.

III

ACCEPTANCE OF THIS CONCEPT usually requires some reorientation of basic philosophy. The American frontier exerted a profound effect on the economic psychology of Americans. People came to believe in the availability of limitless land and resources as long as the frontier was there. It is shifting to one of improved resource management and cost effectiveness in organizational effort. One need only read Secretary Kissinger's "Strategy and Organization" to understand this philosophy and simultaneously to see why Kissinger has been such an influential presidential adviser (17). The entire military establishment is undergoing a managerial revolution to coordinate expenditures with economically relevant strategy (18).

Maximizing 'human capital' production and preservation in the United States requires an integrated awareness of the economic, social, educational, medical and strategic posture of the nation. Anytime a discordant dislocation of resources or effort occurs through unplanned and unrestrained market competition, less than optimum conditions can prevail. Selection of the most economical and effective health strategy is an exceedingly complex undertaking.

As a general principle, health budgeting priorities from the public purse can be ranked in a descending order based on the Pareto improvement in 'human capital' preservation per dollar spent. Or, in a slightly less mercenary vein, the budgeting priorities can be ranked in descending order of preserved functional man-days per dollar spent. The real costs for manpower and facilities required to achieve the various objectives in the rank sequence would have to be related to the relevance of the effort. The entire public system would have to be permeated with effective public education so that each individual, through knowledge, could protect himself from detrimental commercial pressures of all types—again as Thomas Jefferson originally recommended (19).

Cancer Research Center
Columbia, Mo. 65201

1. I have presented this data previously. See J. S. Spratt Jr., "The Measurement of the Value of the Clinical Process to Individuals by Age and Income," *The Journal of Trauma,* 11 (1971), pp. 966–73.

2. An entire article describes this distribution skew. See J. S. Spratt Jr., "The Lognormal Frequency Distribution and Human Cancer," *Journal of Surgical Research*, 11 (1969), pp. 151–57.

3. Vilfredo Pareto, *The Mind and Society: a Treatise on General Sociology* (4 vols. bound as 2), (New York: Dover, 1935), pp. 1733–1912. In order to fully understand Pareto's societal and economic study and the references herein, one should study this two volume set. Pareto integrates his economic theories with his sociological insights throughout this significant study. Also helpful is Raymond Aron's preface to the Swiss edition, Pierre Doven, ed., *Traité de Sociologie Générale* (Geneva: Librarie Droz, 1968), pp. viiff.

4. B. F. Kiker, "Von Thünen on Human Capital," *Oxford Economic Papers*, 21 (1969), p. 339. Kiker cites von Thünen's classic work to illustrate "now quite opportune views on human capital": J. H. von Thünen, *Der Isolierte Staat* (1875), translated by Bert F. Hoselitz (Chicago: Univ. of Chicago Press, no date), Vol. II, Pt. ii, pp. 140–52.

5. W. Petty, "Political Arithmetick," *The Economic Writings of Sir William Petty*, edited by Charles Henry Hull (Cambridge: Cambridge Univ. Press, 1899), Vol. I, pp. 233–313.

6. See B. F. Kiker, "The Historical Roots of the Concept of Human Capital," *Journal of Political Economy*, 74 (1966), pp. 481–99. Semantic purists, of course, object to this approach as popular, not scientific. See R. S. Eckaus, *Basic Economics* (Boston: Little Brown, 1972), pp. 628–29, however.

7. E. J. Mishan explains his theory in the following article: "Evaluation of Life and Limb: a Theoretical Approach," *Journal of Political Economy*, 79 (1971), pp. 687–705.

8. J. Yudkin, *Sweet and Dangerous* (New York: Peter H. Wyden, 1972), pp. 50–141. In chapters 6 to 14, Yudkin discusses the consequences of sucrose consumption, its relation to obesity and to various chronic diseases.

9. A number of studies support this thesis. Among them are J. Bjorksten, "Why Grow Old?" *Chemistry*, 37 (1964), pp. 6–11; B. I. Strehler and A. S. Mildvan, "General Theory of Mortality and Aging," *Science*, 132 (1960), pp. 14–21; J. Bjorksten, F. Andrews, J. Bailey and B. Trenk, "Fundamentals of Aging: Immobilization of Proteins in Whole-body Irradiated White Rats," *Journal of the American Geriatrics Society*, 8 (1960), pp. 37–47; D. Harman, "Prolongation of Life: Role of Free Radical Reactions in Aging," *Journal of the American Geriatrics Society*, 17 (1969), pp. 721–35; H. P. Loomer, "A Philosophy for Geriatric Research," *ibid.*, pp. 406–7; E. Pfeiffer, "Survival in Old Age: Physical, Psychological and Social Correlates of Longevity," *ibid.*, 18 (1970), pp. 273–85; T. H. Howell, "Some Terminal Aspects of Disease in Old Age: a Clinical Study of 300 patients," *ibid.*, 17 (1969), pp. 1034–38; Bjorksten Research Foundation, *Thirteen-year Report (1952–1965) of the Studies on Aging* (Madison, Wis.: published by the Foundation, 1965); "Aging," *Medical World News*, 12 (1971), pp. 46–48, 52–55, 57; J. Bjorksten, "Aging, Primary Mechanism," *Gerontologia*, 8 (1963), pp. 179–92; J. Bjorksten, "Aging: Present Status of Our Chemical Knowledge," *Journal of the American Geriatrics Society*, 10 (1962), pp. 125–39; S. Benet, "Secrets of 100-Year-Old Russians," *St. Louis Post-Dispatch*, January 9, 1972.

10. B. L. Strehler and A. S. Mildvan, *op. cit.*, pp. 14–21. Strehler explains his model in this article.

11. Bjorksten, "Why Grow Old?" *op. cit.*, p. 11.

12. B. F. Kiker and J. Birkeli, "Human Capital Losses Resulting from U.S. Casualties of the War in Vietnam," *Journal of Political Economy*, 80 (1972), pp. 1024–25.

13. B. F. Kiker and J. K. Weeks, "The Value of the Clinical Process: an Economist's View," unpublished paper. For Kiker the upper extreme of the age range is 'retirement age' or age 65.

14. J. S. Spratt, Jr., "The Measurement of the Value of the Clinical Process to Individuals by Age and Income," *op. cit.*, p. 969; U.S. Bureau of the Census: *Consumer Income. Annual Mean Income of Men in the U.S. for Selected Years, 1956 to 1968* (Washington, D.C.: U.S. Government Printing Office, 1969).

15. *Loc. cit.*; U.S. Bureau of the Census: *Statistical Abstract of the United States, 1969* (Washington, D.C.: U.S. Government Printing Office, 1969); U.S. Department of Health, Education and Welfare, *United States Life Tables, 1959–1961*, Public Health Service Publication No. 1252 (Washington, D.C.: U.S. Government Printing Office, 1964), Vol. 1, No. 1.

16. J. S. Spratt Jr., "Thomas Jefferson: the Scholarly Politician and His Influence on Medicine," *Southern Medical Journal*, in press, 1975.

17. H. A. Kissinger, "Strategy and Organization," *Foreign Affairs*, 35 (1957), pp. 379–84.

18. T. Bauer, *Requirements for National Defense* (Industrial College of the Armed Forces, 1970), pp. 90–93, National Security Management Series; F. R. Brown: *Management: Concepts and Practice* (Industrial College of the Armed Forces, 1967), National Security Management Series, p. 180.

19. J. S. Spratt Jr., "Thomas Jefferson: &c.," *op. cit.*

23. Application of Cost-Benefit Analysis to the Health Services and the Special Case of Technological Innovation

HERBERT E. KLARMAN

Reprinted with permission from *International Journal of Health Services* 4. Copyright © 1974, Baywood Publishing Company, Inc. 325-352.

As an economic technique for evaluating specific projects or programs in the public sector, cost-benefit analysis is relatively new. In this paper, the theory and practice of cost-benefit analysis in general are discussed as a basis for considering its role in assessing technology in the health services. A review of the literature on applications of cost-benefit or cost-effectiveness analysis to the health field reveals that few complete studies have been conducted to date. It is suggested that an adequate analysis requires an empirical approach in which costs and benefits are juxtaposed, and in which presumed benefits reflect an ascertained relationship between inputs and outputs. A threefold classification of benefits is commonly employed: direct, indirect, and intangible. Since the latter pose difficulty, cost-effectiveness analysis is often the more practicable procedure. After summarizing some problems in predicting how technologic developments are likely to affect costs and benefits, the method of cost-benefit analysis is applied to developments of health systems technology in two settings—the hospital and automated multiphasic screening. These examples underscore the importance of solving problems of measurement and valuation of a project or program in its concrete setting. Finally, barriers to the performance of sound and systematic analysis are listed, and the political context of decision making in the public sector is emphasized.

The purpose of this paper is to discuss the application of cost-benefit analysis to the assessment of technology in the health services. With the few exceptions that are noted, the focus of this paper is on services, not research.

In carrying out this task, there is no substantial body of empirical research literature to draw upon, analyze, and synthesize. Accordingly, the task will be approached in three distinct steps. First, the theory and practice of cost-benefit analysis in general will be reviewed. Second, applications to the health field will be discussed. Third, the potentialities and limitations of cost-benefit analysis for the assessment of health systems technology will be suggested, using concrete illustrations.

THEORY AND PRACTICE OF COST-BENEFIT ANALYSIS

As a formal and systematic approach to choosing among investments in public projects, cost-benefit analysis is only a generation old. It derives from the marriage of theoretical advances in the new welfare economics and the previously undernourished public expenditures branch of public finance (1). In reviews of the cost-benefit literature, few references are encountered that antedate 1958 (2-4). Most of the theoretical as well

This article is a revision of a paper presented at the Conference on Technology and Health Care Systems in the 1980s in San Francisco in January 1972, sponsored by the Health Care Systems Study Section, National Center for Health Services Research and Development.

as empirical research has been carried out in connection with water resources projects (5-10).

Aims and Criteria of Choice

Cost-benefit analysis aims to do in the public sector what the better known supply-demand analysis does in the competitive, private sector of the economy. When market failure occurs—whether through the absence of a market or through the existing market's behaving in undesirable ways—public intervention comes under consideration (11). Cost-benefit analysis is helpful in determining the nature and scope of such intervention.

The most egregious example of lack of a market is given by the case of the pure public good. Such a good is collective, usually entails governmental action, and is characterized by a particular feature: when more of it is consumed by A, B need not consume less (12). National defense is one example frequently encountered in the literature, and the lighthouse on the shore is another. Certain aspects of basic research and the dissemination of research findings share this feature, since the acquisition of new knowledge by D does not diminish its value for C, the original investigator who developed it.

In the context of cost-benefit analysis the most important cause of market failure is the presence of substantial external effects. Such effects are called economies if positive, and diseconomies if negative. Vaccination against a communicable disease is perhaps the most commonly cited example of benefits accruing to a third party or to the community, in addition to the benefits received by the patient and health worker, who are directly involved in the transaction (13, p. 18). Still another example from the health field is the protection accorded to the community by hospitalizing persons with severe mental illness (14, p. 12).

The goal of public policy is to adopt those projects or programs of service that yield the greatest surplus of benefits over costs. Evaluation of projects is prospective, oriented toward the future. The criterion of choice, analogous to that of maximizing profits in the market economy, is to maximize present value. Stated differently, but meaning the same, the criterion is to equalize marginal benefit and marginal cost. Strictly speaking, as Stigler (15) notes, maximizing present value is also the criterion for optimum behavior in the private sector. As Fuchs (16) pointed out, this criterion is quite different from that of attaining the maximum amount of a particular indicator of benefit.

Of course, the notion of balancing benefits and costs is by no means alien to medicine. Lasagna (17) states, "Since no drug—free of toxicity—has ever been introduced that is effective for anything, those of us who are pharmacologists have learned to live reasonably comfortably with the notion of paying some sort of toxicological price for welfare."

A possible source of misunderstanding about cost-benefit analysis is that benefits are usually costs presently borne that would be averted if the program in question proved to be effective. It is essential to distinguish these present and potentially avertible costs from the resource costs required to conduct that program. Since the two types of cost are not always juxtaposed, this distinction is not obvious, and the failure to draw it is not evident.

There are two essential characteristics of cost-benefit analysis: breadth of scope, and length of time horizon. The objective is to include all costs and all benefits of a program, no matter "to whomsoever they accrue," over as long a period as is pertinent and practicable (3).

Counting, Measuring, and Valuing Benefits and Costs

When an agency wishes to undertake a project or program, it may be tempted to go far afield in counting benefits and to neglect some costs. For example, in water resources projects, certain secondary benefits may be included improperly. In vocational rehabilitation programs both savings in public assistance grants and income taxes on subsequent earnings are sometimes counted as benefits, even though neither item entails a saving in the use of resources. Both grants and taxes are transfer payments, that is, they represent a transfer in command over resources (18, p. 47).

The distinction between costs and transfers is not meant to suggest that the sole justification of public projects or programs is an increase in output or gross national product (GNP). On the contrary, there is increasing recognition that public projects or programs may carry multiple objectives, including income distribution, more jobs, and regional growth (19-22). There is no reason why, for purposes of cost-benefit analysis, earnings on a job cannot be assigned greater weight than the same amount of money received in public assistance grants (18, p. 167). What must be recognized is that such weights are judgmental, are likely to be arbitrary (at least initially), should be derived in the public arena, and, above all, must be clearly stated.

Similarly, as shown by the progressive individual income tax, we seem to act on the belief in the United States that an extra dollar accruing to a low income person is worth more than an extra dollar accruing to a high income person (19). Again, assigning relative weights may help to improve analysis for public policy. There is no reason to believe, however, and no intention to claim, that agreement on such weights is imminent.

On the cost side a good example of the tendency toward understatement is the neglect of compliance costs imposed on individuals and firms in calculating such costs as those of administering the individual income tax, and of Medicare for the aged. Once the installation of seat belts in automobiles is made mandatory, the temptation arises to disregard the cost of seat belts to car owners (23, 24).

Counting benefits and costs involves deciding what to include and what to exclude. When an item that may be properly included can be measured, the next problem is that of valuation. The ease of valuation, indeed its possibility, depends largely on whether the item in question is traded in the market and bears a price. In that case there are many good reasons for simply adopting that price (25). When market price is deemed to be a defective measure of value, however, an attempt is made to estimate an imputed or shadow price (26). One modification of market price that is widely accepted is to set a lower value on unemployed resources; the size of this adjustment may vary not only with the state of the economy at large, but also by geographic region and by occupation (20).

When an item, even an important one, lacks a market price, the tendency is to omit it from calculations. If total benefits are thereby understated, a program may be erroneously deleted. More important, perhaps, programs with a sizeable proportion of unvalued to total benefits stand to lose in competition for funds with programs that have few, if any, unvalued benefits (27). Among the items most likely to be omitted are so-called intangible benefits; such benefits are especially prominent in the health field. It is not that they can never be valued (28). Rather, one may distinguish between intangible benefits that for the time being remain difficult to value and pure public goods, which are not traded on the market and therefore cannot be valued.

The dilemmas of valuation can be escaped by retreating from cost-benefit analysis to cost-effectiveness analysis. The latter is the less demanding approach, since it does not require the valuation of all benefits in terms of a common numéraire. Cost-effectiveness analysis requires only that benefits be measured in physical terms. Once an objective or output is specified, the aim is to minimize the cost of attaining it. The cost data required for cost-effectiveness analysis are, however, the same as for cost-benefit analysis (29).

Retreating from the valuation of benefits to measurement alone entails a substantial loss: analysis can no longer assist in setting priorities among several fields of public activity. The reason is simple. While cost-benefit analysis cuts across diverse objects of public expenditure, cost-effectiveness analysis can only help in choosing among alternate means of achieving a given, presumably desired, outcome (30). It is cost-effectiveness analysis that was incorporated as a major element in the planning, program, and budgeting (PPB) systems of the federal government. After its initial development by the Rand Corporation, PPB was introduced by the Department of Defense in 1961 and extended to other departments and agencies by Executive Order in 1965 (31, 32).

Both cost-benefit analysis and cost-effectiveness analysis imply the measurement of outcomes that are associated with particular projects or programs of service. Presumably there is a link between inputs and outputs that is measurable and known. It does not matter whether behavior follows a deterministic or probabilistic pattern. In the development of water resources the design of a particular project almost guarantees the emergence of certain physical outcomes—so much land will be lost to flooding, so much more land will be protected from flooding, so much land will be irrigated, etc. In national defense the outcome of a proposed course of action is much more uncertain, since other countries can take evasive and retaliatory action. In the health field, as will be shown, the presumed link between inputs and outputs is sometimes tenuous (33). Too often, the task of measurement, which necessarily precedes valuation, has been neglected.

The Rate of Discount

There is wide consensus in economics that a dollar is worth more today than it will be worth a year or two from now; this holds true when overall price level remains constant. As long as assets are safe, consumers are believed to have a positive time preference, that is, prefer to consume now rather than later. For producers investment may be productive through either the lapse of time, as in wine making, or the adoption of more round-about methods of production. Borrowers are therefore willing to pay interest for the use of capital, and lenders, in a capitalist economy, expect to receive interest. In a socialist economy an accounting or imputed rate of interest is employed to help allocate resources over time. The interest rate that calculates the present values of future streams of benefits and future streams of costs for public projects or programs is the well-known discount rate of cost-benefit analysis (18, p. 165).

Although economists agree that a discount rate is necessary for rendering commensurate benefits accruing and costs incurred at different times, they do *not* agree on the size of the discount rate. Marked differences of opinion prevail for a number of reasons. One is that a diversity of interest rate structures exists in the real world, owing to capital market imperfections, differences in risk, and governmental monetary policies (2, 3, 34). There is controversy regarding which imperfections to allow for and how to allow for them. Another reason for differences of opinion, as Musgrave (35) makes clear, is the source of financing—private consumption or investment. Still another reason for differences of opinion is a value judgment: whether the proper measure of the discount rate for public projects is the opportunity cost of capital in the private sector, or, to the contrary, whether it is the social rate of time preference. The private rate may be high, well above 10 per cent, particularly when allowance is made for the corporation income tax of 50 per cent (36). The social rate of time preference is usually much lower, based on a longer time horizon or greater readiness by the community acting together than by individuals to postpone gratification in favor of future generations. The social rate, which has been justified in terms of future risk and uncertainty, probability of personal survival, and the diminishing marginal utility of additional income or consumption as per capita income grows over time, is not a number that we know how to ascertain empirically (34). Accordingly, still another procedure, which combines private opportunity cost and social time preference, is also not measurable.

In practice, the agencies of the federal government have employed a wide range of discount rates, usually without giving a reason (37). Nevertheless, the consequences of choosing a high or a low discount rate are clear. A low discount rate favors projects or programs with benefits accruing in the distant future. In effect, as Boulding (38) has suggested, a high interest rate favors the aged and a low one favors the middle aged. When a project or program is short-lived, with both benefits and costs concentrated in the near future, the choice of discount rate is of minor or no consequence; indeed, for a short-lived program discounting may be dispensed with. Some economists are averse to selecting a particular discount rate, on the ground that they are in no position to choose between generations (13, p. 57). The tendency is to display calculations of the present values of benefits and costs under two or more discount rates. It seems to me that such alternative calculations do not afford helpful guidance to the policy maker, unless he is advised when to employ one or the other.

Even in the present state of the controversy there may be some merit to employing a single number for all public projects or for all public human investment projects. The combined method, recommended by a panel of consultants to the Bureau of the Budget in 1961 (39), and subsequently developed by Feldstein (40), can furnish an adequate rationale even though it does not yet yield a specific number. Such a number admittedly would be arbitrary, a reflection of value judgment (2). Henderson (34) reports that the French have adopted a centrally determined rate of discount of 7 per cent, to be applied to all public enterprises. This rate is higher than that encountered in many American cost-benefit studies.

APPLICATIONS OF COST-BENEFIT ANALYSIS TO THE HEALTH FIELD

The health services literature contains many affirmations of the importance of cost-benefit analysis for improving the allocation of resources to and within the health field. It may prove to be a source of astonishment that relatively few complete cost-benefit studies of health programs have been carried out. Perhaps it is appropriate that fewer cost-benefit studies have been performed than advocated. Where the aim is to minimize the cost of producing a given good or service, or even of constructing a hospital of specified size and with suitable appurtenances, the apparatus of cost-benefit analysis is superfluous (33). It then suffices to compare unit costs.

Criteria for Inclusion

The major reason for the shortness of the list of complete cost-benefit studies is that most studies conducted to date are limited in one or more respects. First, in the 1970s, there seems to be little point to considering nonempirical analyses. Thus, today Mushkin's seminal work (41) in conceptualizing the application of cost-benefit analysis to the health field must be excluded from consideration.

A second, perhaps more critical, requirement for including a study is that both the benefits and costs of specified programs be measured and valued simultaneously, with their respective present values juxtaposed and compared. By this criterion, the majority of empirical studies so far performed in the health field are excluded, including that by Fein (42) on mental illness, by Rice (43, 44) on a number of diagnostic categories, and my own on syphilis (45) and on heart disease (46). While all of these studies attempt to measure and value the cost of a disease, thereby, in effect, measuring and valuing the total benefits of eradicating that disease, none attempts to estimate the costs of conducting programs with specified contents and aims. Although each study has made a contribution to the counting, measurement, and valuation of direct and indirect tangible benefits, and two have explored the valuation of intangible benefits, none has presented a comparison of costs and benefits under a specified set of conditions.

The above two requirements—quantification and juxtaposition of costs and benefits—impress me as being incontestable. A third requirement can be defended as equally necessary: that benefits and costs reflect a known link, alluded to above, between program and outcome, i.e. between inputs and outputs. Such a link should be empirically based. Today, speculative or hypothetical relationships do not suffice (47). To apply economic valuation to hypothetical relationships between programs and outcomes is to indulge in an academic exercise, since the results of such valuation cannot transcend the quality of the underlying measurements. Such an exercise is not only idle, in that it can make no contribution to policy formulation, but it may be counterproductive if it obscures the fact that the relationships between inputs and outputs are not yet known and remain to be ascertained (14, p. 29).

In an article discussing the contribution of health services to the U.S. economy, Fuchs (48) has demonstrated the importance of information concerning the efficacy of health services. The economist can indicate the types of data he requires, but he is seldom in a position to procure them by himself; he must rely on other investigators in health services research to help him to obtain them.

This third requirement implies an important corollary. The size of a problem, as measured by the total costs of a disease, is not a reliable guide for policy (49, 50). Even in communicable diseases, less than eradication may be an acceptable goal. For most diagnostic conditions it is essential to know the extent to which a given program is likely to reduce the size of the problem. This point is often overlooked. It lends itself to oversight particularly when benefits and costs are not juxtaposed. In the early cost-benefit studies in the health field there may have been a further tendency for economists to attribute greater efficacy to medical care than was perhaps warranted (51).

Weisbrod (13) performed the earliest of a small number of such studies and his remains one of the most systematic. He compared the benefits and costs of intervening in three diseases—cancer, polio, and tuberculosis. Drawing in a creative way on Bowen's work in deriving the demand curve for a public good (52), Weisbrod was frequently reduced to obtaining cost data and some notion of the link between inputs and outcomes from personal communications with clinicians and administrators. His threefold classification of benefits–direct, indirect, and intangible–followed Mushkin and has become the convention.

How such benefits are measured and valued, as well as an assessment of the current state of the arts, will be given below. Both accomplishments to date, and possible shortcomings in the accepted procedures will be presented.

Direct Benefits

Direct benefits are that portion of averted costs currently borne which are associated with spending for health services. They represent potential tangible savings in the use of health resources. Certainly in the long run manpower not required to diagnose and treat disease and injury does become available for other uses. It is reasonable to suppose that our economy, like others, has a vast variety of wants in the face of a totality of relatively scarce resources, so that freeing resources for other, desired, objectives represents a contribution to economic welfare.

In the absence of a specific program of services to be evaluated, the measure of direct benefits is usually taken to be total resource costs currently incurred. The appropriateness of this measure as a basis for policy is questionable, as indicated above. Nor is it helpful to take some fraction of the total. In terms of resource use, diminishing marginal productivity is likely to set in as a program expands beyond a certain point. In terms of valuation of benefits, diminishing marginal utility is often a plausible assumption.

While it is usually taken for granted that direct benefits, or the current costs of care that will be averted, can be measured with precision, this is true only when a firm produces a single good or service, such as maternity care in a special hospital. In most instances several goods or services are produced jointly. Under conditions of joint production it is possible to calculate the extra or marginal cost for each product, but not its average unit cost (10, pp. 44-45). When average unit cost figures are presented, they reflect an allocation of overhead and joint costs; and such allocation is necessarily an arbitrary accounting procedure, even where it is systematic and replicable. An alternative procedure, which is no less arbitrary, is to assign to a diagnostic category its proportion of total costs, with the proportion taken from the percentage distribution of patients or services. In the absence of facilities that produce only a single product, it might be helpful to analyze cost data for facilities with varying diagnostic compositions of patient load. However, other factors are also at play, and there is no logical solution to the problem of determining average cost under conditions of joint production of multiple outputs (18, p. 166).

Another complication, which affects the calculation of direct benefits and also of indirect benefits, is the simultaneous presence of two or more diseases in a patient. The presence of disease B when intervention is attempted in disease A serves to raise or lower the costs of intervention and therefore the corresponding benefits (45). The reason that indirect benefits, which represent gains in future earnings, are also affected is that the presence of diseases A and B in a patient may reduce the probability of successful outcome from the treatment of either. The effect is to overstate the benefits expected from reducing the incidence of one or the other disease (51). The magnitude of this effect is not known.

The prevailing tendency is to take direct benefits from a single-year estimate of costs (44). Since survivors will also experience morbidity in the future, some medical care costs are being neglected. Initially this procedure may have been associated with an emphasis on single-year estimates, to the exclusion of present value estimates (50). Once the necessity of present value estimates is recognized, other explanations must be sought for this shortcut. A possible explanation is that survivors will experience only average morbidity in the future; when extra morbidity is absent, there is perhaps no need to deal with morbidity. A more plausible explanation lies in the lack of longitudinal data on the morbidity experience of defined population cohorts.

The fact is that a single-year estimate reflects the prevalence of a disease, not its incidence. It may be that the prevalence figure is sufficiently greater than the incidence figure for chronic conditions, so that it makes ample allowance for future events. Indeed, the prevalence figure in the base year is the same as the sum of the incidence figures for all survivors to this year, if certain factors remain constant, such as the size of population, death rates for the particular diagnostic group, and the incidence rate. When any of these factors follows a rising trend, however, the prevalence figure exceeds the cumulative sum of the past and present incidence figures and falls short of the sum of incidence figures expected in the future.

To the extent that unit costs or prices tend to increase faster in the health services sector than in the economy at large, the value of direct benefits will also increase. In my own work I have incorporated an adjustment for this factor into the discount rate, deriving thereby a *net* discount rate (45, 46). If economic growth were to slow down in this country, the lag in productivity gains of the health services sector behind the economy at large would be reduced, and so would the size of this adjustment.

Transportation expenses for medical care are a resource cost which is disregarded in cost-benefit analysis, although they are allowed as deductions under the individual income tax. When the physician made home calls, his travel expenses were automatically included in health service expenditures. The foremost reason for neglecting them today is, most likely, lack of reliable data. There may be the further, implicit assumption that patients' transportation costs are of a small order of magnitude.

Indirect Benefits

Earnings lost due to premature death or disability, which will be averted, are indirect benefits. Debility as an impairing factor in production has not attained the prominence in empirical studies that Mushkin (41, 51) attached to it from a conceptual standpoint.

Since the publication of Rice's studies (53) it is no longer necessary to estimate loss of earnings on the back of an envelope. Drawing fully on the data resources of the federal government and using unpublished tabulations almost as much as published ones, Rice (43-44) prepared her estimates in systematic fashion. She applied labor force participation rates, employment rates, and mean earnings, inclusive of fringe benefits, to the population cohort in question. For men and women separately, she derived estimates of the present values of lost earnings due to mortality under alternative discount rates and a one-year estimate of lost earnings due to disability or morbidity.

Several elements of the benefit calculation that were still at issue a decade or so ago appear to be more or less settled now, some perhaps prematurely. These can be summarized as follows:

1. Our ordinary concern is with loss in earnings, not income. The latter includes income from property.

2. Consumption by survivors is no longer subtracted from gross earnings in order to arrive at net earnings. Viewed prospectively, everybody is a member of society, including the patient (54).

3. The value of housewives' services is recognized, despite the fact that such services are not traded in the market and are omitted from the GNP. Weisbrod (13, pp. 114-119) developed and applied a complex method for measuring the cost of a substitute housekeeper, but subsequent writers have followed Kuznets (55) in employing a simpler approach, putting the value of the services of a housewife at the level of earnings of a full-time domestic servant. To employ a single number is the more practical procedure by far. The magnitude of that number is a separate question, however. It is increasingly evident that the value given by the earnings of a domestic servant is not adequate (56). Thus, the accepted value of the housewife's contribution would increase substantially if day care centers for working women were expanded at public cost.

An alternative approach is to value the housewife's contribution at the opportunity cost of her staying out of the labor force (45). Implementation of this approach is impeded by two considerations (57). First, the method is complicated, since values would vary with the individual housewife's educational attainments, type of occupation, amount of job experience, full- or part-time employment status, etc. Second, nonpecuniary factors, which certainly influence the labor force participation rates of women, are difficult to measure and may behave erratically. When total family income permits, the pecuniary opportunity cost of the wife's staying home has been known to be as low as zero or even negative.

4. The employment rate has been typically taken at 96 per cent, or an overall level of 4 per cent unemployment at the level of "full" employment (44). In the 1970s the magnitude of this rate is at issue. Whatever the magnitude, Mushkin's argument is accepted that the health services system should not be charged with failures by the economy to provide jobs to all who seek them (41, 58).

What is often not taken into account is the tendency for persons rehabilitated after serious illness or injury to find fewer job opportunities than persons who have remained healthy and on the job. In my study of syphilis (45), I recognized the loss of earnings due to the "stigma" attached to this and similar diseases. When prevention is feasible, it seems appropriate to assign to it an extra weight or bonus for this reason.

5. Calculations of indirect benefits rest on the implicit assumption that the life expectancies of cohorts of potential survivors are known. Usually standard life tables are employed, separately for men and women. For diseases of low frequency it seems reasonable to disregard any effect on the total death rate occasioned by the deletion of a particular cause of death. For major diseases the problem is important, although simple deletion may be incorrect. As Weisbrod (13, pp. 34-35) recognized more than a decade ago, survivors who have avoided a particular cause of death may have a higher or lower susceptibility to other, competing causes of death. I compared the effects of simply deleting heart disease as a cause of death on life expectancy and on work-life expectancy. The former was large—11 to 12 years—and the latter was small—less than a year (46). For a disease with heavier impact at the younger ages, the effect on work-life expectancy would be relatively larger, and correspondingly greater attention would have to be paid to the effect of competing causes of death.

Intangible Benefits

Pain, discomfort, and grief are among the costs of illness currently borne, which constitute the intangible benefits of a program of health services that averts them. The benefits accrue partly to the patients and partly to their friends, relatives, and society at large, to the extent that we take pleasure in the happiness of others. That positive external effects in consumption exist is indicated by personal and philanthropic gifts, to the extent that they are not subsidized by the deductibility provisions of the income tax (59). Looming even larger is the averted premature loss of human life. Since none of these effects is traded on the market, none carries a price tag. In attempting to put a value on averting them the question arises: what would one be willing to pay to avoid them?

In my paper on syphilis (45), I estimated willingness to pay for escaping the early and late manifestations of the disease by examining expenditures incurred in connection with other diseases that met certain conditions. After consultation with clinicians I adopted psoriasis as the analogue for early syphilis, and terminal cancer as the analogue for its late stage. The conditions specified were that the expenditures for medical care represented principally a willingness to pay for freedom from the particular disease, since in neither case could direct or indirect tangible benefits, as defined above, be realized. To the extent that payments were made only by the patient (directly or through health insurance), willingness to pay by others was neglected and total willingness to pay was understated.

Neenan (60) has estimated the consumer benefit of a community chest x-ray program for tuberculosis. With the help of some fee data indicating willingness to pay, he obtained very high estimates of value.

Several years have elapsed since intangible benefits were valued. The analogous diseases approach has not been repeated; this suggests that neither the estimates themselves nor the procedures for obtaining them have been found useful. One reason is obvious: the approach is specific, calling for the development of estimates, disease by disease.

A larger body of literature is devoted to the value of human life than to the other types of intangible health benefit. Life insurance holdings are clearly not applicable to bachelors and jury verdicts are inconsistent (13, p. 37). The implications of public policy decisions or governmental spending are difficult to elicit in the absence of information on the alternatives that faced the decision makers (19). Moreover, such valuation may lack stability and consistency (24, pp. 133-134).

Schelling (61) has proposed a different approach. He would measure the value of human life, as distinguished from livelihood, by the amount people are willing to spend to buy a specified reduction in the statistical probability of death. Acton (24, p. 258) applied this approach, and derived an estimate of the value of human life at $28,000. This amount serves as a substitute for the net value of lost earnings and is not an additional sum.

I am not sanguine about the applicability of Acton's numerical estimate to the evaluation of program alternatives. Acton was the first to criticize the defects in his estimate, including the small size of his sample, and its apparent biases. While these defects can be remedied in the future, what troubles me is the likelihood that respondents to this type of question may not grasp its meaning. Do respondents know the actual probabilities of their dying in the coming year? How is a small—e.g. 1 per cent—reduction in statistical probability perceived? How much more is a 10 per cent reduction worth than a 1 per cent reduction? Is it plausible to postulate a strictly linear relationship between increase in risk and willingness to pay to cover it? (54). Moreover, does not the value of a gain depend somewhat on the starting point? (62). If all payments come from the consumer, the distribution of income must exert a sizeable influence; by how much would willingness to pay change if the task of reducing the death rate were viewed as a collective responsibility that is fully financed from public funds?

Titmuss (63) regards the value of human life as priceless and beyond valuation. Yet implicit values are being placed on human life whenever public policy decisions are made on highway design, auto safety, airport landing devices and traffic control measures, mining hazards, factory safeguards, etc. In emphasizing voluntary giving, the sense of community that the gift relationship in blood both reflects and promotes, Titmuss seems to be pointing to a large external benefits component that is neglected when life-time earnings are taken as the proxy for the value of human life. Although the concern for the altruistic motive is salubrious and appropriate, the conclusion does not follow that human life is priceless.

As Mishan (54) observes, a rough measure of a precise concept is superior to a precise measure of an erroneous concept. It is agreed that the notion of the value of human life, apart from livelihood, is sound. A numerical estimate of this value would be useful in comparing the worthwhileness of alternative programs. Comparisons of programs would gain in relevance and aptness if all benefits were counted, including the saving of human life or improvements in life expectancy. This potential gain is much more likely to be realized if all benefits are entered into the model, rather than if some appear only in footnotes.

I am unable to say at this time how such a number or set of numbers for the several age groups can best be derived. Certainly Schelling's questionnaire method (61) can be improved. Perhaps the implications of past or existing public policies will yield a narrower range than one expects. It is conceivable that a committee can do a better job in the realm of values than in the realm of fact. In any event, the value of human life is probably higher for identified and known individuals than for members of statistical populations. If so, incurring extraordinarily large expenditures in behalf of the former is far from conclusive evidence of irrational behavior.

Weisbrod (13, p. 96) avoided dealing with the problem of valuing intangible benefits by assuming proportionality to tangible benefits. This is an unsatisfactory solution, given the differential impacts of various diseases on life expectancy, disability, and morbidity. However, a solution to this problem was not needed when the emphasis of public expenditures analysis shifted from cost-benefit to cost-effectiveness. To repeat, in cost-effectiveness analysis outcome is expressed in physical terms, e.g. life years gained, and the task of analysis is to discover the program that will yield the desired outcome at the lowest unit cost. In the health services it goes without saying that desired outcome incorporates a constant level of quality of care, or at least an acceptable level.

Cost of Program

The estimate of the cost of a proposed program, with which benefits are compared, poses no special difficulties. A budget is prepared in terms of the market prices of inputs, which may be adjusted by shadow prices when warranted.

If programs vary in size, it is appropriate to examine the possibility that economies of scale exist (14, pp. 82-83). However, since health services are rendered in the local area, the prospects of realizing such economies are much more limited than in the manufacture of goods. Moreover, when the size of a program increases, factor costs may rise. Finally, as the scope of a program approaches the size of the total population at risk, the extra cost of additional units of output increases when increasingly resistant groups are encountered. Conversely, it has been suggested that in the early phases of a program unit cost is likely to be higher than later on, since administrators learn by doing (14, p. 24).

Cost-Benefit Versus Cost-Effectiveness Analysis

Although it is not so difficult to estimate the costs of programs, it is quite difficult to formulate the contents and expected outcomes of programs. In my judgment this has been the chief obstacle to the useful application of cost-benefit or cost-effectiveness analysis in the health field.

Elsewhere I have listed the data required by the economist for valuing outcomes (46). A clear statement of each type of outcome is necessary. Certain events, such as death, disability, extra unemployment, and the use of health services must be entered on a calendar, beginning with the base year, and assigned a duration. The data should extend for a period as close to a person's lifetime as possible, with particular attention to the possible recurrence of illness and its exacerbation.

This list of data requirements implies a degree of knowledge about the effects of health services on the health of a population that is often lacking. The obstacles to the attainment of such knowledge are many. Medicine is not an exact science, and physicians may disagree among themselves and the same physician may disagree with his own past findings. Field studies are complicated by what Morris (64) calls the iceberg phenomenon: members of the designated control group, who are presumably normal, may in fact have the disease under investigation in asymptomatic form. The possibility of inducing iatrogenic disease means that only studies performed on normal populations in the community, which are far more costly than studies of captive clinical populations, can yield valid results (65).

A serious gap in existing data arises from the lack of longitudinal studies of populations. Few investigators possess the requisite patience and dedication, or experience the necessary career stability. The funding agencies, under conditions of budgetary stringency, have even shorter time horizons. Although statistical manipulation of existing cross-section and time-series data is a much cheaper and almost always available approach, it may not afford an adequate substitute in many instances, especially when a high degree of correlation exists among the independent variables under scrutiny. In 1965 I reported that only one study met the longitudinal data requirements listed above—Saslaw's study (66) on rheumatic fever. Unfortunately, the report on this study was truncated in publication. Neenan's study of chest x-rays for tuberculosis (60), conducted in 1964, concentrated on the short term, on the ground that a recovered patient suffers no impairment of earnings while early detection alone does not alter the long-term outlook. No evidence is adduced for these assumptions.

Acton (24) has recently completed a cost-benefit analysis of alternative programs for reducing deaths from heart attacks. He considered five programs: an ambulance with specially trained nonphysician personnel; a mobile coronary care unit with a physician; a community triage center; a triage center combined with the ambulance; and a program to screen, monitor, and pretreat the population. The largest net benefit, whether measured by the number of lives saved, or valued by the criterion of earnings or that of willingness to pay, is given by the screening, monitoring, and pretreatment program. However, the value of personal time lost in screening is neglected, and the screening program seems to display great variability in outcome. Acton's cost-benefit analysis follows his cost-effectiveness analysis, in which lives saved are not assigned a value. The screening, monitoring, and pretreatment program yields the largest number of lives saved, but the average cost per life saved is second from the highest and the marginal cost of saving two additional lives is $24,000 each, compared with the estimated average and marginal cost of $3,200 for saving the first 11 lives under the ambulance program (24, p. 117). Acton's work is noteworthy for the wealth of detail on the epidemiology of heart attacks, physiology, treatment, and delivery systems for treatment or prevention. This economist drew extensively on the expertise of health services specialists and investigators.

The report of the Gottschalk Committee to the Bureau of the Budget (BOB) (67) contains a cost-effectiveness analysis of alternative modalities for treating chronic end-stage kidney disease. The problem facing the BOB, and posed to the Committee, was to define the appropriate role of the federal government in this field. The conclusion that a substantially expanded federal role was warranted was reached on other grounds, which did not entail an economic analysis. These included: some veterans were already receiving free care in veterans administration hospitals; several foreign countries, each poorer than the United States, were committed to delivering this service to all patients; voluntary insurance plans in the U.S. were not paying for the cost of prolonged hemodialysis and their leaders saw no prospect of doing so; the patients requiring treatment largely comprised middle-aged adults; and what was still a unique life-saving measure was available for application to known individuals, persons who would otherwise die in short order. Once the recommendation was made in favor of an expanded role for the federal government and a feasible mechanism was designed to finance the care rendered to individuals, the problem that remained for economic analysis was how best to discharge this responsibility—through hemodialysis in an institution, hemodialysis in the patient's home, kidney transplantation, or some mixture of these modalities.

The cost-effectiveness analysis clearly pointed to the superiority of the transplantation route, which incorporates hemodialysis both for initial and back-up support. When hemodialysis is necessary, doing it at home is much cheaper (29). These findings influenced the Gottschalk's recommendations to the BOB that kidney transplantation be expanded as far as possible. (The best mix of modalities was not solved for because the implied assumptions of constant unit cost and constant utility of a life-year made it unnecessary.) Again, as noted with respect to Acton's study, the economic analysis drew heavily on the underlying epidemiologic, physiologic, and clinical data developed by or in behalf of the Committee.

Had the Gottschalk Committee performed a cost-benefit analysis, it seems plausible to postulate that a shortage of kidneys for transplantation and the relatively greater ease with which hemodialysis facilities can expand might have yielded a higher net benefit value for dialysis, at least in the near future. However, allowance for the superior quality of life under transplantation would constitute a partial offset (29).

Contrary to some impressions (68), the Gottschalk Committee did inquire into available prevention programs and determined that, for the foreseeable future, the number of eligible patients with end-stage kidney disease would not change. The Committee did not inquire into the dispersion of the distribution of life years gained.

Thus, it did not consider whether an average gain of 10 years is worth the same when it is the product of 10 years each gained by 100 per cent of the population at risk, or of 20 years each gained by 50 per cent of the population, or of 40 years each gained by 25 per cent of the population. Can it be said that the marginal utility of an additional year is constant or does the principle of diminishing marginal utility govern?

The Committee did not have to deal with two problems that might arise under different circumstances. One is that even cost-effectiveness analysis is not so simple as it appears to be when two or more types of outcome are sought as goals. If only one outcome, such as life years gained, is preeminent, other outcomes may be neglected. Where all outcomes are important—reduced mortality, lower morbidity, and less disability—it becomes necessary once again, as under cost-benefit analysis, to arrive at common or weighted measures of outcome for alternative programs (69). Only the problem of valuing intangible benefits is escaped. However, in cost-effectiveness analysis the focus is confined to outcomes common to health services programs, and the weighting problem is serious only when the several types of outcome do not occur in the same proportions for every program. The second problem not faced by the Gottschalk Committee is the appropriate role for government to assume if expensive life-saving measures became practicable for other organs of the body. Nor did the Gottschalk Committee attempt to deal with the question of increases in patient load if the very success of the program it sponsored led to the relaxation of criteria governing patient eligibility for treatment. The quantitative effect of such relaxation may be appreciable.

In the years 1966-1967, during the early spread of PPB in the federal government, a number of cost-effectiveness studies were carried out in the Department of Health, Education, and Welfare (23, 49, 68). Although costs and benefits were calculated simultaneously, the link between the inputs and outputs of programs was measured too often by means of hypothetical numbers. Once the relationships were postulated, no effort was made to pursue the measurement problem through empirical inquiry in subsequent budgetary periods. In certain instances only expenditures chargeable to the federal budget were counted as costs, neglecting expenditures incurred by individuals and by other levels of government (23, 24).

PROBLEMS IN ASSESSING HEALTH SYSTEMS TECHNOLOGY

This discussion of the potentialities and hitherto modest achievements of cost-benefit analysis and cost-effectiveness analysis in the health field bears directly on the analysis of the development and spread of health systems technology. However, changes in technology bring to the fore an additional factor: a heightened degree of uncertainty concerning future benefits and costs. According to systems analysis, one appropriate response to the prospect of uncertainty is to perform a sensitivity analysis, concentrating on a few key factors or assumptions to which the measure of costs or benefits appears to be especially sensitive (34, 70). This proposition strikes me to be a formal one, awaiting empirical content.

Nevertheless, within the time frame of a decade, any allowance for uncertainty due to developments in technology may be excessive. It has been suggested that the technology that will be applied in the next ten years is already known, and that the pattern of technologic diffusion is discernible (71). This view may be too sanguine, but it is not contradicted by the record of the Gottschalk Committee. By wisdom or good luck, the

Committee's projections of survivorship of patients with transplanted kidneys and the cost of hemodialysis at home, both of which were originally supported by scanty data, have been borne out (72).

If technologic developments over the next decade are, in effect, already known to those gifted with early recognition, what can be said about prospective benefits and costs? In a plea at a health services research seminar in New York City for more research and development funds, Bennett (73) argued that the half-finished invention is the most costly product, so that technologic progress is bound to bring a lower unit cost of service, as well as improved performance.

In those cases where straightforward development takes place and serious adverse side-effects are not encountered, Bennett's view of the cost-reducing and benefit-enhancing effects of technologic progress is undoubtedly correct. However, in many respects the future is shrouded in uncertainties. Such factors as the size and geographic distribution of population, value structures, and political decisions are uncertain for the future, even if technologic developments are not. Public policies are also known to create unintended and unanticipated consequences. An accepted way to deal with uncertainty is to provide for flexible operation, that is, to avoid a finely tuned operation which yields a minimum cost only for a particular scale of output. Similarly, if manpower is to be used flexibly in the future, it must be endowed with a more general education than otherwise. Thus, flexibility, whatever its cause or source, imposes a modest extra cost over a moderate range of outputs (18, pp. 105, 123-124).

The Historical Record

Rather than pursue this argument of pros and cons, I propose to examine the historical record. What have been the effects of past changes in health systems technology on costs and on benefits? A review of the literature on this subject reveals sharp differences of opinion.

In a monograph on hospital expenditures sponsored by the National Center for Health Services Research and Development, Feldstein (74) attributes most of the postwar increase in hospital cost to an increase in demand, or, more precisely, to an upward shift in the demand curve. To paraphrase his argument, technical change in the absence of scientific progress may occur for two different reasons. Economic analysis has emphasized technical change in response to a shift in the relative prices of inputs (75). If wages rise faster than the prices of other inputs, for example, hospitals will economize on labor by using more disposable items, by automating laboratory procedures, etc. The effect of such substitution is to prevent costs from rising as fast as they otherwise would have.

The second reason for technical change without scientific progress, which Feldstein emphasizes, is a shift in the demand for hospital care. This type of change generally yields a new product. The spreading of high-cost techniques is primarily due to rising income and increased health insurance coverage. As income increases, patients tend to raise the valuation of more costly care by relatively more than the valuation of less costly care. An increase in the proportion of the hospital bill paid by insurance will shift hospitals to more expensive technology, as the out-of-pocket price per unit of benefit is lowered.

Gains in scientific knowledge, including managerial innovations, that have the potential of lowering the cost of care may actually have the opposite effect. This happens again if the new scientific knowledge raises the benefits of expensive care by relatively more than the benefits of inexpensive care. In addition, if patients' real preferences do not prevail but hospitals persist in producing services with the most expensive techniques for which benefits are not less than cost, scientific progress cannot lower cost per patient day.

In a monograph on physician expenditures, Fuchs and Kramer (76) draw a sharp distinction between the effects of demand factors and those of technology. Their arguments concerning technology reflect an historical perspective, and may be paraphrased as follows. The late 1940s and early 1950s were marked by the introduction and widespread diffusion of many new drugs, particularly the antibiotics, which had a pronounced effect on the length and severity of infectious diseases. Since the mid-1950s, advances in medical technology have not brought about a similar improvement in the ability of physicians to improve health. Renal dialysis, cancer chemotherapy, and open heart surgery may achieve dramatic effects in particular cases, but bring about only marginal improvement in general indexes of health. Moreover, the early advances tended to be physician-saving, while the later ones were characteristically physician-using. The improvement in health resulting from the early advances was so great, that it turned the anticipated slight rise in demand for physician services into a slight decline. The reason is, according to Grossman (77), that healthier people have less objective need for physicians' services. By contrast, Fuchs and Kramer conclude that changes in demand factors had little effect on expenditures for physician services before the advent of Medicare and Medicaid in the mid-1960s.

In effect, whereas Fuchs and Kramer view technology and the conventional demand forces as being independent of one another, Feldstein holds that the effects of technology may also be exerted through a shift in demand. Both positions are stated ably and forcefully. As often happens, each raises more questions than it can answer. It would be premature, therefore, to attempt to pass judgment on the validity of the respective findings concerning the effects of technology in the postwar era.

In a study focusing on the marked acceleration in the upward trends of costs and expenditures for hospital and physician services in 1966 (78), I have argued, though by no means conclusively, that the large expansion in cost reimbursement to hospitals and the adoption of a new, previously untried method of paying physicians at reasonable and customary fees, subject to the prevailing distribution of fees in a local area, must have exerted strong effects of their own. In the case of hospitals, cost reimbursement for most patients leads to an impairment of financial self-discipline, since a dollar need only be spent in order to be gotten back. In my judgment, this proposition holds true for any institution, whether it be under voluntary nonprofit, governmental, or proprietary auspices. So far I am not persuaded by the empirical studies that have reached conclusions to the contrary (79, 80).

A number of works have appeared that attempt to explain the behavior of the nonprofit hospital (81-85). They are, for the most part, far-ranging and enlightening. One is also entertaining, positing a theory of conspicuous production, with the hospital's objective taken to be the closing of a status gap (85). None really attempts to deal with the sharp discontinuity in hospital cost and price behavior beginning in 1966.

A rise in personal income may lead to greater reliance on technology for still another reason. For example, many persons are unable to stop smoking. A higher income enables them to pay more for cigarettes with a filter and reduced tar and nicotine contents.

Similarly, a higher income permits people to spend more on automobiles with safety gadgets, reducing the need to exert influence on the behavior of drivers. It may be more effective to operate on impersonal environmental forces than to try to change the behavior of individuals (86).

At this time no general answer is discernible to the question of how changes in health systems technology affect costs and benefits. It happens only once in a generation, perhaps even less frequently, that an idea such as early ambulation after surgery is born of necessity in wartime, effects huge savings in the use of health resources, and also exerts a positive effect on health. In most cases, the effects of technology will be mixed. Often the product is new, in the sense that a treatment is created that was not available previously and therefore could not have been demanded. The decision of whether or not to adopt a piece of technology, and the extent of its spread once adopted, depend on a number of factors, including the values of consumers, the motivations of providers, the availability of funds, methods of provider remuneration, as well as the cost and efficacy of the service in question.

Such a general formulation of the problem of assessing health systems technology, as provided above, affords practically no guidance to decision making. Only the concrete circumstances surrounding a project or program can indicate the special problems of measurement and valuation and the unique opportunities for solving them, what is to be emphasized in the analysis, and what may be neglected with only a moderate degree of trepidation. Accordingly, I will examine two examples in detail: hospitals and automated multiphasic screening (58).

The Hospital

Economists have offered essentially three views concerning capital investment in the hospital. First, hospitals invest too little capital, hence their productivity gains lag behind those of the economy at large (87). Second, hospitals invest too much, because grants and bequests accrue to them at zero price (88). Third, there is no optimum amount of investment in hospital beds, since there is no standard of appropriate hospital use (89). Conceivably, each position may have some merit to the extent that it reflects the situation in different sectors of the hospital.

For simplicity I shall employ a threefold classification of hospital capital investment—patient beds, supporting housekeeping services, and ancillary medical services (82). The unique problems of measurement and valuation facing the application of cost-benefit or cost-effectiveness analysis will be explored for each sector.

Patient Beds. The heart of the exercise in evaluating a project to expand hospital bed capacity, in my judgment, lies in one's explanation of the phenomenon of hospital use. At one pole, if the primary determinants of use are biologic in nature, an increase in bed supply beyond a certain point must result in additional empty beds. If hospitals are paid at stated charges, empty beds inflict a heavy financial burden on each institution (79). The reason is that fixed costs constitute two-thirds to three-quarters of total operating costs (90). Each institution would therefore be subject to financial self-discipline in building beds, and there would be little occasion for outside intervention beyond the provision of information on the plans of other hospitals. The effect of introducing more technology might well be to increase the proportion of fixed costs to total operating costs, thereby reinforcing the efficacy of financial self-discipline.

At the other pole, if all beds built tend to be used under conditions of prepayment, as Roemer (91, 92) first suggested, there is no automatic criterion for an optimum bed supply. In the absence of evidence that low hospital use has an unfavorable effect on health status, the appropriate public policy is to clamp a tight lid on bed supply (79). The application of more or less technology in the hospital is beside the point, although it does seem preferable to operate any extra beds as cheaply as possible.

Patient census is a function of bed supply in the long run; combined with patient mix, it sets the requirement for nursing personnel, which may be viewed largely as a requirement for personal services, with little or no substitution of equipment permitted. However, substitution is possible among levels of nursing personnel. The extent of actual substitution of low-paid for high-paid staff is perhaps overstated by the failure of hospital budgets to incorporate expenditures for special duty nurses.

Housekeeping Services. I do not see any problems of sophisticated analysis in the area of supporting housekeeping services. Here the appropriate criterion for decision making is that of cost minimization. Bed sheets and towels are to be washed as cheaply as possible, for a given specification of whiteness. Patients' rooms and corridors are to be kept clean as cheaply as possible. Meals of a given quality—nutrition, calories, hot or cold—are to cost as little as possible.

Once it is recognized that certain products or services need not be produced by the hospital but can be purchased from the outside, the problem is that of developing valid comparisons of unit cost. In addition, some administrators may wish to allow for certain risk factors. In the absence of competition among suppliers, the sales price may be quoted artificially low at the outset, only to be raised later. Also, in the absence of competition, purchases from the outside may increase the risk of running out of inventory.

Apart from an allowance for lower risk associated with production within the hospital, estimates of internal cost of production should include only differential cost. No portion of overhead cost should be attributed, because this would continue in entirety after internal production ceased. Moreover, top management will perform the same role as coordinator, whether some goods and services are produced inside the hospital or acquired by purchase.

In fact, the rise in hospital wages and gains in productivity attainable in large-scale manufacturing have led hospitals to increase the purchase and use of disposable items and ready packaged supplies. As Flagle (93) reports, gains in productivity from investment in large-scale plant have been achieved outside the health care system, which shares in them through purchase.

If the objective of cost minimization is for a given level of cleanliness or nutrition, how this level is to be determined must be established. I doubt whether much would be accomplished by searching for effects on the health of patients. Rather, the criteria must be either patients' satisfaction or acceptability to management. Expressions of satisfaction are somewhat suspect, since patients are likely to be impressed by any display of interest in their opinions. A more practicable approach would be to compare alternative standards of service, none of them falling below adequacy, with the additional cost of attaining successively higher levels.

In some respects the computer partakes of a supporting housekeeping service and in other respects, when participating in diagnosis, it is akin to an ancillary medical service (94). The computer is a housekeeping service when it processes the payroll and issues bills to patients and insurance plans. As a substitute for older ways of bookkeeping and billing, the evaluation of computer performance is straightforward. Does it reduce costs? If so, by how much?

Medical Services. Even when the computer helps in diagnosis the test is still cost reduction, if an older way of performing the same task is being replaced. There may be a complication, however. The cost of operating the computer falls on the hospital, while savings in physician time accrue to the attending physician. The presence of distributional considerations suggests that the decision reached is not independent of who the decision maker is, or who exerts predominant influence on him.

Apart from the distributional considerations of who pays and who saves, evaluation of the worthwhileness of the computer in assisting in diagnosis is no different from the way another ancillary medical service, the laboratory, is evaluated. With respect to services that were rendered in the past, the test is simple. Does the new equipment save money or does it expand services for the same amount of money? In the laboratory additional and more costly equipment does replace technical personnel. A possible offset is the tendency to prescribe more services (95), although within the limits of existing capacity of equipment and staff the marginal cost of additional units of service is low. What is not known is how much good is accomplished, particularly in the absence of information on the timeliness of delivery of the reports on these services.

Flagle (93) has reported economies achieved in patient surveillance due to continuity of use of the monitoring system in infusing blood. This finding strikes me as analogous to the finding in his early work (96) that a single channel is more efficient than two channels when the demand for services varies stochastically.

The intensive care unit is a more complex operation to evaluate. To the extent that it substitutes equipment for nurses it should cost less. However, the unit is also intended to save lives. The yield in life-years gained is properly subject to more sophisticated analysis.

From this discussion it appears that cost-benefit or cost-effectiveness analysis is a plausible approach only if the service rendered is a new one or if the old product has changed appreciably, gaining new dimensions. When all benefits take the form of savings in health resources, that is, are direct and tangible benefits, the appropriate form of analysis is cost-benefit. When the preponderant benefits are intangible or life-saving, the dilemma is to choose between cost-benefit and cost-effectiveness analysis. On the one hand, cost-effectiveness analysis is easier to perform, since intangible benefits need only be measured but not valued. Indeed, according to Feldstein (97), even the problem of choice of discount rate is simpler in the case of cost-effectiveness analysis, with only the social time preference rate being relevant. On the other hand, to resort to cost-effectiveness analysis is to give up in advance whatever help analysis can offer in choosing among several objectives or program areas. It then becomes necessary to make the choice among programs on other grounds, as the Gottschalk Committee did.

I am unable to discern a general resolution to this dilemma. It is certainly not evident how to establish priorities in a systematic way when cost-benefit analysis is abandoned. Perhaps the choice can still be made in a practicable way, with reasons explicitly stated, when remarkable benefits are under consideration, as in the treatment of end-stage kidney disease. When the benefits in question are modest but difficult to value, how is one to decide whether or not to adopt a particular piece of technology? To follow the lead of pace-setting organizations is almost always to say yes. Perhaps we should put trust in our ability to continue to improve the valuation of intangible benefits in the future (28). Setting standard values on gains in life expectancy at various ages would seem worth exploring. However, I can also see increasing difficulty in the future in valuing direct tangible benefits, if fewer market prices become available for health services in the event that provider reimbursement shifts away from fee-for-service toward capitation and salary methods.

Automated Multiphasic Screening

Often cited and discussed as an example of technologic development in the health field is automated multiphasic health screening (98). The reports issued from the Kaiser-Permanente laboratories in Oakland and San Francisco reveal a good deal about the organization and staffing of such a service and present data on unit costs (99-103). No evaluation akin to cost-benefit or cost-effectiveness analysis was attempted prior to 1973, when a preliminary cost-benefit analysis for middle-aged men was issued (104).

Collen and associates (101) report that total costs for screening an individual are $21.32; which, they note, is only one-fourth or one-fifth of the cost of a periodic health examination employing more conventional modalities. The position of the authors is that this comparison will serve for the time being, pending determination of the efficacy of multiphasic health screening. The fact is that some people do undergo a periodic health examination, whatever its efficacy may be.

Garfield's position (105, 106) differs from that of Collen, in that the effectiveness of screening in arresting or curing previously unknown disease is beside the point. For Garfield, automated multiphasic screening has assumed a useful social function, serving as a sorting mechanism for patients with prepayment who would otherwise flood the health services system.

I have difficulty with both positions. Collen's comparison of cost with that of the periodic health examination reminds one that the latter procedure is notoriously controversial, with the central issue revolving precisely about its effectiveness. Among physicians there appear to be true believers, persistent skeptics, and ambivalent prescribers (107-109). Furthermore, as emphasized in the Nuffield report (110), screening implies an invitation to the patient to come and see the doctor who promises him a favorable outcome. This is in contrast to the more usual visit initiated by the patient who has symptoms and seeks relief.

My criticisms of Garfield's position are more serious, for his view that automated multiphasic screening should be regarded as a sorting mechanism, a substitute for the rationing of services by price, raises a host of questions. Apparently, judging from a more recent presentation of his position (111), much of Garfield's argument is based on an interpretation of what happened under Medicare and Medicaid. To my knowledge, the Medicare program experienced only a modest increase in the use of services and a huge, unexpected, increase in unit cost. There is no way to interpret the unanticipated rise in expenditures under Medicaid in the absence of data on trends in size of the eligible population, per capita use, and unit cost. My own view is that the increase in eligible population may have been the major factor.[1]

Garfield (111) has hypothesized a difference in price elasticity of demand between the sick and his other three categories of patient—the well, the worried well, and the early sick. However, there have been no empirical studies of the demand for physician services

[1] See Klarman, H. E. Major public initiative in health care. *Public Interest* 34: 106-123, 1974.

in which people are so classified. From other studies it would appear that a host of factors, such as health insurance, earnings as an expression of the value of time, age, and the supply of providers, are important determinants of the demand for physician services (112).

The assertion that the supply of services for sick care is inelastic is not unique to Garfield. In the area of trends in the education of physicians, which takes longer and therefore responds more slowly than any other health occupation, my own reading indicates that even this system has been somewhat responsive, even while insisting that class size in medical school must be kept small (18, p. 101), and still more responsive after the policy decision to expand enrollment was made and implemented by funding. Whether the supply response has been sufficient to meet rising demand is, of course, a different issue.

The most serious reservation I have about Garfield's position touches closely on the nature and function of cost-benefit analysis. If complete prepayment serves to create a condition of perpetual excessive demand, then some rationing or control measures are clearly indicated. Why assume, without comparing alternatives, that automated multiphasic screening is the most appropriate instrumentality? It seems to me that when the stated purposes of a program change, so should the menu of alternatives to be considered.

Two reports by Collen (101, 102) on the cost of screening fill a real need. Two measures are presented—cost per test and cost per screening. Cost per test reflects only direct departmental costs, while cost per screening incorporates an allocation of overhead expense. The article published in 1970 (102) offers a costing rule: in order to allow for all costs incurred, double the reported cost per test. The earlier article (101), which appears to present essentially the same data, suggests a blow-up of 50 per cent; I am unable to account for the difference.

Since the screening process is automatic, the capital equipment is indivisible, and all procedures are schedulable, economies of scale are to be expected. The larger the scale of operation, the lower is the average unit cost. However, to achieve the lower cost, full utilization of existing facilities is essential. Accordingly, it is said to be advantageous to have available a source of stand-by patients, such as those awaiting admission to the hospital (103).

Collen's second article (102) goes beyond cost per test or per screening, and reports cost per positive case. For mammography a prevalence rate of 1.2 per cent converts the unit cost of $4.90 into a cost per positive case of $408. Since one-fifth of the women with positive mammograms have cancer of the breast, the screening cost per true positive case is $2,000. His doubling rule would raise the cost to $4,000. The cost of diagnosis for all five women and of treatment for one is still excluded.

The proportion of false positives is a function not only of the accuracy of the screening test but also of the prevalence rate (113, 114). There are two reasons for aiming to keep down the number of false positives: to avoid needless anxiety, and to prevent iatrogenic disease associated with the diagnostic process itself.

The data reported to date from the Kaiser-Permanente laboratories indicate that automated multiphasic screening is both feasible and affordable. The question is whether it is worthwhile. One answer is in terms of its effects on health. The Advisory Committee on Automated Multiphasic Health Testing and Services (AMHTS) (115) states that much of disease uncovered by testing will be chronic or not reversible; it will not yield a saving in the use of services or an improvement in health. There seems to be little point to using multiphasic screening if this is the case.

A second answer is that of Garfield (111), which I have criticized at length. He provides no persuasive reason for choosing this instrumentality to control the use of physician services.

A third answer is possible: that automated multiphasic screening is an integral part of a package of comprehensive health services to which everybody has a right. Usually a service is aspired to by the poor because the middle and upper classes are already getting it. This is not yet the case regarding automated multiphasic screening.

Clearly, a reasonable answer can only be provided through an evaluation of automated health screening for its worthwhileness. The report by the Advisory Committee (115) states, "There are elements of AMHTS that defy cost-effectiveness analysis, but which depend primarily on medical, social, and scientific objectives." If I understand the statement, I disagree with it. It may be, however, that I do not understand it. What are the medical, or social, or scientific objectives that defy measurement?

Following the formulation of data requirements given in the preceding section, I propose that data be compiled to evaluate automated multiphasic screening as follows: the volume of disease detected that was not previously known; what could be and in fact was done about all this disease; what the outcomes in terms of health status and subsequent utilization of services were; and at how much cost, inclusive of diagnosis and treatment, the outcomes were attained (116, 117). It must be added that, as indicated by a recent paper (118) which compares study and control groups for such measures of outcome as work and health services utilization, Collen's group is steadily compiling more and more of the requisite data. Still lacking is information on costs that correspond to the specified benefits.

Barriers to Systematic Analysis

To bring some focus to a discussion of the necessary steps ahead, I have prepared a list of barriers to the systematic and rational analysis of expenditures for health systems technology. At the same time I shall assess the prospects for lowering or overcoming each barrier.

1. When the costs of operation mount beyond all projections, the tendency is to argue that the computer or automated laboratory, as the case may be, is not merely providing services but is performing a research function. Yet doing things we know little about does not define research. Certain features of research, such as formulation of hypotheses, design of study, and capability for statistical analysis of data, are not necessarily available wherever services are rendered. Although some replication of research is desirable, it should be intentional and need not be universal (119). It follows that sources of research funds should exercise discrimination in allocating them. If the absorption of so-called research costs by patients is precluded, this tendency to encourage pseudoresearch will be minimized.

2. A tendency exists to expand the range of functions said to be performed by new equipment. Surely, data on payroll could assist management in controlling cost by department; data on billings could provide a proxy for cost data by diagnosis. The first of these applications can be evaluated according to a strict criterion: is potential cost control

achieved, so that savings are realized? The second application can be judged on its own merits as an intermediate good: of what value is such information and to whom?

3. In the health field there is a tendency to adopt the best available and latest technology in every institution. This drive is promoted by the medical ethic of doing the utmost for the individual patient and reinforced by current methods of paying providers by third parties. The voluntary nonprofit form of organizing hospitals is frequently mentioned as a factor. Still another factor is usually neglected, namely, the nature of the physician-hospital relationship in this country. Physicians who specialize in treating patients with a given disease will not accede to its exclusion from hospital A, where they hold a staff appointment, unless they are granted staff privileges in hospital B, where the planning agency would like to concentrate all facilities for diagnosis and treatment. Only in part are financial interests involved; equally, or even more important, is the preservation and application of professional skills.

4. Economic valuation has no meaning without a firm basis in the underlying data on the link between the inputs and outputs of specific programs. It is not often that economists can develop such data. Other investigators must be persuaded and enabled to do this by investing their time and energies in longitudinal studies.

5. It is discouraging to perform technical analysis, to persuade the decision makers of its usefulness, to have it adopted, and then to discover that funds for health services are cut off because total government spending is being curtailed. Adjusting aggregate demand in the economy through changes in total expenditures is bound to result in the stop-and-go operation of individual programs. This is both wasteful and frustrating, and poses a substantial threat to continuity in the provision of health services through public financing.

6. Since cost-benefit or cost-effectiveness analysis is economic evaluation of public projects or programs, it must inevitably take place in a political climate. While the economic tool of cost-benefit analysis implies a delineation of goals and an articulation of values, the imperatives of the political process may call for a blurring of differences and potential conflicts, in order to facilitate the building of coalitions aimed at the accomplishment of particular ends. Schultze (31) has observed this paradox: PPB has been applied most in an area, national defense, where future uncertainty is greatest but value differences among citizens have been traditionally least; PPB is not applied much in the human resources area, where the problem of uncertainty is not so serious, but differences in values among citizens prevail, as well as a great many vested interests.

Some political scientists, such as Wildavsky (120, 121), would agree with the above description and conclude that such are the facts of life. Most changes in governmental budgets are incremental anyway and do not—indeed cannot—derive from base zero (122). Within the boundaries set by defined political understandings, there are ample opportunities to improve decision making through systematic analysis. There is no reason to believe that politicians prefer to make poor decisions over good ones. In cases that are of vital importance to the body politic, many politicians, when persuaded of the right thing to do, would be willing to use up some of the credit they have accumulated and make the tough, though unpopular, choice. They cannot take such a stand on every issue, however. Therefore, the exceptionally capable practitioner of economic cost-benefit analysis must know how and when to make an allowance for the existence of a political cost-benefit calculus (120).

REFERENCES

1. Haveman, R. H. Public expenditures and policy analysis: An overview. In *Public Expenditures and Policy Analysis*, edited by R. H. Haveman and J. Margolis, pp. 1-18. Markham Publishing Company, Chicago, 1970.
2. Eckstein, O. A survey of the theory of public expenditure criteria. In *Public Finances: Needs, Sources, and Utilization*, edited by J. M. Buchanan, pp. 439-494. Princeton University Press, Princeton, N.J., 1961.
3. Prest, A. R., and Turvey, R. Cost-benefit analysis: A survey. *Economic Journal* 75(300): 683-735, 1965.
4. Steiner, P. O. *Public Expenditure Budgeting*. The Brookings Institution, Washington, D.C., 1969.
5. Eckstein, O. *Water Resources Development*. Harvard University Press, Cambridge, 1958.
6. Hirshleifer, J., DeHaven, J. C., and Milliman, J. W. *Water Supply: Economics, Technology and Policy*. University of Chicago Press, Chicago, 1960.
7. Kneese, A. V., and Smith, S. C. *Water Research*. Johns Hopkins Press, Baltimore, 1966.
8. Krutilla, J. V., and Eckstein, O. *Multiple Purpose River Development*. Johns Hopkins Press, Baltimore, 1958.
9. Maass, A., Hufschmidt, M. M., Dorfman, R., Thomas, H. A., Marglin, S. A., and Fair, G. M. *Design of Water-Resource Systems*. Harvard University Press, Cambridge, 1962.
10. McKean, R. N. *Efficiency in Government Through Systems Analysis*. John Wiley & Sons, Inc., New York, 1958.
11. Arrow, K. J. The organization of economic activity: Issues pertinent to the choice of market versus nonmarket allocation. In *Public Expenditures and Policy Analysis*, edited by R. H. Haveman and J. Margolis, pp. 59-73. Markham Publishing Company, Chicago, 1970.
12. Samuelson, P. A. The pure theory of public expenditure. *Review of Economics and Statistics* 36(4): 387-389, 1954.
13. Weisbrod, B. A. *Economics of Public Health*. University of Pennsylvania Press, Philadelphia, 1961.
14. Sloan, F. A. *Planning Public Expenditure on Mental Health Service Delivery*. The New York City Rand Institute, New York, 1971.
15. Stigler, G. J. *The Theory of Price*, rev. ed., p. 150. Macmillan and Company, New York, 1952.
16. Fuchs, V. R. Health care and the U.S. economic system: An essay in abnormal physiology. In *Technology and Health Care Systems in the 1980's*, edited by M. F. Collen, pp. 169-175. National Center for Health Services Research and Development, Washington, D.C., 1973.
17. Lasagna, L. Quoted in *Decision-Making on the Efficacy and Safety of Drugs*, edited by J. D. Cooper, p. 2. Interdisciplinary Communication Associates, Washington, D.C., 1971.
18. Klarman, H. E. *The Economics of Health*. Columbia University Press, New York, 1965.
19. Freeman, A. M. Project design and evaluation with multiple objectives. In *Public Expenditures and Policy Analysis*, edited by R. H. Haveman and J. Margolis, pp. 347-363. Markham Publishing Company, Chicago, 1970.
20. Haveman, R. H., and Krutilla, J. V. *Unemployment, Idle Capacity and the Evaluation of Public Expenditures*. Johns Hopkins Press, Baltimore, 1968.
21. McGuire, M. C., and Garn, H. A. The integration of equity and efficiency criteria in public project selection. *Economic Journal* 79(316): 882-893, 1969.
22. Weisbrod, B. A. Income redistribution effects and benefit-cost analysis. In *Problems in Public Expenditure Analysis*, edited by S. B. Chase, pp. 177-209. The Brookings Institution, Washington, D.C., 1968.
23. United States Department of Health, Education, and Welfare. *Motor Vehicle Injury Prevention Program; Cancer Control; Arthritis Control; Selected Disease Control Programs*. Office of Assistant Secretary for Program Coordination, Washington, D.C., 1961.
24. Acton, J. P. Evaluation of a Life-Saving Program: The Case of Heart Attacks. Doctoral Dissertation, Harvard University, Cambridge, 1970.
25. McKean, R. N. The use of shadow prices. In *Problems in Public Expenditure Analysis*, edited by S. B. Chase, pp. 33-65. The Brookings Institution, Washington, D.C., 1968.
26. Margolis, J. Shadow-prices for incorrect or nonexistent market values. In *Public Expenditures and Policy Analysis*, edited by R. H. Haveman and J. Margolis, pp. 314-329. Markham Publishing Company, Chicago, 1970.
27. Fein, R. Definition and scope of the problem: Economic aspects. In *Assessing the Effectiveness of Child Health Services*, edited by A. B. Bergman, pp. 44-50. Ross Laboratories, Columbus, Ohio, 1967.
28. Weisbrod, B. A. Concepts of costs and benefits. In *Problems in Public Expenditure Analysis*, edited by S. B. Chase, pp. 257-262. The Brookings Institution, Washington, D.C., 1968.

29. Klarman, H. E., Francis, J. O'S., and Rosenthal, G. D. Cost effectiveness analysis applied to the treatment of chronic renal disease. *Med. Care* 6(1): 48-54, 1968.
30. Gorham, W. Allocating federal resources among competing social needs. *HEW Indicators* pp. 1-13, August 1966.
31. Schultze, C. L. *The Politics and Economics of Public Spending*, pp. 1-34, 77-102. The Brookings Institution, Washington, D.C., 1968.
32. United States Bureau of the Budget. Bulletin 66-3, Supplement, and Bulletin 68-2 on Planning-Programming-Budgeting, October 12, 1965, February 21, 1966, and July 18, 1967. Reprinted in *Planning, Programming, Budgeting: A Systems Approach to Management*, edited by F. J. Lyden and E. G. Miller, pp. 405-443. Markham Publishing Company, Chicago, 1968.
33. Klarman, H. E. Present status of cost-benefit analysis in the health field. *Am. J. Public Health* 57(11): 1948-1953, 1967.
34. Henderson, P. D. Investment criteria for public enterprises. In *Public Enterprise*, edited by R. Turvey, pp. 86-169. Penguin Modern Economics Readings, Penguin Books, Baltimore, 1968.
35. Musgrave, R. A. Cost-benefit analysis and the theory of public finance. *Journal of Economic Literature* 7(3): 797-806, 1969.
36. Baumol, W. J. On the discount rate for public projects. In *Public Expenditures and Policy Analysis*, edited by R. H. Haveman and J. Margolis, pp. 273-290. Markham Publishing Company, Chicago, 1970.
37. *Interest Rate Guidelines for Federal Decision-Making*. Joint Economic Committee, Congress of the United States. U.S. Government Printing Office, Washington, D.C., 1968.
38. Boulding, K. E. Notes on a theory of philanthropy. In *Philanthropy and Public Policy*, edited by F. G. Dickinson, pp. 57-71. National Bureau of Economic Research, New York, 1962.
39. Hufschmidt, M. M., Krutilla, J., and Margolis, J. Standards and criteria for formulating and evaluating federal water resources developments. In *Hearings on Guidelines for Estimating the Benefits of Public Expenditures*, pp. 135-212. Joint Economic Committee, Congress of the United States. U.S. Government Printing Office, Washington, D.C., 1969.
40. Feldstein, M. S. The social time preference discount rate in cost benefit analysis. *Economic Journal* 74(294): 360-379, 1964.
41. Mushkin, S. J., and Collings, F. d'A. Economic costs of disease and injury. *Public Health Rep.* 74(9): 795-809, 1959.
42. Fein, R. *Economics of Mental Illness*. Basic Books, New York, 1958.
43. Rice, D. P. *Economic Costs of Cardiovascular Diseases and Cancer*. Health Economics Series No. 5. U.S. Government Printing Office, Washington, D.C., 1965.
44. Rice, D. P. *Estimating the Cost of Illness*. Health Economics Series No. 6. U.S. Government Printing Office, Washington, D.C., 1966.
45. Klarman, H. E. Syphilis control programs. In *Measuring Benefits of Government Investments*, edited by R. Dorfman, pp. 367-410. The Brookings Institution, Washington, D.C., 1965.
46. Klarman, H. E. Socioeconomic impact of heart disease. In *The Heart and Circulation*, Vol. 2, pp. 693-707. Federation of American Societies for Experimental Biology, Washington, D.C., 1965.
47. Menz, F. C. Economics of disease prevention: Infectious kidney disease. *Inquiry* 8(4): 3-18, 1971.
48. Fuchs, V. R. The contribution of health services to the American economy. *Milbank Mem. Fund Q.* 44(4, part 2): 65-101, 1966.
49. Grosse, R. N. Cost-benefit analysis of health service. *Annals* 399: 89-99, January 1972.
50. Klarman, H. E. Conference on the economics of medical research. In Report of the President's Commission on Heart Disease, Cancer, and Stroke, Vol. 2, pp. 631-644. U.S. Government Printing Office, Washington, D.C., 1965.
51. Mushkin, S. J. Health as an investment. *Journal of Political Economy* 70(5): 129-157, 1962.
52. Bowen, H. R. *Toward Social Economy*. Rinehart and Company, Inc., New York, 1948.
53. Rice, D. P., and Cooper, B. S. The economic value of human life. *Am. J. Pub. Health* 57(11): 1954-1966, 1967.
54. Mishan, E. J. Evaluation of life and limb. *Journal of Political Economy* 79(4): 687-705, 1971.
55. Kuznets, S. *National Income and Its Composition, 1919-1938*, pp. 22-23. National Bureau of Economic Research, New York, 1947.
56. Walker, K. E., and Gauger, W. H. The Dollar Value of Household Work. New York State College of Human Ecology, Cornell University, Ithaca, New York, 1973 (processed).
57. Sirageldin, I. A-H. *Non-Market Components of National Income*. Institute for Social Research, University of Michigan, Ann Arbor, 1969.
58. Gelman, A. C. *Multiphasic Health Testing Systems: Reviews and Annotations*. U.S. Government Printing Office, Washington, D.C., 1971.

59. Vickrey, W. S. One economist's view of philanthropy. In *Philanthropy and Public Policy*, edited by F. G. Dickinson, pp. 31-56. National Bureau of Economic Research, New York, 1962.

60. Neenan, W. B. *Normative Evaluation of a Public Health Program*. Institute of Public Administration, University of Michigan, Ann Arbor, 1967.

61. Schelling, T. C. The life you save may be your own. In *Problems in Public Expenditure Analysis*, edited by S. B. Chase, pp. 127-162. The Brookings Institution, Washington, D.C., 1968.

62. Thurow, L. *Investment in Human Capital*, p. 134. Wadsworth Publishing Company, Inc., Belmont, California, 1970.

63. Titmuss, R. M. *The Gift Relationship*, p. 198. Pantheon Books, New York, 1971.

64. Morris, J. N. *The Uses of Epidemiology*, p. 45. E. & S. Livingston, Edinburgh, 1957.

65. Scheff, T. J. Preferred errors in diagnosis. *Med. Care* 2(3): 166-172, 1964.

66. Saslaw, M., Vieta, A., and Myerburg, R. Cost of rheumatic fever and its prevention. *Am. J. Public Health* 55(3): 429-434, 1965.

67. Report of the Committee on Chronic Kidney Disease (C. W. Gottschalk, chairman). Bureau of the Budget, Washington, D.C., 1967.

68. Grosse, R. N. Problems of resource allocation in health. In *Public Expenditures and Policy Analysis*, edited by R. H. Haveman and J. Margolis, pp. 518-548. Markham Publishing Company, Chicago, 1970.

69. Feldstein, M. S. Health sector planning in developing countries. *Economica*, New Series 37(146): 139-163, 1970.

70. Quade, E. S. Systems analysis techniques for planning-programming-budgeting. In *Planning, Programming, Budgeting: A Systems Approach to Management*, edited by F. J. Lyden and E. G. Miller, pp. 292-312. Markham Publishing Company, Chicago, 1968.

71. Sturm, H. M. *Technology and Manpower in the Health Service Industry, 1965-1975*. U.S. Government Printing Office, Washington, D.C., 1968.

72. Klarman, H. E. Economic Aspects of Chronic Kidney Disease Revisited. Paper presented at annual meeting of American Public Health Association, November 11, 1969 (processed).

73. Bennett, I. L. The Scientific and Educational Basis for Medical Care. Paper presented at New York Health Services Research and Policy Seminar, December 1, 1970 (processed).

74. Feldstein, M. S. *The Rising Cost of Hospital Care*. Information Resources Press, Washington, D.C., 1971.

75. Blaug, M. A survey of the theory of process innovation. In *The Economics of Technological Change*, edited by N. Rosenberg, pp. 86-113. Penguin Modern Economics Readings, Penguin Books, Baltimore, 1971.

76. Fuchs, V. R., and Kramer, M. J. *Expenditures for Physicians' Services in the United States, 1948-1968*, pp. 35-42. National Center for Health Services Research and Development, Washington, D.C., 1973.

77. Grossman, M. *The Demand for Health: A Theoretical and Empirical Investigation*. National Bureau of Economic Research, New York, 1972.

78. Klarman, H. E. Increase in the cost of physician and hospital services. *Inquiry* 7(1): 22-36, 1970.

79. Klarman, H. E. Approaches to moderating the increases in medical care costs. *Med. Care* 7(3): 175-190, 1969.

80. Pauly, M. V., and Drake, D. F. Effect of third-party methods of reimbursement on hospital performance. In *Empirical Studies in Health Economics*, edited by H. E. Klarman, pp. 297-314. Johns Hopkins Press, Baltimore, 1970.

81. Davis, K. A. Theory of Economic Behavior in Non-Profit Hospitals. Doctoral Dissertation, Rice University, Houston, 1969.

82. Ginsburg, P. B. Capital in Non-Profit Hospitals. Doctoral Dissertation, Harvard University, Cambridge, 1970.

83. Newhouse, J. P. Toward a theory of nonprofit institutions: An economic model of a hospital. *American Economic Review* 60(1): 64-74, 1970.

84. Reder, M. W. Some problems in the economics of hospitals. *American Economic Review* (Papers and Proceedings) 55(2): 472-480, 1965.

85. Lee, M. L. A conspicuous production theory of hospital behavior. *Southern Economic Journal* 38(1): 48-58, 1971.

86. Rosenstock, I. M. Why people use health services. *Milbank Mem. Fund Q.* 44(3, part 2): 94-124, 1966.

87. Ginzberg, E. *Men, Money, and Medicine*, p. 55. Columbia University Press, New York, 1969.

88. Long, M. F. Efficient use of hospitals. In *The Economics of Health and Medical Care*, edited by S. J. Mushkin, pp. 211-226. Bureau of Public Health Economics, University of Michigan, Ann Arbor, 1964.

89. Anderson, O. W. Trends in hospital use and their policy implications. In Fifth Annual

Symposium on Hospital Affairs, *Where is Hospital Use Headed?* pp. 2-5. Graduate School of Business, University of Chicago, Chicago, 1964.

90. Feldstein, P. J. *An Empirical Investigation of the Marginal Cost of Hospital Services.* Graduate Program in Hospital Administration, University of Chicago, Chicago, 1961.

91. Roemer, M. I. Bed supply and hospital utilization: A national experiment. *Hospitals* 35(21): 36-42, 1961.

92. Shain, M., and Roemer, M. I. Hospital costs relate to the supply of beds. *Mod. Hosp.* 92(4): 71-73, 168, 1959.

93. Flagle, C. D. Evaluation and control of technology in health services. In *Technology and Health Care Systems in the 1980's,* edited by M. F. Collen, pp. 213-224. National Center for Health Services Research and Development, Washington, D.C., 1973.

94. Shegog, R. F. A. Reviewing some applications of computers to medicine. In *Problems and Progress in Medical Care,* Third Series, edited by G. McLachlan, pp. 145-170. Oxford University Press, London, 1968.

95. Ahlvin, R. C. Biochemical screening—A critique. *New Engl. J. Med.* 283(20): 1084-1086, 1970.

96. Flagle, C. D., Gabrielson, I. W., Soriano, A., and Taylor, M. M. *Analysis of Congestion in an Out-patient Clinic.* Operations Research Division, The Johns Hopkins Hospital, Baltimore, 1959.

97. Feldstein, M. S. Choice of technique in the public sector: A simplification. *Economic Journal* 80(320): 985-990, 1970.

98. National Academy of Engineering. *A Study of Technology Assessment,* pp. 96-104. Committee on Science and Astronautics, U.S. House of Representatives. U.S. Government Printing Office, Washington, D.C., 1969.

99. Collen, M. F. Statement in Subcommittee on Health of the Elderly, Special Committee on Aging, U. S. Senate. *Hearings on Detection and Prevention of Chronic Disease Utilizing Multiphasic Health Screening Techniques,* pp. 214-222. U.S. Government Printing Office, Washington, D.C., 1966.

100. Collen, M. F. Periodic health examinations using an automated multitest laboratory. *J.A.M.A.* 195(10): 830-833, 1966.

101. Collen, M. F., Kidd, P. H., Feldman, R., and Cutler, J. L. Cost analysis of a multiphasic screening program. *New Engl. J. Med.* 280: 1043-1045, 1969.

102. Collen, M. F., Feldman, R., Siegelaub, A. B., and Crawford, D. Dollar cost per positive test for automated multiphasic screening. *New Engl. J. Med.* 283: 459-463, 1970.

103. Collen, M. F. Automated multiphasic health testing: Implementation of a system. *Hospitals* 45(5): 49-50, 56-58, 1971.

104. Collen, M. F., Dales, L. G., Friedman, G. D., Flagle, C. D., Feldman, R., and Siegelaub, A.B. *Multiphasic Checkup Evaluation Study: 4. Preliminary Cost-Benefit Analysis for Middle Aged Men.* Medical Methods Research, Oakland, California, 1973 (processed).

105. Garfield, S. R. The delivery of medical care. *Sci. Am.* 222(4): 15-23, 1970.

106. Garfield, S. R. Multiphasic health testing and medical care as a right. *New Engl. J. Med.* 283(20): 1087-1089, 1970.

107. Ingalls, T. H., and Gordon, J. E. Periodic health examination, 1900-1965. *Am. J. Med. Sci.* 251(3): 123-140, 1966.

108. Siegel, G. S. An American dilemma—The periodic health examination. *Arch. Environ. Health* 13(3): 292-295, 1966.

109. Wade, L., Thorpe, J., Elias, T., and Bock, G. Are periodic health examinations worthwhile? *Ann. Intern. Med.* 56(1): 81-93, 1962.

110. McKeown, T. Validation of screening procedures. In *Screening in Medical Care: Reviewing the Evidence,* pp. 1-13. Oxford University Press, London, 1968.

111. Garfield, S. R. A look at the economics of medical care. In *Technology and Health Care Systems in the 1980's,* edited by M. F. Collen, pp. 169-175. National Center for Health Services Research and Development, Washington, D.C., 1973.

112. Feldstein, P. J. Research on the demand for health services. *Milbank Mem. Fund Q.* 44 (3, part 2): 128-162, 1966.

113. Blumberg, M. S. Evaluating health screening procedures. *Operations Research* 5(3): 351-360, 1957.

114. Thorner, R. R., and Remein, Q. M. *Principles and Procedures in the Evaluation of Screening for Disease.* U.S. Government Printing Office, Washington, D.C., 1971.

115. Report of the AMHTS Advisory Committee to the National Center for Health Services Research and Development, Vol. 1, pp. 29, 31. U.S. Government Printing Office, Washington, D.C., 1970.

116. Pole, J. D. Economic aspects of screening for disease. In *Screening in Medical Care: Reviewing the Evidence,* pp. 141-157. Oxford University Press, London, 1968.

117. Suchman, E. A. *Evaluative Research,* p. 65. Russell Sage Foundation, New York, 1967.

118. Ramcharan, S., Cutler, J. L., Feldman, R., Siegelaub, A. B., Campbell, B., Friedman, G. D., Dales, L., and Collen, M. F. Kaiser-Permanente Multiphasic Health Checkup Evaluation Project: 2. Disability and Chronic Disease after Seven Years of Multiphasic Health Checkups. Paper presented at the Epidemiology Section of the American Public Health Association, October 11, 1971 (processed).
119. Etzioni, A., and Remp, R. Technological 'shortcuts' to social change. *Science* 175: 31-38, January 7, 1972.
120. Wildavsky, A. The political economy of efficiency: Cost-benefit analysis, and program budgeting. *Public Administration Review* 26(4): 292-310, 1966.
121. Wildavsky, A., and Hammann, A. Comprehensive versus incremental budgeting in the department of agriculture. *Administrative Science Quarterly* 10(3): 321-346, 1965.
122. Lindblom, C. E. Decision-making in taxation and expenditures. In *Public Finances: Needs, Sources, and Utilization*, edited by J. M. Buchanan, pp. 295-329. Princeton University Press, Princeton, N.J., 1961.

Manuscript submitted for publication, April 12, 1973

Direct reprint requests to:

Dr. Herbert E. Klarman
Professor of Economics
New York University
Graduate School of Public Administration
4 Washington Square North
New York, New York 10003

REGULATION AND PUBLIC POLICY

24. Effects of Hospital Cost Containment on the Development and Use of Medical Technology

KENNETH WARNER

Reprinted with permission from *The Milbank Memorial Fund Quarterly/Health and Society* 56. Copyright © 1978, Milbank Memorial Fund, 187-211.

O NE OF THE DOMINANT CHARACTERISTICS of modern American medicine is the development and widespread diffusion of sophisticated technology. Originally considered an unequivocal blessing, the technological revolution in medicine has of late acquired something of a bad name. This change reflects a shift in the nature of current technology and its presumed contributions to the costs and benefits of medical care. In the 1940s and 1950s, biomedical science contributed the antibiotics that dramatically reduced the morbidity and mortality associated with a variety of infectious diseases. This true "high technology" of medicine was effective, safe, and inexpensive to administer (Thomas, 1974). Today, however, the public and many professionals view the medical technological revolution as expensive and complex, characterized by resource-intensive capital equipment of unestablished efficacy, which frequently requires hospitalization and serves to inflate the cost of care while delivering little demonstrable health benefit.

Increased awareness of the opportunity costs of resources devoted to expensive "halfway technology" is poignantly illustrated by Gaus and Cooper (1976):

> [W]e spent 4 billion dollars for new technology [for Medicare patients in 1976] and we do not know if it did any good, much less how much . . . .
>
> . . . If we had continued providing hospital services to the aged, as they were in 1967, then we could have spent that 4 billion dollars last year [to] . . . have
>
> • Brought *all* aged persons above the poverty line [with at least 3.3 million currently living below it]; or
>
> • Provided the rent to raise 2 million elderly from substandard to standard housing units; or
>
> • Brought all the elderly above the lowest accepted food budget and more; or

- Provided eyeglasses and hearing aids to all who needed them [estimated at 18 million needing or wearing glasses and over 3 million needing hearing aids], and more.

Which would have helped the most, [medical] technology or food?

The "technology problem" is simply a reflection of the fundamental dilemma of American health care: how to provide accessible, high quality care to all and at the same time restrain inflation in the cost of providing care. The profusion of expensive medical technology has been cited as a cause of rising costs and one of the effects of attempts to provide quality care. The question is how to search for, develop, produce, distribute, and utilize technology that will truly contribute to the higher quality and economic efficiency of health care, and how to simultaneously weed out technologies whose benefits are not commensurate with their costs.

The severity of the inflation problem is reflected in Congress' willingness to seriously entertain proposals for national hospital cost containment.[1] Concern has also been demonstrated recently by several government-sponsored inquiries into diverse technology issues: the deterioration of technology's research base; the safety and efficacy of technology; the role of technology in inflation; and so on (the President's Biomedical Research Panel, 1976; Office of Technology Assessment, 1978; National Academy of Sciences, forthcoming). In this paper we merge these policy interests by asking: How might hospital cost containment affect the development and use of medical technology?

Perspectives on the Technology Problem

The concerns with which different observers voice this seemingly neutral question indicate the diversity of perspectives on "the technology problem." The major perspectives are not inherently incompatible, but they do reflect a tension that pervades the cost containment debate. Proponents of medical technological development ask the question with trepidation, fearful that the economic discipline in cost containment will retard the development of useful medical technologies. These individuals believe that regulatory meddling by government coupled with the inherent public-good problems of research have erected barriers to the pursuit of promising biomedical research and development (R&D). Cost containment might exacerbate the situation, further weakening American

---

[1]The Carter Administration's Hospital Cost Containment Act, as amended in the Subcommittee on Health and the Environment of the House Committee on Interstate and Foreign Commerce, is HR 9717. The Senate version of the bill is S 1391. The competing alternative, S 1470, introduced by Senator Talmadge and others, is limited to Medicare and Medicaid reimbursement. The major provisions of these bills, prior to amendment, are described in Committee on Interstate and Foreign Commerce, 1977.

leadership in biomedical science and restricting productivity growth in the practice of medicine.

Proponents of cost containment generally believe that the current system fosters excessive adoption and use of medical technology. They ask the same question in the hope that cost containment will direct the allocation of medical resources more efficiently, producing more cost-effective technology and reducing the waste they perceive to be associated with much existing technology. The dimensions of that waste include the following:

> The current system fosters the production of too much technology, *i.e.*, technology whose social benefit is not worth its social cost.
>
> New and existing technology is too widely distributed; new technology often diffuses too rapidly and indiscriminately.
>
> Technology is used excessively and in many instances improperly.
>
> The R&D and medical practice systems have led to the production of the wrong mix of cost-saving and cost-increasing technology, with the system heavily biased toward the latter.

The "pro" and "anti" technology views are not necessarily incompatible, because they focus on different stages of the R&D-use spectrum. This difference suggests a subtle but important point that has eluded most discussion of the technology cost issue: while there is general agreement that technology contributes to the medical cost inflation problem (Warner, 1977), there is little consideration of the *mechanism* linking technology to inflation; yet for cost containment to be effective, policy must be tailored to the source of the problem. For example, if the problem results from an excessive stock of capital equipment, policy ought to focus on hospitals' acquisition of equipment, as do Certificate of Need (CON) and a ceiling on hospital capital expenditures. If the problem derives from excessive use of a reasonable stock of equipment, legislators should concentrate on reimbursement policies.

Alternatively, the inflation problem may result from the flow of new technology into the system, namely, the rate of increase in available new technology and the consequent pressures to adopt it. This might call for policy focusing on the medical technology R&D system, and not on hospital or physician behavior *per se*. Finally, it may be that "the tendency to overinvest in and overuse sophisticated services is just part of a larger tendency to overuse health services or to invest too many labor or nonlabor resources in the production of hospital services"(Wagner and Zubkoff, 1978). If this is the case, the contribution of technology to inflation should not be isolated as a "technology problem." Rather, cost containment policy should concentrate on general reimbursement and regulatory mechanisms, without an explicit technology focus. (See also Schroeder and Showstack, 1977.)

Medical technology comes in all sizes and shapes. Similarly, cost containment has many forms, varying from a dichotomous decision on whether to grant a hospital's request for a specific piece of equipment, to a general cap on hospital revenues. Each of the cost containment forms may have different effects on the development and use of medical technology; indeed, a single form may have very different effects on different types of technology. Thus for purposes of analysis it is necessary to define the meanings of both cost containment and medical technology. In this paper, cost containment will refer to a limit on hospitals' inpatient revenues, as proposed by the Carter Administration, with separate consideration of a ceiling on capital expenditures, a second significant component of many proposals. The operation of these limits and details on specific proposals are described elsewhere (see the bills referenced in footnote 1 and Committee on Interstate and Foreign Commerce, 1977). Medical technology will refer to non-labor inputs, with interest focused on sophisticated, high-priced capital equipment, *e.g.*, computerized axial tomography (CAT scanners), and other equipment and supplies having significant implications for hospital costs due to frequency of use, *e.g.*, automated electrocardiography. To an economist, technology means a defined configuration of all inputs, both human and nonhuman, used in a specific production process. The emphasis in this paper on "hardware" reflects the popular usage of the term, and concern about, "medical technology."

The remainder of this paper suggests some tentative answers to the issues raised by our question: How might hospital cost containment affect the development and use of medical technology? We begin by analyzing the environment in which medical technology develops, is adopted, and used. The purpose of this discussion is twofold: to provide a context within which one can understand how hospital cost containment might influence the development and use of technology; and to provide a perspective for assessing the desirability of alterations in the status quo. The following section suggests what some of those changes might be.

Factors Affecting the Development and Use of Medical Technology

Advancement of medical technology depends on a robust system of biomedical R&D and on demand for the products of R&D. In most industrial settings, these two factors are inextricably linked: the nature and amount of R&D depend principally, if not exclusively, on the productivity of firms' R&D departments (measured as contribution to profitability). In contrast, frequently in biomedicine much of R&D appears to function as an entity unto itself, dependent more on the mood of Congress and the public than on its innate productivity. In part, of course, this simply reflects the great difficulty in measuring the productivity of biomedical R&D, especially that of basic research. But it does raise an important point: some aspects of medical technology development and advancement are quite independent of the medical care delivery system and hence are unlikely to be affected by changes in the technology use patterns of hospitals that result from cost containment; other aspects do depend on changes in the delivery system and seem likely to be affected by cost containment. We will discuss these distinctions in the next section of this paper, after briefly examining herein the factors that influence both the development and use of medical technology.

Much of biomedical R&D, including almost all basic research, is the ward of the state. Through the National Institutes of Health and other agencies, the federal government dominates determination of how much and what type of research will be undertaken. Decisions about funding levels, categorical disease emphases, and the mix of fundamental and targeted research all reflect a combination of professional and political influences. Even many of the immediate beneficiaries of the government's largesse—medical schools and biomedical researchers—have little interest in the economic implications of the fruits of biomedical R&D. In short, market forces play only indirect roles in governmental R&D allocations, despite the fact that "Many . . . research funding decisions [which] appear to be million-dollar decisions at the time they are made . . . turn out to be billion-dollar decisions when the outcomes of the funded research reverberate through the health care system" (Gaus, 1975).

Involvement of the private sector in biomedical R&D varies according to the stage of research. Industry supports very little fundamental bioscience, concentrating rather on applied research and, especially, development. This is consistent with the theory of public goods, since the economic benefits of development work are both more certain and more appropriable than those deriving from basic research. Thus, private industry contributes relatively little to the creation of new basic bioscience knowledge but plays a major role in bioengineering and the development and production of hardware.

Both for-profit firms and non-profit researchers have incentives to work toward the solution of unsolved medical problems. There are few incentives to search for less expensive means of accomplishing an existing task, which is the goal of much of private industry's conventional research. The bias toward "new-solution" technology results from the professional prestige associated with developing and using a "new solution" and a reimbursement environment (discussed below) in which adoption and use decisions are effectively free to the decision makers. The consequence, many observers suggest, is that the bulk of the technological innovations that issue from biomedical R&D increase costs; relatively few save costs.

The biomedical R&D enterprise continually presents health care providers with a wide array of innovations. The medical professional environment encourages the adoption and use of innovations. Physicians, it has frequently been claimed, are driven by a "technological imperative" instilled during medical training where the image of high quality medicine is predicated on a scientific approach to problems, with modern technology constituting the instruments with which that approach is practiced. Furthermore, the existence of high-cost, hospital-based technology is considered a factor in the trend toward increasing physician specialization, which in turn reinforces the hospital's growing importance as a source of care and increases the demand of physicians for still more technology. Possession of modern, sophisticated technology confers prestige on physicians, and it often contributes to their economic well-being. As a result, hospital administrators want to acquire sophisticated equipment and facilities, both for their own prestige and to attract and hold high caliber physicians on their staffs. Finally, the public's growing faith in the power of science in general and of curative medicine in particular accelerates the demand for technologically advanced methods of care. In short, technological sophistication is viewed by many—patients, physicians, and administrators—as a surrogate for high-quality care.

The "social contract" binds physicians to provide the "best possible care." This acts as an additional pressure to adopt and use new technology. In medically desperate situations—*i.e.*, where the prognosis is poor and reasonable therapeutic alternatives few— physicians are often encouraged to use experimental innovations in nonexperimental settings. This may result in widespread diffusion of innovations well before their medical efficacy, toxicities, costs, and so on are understood (Warner, 1975), although early diffusion is not restricted to medical crisis situations (Altman and Eichenholz, 1976; Gaus, 1976).

Direct governmental involvement can promote the development and diffusion of technology, as does its support of research, but it can also restrict production and use, principally through regulatory policies. The overall effects of regulation on technology adoption and use are uncertain, although the available evidence is not encouraging: regulation intended to limit the spread of medical capital appears to have been reasonably ineffective (Needleman and Lewin, 1977). For example, where CON has succeeded in limiting growth in hospital bed supply, purchase of other equipment has increased, resulting in no overall savings in capital expenditures (Salkever and Bice, 1976). In contrast, the new medical device regulation procedures (U.S. Congress, 1976), which are intended only to assure the safety and efficacy of medical services, have raised the fear that "over-regulation" will stifle entrepreneurial initiative and thus reduce the discovery and production of new safe and efficacious devices. Certainly the regulatory effects of a ceiling on capital expenditures might be quite significant.

The economic environment of medical care provides some positive incentives and few disincentives to adopt the newest technology. Beginning with the subsidization of research and development, the government pumps considerable money into medical schools and elsewhere to encourage development of new knowledge and technical innovations.

But the most salient feature of the medical technology market is the mixture of the sellers' profit incentive and buyers' relatively unconstrained positions. The sellers' profit incentive has been cited as motivating the rapid and indiscriminate adoption of technology (Fuchs, 1973), but such adoption can occur only because technology buyers and users do not discriminate on the basis of all costs as well as benefits. This applies to each of the groups that buy or use medical technology: physicians, consumers, and hospitals.

As buyers and users of technology, cost-reimbursed physicians are indifferent to costs that are not borne by themselves or by insured patients. As suppliers of services in a fee-for-service setting, physicians often have a positive economic incentive to overutilize tests and other services that can generate personal profit.

Consumers find that increasing insurance coverage and affluence have significantly reduced the real direct (out-of-pocket) cost of much medical care, especially that provided in hospitals. Patients now pay less than one-eighth of the average hospital bill directly, compared with one-half in the early 1950s. In addition, increases in real income over the period mean that patients must now work fewer hours to pay the direct cost of a day of hospital care (Feldstein and Taylor, 1977). The lower real direct cost has increased the demand for care, particularly for the "style" and "high quality" of care (Feldstein, 1971, 1977). The hospital administrators' response has been "improvements," including the acquisition of the "latest" technology, which have driven costs up. Completing the circle is the consumers' response to the higher costs—namely, to buy more insurance (Russell, 1977):

> Thus, as third party payment has increased over the years, the benefit required to justify a decision in the eyes of doctors and patients has declined. This has led to the increased use of resources in all sorts of ways — including the introduction of technologies that otherwise might not have been adopted at all and, more often, the more rapid and extensive diffusion of technologies that had already been adopted to some extent.

Cost or cost-plus reimbursement has two direct influences on hospitals *qua* technology purchasers. First, reimbursement of interest payments lowers the effective cost to hospitals below the true interest rate, encouraging overinvestment in marginal projects. Overinvestment is further encouraged by the relative ease with which hospitals can borrow, a result of the tax-exempt status of many bond issues and the safety associated with third party reimbursement. Thus, hospitals are not forced "to experience the real discipline of the capital market" (Silvers, 1974). This is particularly important if, as some observers argue, the availability of financing governs the rate of adoption of high-cost technology, with the technology's medical efficacy being of secondary importance (Rice and Wilson,

1975), as may be demand or costs (Ginsburg, 1972). Second, the reimbursement mechanism fails to distinguish resource-saving from quality-enhancing or service-expanding projects. Hence the economic system does not counter the non-economic forces that favor adoption of sophisticated and generally costly technology. Both of these consequences are reinforced by the fact that frequent upgrading of existing services and addition of new ones give providers greater leeway in the allocation of overhead, and most cost-based reimbursement schemes probably allow considerable latitude in this area (Silvers, 1974).

"In short, when those making the decisions pay none of the costs, resources are used as though they cost nothing" (Russell, 1976). All of the elements come together here to produce a situation in which the binding constraint may be the state of the art, *i.e.*, the technology itself, and not, as elsewhere, considerations of all costs and benefits.

Likely Effects of Hospital Cost Containment on the Development and Use of Medical Technology

Hospital cost containment is not a panacea in the battle against the rapidly rising costs of medical care. Even if it were thoroughly successful, hospital cost containment would only address the inflation problem in one component of the medical care sector. Medical inflationary pressures might continue unabated outside of hospitals. Indeed, there is considerable concern that hospital cost containment will transfer inflation problems—and technology—to non-hospital settings, conceivably exacerbating overall inflation and making containment of costs within hospitals a Pyrrhic victory. In addition, of course, is the real possibility that a program of hospital cost containment will not work. The ability of such a program to succeed in its principal objective—containing costs—is not the focus of this paper; neither are other, non-technology effects (*e.g.*, effects on employment in hospitals). These concerns are left to other authors (*e.g.*, Congressional Budget Office, 1977; Reinhardt, 1977; Silver, 1977; Zelten, 1977) but are mentioned here to keep the ensuing discussion in perspective.

The immediate target of hospital cost containment is decision-making on resource allocation within hospitals. Changes in the mix of resources within hospitals and in the frequency of their use are the first-order effects of cost containment. The effects on other health care delivery institutions and on the development and advancement of technology—in essence, on public and private sector R & D— are mainly derivative or second-order consequences. We shall examine separately both first- and second-order consequences for each of a general inpatient revenue limit and a ceiling on capital expenditures.

Limit on Total Inpatient Revenues

First-Order Effects: The most direct impacts of an inpatient revenue limit relate to the acquisition and use of technology within hospitals. The following first-order effects can be anticipated:

1. Decreased use of technology already in place.   Staff physicians would be discouraged from ordering procedures perceived to have only marginal value. The recent trend toward more and more laboratory tests per illness (Scitovsky and McCall, 1976) can be expected to be reversed. Increasing input intensity—that is, inputs used per patient with a given diagnosis—has been cited as a major source of hospital cost inflation (Feldstein, 1971; Feldstein and Taylor, 1977; Redisch, 1974).

2. Substitution of existing lower-cost alternatives to tests or procedures of choice.   The cost factor would join the convenience, versatility, or other attributes of procedures that currently dictate preferences.

3. Reduction in the flow of new cost-increasing technology into the practice of medicine, particularly in hospitals.   This reduction would result from both supply and demand factors. Under pressure to contain costs, hospitals would reduce their orders (demand) for new cost-increasing technology. A second-order effect, expanded upon below, would be a reduced supply of cost-increasing innovations unless demand outside of hospitals grows sufficiently to compensate for the loss in hospital-based demand.

4. Increased interest in and consumption of new cost-saving technology.   Obviously, this has implications for R&D, as discussed below.

5. Decreased diffusion of existing technology.

6. Increased hospital and area-wide cooperation and coordination.   This is an obvious desirable outcome of a hospital cost containment program. Empirical studies provide evidence that many service areas currently have unnecessary excess technology and duplication of facilities (Abt, 1975; Roche and Stengle, 1973; U.S. DHEW, 1971).[2] Reimbursement mechanisms foster adoption of such excess capacity, and apparently regulatory efforts have not demonstrably inhibited it (Needleman and Lewin, 1977). Cost containment would put a significant price on duplication of facilities, and should therefore encourage hospital administrators to seek

---

[2]Excess capacity may be justified on the basis of option demand. That is, we are willing to pay a price (*i.e.*, the costs of unutilized capacity) in exchange for the certainty of the ready availability of the technology whenever it might be needed. While option demand is a legitimate basis for unused capacity, the amount of excess capacity often documented considerably exceeds that which option demand would recommend.

means of reducing duplication and excess capacity. An obvious means is the coordination of area-wide facilities planning, which is much more likely to be effective with the support, rather than opposition, of hospitals.[3] In major cities, this might result in specialization in the services offered by hospitals.

Second-Order Effects on Other Health Care Delivery Institutions: The derivative effects of an inpatient revenue ceiling on other health care delivery institutions reflect incentives to shift resource-intensive care to these other settings:

1. The "dumping" of expensive cases on other institutions. Since financially catastrophic cases would reduce the hospital's resources for treating other patients, the hospital would have an incentive to send expensive cases to other institutions, including public (*e.g.,* state) hospitals and nursing homes. While this might be within the letter of the law, it would certainly violate the spirit, since the cost would have been transferred, not contained. Whatever technology must be applied to expensive cases — and expensive cases are often technology-intensive — would probably move with the patients to these alternative institutions.

2. Shift in the use of cost-increasing technology from hospitals to private physicians' offices. As long as cost containment is limited to hospitals, there would be incentives for technology suppliers and physicians to locate technology in private practices. Both public and private organizations have called for extension of regulatory authority (especially for CON) to private non-hospital settings (Iglehart, 1977b; Institute of Medicine, 1977). Needless to say, such an extension would be politically difficult, but without it some cost problems might simply be transferred from hospitals to other delivery settings. Indeed, with physicians having a greater financial interest in the use of such technology in their own offices, additional unnecessary uses of technology might result. The danger of transfer of technology is exacerbated by the growth of Medical Service Plans (MSPs), groups of private physicians who contract with hospitals to staff specific services. Such groups are not covered in most hospital cost containment proposals, yet they are in an ideal position to purchase and use technology normally employed only in hospitals. Thus, hospital cost containment raises the spectre of the following scenario. Cost containment makes technology usage in hospitals "expensive" to medical decision-makers; *i.e.,* it limits the resources

---

[3]Area-wide planning has met with limited success. The Comprehensive Health Planning Agencies, which preceded the new Health Systems Agencies (HSAs), were viewed as generally ineffective in this capacity. The National Health Planning and Resources Development Act of 1974 (PL 93-641) put some teeth into the HSAs created by the Act. However, active and cooperative involvement of hospitals and the medical profession in area-wide planning would certainly facilitate this process. Hospital cost containment would appear to encourage such constructive involvement.

available for other inputs. Consequently, it provides an incentive to remove such technology use from the hospital's class of costs that are subject to the revenue ceiling. Private groups (*e.g.*, MSPs) then form, leasing or purchasing the technology in question, charging patients for its use, independent of their hospital bills, despite the fact that the technology is employed in the hospital in the care of inpatients. The cost of the technology is transferred through an accounting trick—it is not contained—and as observed above, use and hence cost actually increase with private groups now possessing a profit motive. This is not a certain consequence of an inpatient revenue ceiling, but neither is it a logical impossibility.

3. Shift in the use of technology from an inpatient to an outpatient basis. With the revenue limit applying only to inpatient care, there might be a wholesale shifting to outpatient care, according to opponents of this form of hospital cost containment. However, the question of the net effects of such shifting on both technology use and cost remains unresolved. Much hospitalization and inpatient use of technology result from an insurance system that favors these over ambulatory care. Thus, the cost containment incentive favoring outpatient care may simply balance the insurance system's inpatient bias.

Second-Order Effects on Development of New Technology: The effects of an inpatient revenue ceiling on the development of new technology derive from the effects on the use of technology by health care providers. The greater the distance between the stage of development and the application of technology, the less consequential should cost containment be. Thus, in general, basic research should be little affected, while some applied research and developmental work might respond significantly. The differential effects on private and public sector activity relate principally to the R&D stages upon which these sectors focus their efforts and on the financial dependence of the sectors' R&D on the use of technology.

The most profound consequences are likely to be experienced by private firms engaged in applied R&D, where most private sector R&D activity is concentrated. The dependence of such firms on the successful marketing of their R&D products is clear. If a revenue cap diminishes the market for cost-increasing technology,[4] one would expect to see:

1. Reduction in private sector R&D activity directed toward cost-increasing technology; decrease in the production of cost-increasing technological innovations; reduction in the number of firms engaged in the development and supply of such medical technology. This is a simple and direct response to the change in market conditions.

---

[4]The "if" relates to the question of how much technology demand would be transferred to non-inpatient settings rather than simply "drying up."

2. Greater price competition among suppliers and lowered hospital costs.   With the economic discipline imposed on hospitals, administrators and department heads would be forced to shop around. Hence cost containment would have a double-dose effect on hospital costs, inducing price competition among suppliers and encouraging frugality in the use of existing resources within hospitals.

3. More R&D and production of cost-saving technologies. Hospitals' incentive to constrain costs would create a significant new demand for cost-saving technology. Coupled with decreased demand for cost-increasing technology, this new demand would provide a powerful incentive for private firms to aggressively enter this new market. It is conceivable that hospitals' demand for cost-saving technology and the potentially large, relatively untapped reservoir of research ideas would combine to produce an even more robust medical technology market than currently exists. To be sure, the character of that market and its product would differ substantially from that which exists today, but the possibility remains that there would be active, imaginative R&D into a wealth of technological possibilities yet to be unearthed simply because the system has not previously offered professional or economic rewards for such products. If this accurately characterizes the situation, applied R&D might prove extremely productive in an era of cost containment.[5]

4. Little effect on basic bioscience research.   As noted above, the amount and nature of basic research are principally a function of federal funding. The incentive for researchers is to produce new knowledge, not to develop and sell a physical product. If anything, there has been a concern that fundamental biomedical research and medical practice are so dissociated that the fruits of research are not diffused sufficiently rapidly or widely into practice (Gordon and Fisher, 1975). If cost containment did have an undesirable effect on this most basic stage in the advancement of medical technology, research funding policies could be adjusted to compensate. Because there is likely to be a limited effect on basic research and a more significant effect on targeted R&D, one might anticipate a relative shift away from big capital-intensive technology toward knowledge-intensive "soft" technology. Much of the cost-increasing equipment

---

[5]This theoretical conclusion is supported by the analysis of a major private sector supplier of hospitals. Becton Dickinson, a firm with nearly $600 million in sales last year, believes that the struggle to hold down costs "can open up a relatively new area of product opportunity in the hospital for supplies primarily designed to reduce the cost of procedures. Historically, most new supply items have been sold on the basis of improvement in medical care . . . . The system . . . has not been receptive to cost reduction as a sales tool.

"Given a receptive, cost conscious environment, cost-reducing supplies represent a truly new class of products. Such items will be less expensive to develop and market and involve significantly less regulatory delay and risk than the medically more innovative products." (Blue Sheet, 1978)

embodied technology—the centerpiece of the current cost of technology debate—arises from the applied R&D work of the private sector. If this work declines due to a hospital cost containment program, the product of biomedical R&D will shift toward that which is least affected by the program, namely, the outcomes of basic science research.

A revenue limit program will not take place in what is otherwise a regulatory vacuum. Changes in the regulatory environment may have as much effect on the development of technology as do the explicit cost containment provisions. In addition to professional ethics, government policy and regulation are the only major hindrances to the development, adoption, and use of technology.[6] Cost containment could replace or eliminate the need for certain types of regulation that have had a repressive effect on the advancement of technology due to the maze of bureaucratic red tape they have constructed. Any diminution of such regulation would encourage exploration of new technological possibilities, even cost-increasing ones, thus partially offsetting the deterrent effects of cost containment *per se*.

Ceiling on Capital Expenditures

A ceiling on total capital expenditures would have many of the same effects as that on total revenues, but it would also have some quite distinct impacts resulting from concentration on a particular class of inputs, with exclusive focus on the capital costs of those inputs. The latter differentiates a dollar spent on acquisition of technology from one devoted to its use. Under a capital limit, a hospital faces real penalties for acquiring high-cost capital equipment, but virtually none for using equipment once it is in place.[7]

Were high-cost capital-intensive technology perceived to be simply another input responsive to the same incentives as other inputs, there would be no reason to have a ceiling on capital expenditures in addition to one on overall revenue if the revenue ceiling were applied to both equipment acquisition and all operating activities. The economic discipline inherent in the revenue limitation

---

[6]Regulation can retard or prevent development, adoption, or use, either directly or indirectly. Examples of direct effects include: on development, restrictions on recombinant DNA research; on adoption, CON for high-cost technology; and on application, FDA approval of drug uses. Indirect effects are illustrated by the development penalties of added delays and other costs in the research-to-market process due to medical device certification of safety and efficacy. Policy decisions not to reimburse for use of a technology for specified purposes obviously will have strong deterrent effects.

[7]To the extent that physical depreciation of equipment is positively associated with use, increasing usage leads to an earlier need for replacement, and hence to capital expenditure. This would seem to be a very minor consideration relevant to frequency of use, particularly given that much medical equipment is scientifically obsolete well before it has physically deteriorated to the point where replacement is necessary.

would be relied upon to produce a rational allocation of the limited resources across all inputs. The fact that major legislative proposals include a separate capital expenditure ceiling suggests that policy makers do perceive a distinct "technology problem," and do believe that, under a general revenue limit alone, high-cost technology would continue to flow into the hospital sector at rates disproportionate to the true relative value of such technology. Although politically prominent, this view is far from universally accepted in academic circles. Indeed, a separate capital ceiling might be considered counterproductive, for reasons suggested below.

First-Order Effects: The direct results of a capital expenditure ceiling on the acquisition and use of technology within hospitals would include the following:

1. Decrease in the acquisition by hospitals of expensive capital-intensive technology.   Both acquisition of new technology and diffusion of established high-cost technology would decrease. Furthermore, the ceiling would not distinguish between cost-increasing and cost-decreasing technology. Unlike the general revenue limit, which would encourage acquisition of the latter, the capital expenditure ceiling would discourage all forms of capital acquisition, irrespective of ultimate operating cost. Implicit in the incentive to avoid high-cost capital technology is decreased use of such technology in the aggregate, with the possibility of more intensive use of acquired technology. Obviously, a capital expenditure ceiling would combat the purported unnecessary duplication and consequent underutilization of capital-intensive facilities. The danger is a reversal of the problem: a very restrictive ceiling might lessen the optimal availability of facilities and impose excessive burdens on existing technology, leading to reliance on second-best alternatives instead of capital-intensive technologies.

2. Search for diagnostic and therapeutic alternatives with lower component prices.

Second-Order Effects on Other Health Care Delivery Institutions: The derivative effects of a capital expenditure ceiling on other health care delivery institutions are similar to those associated with the overall limit. One would anticipate some shifting of capital-intensive technology and associated care to non-hospital settings, including to the offices of private medical group practices.

Second-Order Effects on Development of New Technology: The effects of the capital ceiling on the development of medical technology are also similar to the effects of the revenue limit, although certain effects are exacerbated by the capital ceiling and at least one effect is quite distinct:

1. Decrease in technology-oriented applied R&D.   This effect is exacerbated by the capital ceiling.

2. Decrease in the development of all high capital cost technology. This impact is distinctive because it will occur irrespective of the technology's implications for hospital operating costs. Unlike the general limit on inpatient revenue, the capital expenditure ceiling will work against the search for capital-intensive cost-saving technologies. This has obvious implications for the medical technology industry.

3. Little effect on basic bioscience research. Like the revenue limit, the capital ceiling should have little impact on fundamental research.

Conclusions

Hospital cost containment will restrict the flow of resources into medical care, assuming that "contained" costs are not transferred *in toto* to non-inpatient medical care. Containment may inhibit research into and the development of cost-increasing technology; a capital expenditure ceiling would also discourage R&D related to certain cost-decreasing technologies. Evaluation of the desirability of these consequences may ultimately rest on one's subjective opinion, but an informed judgment will include appreciation of the economic context in which such changes will take place. These are not changes from a position of social optimality. If they were, there would be no need to consider a policy of containing hospital costs.

The fundamental economic truism is that resources are scarce and have alternative uses. The true cost of an activity is the benefit that the resources consumed would have produced in their best alternative use(s). In a market economy, prices reflect these opportunity costs: to acquire a resource or commodity, one must be willing to pay at least what that good is worth to others. The assurance of the value of the good lies in the sacrifice the purchaser must make: by willingly sacrificing the price of the good — and hence foregoing alternative purchases — the buyer is demonstrating that the benefit of the good is at least commensurate with its cost and exceeds the benefits that would have been derived from the alternative purchases.

In medical care, the absence of direct financial liability for the consumption of many services implies that neither patients nor providers need be concerned with the economic value of the medical resources consumed. Hence, the true social cost of utilizing the resources can exceed the benefit that induced their consumption. Providers' profit incentives may exacerbate the situation. The logical outcome is excess and possibly inappropriate use of resources. The problem is most acute where the vast majority of costs are assumed by third party payers, as in the case of hospital care.

The existence of widespread and deep insurance coverage reflects a variety of factors. In the private sector, both the depth of coverage—the small deductibles and low copayments—and the extensiveness of employer provision of coverage reflect in part the preferential tax treatment of medical insurance premiums (Ehrbar, 1977; Havighurst, 1977). In addition to performing the true insurance function—providing protection against unforeseen financial catastrophes—relatively complete coverage becomes a form of prepayment, significantly lowering the out-of-pocket cost of care and hence encouraging increased consumption. Increased demand leads to higher prices, which in turn increase the demand for insurance.

Public insurance programs are a positive reflection of the nation's social conscience in general and specifically of the attitude that money should not be a barrier to the receipt of necessary high-quality medical care. The inflationary implications of Medicare and Medicaid are the price society has been paying for the equity these programs have delivered. Herein lies the problem: in both the private and public sectors, we have been attempting to implement the principle that health care is a right, by incrementally decreasing the out-of-pocket cost of care. In essence, we have been "freeing up" and "nationalizing" the demand side of the economic equation while struggling to preserve the free enterprise character of the supply side. Any student of elementary economics could predict the effects; any literate citizen can read about them daily.

Cost containment represents an attempt to preserve the distributional equity gains of the past decade while reintroducing an economic discipline into the provision of care, at least in hospitals. The objective is to counteract the consequences of the removal of financial barriers to care: inflation and the less understood problem that excess resources devoted to medical care deprive people of greater benefits from alternative uses of the resources. Conceptually, cost containment is a step in the right direction, attuning decision makers in the health care system to the cost implications of resource consumption. Furthermore, one group of hospital cost containment proposals—those which constrain overall revenues or expenditures but leave individual resource decisions to physicians and administrators—forces knowledgeable decision makers to confront alternatives directly: purchase of a CAT scanner would no longer simply require CON approval; now it would imply that a hospital could *not* purchase machines X, Y, and Z.

Many health care professionals argue that putting a cap on hospital revenues will unduly restrict the provision of services, possibly decreasing both the quality and quantity of care (Silver, 1977). If it is assumed that physicians and administrators will learn to make wise choices, damage can be minimized. Services of marginal effectiveness should be the ones reduced, and decision makers should learn to provide services more efficiently. Again, from the social perspective, resources not consumed in medical care will be used in other activities, possibly with more beneficial implications for health (*e.g.*, pollution control). Indeed, if the previous characterization of the medical market is accurate—namely, that the relative absence of economic constraints has led to an overproduction of services, to excessive and inefficient use of resources—then an absolute *decrease* in resources devoted to medical care might actually be socially desirable. However, hospital cost containment calls only for *relative* belt-tightening, *i.e.*, a decrease in the rate of growth of hospital expenditures.

Needless to say, it is a long way from the concept of cost containment to the implementation of an effective program. Regulation is pervasive in health (Iglehart, 1977a); based on past experience in this and other fields (Havighurst, 1977; Noll, 1975), one should not feel entirely sanguine about the prospects for success. Hospital cost containment is not synonymous with medical care cost containment. As noted above, a principal concern is that costs intended to be contained will simply be shifted from inpatient to outpatient status or from hospitals to other delivery settings. To the extent that this occurs, the predicted effects on the development and use of technology would be diminished.

The discussion above should place in perspective the effects on technology development and use of two major cost containment proposals. A ceiling on capital expenditures appears to be a means of supplementing relatively ineffective regulatory apparatus (*e.g.*, CON) with some policy muscle. A truly restrictive ceiling, such as that proposed by the Carter Administration, would have clear and strong implications for both the development and use of capital-intensive medical technology, particularly if combined with equipment- and service-specific national guidelines on appropriate maximum supplies, as defined in the Administration's bill (HR 9717, Sec 302). Put simply, the acquisition of such technology would be discouraged and hence so would be related research and development. Unfortunately, the ceiling fails to distinguish cost-saving from cost-increasing capital expenditure. Thus, to the extent that cost-saving capital-intensive technologies might be developed, the proposal is partially self-defeating.

The general inpatient revenue limit might adequately serve the cost containment objective independent of the capital expenditure ceiling, assuming that the revenue limit was structured to relate to reimbursement for all costs and not simply operating costs. This is especially true if, as suggested earlier, excess investment in and use of technology are simply a reflection of the general problem of excess use of resources in medical care. Even if sophisticated technology is currently treated preferentially, the revenue limit's imposition of an effective budget constraint would force reevaluation of such preferential treatment.

Under a general inpatient revenue limit, the demand in hospitals for certain types of technology would slacken, and overall demand would cease to grow as rapidly as it has in recent years. Both of these factors could be viewed as deterrents to the development and adoption of technology. However, both can also be viewed as bringing the demand for cost-increasing technology, and hence for related research, more into line with the reality of the opportunity costs associated with them. Significantly, under a revenue limit, the new economic environment for hospital-based care would produce incentives for technology researchers and developers to channel their creativity into the search for and development of cost-saving technology. Such technology could expand the capability of the health care industry to deliver care with a given amount of resources. The relative absence of research effort in this area suggests the possibility that it might have a high and rapid pay-off. A shift in the mix of technology from cost-increasing toward cost-saving would represent a significant change in the delivery of medical care, and it might augur a new golden age of medical technology.

Much of the impact of cost containment on the improvement of health through new technology depends on the research origins of real breakthroughs. If future medical progress lies in the development of sophisticated capital equipment, with the private sector playing a leading role in the design and production of such equipment, hospital cost containment could significantly slow the advancement of medical science. If, by contrast, the true high technology of medicine is simple, inexpensive, and derived from basic research, cost containment seems unlikely to jeopardize medical scientific progress.

Hospital cost containment represents an attempt, albeit imperfect, to reduce or compensate for the discrepancy between the private decision-making costs and the social costs of medical care. Any serious and effective cost containment policy will have a substantial impact on the quantity and use of resources devoted to hospital-based care. The likely effects on medical technology are numerous and significant, although as a price to pay for controlling the ever-inflating costs of care, they do not necessarily appear to be intolerable. Some, in fact, should prove to be desirable.

References

Abt Associates, Inc. 1975. Incentives and Decisions Underlying Hospitals' Adoption and Utilization of Major Capital Equipment. HRA contract no. HSM 110-73-513. Cambridge, Mass.

Altman, S., and Eichenholz, J. 1976. Inflation in the Health Industry—Causes and Cures. In Zubkoff, M., ed., *Health: a Victim or Cause of Inflation?*, pp. 7-30. New York: PRODIST.

Blue Sheet, The Drug Research Reports. 1978. Hospital Supply Firm Sees New Sales Opportunities in Cost Control Effort; Shift to Preventive Medicine, Use of Paraprofessionals to Open New Markets? Washington, D.C. 21 (January 11): 6-7.

Committee on Interstate and Foreign Commerce, U.S. House of Representatives. 1977. Selected Hospital Cost Containment Proposals: Major Provisions (September 9). Washington, D.C.: U.S. Government Printing Office.

Congressional Budget Office. 1977. *The Hospital Cost Containment Act of 1977: An Analysis of the Administration's Proposal.* Report prepared for the Subcommittee on Health and Scientific Research of the Committee on Human Resources, U.S. Senate. Washington, D.C.: U.S. Government Printing Office.

Ehrbar, A. 1977. A Radical Prescription for Medical Care. *Fortune* XCV (February): 164-172.

Feldstein, M. 1971. *The Rising Cost of Hospital Care.* Washington, D.C.: Information Resources Press.

———. 1977. Quality Change and the Demand for Hospital Care. Paper written for the Council on Wage and Price Stability, Executive Office of the President.

Feldstein, M., and Taylor, A. 1977. *The Rapid Rise of Hospital Costs.* Staff Report of the Council on Wage and Price Stability, Executive Office of the President. Washington, D.C.: U.S. Government Printing Office.

Fuchs, V. 1973. Health Care and the U.S. Economic System. In Collen, M., ed., *Technology and Health Care Systems in the 1980's,* National Center for Health Services Research. DHEW Pub. No. (HSM) 73-3016. Washington, D.C.: U.S. Government Printing Office.

Gaus, C. 1975. Biomedical Research and Health Care Costs. Testimony of the Social Security Administration before the President's Biomedical Research Panel.

———. 1976. What Goes into Technology Must Come Out in Costs. *National Leadership Conference on America's Health Policy,* April 29-30, pp. 12-13.

Gaus, C., and Cooper, B. 1976. Technology and Medicare: Alternatives for Change. Background Paper for Conference on Health Care Technology and Quality of Care, Boston University Health Policy Center, November 19-20, at Boston, Mass.

Ginsburg, P. 1972. Capital Investment by Non-Profit Firms: the Voluntary Hospital. East Lansing: Michigan State University, Econometrics Workshop Paper No. 7205.

Gordon, G., and Fisher, G., eds. 1975. *The Diffusion of Medical Technology: Policy and Research Planning Perspectives.* Cambridge, Mass.: Ballinger.

Havighurst, C. 1977. Controlling Health Care Costs: Strengthening the Private Sector's Hand. *Journal of Health Politics, Policy and Law* (Winter) 1: 471-98.

Iglehart, J. 1977a. The Cost and Regulation of Medical Technology: Future Policy Directions. *Milbank Memorial Fund Quarterly/Health and Society* (Winter) 55: 25-59.

———. 1977b. Stemming Hospital Growth—the Flip Side of Carter's Cost Control Plan. *National Journal* 9 (23): 848-52.

Institute of Medicine. 1977. *Computed Tomographic Scanning—a Policy Statement.* Washington, D.C.: National Academy of Sciences.

National Academy of Sciences. (Forthcoming). Report of the Committee on Technology and Health Care. Washington, D.C.

Needleman, J., and Lewin, L. 1977. Impact of State Health Regulation on the Adoption and Utilization of Equipment-Embodied Medical Technology. Paper prepared for Committee on Technology and Health Care, National Academy of Sciences. (Forthcoming in the Committee's Report.)

Noll, R. 1975. The Consequences of Public Utility Regulation of Hospitals. In *Controls on Health Care,* pp. 25-48. Washington, D.C.: National Academy of Sciences.

Office of Technology Assessment, U.S. Congress. 1978. Efficacy and Safety of Medical Technology. Draft Report.

President's Biomedical Research Panel. 1976. Report of the President's Biomedical Research Panel. Washington, D.C.: U.S. Government Printing Office.

Redisch, M. 1974. Hospital Inflationary Mechanisms. Paper presented at Western Economics Association Meetings, Las Vegas, Nevada, June 10-12. Revised October, 1974.

Reinhardt, U. 1977. The Role of Health Manpower and Education in Cost Containment. Paper prepared for Project HOPE Committee on Health Policy Meeting, Washington, D.C., October 30-November 1.

Rice, D., and Wilson, D. 1975. The American Medical Economy—Problems and Perspectives. Paper prepared for International Conference on Health Care Costs and Expenditures, Fogarty International Center, Bethesda, Maryland, June 2-4.

Roche, J., and Stengle, J. 1973. Facilities for Open Heart Surgery in the United States: Distribution, Utilization, and Cost. *American Journal of Cardiology* 32 (August): 224-28.

Russell, L. 1976. Making Rational Decisions about Medical Technology. Paper presented at meeting of the AMA's National Commission on the Cost of Medical Care, Chicago, Ill., November 23.

———. 1977. How Much Does Medical Technology Cost? Paper presented at Annual Health Conference of the New York Academy of Medicine, New York, April 29.

Salkever, D., and Bice, T. 1976. The Impact of Certificate-Of-Need Controls on Hospital Investment. *Milbank Memorial Fund Quarterly/Health and Society* 54 (Spring): 185-214.

Schroeder, S., and Showstack, J. 1977. The Dynamics of Medical Technology Use: Analysis and Policy Options. Health Policy Program Discussion Paper. San Francisco: University of California, School of Medicine.

Scitovsky, A., and McCall, N. 1976. Changes in the Costs of Treatment of Selected Illnesses 1951-1964-1971. Washington, D.C., National Center for Health Services Research, DHEW Pub. No. (HRA) 77-3161.

Silver, G. 1977. Hospital Cost Control: Implications for Access and Quality for the Poor. Paper prepared for Project HOPE Committee on Health Policy Meeting, Washington, D.C., October 30-November 1.

Silvers, J. 1974. The Impact of Financial Policy and Structure on Investments in Health Care. In Abernathy, W., Sheldon, A., and Prahalad, C., eds., *The Management of Health Care.* Cambridge, Mass.: Ballinger.

Thomas, L. 1974. The Technology of Medicine. In *Lives of a Cell,* pp. 31-36. New York: Viking Press.

U.S. Congress. 1976. Medical Device Amendments of 1976. *Congressional Record-House,* March 9, pp. H1719-H1759.

Wagner, J., and Zubkoff, M. 1978. Medical Technology and Hospital Costs. In Zubkoff, M., Raskin, I., and Hanft, R., eds., *Hospital Cost Containment: Selected Notes for Future Policy.* pp. 263-289. New York: PRODIST.

Warner, K. 1975. A "Desperation-Reaction" Model of Medical Diffusion. *Health Services Research* 10 (Winter): 369-83.

———. 1977. The Cost of Capital-Embodied Medical Technology. Paper prepared for Committee on Technology and Health Care, National Academy of Sciences. (Forthcoming in the Committee's Report.)

Zelten, R. 1977. Hospital Cost Containment and Hospital Fiscal Management. Paper prepared for Project HOPE Committee on Health Policy Meeting, Washington, D.C., October 30-November 1.

This is a revised version of a paper submitted to the Project HOPE Committee on Health Policy and does not necessarily express the views of that organization, nor those of Project HOPE or its cooperating organization, the University of Southern California Center for Health Services Research.

The helpful comments of the referees are gratefully acknowledged.

Address correspondence to: Kenneth E. Warner, Ph.D., School of Public Health, University of Michigan, Ann Arbor, Michigan 48109.

25. National Health Insurance—Memorandum for Secretary Califano

ALAIN ENTHOVEN

Reprinted from unpublished research report. HEW, 1977, 1-29.

. . . We must have a comprehensive program of national health insurance. . . . The coverage must be universal and mandatory . . . freedom of choice in the selection of a physician and treatment center . . . will always be maintained. . . . We must phase in the program as rapidly as revenues permit, helping first those who most need help, and achieving a comprehensive program well-defined in the end. . . . We must encourage . . . alternative delivery systems such as health maintenance organizations and rural group practices. . . . I support organized approaches to delivery of services. . . . Incentives for reforms in the health care delivery system and for increased productivity must be developed. . . . Incentives for the reorganization of the delivery of health care must be built into the payment mechanism. . . . It is not required that the government run the entire health care program in our country—I would not favor that.

Jimmy Carter
April and October, 1976

Editorial Note: The appendixes referred to in this memorandum are not included in this publication.

I. GOALS

This memorandum outlines what I believe is the best strategy to move us toward the goal of access (financial, geographic, and social) for every American to comprehensive health care services of good quality, willingly provided, and with freedom of choice that respects each person's preferences. Our society also has other pressing needs: helping the poor, rebuilding cities, energy conservation, environmental protection, and investment incentives to create jobs. So the care we seek must be cost-effective.

To achieve our health care goals at a cost in balance with other goals, we need to reorganize the delivery system. The Government cannot do that directly. People would resist such changes involuntarily imposed. But Government can change the underlying economic incentives so that consumers and providers of care can benefit from seeking out and joining cost-effective organized systems (e.g., Health Maintenance Organizations and the like). The delivery system would then be forced to reorganize itself in response to a market of consumers who are seeking out and choosing what is in their own best interest. Because the distinctive idea of this NHI proposal is to let consumer preferences guide the reorganization of the system, I have called it "Consumer Choice Health Plan (CCHP)."

II. INFLATION AND INEQUITY TODAY

1. *Main Problems.* Real (i.e., net of general inflation) per capita spending on health care increased 79 per cent from 1965 to 1976; on hospital care it increased 110 per cent. As a per cent of GNP, health care went from 5.9 to 8.6 per cent. There are good reasons for much of this: the growth in public and private insurance coverage brought access to many who previously did not have it, especially the aged and the poor; advances in technology increased the power of medicine to prolong life and enhance its quality; the population aged; the health care system took on new assignments (e.g., in mental health, alcohol and drug abuse); the pay of health care workers was brought up to the level of other industries; rising incomes and expectations increased consumer demand for health care services. Our present concern with the growth in spending should not mislead us into thinking it is all bad.

But, especially in recent years, the increase has far exceeded what could be justified on these grounds. Hospital charges and physician fees rose faster than the CPI. Health workers' pay overshot equality with other industries.[1] There is great inefficiency, e.g., duplication of costly underutilized facilities. Wide variations in the per capita consumption of various costly health services (e.g., hospitalization and surgery) among similar populations, without any apparent difference in medical need or health outcome, suggest that there is much spending that yields no significant benefit in terms of health.[1] People might be just as healthy with half as much hospitalization.

While the nation is spending more, some people are enjoying the benefits less. Gaps in coverage leave some unprotected from heavy financial burdens, others protected only after medical costs have made them poor. Public funds (including tax subsidies) do more for the well-protected well-to-do than for the working poor who need help more. Also there is uneven geographic distribution, leaving many rural and inner-city residents poorly served while there are too many doctors in some well-to-do areas.

2. *Causes of Inflation and Inequity.* The main cause of the unjustified and unnecessary increase in costs is the complex of perverse incentives inherent in the tax-supported system of fee-for-service for doctors, cost-reimbursement for hospitals, and third-party intermediaries to protect consumers. Fee-for-service rewards the doctor for providing more and more costly services whether or not more is necessary or beneficial to the patient. Cost-reimbursement rewards the hospital with more revenue for generating more costs. Indeed, a hospital administrator who seriously pursued cost cutting, e.g. by instituting tighter controls on surgery and laboratory use and avoiding buying costly diagnostic equipment by referring patients to other hospitals, would be punished by a loss in revenue (Medicare and Medicaid would cut him dollar for dollar), and a loss in physician staff and, therefore, patients. Third-party reimbursement leaves the consumer with, at most, a weak financial incentive to question the need for or value of services or to seek out a less costly provider or style of care.

These incentives are reinforced by the demands and expectations of anxious patients, the prestige associated with costly technological care, the malpractice induced need for "defensive medicine," and the government-inspired proliferation of health manpower—especially physicians. Thus, the financing system rewards cost-increasing behavior and provides no incentive for economy. At the same time, it is inequitable. Medicare and Medicaid are among the worst offenders.

1. Medicare pays more on behalf of the people who choose more costly systems of care. For example, in 1970,

Medicare paid $202 per capita on behalf of beneficiaries cared for by cost-effective Group Health Cooperative of Puget Sound, but paid $356, or 76 per cent more, on behalf of similar beneficiaries in the same area who got their care from the fee-for-service sector. Medicare pays more to doctors who charge more and more to hospitals that cost more. At the same time, Medicare pays more on behalf of rich than poor (because they live in better-served areas and can more easily afford the coinsurance), white than black, well-served than underserved.

2. Medicaid, which also relies almost entirely on third-party, fee-for-service and cost-reimbursement, is particularly vulnerable to fraud and abuse. Its beneficiaries are particularly unlikely to be able to judge the need for or value of services provided to them, and are less motivated to weigh the value against the cost because they are not spending their own money. As President Carter said last year, "Medicaid has become a national scandal. It is being bilked of millions of dollars by charlatans."

3. Tax-subsidized private insurance, with no limit on tax-free employer contributions, subsidizes employee decisions to select more costly health care systems, and encourages employee pressure for rich employer-paid benefits. (Most of the roughly $10.1 billion FY 1978 "tax expenditures"—including payroll taxes—is about a 30% subsidy of health insurance.[21]) This tax system also provides more subsidy for better paid and covered than for poorly paid and covered people.

These incentives also help to defeat regulation and local efforts at cost containment. Why should a Health Systems Agency or a Board of County Supervisors defy local pressures and force the closing of an unneeded hospital, with loss of jobs, when most of the extra costs of keeping it open are paid from outside their area?

Thus, the increase in health care spending is a serious problem, but not because more spending is bad in itself. Indeed, if the spending were all on necessary, cost-effective care yielding significant benefits for the quality of people's lives (and much of it is), we would be celebrating it. Rather, it is a problem because:

1. The financing system does not inspire confidence that resources are being used wisely, and examples of waste abound; and

2. Medical care costs are straining public finances at every level of government, and are forcing cutbacks in services to the needy. Public sector spending rose from $9.5 billion, or 25 per cent of the total, in 1965 to $59 billion, or 42 per cent of the total, in 1976. More than half of this is in open-ended, third-party reimbursement programs in which government spending is not controllable. Medicare outlays are increasing 47 per cent from FY 1976 to FY 1978.

3. *Lack of Competition and Choice.* There are competitive elements in the health care industry. For example, insurance companies compete with each other, and with self-insurance, for group contracts, by offering lower administrative costs. But there is very little competition to produce services more efficiently or offer a less costly style of care, and pass the savings on to consumers. Most workers are offered a single health insurance plan by their employer or Health and Welfare Fund (HWF), usually a third-party reimbursement plan. (The Health Maintenance Organization Act was intended to open up employee groups to HMOs by mandating dual choice, but the qualification process has been bogged down in HEW, and many employers are holding back on offering HMOs until they are qualified.)[18]

The Medicare law has a complex provision for paying HMOs, but it is based on retrospective cost-finding, includes an implicit tax on HMOs, and has not been put into operation. So Medicare beneficiaries are stuck with a third-party, cost-reimbursement system; they cannot choose a more efficient system and realize the savings for themselves.

While the fee-for-service, third-party reimbursement system offers the patient a free choice among doctors and hospitals in his community, it does not offer him the alternative of keeping much of the savings he would generate by choosing effective but less costly care. The premiums and charges he must pay reflect the cost-generating behavior of doctors and hospitals in his community and the experience of his insured group. His choice of doctors and hospitals is generally limited to those who work within the framework of the cost-increasing incentives. If he would prefer, for example, a system that used half as much hospitalization per capita, in exchange for more home care or better access to ambulatory care, at an equal per capita cost, the third-party, fee-for-service system would not be able to offer it to him.

4. *Other Market Imperfections*. In addition to these barriers to desirable competition, consumers today generally have poor information about health care alternatives. They must rely on physicians, who often have a financial interest in more costly care, for information on benefits of proposed treatments. There is great uncertainty about these benefits in many cases. There are many restrictive laws and practices.

Geographic and specialty maldistribution of physicians are exacerbated by third-party, fee-for-service financing, which creates an open-ended demand for subspecialty care in well-to-do areas, and little incentive to offer primary care in inner city or rural areas.

5. *The Physicians' Role*. Physicians receive only about 20 per cent of the health care dollar, but they control or influence most of the rest. Even though it may not appear so on an organization chart, physicians are the primary decision-makers in our health care system. But the present structure of the industry imposes very little responsibility on them for the economic consequences of their health care decisions. Their education and professional attitudes combine with the financial incentives and other factors such as the malpractice threat, to minimize concern over cost and to foster cost-increasing behavior. If the managers of a system are not concerned with cost-effectiveness, the system will not be cost-effective.

6. *Discontinuities in Coverage*. Most private health insurance is provided as an employment-related fringe benefit—a system that works reasonably well for a large portion of our economically self-sufficient population with job stability (except that, as noted above, the limit on employer health plan offerings is a key barrier to competition and consumer choice). However, the employment health insurance linkage is not compatible with an effective universal system because: people lose their coverage when they lose their jobs; job changes commonly require health coverage changes, with breaks in continuity of coverage and care and nonproductive administrative costs; it is very difficult to arrange good coverage for persons in marginal industries or with seasonal, intermittent, or otherwise unstable employment; employer-employee financing is regressive; without mandated coverage the low-paid who often need the most protection get the least; and with mandated coverage, in addition to great administrative problems for workers with unstable employment, the economic burden would fall heaviest on the lowest paid and provide a strong disincentive for employing marginal workers.

In a society that agrees that everyone should have financial access to a decent level of health care, it makes no sense to have a system in which many people lose their coverage when they lose their jobs, while many others lose their Medicaid eligibility when they get even a poorly paid job. Cycling in and out of Medicaid eligibility with income changes produces hardship and work disincentives for the poor, and heavy non-productive administrative burdens for States, counties, and providers. As incomes fluctuate, contributions, not eligibility, should vary with ability to pay. Everyone's health care coverage should be continuous.

7. *Regulation Won't Make Things Better.*[2] In recent years, the main line of Government policy has been to attack the problems created by inappropriate incentives with various forms of regulation, e.g., planning controls on hospital capacity, controls on hospital prices and spending, controls on hospital utilization, and controls on physician fees. The weight of evidence, based on experience in many other industries, as well as in health care, supports the view that such regulation is likely to raise costs and retard beneficial innovation.

A great deal of regulation of health services is inevitable. And in some fields, regulation is used to maintain competition, e.g., the Securities and Exchange Commission. Indeed, a key part of CCHP is pro-competitive regulation. The issue, then is not regulation in general; it is the specific types of regulation and their likely consequences. The point here is that direct controls on costs, in opposition to the basic financial incentives, are not likely to make things better.

In the long run, price regulation amounts to cost-reimbursement and has the same incentives. Regulation tends to protect regulated firms whenever competition or technological change threatens established positions within the industry. Regulators often see the purpose of the price structure as providing a mechanism for subsidizing some groups at the expense of others, rather than as a mechanism for offering incentives to buyers and sellers to make economical choices. The main reason hospitals favor regulation is that it would function as a cartel to protect them from buyers who want to cut costs; they know that the approved rates will be based on their costs.

Medical care has many characteristics that make it a particularly unsuitable candidate for successful economic regulation. Basic to the problem is the subtle, elusive, and indeed almost indefinable nature of the product. In the health care sector to date, the only economic regulation that has been thoroughly tested is regulation of hospital capacity. And it is clear that certificate-of-need regulation has not helped control the problem of overbedding. A fixed legislated limit on total capital spending by hospitals might offer a temporary illusion of effectiveness, but it is vulnerable to a number of counter-measures such as "unbundling."

Physician fee controls have been advocated, and were tried in the Nixon Administration. In judging their likely value as a cost control device, one should be aware that the "doctor visit" is highly compressible. And the need for doctor visits is impossible to test objectively except in extreme cases.

Overall controls on hospital spending face similar prospects: circumvention, unbundling, exceptions. The Administration proposal has already been emasculated by the wage pass through, despite the fact that hospital workers now earn more than their counterparts doing similar jobs in other sectors.[1] But even if it were ultimately successful at controlling total hospital spending at the stated growth rate, there would be no force in the system to assure efficiency or equity in the allocation or production of services. At best, we would have frozen the hospital industry in its present wasteful and inequitable pattern.

If you are interested in motivating efficiency and equity, you must address the fundamental financial incentives in the system.

8. *NHI Is Already Here.* We have a sort of NHI system, with separate programs for the aged, poor, employed middle class, veterans, military dependents, etc. So the issue

is not "whether NHI." It is "what kind of NHI." I do not accept the view that we cannot afford NHI now, and that we must wait for it until we get costs under control. On the contrary, we are already paying for NHI, but we are not getting the benefit because we have an inefficient inequitable system that results from historical accident and interest group pressure. Some groups remain unprotected; prompt action is needed to assure universal coverage. But an equally urgent reason for NHI today is the need to find good ways to reorganize the system and build in incentives for equity and cost-effectiveness.

III. CONSUMER CHOICE HEALTH PLAN (CCHP)

A. Main Ideas

1. *Reform Through Incentives*. To achieve good quality comprehensive care for all, at a cost we can afford, we must change the fundamental structure of the health care financing and delivery system. Instead of today's fragmented system dominated by cost-increasing incentives, we need a health care economy made up predominantly, though not exclusively, of competing organized systems. In such systems, groups of physicians would accept responsibility for providing comprehensive health care services to defined populations, largely for a prospective per capita payment, or some other form of payment that rewards economy in the use of health care resources.

Today we cannot see very clearly what such an economy would look like. We should seek to find our way there by a fair market test among competing alternatives in which systems that do a better job for a lower cost survive and grow. Many types of systems might succeed in such a competition, including not only Prepaid Group Practices (PGP) and Individual Practice Associations (IPA), the two "official" types of HMO, but also "Health Care Alliances" as

proposed by Ellwood and McClure and "Variable Cost Insurance" as proposed by Newhouse and Taylor in which premiums reflect the cost-control behavior of providers. There would be a substantial role for pure insurance and for traditional fee-for-service practice. CCHP seeks to accomplish this transformation by voluntary changes in a competitive market.

2. *Informed Choice among Competing Alternatives*. CCHP is designed to assure that all people have a choice among competing alternatives, that they have good information on which to base their choice, and that competition emphasizes quality of benefits and total cost (as opposed to today's emphasis on preferred risk selection, minimizing only administrative cost, etc.). CCHP would resemble the Federal Employees Health Benefits Program (FEHBP) and other conceptually similar plans. It would extend to the whole population and to all qualifying health plans its proven principles of competition, multiple choice, private underwriting and management of health plans, periodic government-supervised open enrollment and equal rates for all similar enrollees selecting the same plan and benefits.

3. *Equity and Incentives for Economizing Choices*. CCHP seeks to correct inequities and cost-increasing incentives in the tax laws and Medicare. The present exclusion of employer and deduction of employee premium contributions would be replaced by a refundable tax credit based on actuarial category. Medicaid would be replaced by a system of vouchers for premium payments, integrated with reformed welfare, and reaching 100 per cent of Actuarial Cost for basic benefits in the case of the poor. Medicare would be changed to give each beneficiary the freedom to have his Adjusted Average Per Capita Cost (AAPCC) paid to the qualified plan of his choice as a fixed prospective periodic payment. Thus, CCHP takes money now used to subsidize people's choice of more costly systems of care, and uses it to raise the floor under the least well

covered. It gives people an incentive to seek out systems that provide care economically by letting them keep the savings. While Government assures that people have enough money to join a good plan, at the margin people are using their own (net after-tax) money, which should motivate them to seek value for it. These changes would permit continuity of coverage regardless of job status.

4. *Incremental Changes.* CCHP is not an immediate radical replacement of the present financing system with a whole new one. Rather, it is a set of incremental "midcourse corrections" in the present financing and regulatory system, each one of which is comparatively simple and familiar taken by itself, but whose cumulative impact is intended to alter the system radically, but gradually and voluntarily, in the long run. CCHP corrects the faulty incentives produced by present government programs, and seeks to correct known market imperfections. CCHP preserves flexibility. If these changes do not produce the desired results, after experience has been gained, more corrections can be made. CCHP recognizes that there is no "final solution" to health care financing problems, as experience in countries with NHI clearly demonstrates. CCHP is not necessarily incompatible with some proposed regulation such as health planning, hospital cost controls, and physician fee controls. On the contrary, CCHP would increase the effectiveness of the Health Systems Agencies by giving them incentives to control costs they now lack. And competing private plans with the right incentives might enforce a fee schedule far more effectively than a government agency could.

B. The Financing System

1. *Actuarial Categories and Costs.*[3] The flow of funds in CCHP is based on Actuarial Cost (AC), i.e., the average total costs of covered benefits (insured and out-of-pocket) in the base year, updated each year by a suitable index, for persons in each actuarial category. For persons not covered by Medicare, the actuarial categories might be the simple and familiar three-part structure of "individual, individual plus one dependent, and individual plus two or more dependents." However, in a competitive situation, this might give health plans too strong an incentive to attempt to select preferred risks by design of benefit packages (e.g., good maternity benefits to attract healthy young families), location of facilities, or emphasis in specialty mix (strength in pediatrics, weakness in gerontology and cardiology). Carried to a logical extreme, such a system could lead to poor care for high-risk persons (though open enrollment—described below—would always assure the right of high-risk persons to join any qualified health plan). So experience might show that a more complex set of actuarial categories is desirable. For example, the three-part structure might be supplemented by special categories for persons aged 45–54 and 55–64. In the limit, one might go to a structure based on individual age (e.g., in 10-year steps) and sex, though I doubt this would be necessary.

Actuarial Cost would also reflect location, because there are large regional differentials in health care costs. The appropriate geographic unit would probably be the State. However, regional differences in real per capita subsidies based on AC would be phased out over a decade.

The appropriate index for updating AC would probably be the "all services" component of the Consumer Price Index (CPI).

Assume, for the sake of illustration, that the AC for a "typical" family of four is $1,350 per year. (This happens to reflect the approximate average per capita cost for hospital and physician services for children and working-age persons in FY 1978.)[21]

In CCHP, premiums would be set by each health plan for each actuarial category and benefit package, based on its own costs and its own judgment as to what it can charge in a competitive market. Thus, persons in more costly actuarial categories would pay higher premiums. This is desirable because we want competing plans to be motivated to serve them. This is made socially acceptable by giving such people higher subsidies through the following mechanisms.

2. *Tax Credit.* The present exclusion of employer and health and welfare fund (HWF) contributions from taxable income, and the deductibility of individual premium payments would be replaced by a refundable tax credit equal to some predetermined percentage (call it "X%") of the family's AC. (The deductibility of direct medical expenses would be limited to those in excess of 10% of Adjusted Gross Income.) Employers and HWFs would continue contributing to employee health insurance under existing agreements, but they would report such contributions as a part of total pay on W-2 forms. The tax credit is allowed only if spent on premiums for a *qualified* health plan. To the ordinary employee, then, CCHP would appear initially as a quite simple change in the way his compensation is taxed.

The appropriate level of "X" requires a policy judgment that balances a number of factors. Too low a level (e.g., below 30%) would leave too weak an incentive for plans to qualify. Too high a level (e.g., about 70%) would set the subsidy at a level above that needed for a truly efficient plan, and would weaken incentives for economy. Within this range, a lower "X" targets a higher percentage of the available funds on the poor through the voucher system. A level around 30% would make the tax credit approximately offset the tax increase caused by repeal of the exclusion of employer contributions for most employed middle-income people—thus helping to minimize political opposition. (Those whose marginal tax-rate times employer contribution exceeded the tax credit would lose.) A greater "X" means more cost to the Federal budget, more income redistribution and less of the total to be in means-tested vouchers. A greater "X" would reduce the incentive for the non-poor to buy high deductible "catastrophic"

insurance, and would reduce the potential for people to manipulate the system to their advantage, taking a minimum cost catastrophic plan when they expect to be healthy, then switching to a full-benefit plan when they anticipate elective surgery or pregnancy. In my judgment, an "X" around 60 per cent, approximating the FEHBP contribution level, would make the system work best. However, CCHP could start with a tax credit equal to 30%, at a comparatively low cost (see below), with higher levels phased in as revenues permit. In what follows, I will assume a 50% tax credit for illustration.

3. *Vouchers for the Poor.*[5] The poor need more subsidy to assure their access to an acceptable plan. CCHP would provide them with a voucher usable only as a premium contribution to the qualified plan of their choice. It should be administered through the reformed cash-assistance system and designed according to the same principles. The voucher's value would be means-tested on the same basis as cash income supplements. The exact choice of formula requires analysis and judgments similar to those that went into welfare reform. Here is one example: Reformed welfare guarantees a family of four a minimum cash income of $4,200; the income supplement is reduced 50 cents for each dollar of earned income until it reaches zero at a family income of $8,400. Related to this, one could set the voucher at $1,350 for a family with a total income, including cash assistance, of $4,200, and phase it down to $625—the tax credit level for non-poor families—at a "benefit reduction rate" of 15 cents for every dollar of income. In this particular case, the voucher would reach $625 at a total family income of $8,367. (This would raise the total Federal "benefit reduction rate" to 59%, a possibility that was anticipated in the analyses leading to welfare reform.)

The voucher system can be integrated with the tax system and the unemployment insurance system.[6]

4. *Medicare* would be retained for the aged, disabled, and victims of end-stage

renal disease (ESRD). Eligibility would be expanded to all legal residents aged 65 and over for Part A (institutional services) and Part B (physicians' services). The benefits should be expanded to conform to the benefits for the rest of the population. The 150-day limit on hospital days should be removed—in effect providing catastrophic coverage. Better still, an annual limit on out-of-pocket expenses on covered benefits by any individual should be enacted.

The most important change needed in Medicare is a "freedom of choice provision" that would permit any beneficiary to direct that the "Adjusted Average Per Capita Cost" (AAPCC) to the Medicare program for people in his actuarial category be paid to the qualified plan of his choice in the form of a fixed prospective periodic payment. If done properly, this would end the Medicare subsidy to those who choose a more costly system of care, and would permit beneficiaries to reap the benefit of their economizing choices in the form of reduced cost-sharing or better benefits.

In addition, about 7.7 million aged, blind, and disabled receive Medicaid supplements to assist with costs not covered by Medicare. CCHP would replace this part of Medicaid, as far as acute care is concerned, with a voucher, comparable to the voucher for the non-aged poor, for premiums for a policy to supplement Medicare. In FY 1978, the average per capita hospital and physician costs for the aged not covered by Medicare will be about $385. This would be an appropriate level for the voucher.

C. Pro-Competitive Regulatory Framework

In order to qualify to receive tax credits, vouchers, or Medicare payments, a health plan would have to operate by the following rules for a fair and socially desirable competition based on quality and cost-effectiveness.

1. *Open Enrollment.*[9] Each plan would participate in a periodic government-run open enrollment in which it must accept all enrollees who choose it, without regard to age, sex, race, religion, national origin, or, with possible minor exceptions, prior health conditions. Each September, for example, every family would receive an informative booklet published by the administrative agency. During October, each head of household would make an election for the coming year, through his employer, welfare office, or local office of the administrative agency. This would greatly enhance competition by giving each person a choice from among competing plans, and it would assure that every person could enroll in a qualified plan.

2. *Community Rating.* A qualified plan must charge the same premium to all persons in the same actuarial category enrolled for the same benefits in the same area. (Nominal differentials might be allowed to reflect differences in costs of collecting premiums from different sized groups.)

Open enrollment and community rating are essential features of CCHP.

3. *Rating by Market Area.* Qualified plans must set community rates by market area (such as Health Service Areas or groups of contiguous HSAs). This is to prevent anti-competitive cross subsidies from one area to another, and to "internalize" the costs of health services by Health Service Area so that a decision by a Health Systems Agency to permit construction of a new health facility will be fully reflected in the premiums paid by citizens in that area, thus giving the HSA a more balanced set of incentives to control costs.

4. *Low Option.* Qualified plans must offer a "low option" limited to the basic benefits defined in the NHI law. This is to prevent plans from limiting membership to the well-to-do offering only plans with costly supplemental benefits.

5. *Maximum on Out-of-Pocket Costs.* Qualified plans must publish a clearly stated maximum on individual (or family) out-of-pocket outlays over a one or two-year period (e.g., $1,500 in one year, $2,500 in any two consecutive years). Beyond that

amount, the plan must pay all costs for covered benefits. This would help assure that plans do not compete by offering "thin" benefits that would leave the seriously ill uninsured and a burden on the public sector. It is appropriate to limit consumer choices in this respect because, in the case of nonpoor families, society's primary objective is to protect everyone in case of serious illness. (I would leave the amount to be set by each plan. It is likely to become an important competitive variable. But it could be set by regulation.)

6. *Health Plan Identification/Credit Card.* Every qualified plan would issue each member a card which would inform providers of each person's coverage and which would serve as a credit card for covered services for eligible providers. This would virtually eliminate questions of payment at the provider's office, and it would put the burden of credit and collection on the financial intermediary, the agency best equipped to handle it. Revolving credit at regulated interest rates would ease the cash flow problem for persons facing large out-of-pocket payments. The intermediary's computer could figure out the copayments and deductibles—a great convenience for the consumer. And the credit card would allow the intermediary to capture total cost information—allowing it to report total per capita cost for covered benefits as discussed below. Special measures would be required to assure the ability of health plans to collect debts and to finance the large float.[10]

7. *Information Disclosure* is an essential part of CCHP to help consumers judge the merits of alternative plans and to help assure public confidence in the plans. Uniform financial disclosure would be required, comparable to what the SEC requires of public companies. Data on patterns of utilization, availability and accessibility would be required, as is required of HMOs in the HMO Act. Data should also be developed and published on qualifications of providers and on indicators of quality of care and consumer satisfaction such as rates of medical injuries, complaints, etc. To aid consumer choice, each plan would be required to publish total per capita costs, including premiums and out-of-pocket costs. The administrative agency would have authority to review and approve (for accuracy and balance) promotional materials, including presentations to be included in the booklet available to all eligibles at "open season"— as the Civil Service Commission does for the FEHBP. The administrative agency would also have authority to review and approve "endorsed options" and contract language such that all options offered would either conform to a standard contract or be able to be described by a standard contract and a manageable number of additions and exclusions. This would force plans to publish their terms in a format that is understandable to consumers and that facilitates direct comparison among plans without the consumer having to master and compare a lot of fine print.

8. *CCHP and Direct Controls.* CCHP is not necessarily incompatible with some proposed regulation such as health planning, hospital cost controls, and physician fee controls. Compliance with controls can be made a condition for a plan to be qualified. CCHP would increase the effectiveness of the Health Systems Agencies by giving them incentives they now lack to control costs. Moreover, the present structure of physician fees has perverse incentives. A system of controls on the fee-for-service sector might improve this situation and also encourage physicians to join cost-effective organized systems. Competing private plans with incentives to control total costs would probably be able to enforce such controls more effectively than could a government agency. Controls on the fee-for-service sector from which cost-effective organized systems were exempted might encourage the restructuring of the delivery system. However, experience with regulation in health care and elsewhere suggests that the regulatory process usually protects established provider interests from competition. So the

purposes of CCHP could be defeated by conventional regulation. The burden of proof must be placed on the proponents of controls to show that the controls will not have their usual effect of retarding cost-reducing innovation.[20]

9. *Other*. In CCHP, as in any NHI system, there would be requirements for grievance procedures, and safeguards for civil rights and against fraud and conflict of interest. Also, some changes in selected State laws would be useful.[12]

D. Benefits and Eligibility

Any NHI plan must include definitions of covered benefits and eligible persons. The choices are largely political judgments. However, there are economic considerations. For example, the use of prescription drugs is strongly influenced by physicians, and it would be desirable for health plans to be at risk for prescription drugs to give physicians an incentive to prescribe carefully. The principles of CCHP can be applied to any of a broad range of benefit packages and eligibility criteria, including coverage of essentially every legal resident of the United States. The philosophy of CCHP suggests that, beyond the essentials, what is included in health benefits plans should be determined by consumer desires expressed in the marketplace, rather than by provider interests.

E. Federal-State Roles in Financing and Administration

CCHP is compatible with many possible ways of splitting Federal and State financing responsibilities. The choice must be considered in the context of Federal-State burden sharing in general—of which acute medical care financing is only one piece—and it must rest largely on political judgments. One illustrative possibility is as follows. First, about 35% of Medicaid pays for long-term care. About 58% pays for acute medical care and prescription drugs and sun-

dries. In Fiscal 1976, the Federal Government paid 55% of Medicaid. The Federal Government might pay 100% of the cost of the health insurance premium vouchers, i.e., the replacement of the acute care paid for by Medicaid, in return for which the States might take on an increased share of the financing of long-term care, supplementary payments to low-income families in high-cost areas where the vouchers do not pay for adequate health care coverage, and assistance with such benefits as dentistry and the part of mental health not financed through NHI. Because States are potentially important factors in health facilities planning and cost controls, the Federal Government should not pay more on behalf of States that have higher real per capita health care costs in such a way as to weaken their incentive to control costs.

CCHP could be administered entirely by the Federal Government or jointly by the Federal Government and the States under Federal standards.

F. Role of Employers, Unions, and Labor-Management Health and Welfare Funds (HWF)

Employers, unions, and HWFs would continue to play a significant, though modified, role in CCHP. They would continue to serve as the main vehicles for collecting the funds for workers' health insurance premiums. There would be no sudden change with enactment of CCHP; merely a change in the way employees are taxed on a fringe benefit. Because additional health benefits would no longer receive preferred tax treatment, one can expect that in the future employees would demand more of their compensation in wages, less in health benefits. If we wish to curb the growth in health spending, that is a desirable result. Open enrollment in all qualified health plans might reduce what little bargaining power employers and HWFs have with respect to providers; it would increase the role of individual choice by consumers. HWF and employer bargaining power would be based on advice, not on their power to limit the choices of their workers. So far, employers and HWFs have not been very successful in bargaining with providers for cost control.

In addition to their key role in aggregating funds for the efficient purchase of health benefits, employers and unions would have two very important roles to play in CCHP. The first would be to organize the provision of information, advice, and voluntary evaluation for their workers. Under CCHP, there might be more than a dozen qualified health plans in operation in some areas. Busy workers would need help in knowing on which few they should focus attention, and the relative merits of each as discovered, in large part, by the experience of their coworkers. Unions and employers could organize committees, hire experts, take surveys of member satisfaction, and publish "consumer reports" to help their workers find their way through the market. Such private voluntary agencies are in a much better position to provide information that depends on value judgments than are government agencies. Government agencies are usually hamstrung by legal requirements of proof and objectivity and by well-focused pressures from providers.

The second role would be direct action to help reorganize the health care delivery system. Under CCHP, it would be even more advantageous for an employer and for union members to have lower health care costs in their area than is the case today. Thus, employers and unions could contribute to the goals of CCHP and serve their own interests at the same time by taking the initiative to organize cost-effective systems of care.

G. Special Categories: DOD (CHAMPUS), Veterans, Indians, Migrants, Derelicts, Underworld, Illegal Aliens, Non-Enrollers, etc.

Special measures can be designed for the special problems of each of these categories

within the context of CCHP. CCHP will not, of itself, solve these problems, but it does provide a framework that helps.[7]

H. Delivery System Reform[14]

CCHP creates a framework of financial incentives that is favorable to the growth of cost-effective organized systems. But it does not, in itself, create those systems. If such systems are to come into being, many local efforts to organize them will be required. Public policies to encourage such efforts should be the subject of separate legislation.

I would not recommend more special grants and subsidies for HMOs because (a) experience with the HMO Act shows that they come at an extremely high political price, and (b) given a truly fair market test, those demonstrating the economic superiority of the best HMOs will prosper without help (though getting started is another matter). The HMO Act promised grants and loans, on the basis of which many costly restrictions were justified. The costly restrictions were enacted; the financial help actually delivered fell far below the amounts originally authorized. Advocates of more "help for HMOs" should remember what happened last time. I am much more impressed by the economic superiority of the best prepaid group practice plans than by unenforceable promises of generous public subsidies for HMOs. Experience suggests that the soundest public policy would be firm adherence to the principle of a fair market test among competing alternatives.

An antitrust strategy specifically designed for the peculiar economics of the health care industry is needed. Ordinary antitrust theory, developed for other industries, does not fit very well in health care. It is easy to imagine some non-competitive outcomes in CCHP. For example, a county medical society might form an IPA and use it as a price-fixing arrangement, and keep out would-be competing physicians through control of hospital privileges. Or a market might continue to be dominated by multiple third-party plans, all paying the same providers the same fees and costs. Continuing research, policy analysis, and possibly more legislation would be needed.

I. Presidential Leadership.

The effectiveness of CCHP could be enhanced considerably by strong Presidential leadership on at least two points. First, the average American needs to be reminded that, ultimately, he will pay the costs of health care, and the costs will be lower and the quality better if many Americans will get involved personally in the cost-effectiveness of their own health plan. Existing laws and financing patterns have created the illusion for most people that health care is being paid for by somebody else. And much NHI rhetoric that is strong on the benefits and quiet about the revenue sources serves to foster that illusion. Second, Presidential encouragement of local voluntary actions to start cost-effective organized systems could be of great value.

J. Costs and the Federal Budget

1. *The Estimating Problem*. Before considering estimates of the costs of NHI, consider the inherent limitations in the estimating methods. Costs are estimated by multiplying recent prices of services by recent utilization rates by the size of the covered population. To that is added an estimate of "induced demand," i.e. the short-term increase in demand attributable to improved coverage. The calculation uses assumptions about elasticity of demand—a measure of utilization increase when price to the consumer is reduced by insurance. There is no firmly based estimate of demand elasticity for health services. But assumptions are made by actuaries that experts agree are reasonable.

But the methods totally lack any scientific way of forecasting the long-term effect of the incentives on unit costs, utilization, and standards of care. Hence, the estimators are forced to make assumptions with very little but judgment to go on. The history of programs like Medicare has been one of consistent large underestimation in the long run. For example, in 1965, the 1975 costs of hospital insurance were projected at $4.3 billion; the actual was about $11.7. Deflate this for the 71 per cent increase in general price levels and you still get about a 60 per cent overrun. Comparing cost estimates as a per cent of taxable payroll allows for inflation. In 1965, the 1971 costs were projected at .95 per cent of taxable payroll; the actual turned out to be 1.30 per cent or 37 per cent higher. There was a similar history in the renal dialysis program. But the problem is potentially far more serious in NHI because the size and impact of the program are larger.

Compounding the effects of a lack of reliable estimating methods are the incentives and optimism of proponents of social insurance programs, similar to the causes of understatement in costs of weapon systems. Few, if any, people may be seriously interested in realistic estimates at the time of program inception. What reward is there for realism?

The best you can do is to start with the judgment of reputable actuaries whose concern for professional reputation gives them an incentive to be accurate. But the assignments given to them may include the directed use of assumptions—such as that hospital cost controls will be effective—chosen by advocates of certain NHI approaches to make the costs of their proposals appear acceptable. Because many assumptions must be made to produce a NHI cost estimate, some important assumptions may not be called to your attention in the summary document.

The key factor in long-run costs is the effect of the incentives in the NHI system on unit costs, utilization, and standards of medical care. A key factor in costs to the Government is whether the system makes them "controllable" or open-ended and uncontrollable. A key feature of CCHP is that, with the exception of the costs of those Medicare beneficiaries who remain with conventional Medicare, CCHP's costs to the Federal Government are "controllable" and can be estimated with far greater reliability than the costs of an open-ended third-party reimbursement system. On the cost issue, these are the points on which you should focus your judgment.

2. *CCHP Cost Estimate*. With respect to the costs of CCHP to the Budget of the Federal Government, Appendix 21 contains detailed illustrative calculations of what the impact on the FY 1978 budget would have been had CCHP been in effect.[21] In each case, the calculations assume:

1. Actuarial Cost (AC) is $200 for a person under 19, $475 for a person 19–64, and therefore $1,350 for a "family of four." (That compares, for example, to annual dues of $1,284 in 1978 for a family in Washington D.C. to join Georgetown University Community Health Plan.)

2. AC for a Medicare beneficiary will be $1,150, all but $385 of which, on average, will be paid by Medicare. Therefore, a 100% of AC voucher for a poor Medicare beneficiary is $385.

3. Offset against the cost of the tax credits and vouchers are the "Federal Income Tax Expenditures of $8.7 billion, Federal Medicaid of $11.8 billion, "Social Security Tax Expenditures" of $1.4 billion, and other programs of $1.9 billion, for a total of $23.8 billion.

4. No changes in the net cost of Medicare.

If the tax credit for the non-poor were 30% of AC (i.e., $405 for a family of four), and the voucher for the poor were 100% of AC at the income guarantee level (e.g., $4,200 for a family of four), reduced 20 cents for each dollar of family income (including cash assistance) above that, the gross cost

of the tax credit/vouchers would be $26.9 billion; the net cost to the Federal budget $3.1 billion.

If the tax credit for the non-poor were 50% of AC, and the voucher for the poor were 100% of AC at or below the cash assistance breakeven level (i.e., $8,400 for a family of four), reduced 25 cents for every dollar of income above the breakeven, the gross cost of the tax credit/vouchers would be $44.6 billion; the net cost to the Federal budget would be $20.8 billion. This would be an extremely generous voucher program; 33% of the population would be receiving voucher payments.

A "full" CCHP program might include a 65% of AC tax credit for the non-poor (i.e., $878 for a family of four), a voucher bringing the total to 100% of AC at the income guarantee level, reduced 10 cents for every dollar of family income above that. The gross cost would be $49.8 billion; the net cost, $26 billion.

As for how to pay for CCHP, I assume that the Administration, which has promised a NHI proposal, is considering this problem in the context of its overall tax reform proposals. Obviously CCHP can cost much less than alternative NHI proposals (see below).

From a fiscal point of view, CCHP would make the Government's contribution to personal health services a "controllable" expenditure that could be set at a level in balance with other priorities, instead of today's open-ended commitments through the third-party intermediary system. Moreover, in CCHP, those who want more health services have the option of using their own net-after-tax income to buy them, which would result in less pressure on the Congress than would be the case, e.g., under Health Security.

Most important, by establishing strong incentives for cost effectiveness, CCHP promises in the long run to be less costly for any given level of coverage.

IV. WHY CCHP? SOME ISSUES

1. **Will the desired reorganization of health services take place fast enough?** Reorganization of health services will take a long time—a very long time by political standards—a decade or more, even under the most favorable conditions, before half the population is served by some kind of organized system with incentives for economy. The Medical Profession is very resistant to organizational change. There are powerful vested interests throughout the health services industry, institutions with long traditions and deep roots in their communities. Many people will change their health plans and providers only reluctantly and slowly. There are no easy routes to health services reorganization. It will take a great deal of effort by many people in many localities.

Direct regulatory approaches to reorganizing health services promise fast results—but all the evidence shows that the promises are false. Health security and universal third-party insurance would freeze the system in its present patterns. (See Section VI below.) A judgment in favor of the CCHP approach must be based, in part, on a realistic appraisal of the alternatives.

The main reason for optimism about the prospects for a reorganization, given a fair market test among competing alternatives, is that the economic advantage of organized systems can be large. A recent review of the many comparison studies over the past 25 years concluded, "The evidence indicates that the total costs (premium and out-of-pocket) for HMO enrollees are 10–40 per cent lower than for comparable people with health insurance." A Social Security Administration comparison of Medicare reimbursements for beneficiaries served by six group practice prepayment plans and a matched sample served by fee-for-service in 1970 found the former cost 73% of the latter. The point is not that *all* HMOs cost a lot less; in any industry there will be more and less efficient producers. The point is that a substantial number of HMOs have shown that the savings can be large. Moreover, these HMOs have achieved large savings even in the absence of real competition from similar organizations.

The creation of organized systems of care would not have to take the many years of institution and facilities building characteristic of the leading Prepaid Group Practice (PGP) plans. If there were a market, simpler organizations, based on existing institutions, facilities, and practice styles, might be developed fairly quickly on the Individual Practice Association (IPA) model, the Health Care Alliance (HCA), or other broadened definition of HMO. In an IPA, the physicians agree to provide comprehensive benefits, largely for a fixed prospective periodic payment, under the following arrangements. First, they agree among themselves on a fee schedule. When they render a service to a member of the plan, they bill the plan, not the member. Second, they accept peer review of the appropriateness of services. Third, they agree to accept a pro rata reduction in fees if the money runs low. Fourth, they team up with an insurance company that offers a hospital insurance policy. The premium for that policy reflects the hospitalization experience of the members of that plan, which is, of course, controlled by the doctors in the IPA. So if the total premium for physician and hospital services is determined by the market, the less the hospitalization, the lower the insurance premium, and the more is left over for the doctors. HCAs have similar characteristics.

IPAs, like other HMOs, have not grown rapidly in the past for reasons explained below. Moreover, there is evidence that IPAs have been less effective than PGPs at control of hospital utilization. I believe the reason for this has been a lack of competitive necessity. If they had to develop good utilization controls to survive, I believe they would do so.

IPAs like this could be operative within a fairly short period of time. They can start with physicians already established in fee-for-service solo practice, with existing doctor-patient relationships, existing facilities, and without the need for large front-end investments. I believe that, to survive in the long run, they would have to strengthen internal controls, carefully balance specialty mix, etc. But these changes could come gradually.

In CCHP, physicians would be under strong economic pressure to sign up with or form qualified plans. This will be intensified by the coming doctor surplus.

Thus, I do not believe that one should estimate future HMO membership in a CCHP world by applying some plausible compound growth rate to present HMO membership. Rather, there is reason to expect that many new organizations would be formed quickly.

2. If HMOs are superior, why haven't they grown faster? The main answer is the strong and pervasive anti-HMO bias in the policies of the Federal Government and the consequent lack of incentives for consumers and providers to join HMOs under existing financial arrangements. The tax laws, the Medicare law, the Planning laws, and the HMO Act all have important anti-HMO biases. And the anti-HMO bias in State laws is notorious. Most people do not have a choice between an HMO and a third-party, fee-for-service plan, or if they do, the tax laws, Medicare, and employer financing arrangements do not let them keep the savings. HMOs have done very well in competitive multiple-choice situations. For example, Kaiser-Permanente of Northern California serves 37% of the Federal employees, 43% of the State of California employees, and 37% of the University of California employees in its service area. And, despite the obstacles, HMOs' growth rates in areas where they are established is impressive. From 1960 to 1976, Kaiser's

California membership increased from 720,000 to 2,617,000, a compound annual growth rate of 8.4%, despite the fact that in many years, they had to limit new enrollments because of the time and cost required to plan, build, and staff new facilities.

3. Is health care financing more appropriately organized as a Government monopoly, or through private markets?[17] Much of the case for NHI rests on "private market failure." And there is no doubt that the private market for health insurance, as presently constituted and shaped by numerous government policies, does a poor job of allocating resources. The main idea of CCHP is that the private market needs to be restructured, and that a reconstituted private market can do a better job than a government monopoly of health insurance.

Consideration of private market failure needs to be balanced by an appreciation of some of the characteristic limitations of government. The following generalizations, while obviously not true in every case, summarize important insights that must be considered in deciding whether NHI should be based mainly on private markets or on a government monopoly. They are stated here baldly and without applicable qualifications to save time. The point of what follows is not to imply that government is "bad" compared to private enterprise, or that government people are better or worse than private enterprise people. Rather, the point is that government has certain limitations that are deep rooted, if not inherent. Government is good at some things such as taking money from taxpayers and paying it to social security beneficiaries, and maintaining competition in many industries; it performs badly at other things. The problem of public policy design is to define the appropriate role for government to achieve desirable social purposes most effectively.

1. Government responds to well-focused producer interests; competitive mar-

kets respond to broad consumer interests. People specialize in production, diversify in consumption. They are therefore much more likely to pressure their representatives on their producer interests than on consumer interests.

2. "The rule of 'Do no direct harm' is a powerful force in shaping the nature of social intervention. We put few obstacles in the way of a market-generated shift of industry to the South . . . but we find it extraordinarily difficult to close a military base or a post office." (Schultze) Thus, a government-run or regulated system must be very rigid.

3. When every dollar in the system is a Federal dollar, what every dollar is spent on becomes a Federal case. Abortion illustrates the point.

4. Equality of treatment by Government tends to mean uniformity. The uniform product is often a bargained compromise that pleases no one.

5. Government generally does a poor job providing services to individuals.

6. The Government performs poorly as a cost-effective purchaser. Think of the Rayburn Building, the South Portal Building, Medicaid, and the C-5A. If a government agency gets tough with suppliers, the suppliers can bring pressure to bear to get the rules changed. Government purchasers are surrounded by many complex procedural rules; they cannot use nearly as much judgment as their private sector counterparts. The Government seems addicted to cost-reimbursement despite its notorious record for generating cost overruns. Cost-reimbursement protects providers.

7. The Government has a much harder time than the private sector in attracting and retaining the best operating management talent on a career basis. Government attracts many of the best people—usually for two to four-year tours. But building an effective, economical operating organization usually takes years of dedicated effort; it cannot be done on revolving two or four-year stands.

8. The political system is extremely risk averse. This makes it very difficult to innovate in a government-regulated environment.

The financing of individual health care services does not need to be a monopoly. There is no technical or economic factor that must make it a "natural monopoly" like a public utility. Nor is personal health care a "public good" like defense or police protection. The benefits of individual health care services are enjoyed primarily by the individual and his family, and he should be allowed a large measure of choice concerning it. The important public purposes of universal access to good quality care can be pursued most effectively in a decentralized private system guided by an appropriate structure of incentives and pro-competitive regulation.

4. The "Consumer Choice" Issue. Proposals to rely on consumer choice to guide the health services system are invariably subjected to the attack that "consumers are incapable of making intelligent choices in health care matters." So it seems worthwhile to make clear exactly what is being assumed. Admittedly, the element of ignorance and uncertainty in health care is very large; that is true for physicians and civil servants as well as ordinary consumers. CCHP does not assume that the ordinary consumer is a *good* judge of what is in his own best interest. Consumers may be ignorant, biased, and vulnerable to deception. CCHP merely assumes that, when it comes to choosing a health plan, the ordinary consumer is the *best* judge of it. The theory of optimum allocation of resources through decentralized markets does not assume that every consumer is perfectly informed and economically rational. Markets can be policed by a minority of well-informed rational consumers. And we are seeking merely a good and workable solution, not a theoretical optimum. CCHP provides consumers with substantially better information than they get now and much stronger incentives to use it. If there were a demand for it, much could be done to organize better consumer information. In any case, the key factor is the incentive CCHP gives to providers, i.e., provider systems will get their money from satisfied consumers rather than from the Government. In CCHP, above the tax credit/voucher level, consumers would be working with their own money, not somebody else's.

Critics of the consumer choice position usually are not very explicit about whom they consider to be better qualified than the average American to choose his health plan for him. In reality, the alternative to a consumer choice system is a provider-dominated system.

Presumably *every* NHI scheme under consideration would allow each consumer choice of physician and free choice as to whether or not to accept recommended medical treatment—decisions that could be aided by technical knowledge. *What distinguishes CCHP from the others is that it seeks to give the consumer a choice from among alternative systems for organizing and financing care,* and to allow him to benefit from his economizing choices. The issue then is whether consumers can be trusted to choose wisely when it comes to picking a health plan—some of which cost less than others.

Part of the "consumer choice" issue is resistance to the idea of letting the poor, because of their poverty, choose a less costly health plan that might not meet their medical needs. There is appearance of a conflict here with the principle of CCHP that people must be allowed to benefit from their economizing choices. (There is, of course, an issue as to how much the poor should be forced to accept their share of society's assistance in the form of costly medical technology of doubtful value, as opposed to leaving them free to spend the resources on other things like food and housing known to be good for health.) The problem can be resolved in CCHP by setting the premium vouchers (usable only for health insurance), at a high enough level to assure access to a plan with adequate benefits—always letting plans that do a better job attract members by offering less cost sharing or more benefits.

5. **Equity Issues.**[19] CCHP uses the most effective way to redistribute income, i.e., directly. It takes money from the well-to-do and pays it to lower-income people in the form of tax credits and vouchers. By this method, the amount of redistribution is clearly visible, and one can be sure the money reaches its intended target. CCHP can thus be used to bring about whatever income redistribution for medical purchases our political process will support. I suspect the reason some will criticize CCHP on equity grounds is because they think that the amount of redistribution Congress will be willing to vote is less than their own personal preferences. So they seek indirect methods of redistribution that may be supported on other grounds. A major trouble with this approach is that third-party insurance systems are an exceedingly ineffective way to redistribute income. Medicare pays more on behalf of rich than poor. In a bureaucratic system, such as would be created under Health Security, individuals and organized groups who are forceful and skillful at getting their way come out ahead.

The equity of CCHP ought to be compared with where we are today and where we are likely to go as a society. It is useless to compare it to some hypothetical egalitarian ideal that has never been attained in any society and is surely not supported by the American people today.

6. **Is a multiple-choice system feasible?** The feasibility of a competitive model for NHI has been demonstrated by the Federal Employees Health Benefits Program (FEHBP) and numerous other choice-of-

plan systems. The FEHBP was authorized in 1959. It now provides health benefits for 10.5 million people. A 1964 report on the FEHBP noted, "The program finally authorized by Congress permits a wide range of choice of plans by all employees and was, in effect, a negotiated compromise among many divergent and highly organized interests. It was the only approach which at any time during the legislative process gained acceptance by all of the principals: the American Medical Association, Blue Cross-Blue Shield, insurance companies employee unions, group and individual practice prepayment plans, and the Federal Government as the employer. Although there can be no doubt that the 'single plan' approach would have been most desirable from the standpoint of administrative simplicity, now that we have learned to live with the administrative problems which stem from multiple choice, it becomes equally clear that the wide choice of plans has produced a program which is more effective in meeting the needs of Federal employees and their dependents. . . . It was anticipated by many that serious administrative problems would develop that would require continual legislation of a perfecting and remedial nature. This has not been the case."

The California State Public Employees' System has been in operation for almost as long as the FEHBP. It provides benefits for about 175,000 people. It has proved so successful that non-State public employee groups are now joining it. And it has been a significant factor in the growth of HMOs in California.

7. Some Other Problem Areas. a. *Underserved rural areas*. CCHP would not "solve" the problem of underserved areas, but it should help. It would provide assured medical purchasing power to people in rural areas, many of whom have low incomes, and by ending the open-ended tax subsidy in the well-served areas, it will put some financial pressure on physicians to relocate.

The best way to provide good care in rural areas is through organized systems that can provide outreach, e.g., through physician extenders, and that can provide financial and professional support to physicians working in such areas. For example, Kaiser-Permanente operates remote outposts in Hawaii, including a single-physician clinic on the northern shore of Oahu. Though far from the main Medical Center, this doctor can easily consult with his specialist partners by telephone, and can refer patients if necessary.

b. *Malpractice*. CCHP will not "solve" the problem of malpractice. But the growth of competing organized systems should help. An important part of the malpractice problem is the frequency of medical injury and the lack of quality control of physicians operating in solo practice. Good physicians in the fee-for-service sector complain of their inability to stop the bad ones from practicing because of the complex legal procedures involved. In an organized system, on the other hand, the physician group has direct professional and financial incentives to control the quality of its membership. Perhaps even more important than the ability to expel the bad actors is the ability of physicians in the Prepaid Group Practice setting to limit the activities of a physician who has passed the peak of his proficiency to tasks that remain within his competence, without threatening his livelihood. In such a system, quality control need not be an "all or none" determination of whether or not a physician should be allowed to practice. It can be a careful delineation of which tasks he is and is not currently qualified to perform. In such a setting, there is no financial incentive for a physician to practice beyond his level of competency.

c. *The "HMO underservice" issue.* Some allege that HMOs achieve financial success by underserving their members. The established HMOs like Kaiser-Permanente and Group Health of Puget Sound, etc., have for many years served such educated middle class groups as Federal and State employees, university faculties and other teachers. If there were a significant amount of under-service, one would think that the word would get around and that these people would switch at the next open season. I have been unable to find any documented case of a pattern of underservice among such HMOs. On the contrary, the main selling point of such organizations is usually improved accessibility. A recent study compared patterns of ambulatory use in five health care delivery systems in Washington D.C. and found ". . . (1) for preventive use, rates are lowest in OPD/ERs (outpatient department/emergency rooms) and highest in the prepaid group (Group Health Association, a Prepaid Group Practice), with both being significantly different from solo practice; (2) for initiation of care, rates are significantly and consistently highest in the prepaid group, . . . ; (3) for follow-up care, rates are highest in fee-for-service groups and moderate in the prepaid group . . . it is clear that services are more equitably distributed in the prepaid system than in the fee-for-service systems, for every use measure." The allegations of underservice arose in the case of the Medicaid Prepaid Health Plans, mainly in Southern California. There, a State government was trying to cut short-run costs in a hurry, and accepted unrealistically low bids for Medicaid contracts, and enrollment practices that interfered with free choice. The underservice problem arose from the State government's politically motivated purchasing policies, not from the nature of HMOs. If you assure that every family has the purchasing power to buy membership in a good plan, and a free choice among competing plans, organizations that make a practice of underserving members will not last long.

This is not to imply that the financial incentives in the existing HMOs are perfect or that their performance is without shortcomings. We simply do not know what are the "right" financial incentives; there is no logical or empirical basis for such a determination. CCHP proposes to find out what

are good incentives through experience in a competitive market. And good incentives do not guarantee good performance. Medical care is full of judgment and uncertainty; mistakes are made in any setting, including HMOs. HMOs may have replaced financial barriers with institutional barriers to care. The most effective pressure to perform to satisfy consumers is competition.

V. PHASING AND PART-WAY STEPS

Section III described the complete CCHP proposal. To have maximum impact, the whole plan should be adopted. But CCHP is not an "all or none" proposal. It can be viewed as a menu of individual proposals, many of which would improve the market, even if adopted alone or in groups. Or it can be seen as a direction—a strategy to be implemented as political and economic realities permit. *It can be phased in.*

1. *Phasing the Tax-Credit Voucher.* As indicated above, a version of CCHP with a tax credit equal to 30% of Actuarial Cost for the non-poor, and a voucher equal to 100% of AC at the income guarantee level ($4,200 for a family of four) and a 20% "benefit reduction rate" would have a net FY 1978 cost of $3.1 billion. The breakeven income for the voucher would be $8,925 for a family of four, and about 24% of the population would receive vouchers. Alternatively, CCHP with a 60% tax credit, and a voucher with a 12% benefit reduction rate would have a net FY 1978 cost of $22.4 billion.

CCHP might be started with a 30% tax credit for the non-poor, with the breakeven point at which the voucher is phased out held constant at $8,925 in 1978 prices, and with an increase of 2.5 percentage points per year in the basic tax credit over 12 years, until the tax credit for the non-poor reached 60% of AC. Thus, the net budgetary outlay would be increased an average of about $1.6 billion per year.

The attractive and unique feature of this approach is that it enables the Government to address the basic financial incentives in the whole system at a net budgetary outlay of several billions in the first year.

2. *Cap the Exclusion of Employer Contributions*. If the above phasing is not acceptable, at a minimum, the Administration should propose to cap the exclusion of employer contributions from taxable income at a level high enough so that few suffer a loss today, but low enough that in the future many people will start paying the extra costs of health insurance out of their own net-after-tax incomes. A level of about $1,500 per year for the sum of employer contributions and premium deductibility would seem about right. Such caps exist in the tax laws now (e.g., on group life insurance).

3. *Amend Section 1876 of Medicare*. The freedom of choice provision in Medicare described above should be enacted whether or not other parts of CCHP are proposed. A similar principle should be applied to Medicaid.

4. *Dual Choice*. Section 1310 of the Public Health Service Act ("the HMO Act") requires any employer of 25 or more who is subject to the minimum wage requirement under the Fair Labor Standards Act to include in his employee health benefits plan the option of joining one group practice HMO and one IPA HMO if such are available in the same area where 25 or more of his employees reside. This requirement might be broadened, all at once, or in steps. In the interest of enhancing competition, employers might be required to add one plan a year up to a maximum of five or six. To this should be added the right of any employee to "carry his health plan membership with him" as he changes job but maintains the same residence.

5. *Premium Rating by States*. The market would be improved if the FEHBP asked its carriers to adopt a system of premium rating by States. The carriers have the information needed to do this, and could do so at a nominal cost. A similar practice would be in the interest of any multi-division or multiplant company that wanted to know its costs

accurately by location. Some carriers offer this as a service to some multi-plant companies now. So it is not clear why this even needs to be required. I recommend that the Federal Government show the way by modifying the FEHBP.

6. *Allow Others to Join the FEHBP*. The California law authorizing the health benefits part of the Public Employees Retirement System allows local government agencies to participate in the State employees system by contract. Would it not make sense to allow other Federal, State, and local government agencies to buy into the FEHBP? (This assumes the premium rating by State outlined above is enacted.) To begin with, some of the seven million civilian CHAMPUS eligibles might be included, e.g., in areas where military facilities are not available. (To include all of them would require resolution of some complex problems of coordination with the military direct care system and the health plans offered by the civilian employers of some of the beneficiaries.)

7. *Should CCHP be tried first in one or a few States?* The answer depends on the purposes of the trials and how they are done. I do not believe that the long-term efficacy of CCHP in motivating delivery system reform can be tested in an "experiment." Experiments may be quite useful in producing information on individual responses to cost-sharing formulas, income subsidies, and the like. But people are not likely to make the kind of effort and long-term commitment required to build institutions for an experiment. However, it could be very useful to use one or a few States as pilot models to test and evaluate rules and procedures in the context of a national decision to follow a CCHP strategy.

Some aspects of CCHP, such as changes in the Federal Income Tax law, would be hard to try on a State basis. Others, such as "freedom of choice" for Medicare beneficiaries should not be turned on and off. These changes would need to be made nationally at the outset and can be justified on their own merits. Many parts of CCHP have been in practice for years on a limited basis. Multiple-choice has been demonstrated in the FEHBP, in the California Public Employees' plan, Medicaid in Oregon, and elsewhere. Congress was sufficiently persuaded of the merits of open enrollment and community rating that it imposed them on HMOs. CCHP merely extends these principles to all qualified health plans. Operational test and evaluation would probably be wise. But those proposing it should specify what questions the test will answer and how.

VI. ALTERNATIVES TO CCHP

There are two broad alternatives to CCHP, each of which can be designed to cover the same people and benefits. The stated goals of their proponents are the same, i.e., access for every American to comprehensive health care services of good quality. The essential differences are in their financial and organizational structures, in the incentives they provide and in the way resources would be allocated.

1. *Universal third-party insurance* is the most familiar approach, i.e., a program that sees to it that, by one means or another, everybody is insured. This would generalize the financing principle that dominates our health care economy today. There are many variations on the theme, i.e., different mixes of public and private insurance and different schedules of copayments and deductibles. Most of the perennial NHI bills are in this group, including "Kennedy-Mills," "Long-Ribicoff," "CHIP" and proposals by the industry groups (AMA, AHA, and HIAA). For purposes of policy analysis, their common reliance on the third-party reimbursement principle is more significant than what distinguishes them from each other.

At least in concept, the simplest way to achieve universal coverage is for the Federal Government to serve as the insurer for everybody, as proposed, for example, in the "Kennedy-Mills" bill in 1974, a sort of "modified Medicare for everybody." The industry group bills seek to assure universal coverage through a mix of private and public programs. Long-Ribicoff would seek to close two of the main gaps in present coverage by a catastrophic illness plan for everybody and a medical assistance plan for the poor. The Nixon Administration proposed the Comprehensive Health Insurance Program (CHIP), essentially (1) mandated employer-employee private insurance meeting certain standards, (2) a State-operated assisted health care program for low-income and high-risk families, and (3) expanded Medicare.

My criticisms of universal third-party reimbursement insurance are several. The essential point is that, from the point of view of economic incentives, the third-party reimbursement principle is not a rational way to finance medical care. Like the cause of air pollution, third-party reimbursement insurance gives people economic incentives to abuse a scarce resource. Third-party reimbursement insurance relieves the consumer of the additional cost of the services he receives, and therefore the incentive to conserve resources, without putting the incentive on the provider. On the contrary, fee-for-service and cost reimbursement reward providers for rendering more services, and more costly services, whether or not they are necessary, effective, or best for the patient. A rational economic system of health care financing would tie the physicians to the economic consequences of their decisions and hold them responsible for using total health care resources wisely. It would also allow consumers to realize the full benefits from choosing less costly systems of care.

The worst effect of universal third-party insurance would be to destroy the incentive of consumers and physicians to reorganize the delivery system in more cost-effective ways. It would deny consumers the opportunity to reap the benefit from choosing less costly systems or styles of care. Consumers would be relieved of most of the costs implicit in their choices, and larger reimbursements would be made on their behalf if they chose more costly providers. Similarly, with government-financed, open-ended demand for services where and when they want to deliver them, physicians would see little gain from accepting the discipline of an organized system.

If you must go along with universal third-party insurance, at a minimum you should be sure that there is a "freedom of choice" provision similar to what I have recommended for Medicare.

A universal third-party system operated by the Government would add roughly $60 billion to Federal outlays, or a net budgetary cost of $50 billion, with no good way of phasing it in. (Estimate based on Kennedy-Mills.[15])

2. *The Health Security Act* is designed to get away from third-party reimbursement and to shift health care financing to a per capita and prospective budgeting basis within a publicly determined total. The Act would assign the entire financing and management of NHI to the Federal Government. It would create a Health Security Board in DHEW to administer the program. It would levy taxes on payrolls, self-employment and unearned income, and match this with an equal sum from general revenue. The Board would establish an annual national budget, based on the cost of the program in the preceding year, adjusted for changes in prices, population and number of providers, not to exceed total receipts. Thus, there would be a firm lid on total health care spending. The Board would allocate the budget to each DHEW region on a per capita basis in categories for institutional services, physicians' services, dental services, drugs, appliances, etc. Within these totals, the Board would then contract for covered services with participating providers, i.e., providers who agree to make no charge to the patient for covered services. In brief, Health Security would create a system that is centrally and politically controlled, in which every participating provider gets all his money from the Federal Government. Spending for personal health care services would be set in the political process on the basis of national priorities rather than in the marketplace based on individual priorities.

Health Security has important strengths. It recognizes that the third-party reimbursement principle provides inappropriate economic incentives in medical care. It seeks to restructure health services into organized systems. Capitation financing, which it emphasizes, gives incentives for economic efficiency in use of total resources. Health Security seeks equity in the use of public funds. And it seeks to equalize per capita spending among regions and between HMOs and the fee-for-service sector.

Many of Health Security's weaknesses are summarized in the discussion of government monopolies and private markets.[17] But the main criticism of Health Security is that it cannot achieve its goals.[16] The Government cannot restructure the system by direct controls. Experience with other regulated industries, and with NHI in other countries, suggests Government would freeze the system in its existing patterns. The "Do no direct harm" rule has prevented the Government for years from closing unneeded PHS hospitals and military bases. Government attempts to close hospitals in obviously overbedded areas drown in a deluge of lawsuits and pressure from employee groups. Imagine the vested interests and the rigidity surrounding the history-based allocations among hospitals, doctors, dentists, etc. It would become much more important to provider groups to defend their allocation than to serve patients. The Health Security Act seems almost designed to freeze existing allocations and to protect existing jobs.

Further reason to doubt the ability of the Government to restructure the system comes from the recognition that the Federal Government has proved itself to be the enemy of HMOs. The list of counter-productive actions and policies is long and impressive. The anti-HMO bias has persisted too long and is too broadly based for it to be able to be written off as "another abuse of the Nixon Administration."[18] The experience suggests that the advocates of Health Security must be required to provide a realistic explanation of how the Government will actually function to restructure the system. They should not be permitted to claim good results based on good intentions and some abstract conception of what government ought to be.

The Health Security Act proposes to bring total spending under control by "top-down budgeting." Top-down budgeting may indeed bring total spending under control, but of itself, without competition, the mechanism has no built-in means for assuring that much useful output is produced. This is especially true of a medical care program whose output cannot be measured in any simple and adequate way. Look at the experience in our largest public health care systems. At least by civilian standards, the Defense Department operates and fills far too many beds. A recent study of the VA system concluded, ". . . there are too many acute beds being operated in the system . . . about half the patients in acute medical beds, one-third of the patients in surgical beds, and well over half the patients in psychiatric beds do not require—and are not receiving—the acute care services associated with these types of beds. These data provide additional evidence that many more VA hospital beds are being operated than are required to meet the needs of veterans . . . The VA has installed many expensive specialized medical facilities that, in many hospitals, are used at rates far below their capacity."[16] The point is that in the bureaucratic budgeting system, one strengthens one's case for more by doing a poor job with the budget one has. If the budgeting system at the institutional level is based on workload rather than capitation, it gives physicians and administrators incentives with respect to utilization that are similar to fee-for-service.

The Government is simply incapable of managing the Health Security Program. It does not have the organization and it cannot acquire the management capability on a *sustained* basis. To illustrate one of the problems, the Act provides that members of the Health Security Board will be paid at Executive Level IV. This means that the top management of the Program would be paid about 25% less than the *average* doctor. The Board might attract outstanding management talent to begin with, based on dedication to public service. But when it becomes clear what doing an effective job means, e.g., closing excess acute hospitals in some areas to pay for needed facilities in others, and Board members start feeling the wrath of citizens expressed through their Congressmen, and seeing the implementation of their plans tied up in court, the 2-year turnover typical of Assistant Secretaries in DOD and DHEW is sure to emerge. Running a large organization effectively requires long-term commitment by its managers; it cannot be done well on revolving two to four-year tours.

Finally, Health Security would add roughly $100 billion to Federal outlays in FY 1978 costs, or a net budgetary cost of $90 billion.[16] (Alternatively, it would add roughly $90 billion to public sector outlays.) And there is no way to phase it in. Health Security is an "all or none" proposal.

26. Cost Containment

IRA E. RASKIN, ROSANNA M. COFFEY, and PAMELA J. FARLEY

Reprinted from *Health: United States 1978*, DHEW Publication No. (PHS) 78-1232, 3-10.

During the last 25 years, the health industry in the United States has grown much more rapidly than the economy as a whole. Health expenditures as a percentage of the Gross National Product have doubled from 4.5 percent in 1950 to 8.8 percent in 1977 (Part B, table 146). Such a substantial shift in the resources allocated to health care has not been accompanied by comparable increases in the basic utilization of the health system, but rather, by continuing changes in the size, complexity, and cost of the service package represented by a day of hospital care or a physician visit. Per person utilization of hospital days increased only 6 percent between 1965 and 1975 (NCHS, 1977a), and the national physician-visit rate for 1976 exceeded the number of physician visits per person in 1966 by only 14 percent (NCHS, 1977b; NCHS, 1968). However, the price of a semiprivate hospital room more than tripled from 1965 to 1975. Physician fees nearly doubled over the 10-year period, rising slightly faster than the rate for all items in the Consumer Price Index (Part B, table 171).

The rapid inflation of health care costs, and of hospital costs in particular, has alarmed both government officials and the American public. As noted in testimony to the U.S. Council on Wage and Price Stability (1976), health care has come to represent a heavy burden for the private sector. Government health budgets are being squeezed between the pressure of inflation and the pressure from taxpayers to reduce public expenditures. At a time when the annual increase in the total Federal and State cost of Medicare and Medicaid will amount to about 15 percent in fiscal year 1978 (Office of Management and Budget, 1978), cost containment has emerged as a nearly essential prerequisite for continued pursuit of the positive goals of public health policy (Rosenthal, 1978).

The country's deep, historic commitment to health care is reflected in institutional arrangements that encourage its continued growth and development, including personal income tax deductions for medical expenses and insurance premiums, provision of health insurance as an employment benefit, public subsidies for health manpower training and research and development, and government financing of health care for the poor and elderly. However, this commitment has now come to represent such a substantial claim on the Nation's resources as to arouse concern that other public and private priorities are being threatened.

There are two aspects of the cost-containment issue that ought to be distinguished. The first is one of efficiency. Can the upward trend in health costs be slowed by encouraging greater efficiency in the health system's use of resources? If such economies could be realized, then further increases in the consumption of health care need not necessarily require the sacrifice of alternative goals and consumer demands. At a higher level of discussion, this question even extends to con-

ᵃ Prepared by Ira E. Raskin, Ph.D., Rosanna M. Coffey, and Pamela J. Farley, National Center for Health Services Research.

533

sideration of the relationship between health care and health itself. It is possible that there are more cost-effective ways to improve the health status of the population than to spend more money on medical care services.

The second aspect of the cost-containment issue deals with total resource allocation. Does the allocation of 10 percent of the country's resources to health care accurately reflect the importance of health among national consumption priorities? For many other services, this issue can be resolved satisfactorily in the marketplace; people simply reveal their preferences by the way they spend their money. In the health industry, however, it is often the case that the providers and consumers who make the consumption decisions do not bear the immediate financial consequences. Because of insurance coverage and government and employer subsidies, there is a tendency to undervalue the real costs of health services that are consumed and, as a result, to consume perhaps more than is truly warranted. However, the relative growth of health expenditures is at least in part a reflection of genuine social preferences that arise from such factors as the aging of the U.S. population and rising real incomes.

The main purpose of this chapter is to identify the cost-containment strategies that have been proposed and to report on findings from the research literature that may be helpful in evaluating their effectiveness. In order to set the stage for this presentation, the structural peculiarities of the health sector that tend to interfere with the satisfactory resolution of the efficiency and resource allocation issues implicit in cost containment must first be discussed.

EFFICIENCY, RESOURCE ALLOCATION, AND PECULIARITIES OF THE HEALTH SYSTEM

Perhaps the most significant peculiarity of the health care system is the infinite complexity of the service that it offers. Among its many dimensions are prevention, treatment, and cure of injury and disease; maintenance of patients with incurable and chronic illnesses; caring and reassurance; reduction of risk; and resolution of diagnostic and prognostic uncertainties.

Given the practical impossibility of defining a standard unit of health care which encompasses all of these considerations, it is also very difficult to monitor the efficiency of health care providers. Attempts to constrain the costs of a service, as measured along one dimension, are likely to produce cutbacks in some other aspect of care. As a result, service providers are traditionally reimbursed for whatever costs are incurred rather than on the basis of a standard rate. Such a system, unfortunately, neither rewards efficiency nor penalizes waste. Hospitals, for example, which are automatically reimbursed for all allowable expenses incurred during the previous year, are largely assured that new equipment and expanded facilities will be paid for, no matter how excessive their cost.

Physician reimbursement, whether from commercial insurance carriers, government intermediaries, or Blue Cross/Blue Shield insurers, is generally based on "customary, prevailing, and reasonable charges." The actual reimbursement rate, known as the reasonable charge, is equal to the lowest of one of three figures—the charge actually billed by the physician, the physician's customary charge, or a specified statistical combination of the prevailing charges of all physicians in the local area (Burney and Gabel, 1978). Hence, it does not pay for a physician to charge any less than other physicians in the area. Since the actual rate reimbursed by insurance carriers increases as the fees of all physicians in the area are raised, such reimbursement practices are ineffective in restraining costs (Holahan et al., 1978).

A second implication of the complex and multidimensional nature of health services is that there are many possible avenues of technological advancement. It has been estimated that approximately 75 percent of the increase in hospital costs, relative to general inflationary trends in the economy, can be attributed to the increased resource intensity of a day of hospital care (Feldstein and Taylor, 1977). New technology is one of the factors responsible for this trend (Redisch, 1978), although its net impact on health costs has yet to be accurately measured (Wagner and Zubkoff, 1978).

The significant feature of technical change in the health care market is that it may be worthwhile without having a clear, demonstrable impact on health outcomes or on treatment costs. For instance, the benefits of a new technology may be in a higher level of diagnostic certainty or in a reduction of danger or discomfort to the patient. Additionally, technological innovations are often cost raising rather than cost reducing. There is little question that the introduction of antibiotics and other drugs prior to 1950 was cost effective in terms of the lives that were saved. The major costs of these advances were for research and development and marketing. Yet other technological developments such as chemotherapy, organ transplantation, and intensive care facilities for heart attack and burn victims require extensive outlays for equipment and skilled personnel (Rice and Wilson, 1976), and are often more important in prolonging life or in reducing the risk of complication than in producing an outright cure.

How such changes impact on the cost of treating selected illnesses has been examined in a research study conducted by Scitovsky and McCall (1976). According to the study, changes since 1951 in treatment methods for specific illnesses have raised per-patient costs in some instances and saved money in others; however, the overall net effect of changing medical technology has been to make treatment more expensive. Cost increases can be attributed to greater use of diagnostic tests, more frequent use of specialists (particularly in hospitals), and the more costly nature of medical and surgical procedures. The notable increase in the cost of treating heart attacks has largely been a result of the use of intensive care units and other special facilities. Yet the present method of treating heart attacks is an example of a medical innovation that should perhaps be examined more carefully. One recent study of the effectiveness of early home care versus extended hospital stays for heart attack victims suggests that there is no difference in outcomes for low-risk patients who are released early and spared the economic expense of hospital care (McNeer et al., 1978). Such conclusions, of course, are tentative and require further validation.

All in all, technological change seems to present more of a chance to expand the capabilities of the health system at significantly increased cost, than to economize on the intensity of its resource use. As in the case of coronary care units, the system is constantly confronted with the problem of weighing all too obvious costs against benefits that are often more a matter of subjectivity and risk than tangible outcome. Were it not for the additional complication introduced by institutional arrangements that often divorce health care purchasing decisions from the responsibility for payment, it would not be so important for policymakers and researchers to try to assess these trade-offs. In other areas, a simple test is available for determining whether even intangible benefits are worth their cost: Are consumers willing to pay the price? Unfortunately, this test gives false readings in regard to health care.

First of all, the scientific and technical content of health services is often so great that patients are not able to make fully informed choices. There is even a tendency to view the costliness and technical sophistication of various services as a signal of their quality. Particularly in regard to hospital services and diagnostic tests, patients depend on the services of a skilled and highly trained "purchasing agent" (i.e., a physician) to assist them in their utilization decisions. In discharging their professional responsibility for safeguarding the welfare of their patients, physicians are not likely to economize on services that offer even the smallest chance of benefit, particularly since they bear none of the cost and are trained to focus on patient needs. One research study uncovered a 17–fold variation in laboratory test costs that could not be explained by the type or severity of the medical conditions seen by the internists involved (Schroeder et al., 1973). The same evaluation demonstrated that the cost of laboratory tests could be reduced 29 percent by simply informing the physicians of the wide disparities in their behavior.

It was observed in a theoretical discussion of this issue that the cost of the resources consumed in a day of hospital care is neither fully apparent to the physician nor fully reflected in the patient's bill (Redisch, 1978). Institutional health care settings base their prices on average costs; prices are calculated by dividing direct operating costs and overhead expenses by the number of patient days an institution expects to provide. Such pricing policies spread the cost of the hospital's services across all patients, protecting the more expensive patients from the full cost of the resources used.

An even more significant feature of the health system which separates the payment responsibility from the decision to seek care is the widespread coverage of health expenses by public and private insurance programs. In fiscal year 1950, only 31.7 percent of all personal health care expenditures were paid by private health insurance, government programs, and philanthropy; in fiscal year 1977, 69.7 percent of health expenditures were covered by third parties (Part B, table 153). Hospital expenses in particular were almost completely covered by third parties— 94.1 percent in fiscal year 1977 (Part B, table 162).

Since 1950, the average cost in real resources of a day in the hospital has increased almost 5 times, but the out-of-pocket cost to the consumer has hardly changed in real terms (i.e., in relation to the prices of all other goods and services) (Feldstein and Taylor, 1977). Although these greatly increased costs are paid by individuals and their employers as health insurance premiums, they do not affect the demand for services at the time of purchase. Any individual's use of health services has such a tiny effect on his or her insurance premium that there is no incentive to economize. Furthermore, having already paid for the insurance, patients are inclined to get their money's worth. The subsidization of health insurance premiums and related employer contributions through the present tax system further disguises the real costs of health care (Feldstein and Taylor, 1977; Mitchell and Phelps, 1976).

COST-CONTAINMENT STRATEGIES

The preceding section highlighted the major reasons for believing that the health system tends to be wasteful in its use of resources and for questioning the reliability of the marketplace as an institution for organizing decisions about the allocation of resources for health care. Yet there is no certain way to go about containing the inflationary growth of health expenditures and still ensure an equitable and efficacious system of care (Rosenthal, 1978). What is even less certain is how to accomplish this objective in a manner that is acceptable to the many different interests that are involved. The multiplicity of competing interests, the decentralization of decisionmaking, and the incentives to resist cost controls in the health industry may be forces too powerful to permit success (Hanft, Raskin, and Zubkoff, 1978).

Even if a compromise could be reached, the appropriate direction for government intervention to take is hardly clear. Many cost-containment proposals are directed at the hospital sector, where the rate of inflation has been most severe. It might be easier to intervene in the health system through a limited number of institutions than through some 360,000 physicians. On the other hand, the advocates of policies directed at medical care providers argue that the physician's role in influencing the content and level of service is too important to ignore.

An alternative approach would be to avoid direct intervention and instead to develop policies to restructure the health care market in ways that would promote efficiency and more careful consideration of the costs and benefits of expanded service. Some combination of these two strategies would be another possibility (National Commission on the Cost of Medical Care, 1978).

In the following sections, the lessons that have come from experience with a variety of cost-containment strategies will be described and analyzed. The unintended, sometimes perverse effects of intervention will also be discussed, with a special effort made to underscore the evidence suggesting that cost-containment instruments are often most effective when combined.

First to be considered are a number of regulatory strategies which would abandon any further reliance on the marketplace as a mechanism for setting the level of health care spending and would instead plan such allocation decisions explicitly and on the basis of political and technical determinations. These strategies include regulation of new investment in institutional facilities, programs to evaluate the existing supply of hospital beds with an eye to their closure or conversion to other uses, the establishment of ceilings on hospital capital expenditures and revenues, and policies to limit the supply of physicians.

It has been argued that limiting the available supply of health services will not only establish control over the total amount of health spending, but will also cause the allocated resources to be utilized more efficiently. Underlying this argument is a growing conviction that whatever the amount of health services available, they tend to be utilized. In hospitals, for example, physicians seem to be under pressure to maintain utilization rates by adjusting admissions and lengths of stay and by making use of expensive equipment that has been installed (Schweitzer, 1978; Roemer and Shain, 1959;

May, 1975; Klarman, 1978; Institute of Medicine, 1976b; McClure, 1976).

A second set of regulatory strategies is concerned with the development of reimbursement or rate-setting policies that will induce service providers to devote greater energy and attention to maximizing the efficiency of their operations. As was noted earlier, the prevailing system of cost-based reimbursement has exacerbated the expansionary trend in health spending by failing to reinforce a cost-conscious attitude on the part of providers.

Finally, consideration is given to a set of cost-containment strategies that would strengthen the marketplace as an instrument for imposing discipline on health care costs by bringing the financial and decisionmaking responsibilities closer together and by fostering competition among service providers. Proponents of these less regulatory strategies note that direct public controls necessarily involve the explicit rationing of a restricted supply of health services among competing uses, all of which are potentially worthwhile. They argue that the traditional reluctance of our society to weigh the benefits of more and better health care against its cost in monetary terms is no more likely to be challenged in the political arena than it has been in the health care marketplace (Havighurst, 1977). Market reforms, such as the introduction of more extensive consumer cost sharing in the health insurance system or the promotion of prepaid group practice, are proposed as a way of allowing for subjective valuation of the benefits of health care, while assuring that patients and providers are more fully conscious of their true costs.

Supply Controls

Hospital certificate of need.—Certificate-of-need programs institute public control over the expansion of hospital capacity by requiring formal justification and review of proposed investment projects with costs in excess of a specified dollar amount. The National Health Planning and Resources Development Act of 1974 (Public Law 93–641) requires that all States receiving Federal funds under the law introduce certificate-of-need programs by 1980. Certificate of need was in limited operation even before the passage of Public Law 93–641, with several States having already initiated their own programs; in ad-

dition, Section 1122 of the Social Security Act Amendments of 1972 (Public Law 92–603) required controls of this type under the Medicare, Medicaid, and Maternal and Child Health reimbursement programs.

Descriptive and empirical studies of experience with certificate-of-need and Section 1122 programs have documented a number of problems with the approach. A major difficulty has been the impossibility of specifying objective, quantifiable standards of "need" (Klarman, 1978; Leveson, 1978). In light of the highly emotional, political, and technical considerations involved in assigning a monetary value to the benefits of lifesaving services, planning agencies face a difficult task in reviewing proposals for new equipment (Klarman, 1978). Furthermore, inadequate funding, staffing, and review standards may cause regulators to depend too heavily on information and technical expertise from the service providers that they are supposed to control (Noll, 1975; Salkever and Bice, 1978; Havighurst, 1975).

A second difficulty is that the effect of certificate of need in protecting existing hospitals from new competition removes one potential incentive for efficiency. It has also been observed that, because there is no upper limit on the total amount of investment that can be approved and because they control only new facilities, current certificate-of-need programs are neither compelled to weigh alternative investment priorities nor empowered to rechannel resources into uses more desirable than the projects that happen to be proposed.

The most widely publicized empirical study of the certificate-of-need process examined State programs in operation from 1968 to 1972, a period of time that preceded the enactment of Public Law 93–641 (Salkever and Bice, 1978). This study corroborated other tentative, empirical evidence that certificate-of-need and Section 1122 programs were effective in curtailing bed expansion (Rothenberg, 1976; Bicknell and Walsh, 1975). However, additional analyses indicated that certificate of need was not an effective instrument for containing total hospital costs. It appeared that certificate-of-need programs had induced a shift in the composition of hospital investment away from new beds and into other types of facilities and equipment, with the composition of annual expenditure increases affected but not the rate of increase in hospital cost (Salkever and Bice, 1978).

Further research on five States with early certificate-of-need programs (New York, California, Connecticut, Maryland, and Rhode Island) showed no consistently significant effect of certificate of need on hospital investment. Although some positive findings were observed for New York, the interpretation was clouded by the Economic Stabilization Program and by the fiscal restraint that affected New York State's public expenditures (Salkever and Bice, in press). This suggests that the effect of certificate of need on costs is an issue that has not yet been satisfactorily resolved. It may be that the effectiveness of certificate-of-need agencies may improve with time. Program maturity has been identified elsewhere as one of the factors which seems to influence the effectiveness of investment controls (Howell, 1977).

There are other reasons that these evaluations of the long-run impact of certificate-of-need programs are inconclusive. Because certificate of need was most likely to be instituted before Public Law 93–641 in States where the pressures for expansion were most intense, one might have expected to observe a relatively greater increase in nonbed investment in those particular States anyway. Furthermore, prior to and in anticipation of the regulatory program, hospitals may have committed themselves to a plan of accelerated investment and construction that carried over into the early period of regulation (Hellinger, 1976).

Whatever the experience with certificate of need so far, the effectiveness of such programs may be enhanced in the future. For example, the Carter Administration has proposed a limit on capital expenditures to be allocated among the States as part of a national hospital cost-containment policy (Title II, H.R. 6575). Each State would be limited to a federally determined ceiling on certificate-of-need approvals, thereby establishing a national limit on annual hospital investment. Presumably, imposition of these ceilings would force local planning agencies to evaluate the trade-offs among various investment proposals rather than review each certificate-of-need application in isolation from the others received over the course of a year.

The continuing development and application of supply and utilization standards, such as those provided in the recently published **National Guidelines for Health Planning** (Public Health Service, 1978), should also improve certificate-of-need programs. Generally, there may be serious limitations to using standards of need that may not adequately reflect local preferences and that, if expressed in simple arithmetic formulas, cannot capture the peculiar health problems and resource configurations of different communities. Nevertheless, the imposition of a hospital-supply ceiling (4 beds per 1,000 population) and an occupancy standard (80 percent) has been proposed in hospital cost-containment legislation for use in conjunction with certificate of need (Title II, H.R. 6575). Specifically, areas not meeting these standards would be prohibited from granting certificate-of-need approval unless two old beds were removed for each new one added. Only 17 of 212 Health Service Areas would have qualified to expand bed capacity in 1974 under these standards (Dunn and Lefkowitz, 1978).

In addition to more formal linkage of planning agencies and rate-setting authorities, a set of controls complementary to certificate of need might also include utilization review, limits on the supply of physicians, and various forms of investment planning (Hanft, Raskin, and Zubkoff, 1978; Dowling, 1974; Bauer, 1978).

Hospital conversion and closure.—Certificate of need in its present form is a strategy limited to controlling the growth, and not the current availability, of the supply of hospital beds. Studies have estimated that current excess hospital capacity in this country is between 60,000 and 100,000 beds (Institute of Medicine, 1976b). The elimination of this excess capacity could offer potential savings on the order of $.5 to $5 billion depending, respectively, on whether portions of existing facilities or entire hospitals were closed (McClure, 1976). It is not surprising, therefore, that proposals have been advanced to offer Federal incentive payments for closure of unnecessary inpatient facilities or their conversion to some other use. Under the supervision of State and local health planning agencies, these payments would cover the costs of merging with other facilities, outstanding hospital debts, and new capital funds for conversion.

An alternative to offering financial rewards for the closure of unnecessary facilities is the adoption of a more punitive approach. It has been proposed, for example, that planning agencies should designate those institutions that ought to cease operations because of their "inappropriateness" (Title III, H.R. 9717). Financial sanctions, that is, the withholding of a specified percentage of the hospital's reimbursement under Federal financing programs, would penalize any failure to comply.

It is to be expected that attempts to close hospitals will meet stiff community resistance, as was the case in Canada (Armstrong, 1978). Closing hospitals will impose losses in employment, community prestige, and other aspects of social welfare that have not, and perhaps cannot, be measured (Hanft et al., 1978). Unless new hospital staff privileges for physicians are arranged elsewhere, the potentially serious impact on both their incomes and the quality of their services may also generate considerable resistance to hospital closure (Klarman, 1978).

The political viability of closing community hospitals is likely to depend on whether or not compensation is offered in the form of new, less costly health facilities or funds for other desired services. Cost consciousness involves making explicit choices between alternative uses of scarce resources. Unless the affected communities are given a share of the savings to be realized from closing unneeded facilities, they are not likely to either make or accept such difficult decisions.

Mandatory hospital revenue ceilings.—The Economic Stabilization Program of 1971–74 and the hospital cost-containment legislation proposed in Title I of H.R. 6575 are illustrative of a cost-containment strategy in which each institution is required to spend against a fixed and predetermined revenue limit. A distinguishing feature of this approach, in contrast to various reimbursement strategies, is that it breaks the usual connection between the hospital's revenues and its costs (Congressional Budget Office, 1977; Altman and Weiner, 1977). Furthermore, it is not the price of a hospital day that is regulated, but rather the total revenues that a hospital may receive over the course of a year.

Phase II of the Economic Stabilization Program limited the rise in total hospital revenue because of price increases to 6 percent more than the previous year, a total increase of approximately 8 percent after adjustment for increased service intensity. While the program, administered by the Cost of Living Council, was apparently effective in reducing the wage increases of hospital employees, it did not seem to have the same effect on overall hospital costs. The explanation for the program's minimal impact seems to have been a combination of the ambiguity of the regulations, perverse incentives to increase hospital admissions and lengths of stay, and the expectation that controls would be short-lived and would not, therefore, require cost-saving managerial changes (Ginsburg, 1978; Lipscomb, Raskin, and Eichenholz, 1978). Although the inflation of the hospital component of the Consumer Price Index did slow during the program, this trend began prior to the initiation of controls and, therefore, cannot be clearly attributed to their presence. The acceleration of hospital inflation subsequent to the termination of Cost of Living Council controls would nevertheless suggest that the program did have a significant influence (Lave and Lave, 1978). In any event, it would be fair to say that evaluation of the Phase II experience has not produced definitive conclusions.

The recently proposed hospital cost-containment legislation (Title I, H.R. 6575) bears a close similarity to the final version of the Economic Stabilization Program, Phase IV, which was never implemented. In contrast to Phase II, Phase IV would have rewarded shorter lengths of stay by regulating revenue increases on the basis of patient admissions rather than patient days. Also, Phase IV would have restricted reimbursement per case to a declining rate beyond a specified increase in admissions, thereby eliminating the incentive under Phase II to obtain more revenue by raising the admissions rate (Lipscomb, Raskin, and Eichenholz, 1978).

Restricting the number of physicians.—The physician's key role in determining the level and mix of resources employed in the delivery of health care was referenced earlier. It has been estimated that 70 percent of personal health care expenditures are controlled by physicians (Blumberg, to be published). Since physicians utilize other health services such as hospital facilities and laboratory services, they have a multiplicative effect on total expenditures. On the basis of data for medical internists, it could be estimated that in 1972 a physician generated an average expenditure of $240,000 (Lyle et al., 1974). Accounting for inflation, this effect would have amounted to approximately $370,000 in 1977.

By 1980, the number of physicians graduating from medical and osteopathic schools will have doubled since 1966. If the current growth rate in the number of graduating physicians and the inflow of foreign medical graduates is maintained, the supply of physicians will have increased another 50 percent by the year 2000. Similar increases are expected in the numbers of other allied health workers (Morrow and Edwards, 1976).

Theoretically, such increases in the supply of providers should produce increased competition for customers and subsequent reductions in price. Physicians, however, are in the peculiar position of being able to influence the demand for their own services. Furthermore, the usual predictions of economic theory do not apply to situations where the public's demand for a service is practically insatiable in the aggregate, as sometimes seems to be the case with health care. As a result, it may be that the current rate of increase in the availability of physicians is a factor directly responsible for placing additional pressure on health care costs.

By limiting the entry of foreign medical graduates into this country, the Federal health manpower legislation enacted in 1976 (Health Professions Educational Assistance Act of 1976) signaled a major shift away from traditional policies of encouraging increases in the supply of physicians to a policy of curtailing such increases. Other restrictions that have been proposed would limit programs that presently offer support to medical schools on the basis of the number of students they enroll (i.e., capitation payments), or would require an American undergraduate degree as a prerequisite for physician licensure (Congressional Budget Office, 1977).

The major unresolved problem with limiting the future supply of physicians involves a trade-off between controlling health expenditures and correcting the existing geographic and specialty maldistribution of physicians (Congressional Budget Office, 1977). It is likely to be much easier to redistribute the country's physician resources by redirecting the flow of newly trained physicians than by rearranging the existing supply. For example, by linking institutional support to increased training opportunities in family practice or other primary-care specialties, it should be possible to increase the proportion of physicians in primary care. Similarly, the National Health Services Corps has been developed as a strategy for influencing the geographic distribution of physicians by offering scholarships with the obligation of a payback of service in underserved areas. Yet, unless a large percentage of these graduates do indeed select and stay in the geographical areas and types of practice where they are most needed, these redistributional objectives may not be achieved.

Incentive Reimbursement

Prospective institutional rate setting.—In contrast to traditional, retrospective methods of cost-based reimbursement, prospective rate setting establishes the level of third-party payment in advance and without regard to the costs actually incurred by the institution. The presumption is that hospitals are thereby forced to make more efficient use of the resources under their control. A variety of approaches (based on formulas, budget review, and budget negotiation, for example) have already been tried by different States (Dowling, 1974), and evaluations of several experiments in rate setting have been reported (Hellinger, 1978). A new round of federally sponsored evaluations of prospective reimbursement has also been initiated recently (Hellinger, 1978). Consequently, it seems best to record here only some tentative conclusions about the country's experience with rate setting to date.

Although some rate-setting commissions recently have claimed success in holding down hospital-cost inflation, scientific evaluation of these programs has just begun. However, none of the early rate-setting experiments appear to have had a demonstrably significant effect on hospital costs (Hellinger, 1978). Setting a prospective rate on the basis of the previous year's actual costs only tends to reinforce existing inflationary trends. A successful program would have to separate allowable rates from actual costs in order to encourage cost-saving innovations. Hospitals also have an incentive to spend as much as the budget allows for the year, since this would maintain the expenditure base upon which future rates would be calculated (Bauer, 1978; Worthington, 1976).

Perverse incentives have also been created by the unit of payment specified for reimbursement rates. By encouraging longer lengths of stay, the per diem rates employed in early rate-setting experiments reduced the average cost of a hospital day but led to greater total revenues for the hospital (Congressional Budget Office, 1977). Shifting the focus to the cost per case and total revenues would discourage such adjustments in utilization (Hellinger, 1978).

Some observers of the rate-setting process have criticized its emphasis on the determination of prices, rather than the development of new incentives to modify the decisionmaking and behavioral patterns within hospitals (Altman and Weiner, 1977). However, many of the essential features of rate-setting programs (e.g., the need for uniformity in hospital accounting and budget information, the submission of detailed cost and budget analyses, the fact of external review, the active participation of third-party payers and the planning agencies, and long-range capital planning) may serve to strengthen internal management and facilitate the setting of internal hospital priorities (Bauer, 1978).

Reimbursing physician services.—It is often argued that the prevailing, fee-for-service system of reimbursement has encouraged a lack of concern among physicians for the costliness and efficiency of the services they provide. One proposed solution is to confront physicians with a fee schedule that constitutes the maximum allowable charge to the patient and is subject to modification only on the basis of negotiation with third-party payers (Glaser, 1976; Somers, 1978). Presumably, these prices would be established at a level that was equitable, but would encourage efficiency.

There is a possibility, however, that some physicians may circumvent such controls and attempt to maintain rising incomes by billing separately for items that were previously included in other charges, or even perhaps by expanding the volume of services (Holahan and Scanlon, 1977). A more appropriate test of the effectiveness of controls on physician fees is, therefore, the effect on total physician earnings and not simply on prices.

The Economic Stabilization Program (ESP) of the early 1970's has provided researchers with an opportunity to study the effects of regulating physician fees. Although the mechanism for limiting fees was essentially voluntary, with consumers and third-party payers reporting violations, the rate of increase in fees was cut approximately in half during the time of the program. The ESP was initiated in August of 1971, a year in which the average net income of physicians increased 8.3 percent (American Medical Association, 1977). This rate was reduced by half in the following year, and was even lower in 1973. According to data from the National Center for Health Statistics, there was no apparent acceleration in the growth of aggregate utilization in compensation for the price controls; the number of physician visits per person jumped 6.5 percent in 1971, but rose by less than 1 percent annually in subsequent ESP years. However, despite such evidence that physicians responded to the ESP with economic restraint, the growth of personal expenditures for physician services actually accelerated from 1972 to 1973 when measured in real terms (Part B, table 148). The reasons why aggregate expenditures on physician services were accelerating under these circumstances have not been clearly delineated.

More detailed analyses of the effect of the ESP on physician reimbursement patterns have been conducted using California Medicare data (Holahan et al., 1978; Hadley and Lee, 1978). During the first and second years of the ESP, when physician fees grew at half their earlier rate, the volume of physician services provided to the elderly in California rose about 4 times faster than the rate of Medicare enrollment increases. After controls were removed and inflation of fees resumed, the rate of increase in services was even less than the expansion of Medicare enrollments. This again raises the question of whether physicians maintain increases in their level of earnings, despite fixed fees, by expanding the volume of services.

The California study was hampered, however, by the lack of data on physician services that were privately reimbursed. There was some tentative evidence to suggest that the increase in services to the elderly represented a substitution of Medicare for private patients because of a narrowing of the differential between Medicare rates and private charges. Therefore, the increased volume of Medicare services under the ESP may not have been representative of an overall trend in physician utilization.

Canada's experience with uniform, fixed fees for physician services under national health insurance seems to demonstrate that limits on physician fees do tend to slow the growth of physicians' net earnings (Hadley, 1977). There may even be some reason for optimism with regard to the wider effects on total health expenditures. The notable increase in health care expenditures that was experienced in Canada after the introduction of national health insurance is not so alarming if the one-time improvement in coverage is isolated from the long-run impact of the program. In fact, when expenditures prior to national health insurance, during the transition to the program, and 1 year after its introduction are examined separately, the later period exhibits an even slower increase in real health care expenditures than occurred before universal coverage (Hadley, 1977).

In the past, public regulation of physician reimbursement in the United States has usually been restricted to public programs, in contrast to more universal controls. One of the dangers of an outright restriction on physician reimbursement levels that applies to public medical care programs while leaving private charges unregulated is that doctors will refuse to accept such program payments as full reimbursement for their services or even to participate in service-benefit programs. When an attempt was made to reduce Medicare reimbursements, patients either paid additional charges out-of-pocket or were denied service (Gornick, 1976). Generally, the extent of physician participation in programs such as Medicare and Medicaid increases as the fee schedule does (Sloan and Steinwald, 1978). Therefore, policies to limit Medicare or Medicaid reimbursements may have an adverse effect on the accessibility of medical services to the low income population. However, willingness to participate in Medicaid is also related to the amount of "red tape" that physicians are required to handle (Cromwell, Mitchell, and Sloan, 1978). This suggests that as another way of securing greater physician participation, the government and other third-party payers might reduce the complexity and time costs of reimbursement procedures.

Other innovations in physician reimbursement have been proposed, in addition to setting maximum allowable fees. To reduce the financial incentives which presently reward the physician who selects more expensive treatment methods, the suggestion has been made to reimburse physicians for time they spend with patients at a higher rate than that allowed for lab tests and medical procedures. To pay physicians a salary is another alternative that would tend to eliminate the undesirable financial incentives influencing physicians and to restrict their autonomous control over expenditures (Redisch, 1978). However, there is evidence to suggest that physicians work fewer hours when they are paid on a salaried basis than when self-employed (Sloan, 1975; Schweitzer, 1978). The Europeans have enjoyed relative success with a system which employs a blend of capitation and fee-for-service reimbursement (Schweitzer, 1978; Redisch, 1978). Specialists generally work as the salaried employees of hospitals, and primary-care practitioners operate in office settings under a combination of capitation and fees for selected services. As discussed later in the chapter, the Health Maintenance Organization is another arrangement that seems to restructure the economic incentives of physicians in ways that encourage a greater degree of cost consciousness on their part.

Market Reform

Consumer cost sharing.—One of the strategies for instilling a greater level of cost consciousness in the health care marketplace is to introduce more deductibles, coinsurance, and copayments into the health insurance system. Research has shown that when consumers are immediately at risk for part of the cost of additional services, they choose to utilize fewer services than when fully insured (Newhouse and Phelps, 1976; Ginsburg and Manheim, 1973; Beck, 1974; Scitovsky and McCall, 1972).

The political feasibility of instituting a system of extensive cost sharing has been questioned, however, as a policy that is in direct contrast to the present trend towards universal first-dollar coverage. This problem was in evidence in the recent bargaining over the United Mine Workers' contract, when a proposal to replace the traditional system of complete health care coverage with a system that insured only expenses in excess of an annual family deductible caused a serious impasse in the negotiations. Cost sharing has not been used extensively in other countries either, where the trend toward first-dollar coverage has also been powerful (Blanpain et al., 1976; Altman and Weiner, 1977).

The political argument against cost sharing is based on a conviction that the level of out-of-pocket expenditure required to instill an effective level of cost consciousness in patients and providers would discourage lower income individuals from making appropriate use of needed services (Altman and Weiner, 1977; Marmor, 1977). Such problems could perhaps be avoided, however, in an income-related, cost-sharing arrangement or in a system that was directed at only "nonessential" services (Schweitzer, 1978; Stevens, 1976).

Experience with the 20–percent coinsurance provisions of Medicare, Part B, also suggests that consumers are likely to subvert a cost-sharing system by purchasing additional, "front-end" insurance to cover these out-of-pocket costs (Stevens, 1976; Keeler, Morrow, and Newhouse, 1977). Therefore, it has been suggested that any national health insurance plan that includes cost sharing would have to reimburse medical care expenditures only after private insurance reimbursement was taken into account and cost-sharing provisions of national health insurance were satisfied (Keeler et al., 1977). The present tax laws, in fact, subsidize purchases of "front-end" health insurance, as they do all other types of health insurance. To make cost sharing an effective cost-containment strategy would require a change in policy that would put a stop to subsidizing all health insurance purchases, or perhaps even ban purchases of supplementary, "front-end" health insurance.[1]

Utilization review and PSRO.—Utilization review and the Professional Standards Review Organizations (PSRO's) represent an attempt on the part of the Federal government and other third-party payers to oversee more closely the quality and cost effectiveness of the services they pay for. Such programs are, in this sense, designed to provide more decisionmaking control for the parties that bear the financial responsibility for health care utilization.

The PSRO program, one form of utilization review, was mandated by the Social Security Act Amendments of 1972, and calls for groups of community physicians to review the medical services provided under Medicare, Medicaid, and the Maternal and Child Health programs. These services are to be reviewed for their compliance with professionally recognized standards of quality, and to assure that they are medically necessary and are provided in an economical fashion. Although it is too soon to draw any firm conclusions (Institute of Medicine, 1976a), the tentative evidence does not provide a very optimistic picture of the potential contribution of PSRO's to cost containment.

An evaluation of the performance of 18 out of 172 PSRO's from 1974 to 1976 suggests that the PSRO program compared with other utilization review systems did not produce any significant effect on overall hospital utilization or admission rates (Health Services Administration, 1977). The findings indicate that the program did not reduce utilization rates by the 1.6 to 2.1 percent required to recover even its administrative costs. This study was conducted at the beginning of the PSRO program and does not necessarily reflect the experience of well-established programs. Although other studies have sometimes shown that cost savings were associated with preadmission review programs in operation prior to the 1972 Social Security Amendments (Congressional Budget Office, 1977), the more recent programs, which have yet to be deemed cost effective, typically rely upon concurrent review, or review just after admission.

There are a number of features of PSRO programs which may lead to an overly conservative, rather than a cost-conscious definition of acceptable patterns of care. Rather than falsely accuse physicians of poor or inefficient practices, particularly in light of the difficulty of developing objective criteria that take into account the many variables that impinge upon utilization decisions, PSRO's are likely to identify only the most obvious errors in judgement (Schweitzer, 1978). The self-interest of providers who practice on a fee-for-service basis and participate in PSRO review also argues against the establishment of cost-oriented norms which might reduce Medicare and Medicaid reimbursements (Gosfield, 1975). Furthermore, patients are also likely to be upset by medical bills for which they are refused coverage (Blumstein, 1978). Despite this, there are no provisions in the PSRO program to compensate for these perverse financial incentives. Department of Health, Education, and Welfare funding is independent of review performance, and the savings generated by more cost-effective standards of care do not necessarily accrue to the community responsible for curtailing utilization (Blumstein, 1978).

Promoting alternative modes of care.—One of the most potentially significant strategies for modifying the present structure of the health care marketplace is encouragement of the prepaid group practice mode of delivery, the Health Maintenance Organization (HMO). A number of national health insurance plans include incentives for HMO development (Davis, 1975; Roy, in press). In contrast to the fee-for-service system, HMO's provide a comprehensive set of health care services in return for a predetermined, prepaid charge for each person enrolled in the group. They consequently operate under strong financial

---

[1] A more extensive discussion of the issues involved in cost sharing is to be found in the previous edition of this volume (NCHS and NCHSR, 1977).

incentives to economize on the use of the limited financial resources at their disposal. In addition to removing the expenditure-increasing financial incentives inherent in fee-for-service arrangements, the HMO approach also tends to reduce physician autonomy in controlling the utilization of the delivery system (Gaus, Cooper, and Hirschman, 1976; Redisch, 1978).

There is extensive empirical evidence to demonstrate that HMO's tend to experience lower hospital costs, but these favorable findings are not open to simple interpretation. Since they may reflect a bias in the types of patients who choose to enroll in HMO's, it is possible that the cost differentials estimated by various research studies would not apply to a system which covered the entire population (Mechanic, 1976; Riedel et al., 1975; Havighurst, 1975; Gaus, Cooper, and Hirschman, 1976; Schlenker and Ellwood, 1973). Other major questions have yet to be answered with regard to differences between fee-for-service and prepaid arrangements in the quality of care provided and with regard to the economic viability and consumer acceptance of the HMO concept.

Under more conventional financing arrangements, broader coverage of outpatient services would perhaps encourage their substitution for more expensive inpatient care. Yet, the evidence to suggest that such a substitution would in fact take place is sketchy. Despite some positive indications from analyses of the Medicare program and other U.S. data (Russell, 1973; Davis and Russell, 1972; Huang, 1975), the Canadian experience does not provide much support for this strategy. The substitution of extended care for hospital utilization in Canada did not save money; the savings from reductions in acute care per illness episode were lost to longer stays in extended care facilities (Evans, 1976). Evidence from Canada also supports the paradoxical conclusion that extended insurance coverage of ambulatory medical care may increase hospital utilization by promoting greater detection of medical problems. This may or may not represent a cost-effective improvement in the efficacy of treatment or in health outcomes (Lewis and Keairnes, 1970; Newhouse and Phelps, 1976; Freiburg and Scutchfield, 1976).

Other proposals.—A variety of other structural reforms have been proposed for which there is even less empirical information to report. One idea that has aroused substantial interest is to provide coverage under reimbursement programs for the cost of consulting a second specialist on the need for elective surgical procedures. Experimentation with one such voluntary "second opinion" program in New York City demonstrated that the initial recommendation for surgery was not confirmed by the second specialist approximately 30 percent of the time (McCarthy and Widmer, 1974). Although such statistics indicate a substantial level of disagreement among surgical providers, there is unfortunately no way to know whether the second opinion in such cases was any more valid than the first. Nor should contradictory second opinions necessarily be viewed as evidence that the subsequent costs of treating these patients were reduced. A followup to the New York study showed that 12 percent of the patients for whom surgery was not recommended by the second specialist had to have the operation at a later date; 5 percent had the surgery anyway; and 31 percent received some kind of medical treatment for their condition (McCarthy, Finkel, and Kamons, 1977).

Another problem that has created a great deal of discussion is the need for patients to be more actively involved in making utilization decisions and to have easier access to information about the costs and quality of the services they receive (Ingbar, 1978; National Commission on the Cost of Medical Care, 1978). Possible corrective strategies range from the development of consumer education programs to such initiatives as those recently undertaken by the Federal Trade Commission to remove the professional ban on advertising of physician and optometric services.

Other reform proposals are directed at the physician's awareness and understanding of health care costs. For example, the National Commission on the Cost of Medical Care has urged that professional training include coursework in the economics of health care and that hospitals provide physicians with a list of prices for the inpatient services that they order on behalf of their patients (National Commission on the Cost of Medical Care, 1978).

In addition, the development of systematic technology assessment to address the effects of medical technologies on the cost and efficacy of care should be considered. It may be a means of providing information for objective decisionmaking on the benefits and costs of new and existing technologies.

BIBLIOGRAPHY

Altman, S., and Weiner, S.: Constraining the Medical Care System, Regulation as a Second Best Strategy. Paper presented at the Federal Trade Commission Conference on Competition in the Health Care Sector. Washington, D.C., June 1977.

American Medical Association: *Profile of Medical Practice 1977.* Chicago. American Medical Association, 1977. p. 184.

Armstrong, R.: Canadian lessons about health-care costs. *Bulletin of the New York Academy of Medicine* 54(1): 84–101, Jan. 1978.

Bauer, K.: Hospital Rate Setting—This Way to Salvation?, in M. Zubkoff, I. Raskin, and R. Hanft, eds., *Hospital Cost Containment, Selected Notes for Future Policy.* New York. Prodist, 1978. pp. 324–369.

Beck, R.: The effects of co-payment on the poor. *Journal of Human Resources* 9(1): 129–142, Winter 1974.

Bicknell, W., and Walsh, D.: Certificate of need, the Massachusetts experience. *New England Journal of Medicine* 292(20): 1054–1061, May 15, 1975.

Blanpain, J., Delesie, L., Nys, H., Debie, J., and Lievens, J.: *International Approaches to Health Resources Development for National Health Programs.* Executive Summary, Contract No. HRA–230–75–0108, National Center for Health Services Research, Public Health Service. Hyattsville, Md., Sept. 1976.

Blumberg, M.: Rational Provider Prices, An Incentive for Improved Health Delivery, in G. Chacko, ed., *Health Handbook, 1978.* Amsterdam. North Holland Publishing Company. To be published.

Blumstein, J.: The Role of PSROs in Hospital Cost Containment, in M. Zubkoff, I. Raskin, and R. Hanft, eds., *Hospital Cost Containment, Selected Notes for Future Policy.* New York. Prodist, 1978. pp. 461–485.

Burney, I., and Gabel, J.: Reimbursement Patterns under Medicare and Medicaid. Prepared for the Conference on Research Results from Physician Reimbursement Studies, sponsored by the Office of Policy, Planning, and Research, Health Care Financing Administration. Washington, D.C., Feb. 1978.

Congressional Budget Office: *Expenditures for Health Care, Federal Programs and Their Effects.* Congress of the United States. Washington. U.S. Government Printing Office, Aug. 1977.

Cromwell, J., Mitchell, J., and Sloan, F.: A Study of Administrative Costs in Physicians' Offices and Medicaid Participation. Prepared for the Conference on Research Results from Physician Reimbursement Studies, sponsored by the Office of Policy, Planning, and Research, Health Care Financing Administration. Washington, D.C., Feb. 1978.

Davis, K.: *National Health Insurance—Benefits, Costs, and Consequences.* Washington. The Brookings Institution, 1975.

Davis, K., and Russell, L.: *The substitution of hospital outpatient care for inpatient care. Review of Economics and Statistics* 54(2): 109–120, May 1972.

Dowling, W.: Prospective reimbursement of hospitals. *Inquiry* 11(3): 163–180, Sept. 1974.

Dunn, W., and Lefkowitz, B.: The Hospital Cost Containment Act of 1977, An Analysis of the Administration's Proposal, in M. Zubkoff, I. Raskin, and R. Hanft, eds., *Hospital Cost Containment, Selected Notes for Future Policy.* New York. Prodist, 1978. pp. 166–214.

Evans, R.: Beyond the Medical Market Place, Expenditure, Utilization, and Pricing of Insured Health Care in Canada, in R. Rosett, ed., *The Role of Health Insurance in the Health Services Sector.* New York. National Bureau of Economic Research, 1976. pp. 437–492.

Feldstein, M., and Taylor, A.: *The Rapid Rise of Hospital Costs.* Staff Report for the Council on Wage and Price Stability. Executive Office of the President. Washington, D.C., Jan. 1977.

Freiburg, L., Jr., and Scutchfield, F.: Insurance and the demand for hospital care, an examination of the moral hazard. *Inquiry* 13(1): 54–60, Mar. 1976.

Gaus, C., Cooper, B., and Hirschman, C.: Contrasts in HMO and fee-for-service performance. *Social Security Bulletin* 39(5): 3–14, May 1976.

Ginsburg, P.: Impact of the Economic Stabilization Program on Hospitals, An Analysis with Aggregate Data, in M. Zubkoff, I. Raskin, and R. Hanft, eds., *Hospital Cost Containment, Selected Notes for Future Policy.* New York. Prodist, 1978. pp. 293–323.

Ginsburg, P., and Manheim, L.: Insurance, copayment, and health services utilization, a critical review. *Journal of Economics and Business* 25(2): 142–153, Spring-Summer 1973.

Glaser, W.: Controlling Costs Through Methods of Paying Doctors, Experiences from Abroad. Paper presented at the Fogarty International Center Conference on Policies for the Containment of Health Care Costs and Expenditures. Bethesda, Md., June 1976.

Gornick, M.: Ten years of Medicare, impact on the covered population. *Social Security Bulletin* 39(7): 3–21, July 1976.

Gosfield, A.: *PSROs: The Law and the Health Consumer.* Cambridge. Ballinger, 1975.

Hadley, J.: National Health Insurance and the Health Labor Force, Physicians. Working Paper 5057–5, The Urban Institute. Washington, D.C., Aug. 1977.

Hadley, J., and Lee, R.: Toward a Physician Reimbursement Policy, Evidence from the Economic Stabilization Period. Working Paper, The Urban Institute. Washington, D.C., July 1978.

Hanft, R., Raskin, I., and Zubkoff, M.: Introduction, in M. Zubkoff, I. Raskin, and R. Hanft, eds., *Hospital Cost Containment, Selected Notes for Future Policy.* New York. Prodist, 1978. pp. 1–30.

Havighurst, C.: Federal regulation of the health care delivery system, a foreword in the nature of a "package insert." *University of Toledo Law Review* 6(3): 577–590, Spring 1975.

Havighurst, C.: Health care cost-containment regulation, prospects and an alternative. *American Journal of Law and Medicine* 3(3): 309–322, 1977.

Havighurst, C., and Blumstein, J.: Coping with quality/cost trade-offs in medical care, the role of PSROs. *Northwestern Law Review* 70(1): 6–68, Mar.-Apr. 1975.

Health Services Administration: *PSRO, An Evaluation of the Professional Standards Review Organization, Volume 1, Executive Summary.* Report No. OPEL 77–12. Office of Planning, Evaluation, and Legislation. Rockville, Md., Oct. 1977.

Hellinger, F.: The effect of certificate-of-need legislation on hospital investment. *Inquiry* 13(2): 187–193, June 1976.

Hellinger, F.: An Empirical Analysis of Several Prospective Reimbursement Systems, in M. Zubkoff, I. Raskin, and R. Hanft, eds., *Hospital Cost Containment, Selected Notes for Future Policy*. New York. Prodist, 1978. pp. 370–400.

Holahan, J., and Scanlon, W.: Price Controls, Physicians' Fees, and Physicians' Incomes. Working Paper 998–05, The Urban Institute. Washington, D.C., Nov. 1977.

Holahan, J., Scanlon, W., Hadley J., and Lee, R.: The Effect of Medicare/Medicaid Reimbursement on Physician Behavior, A Summary of Findings. Presented at the Conference on Research Results from Physician Reimbursement Studies, sponsored by the Office of Policy, Planning, and Research, Health Care Financing Administration. Washington, D.C., Feb. 1978.

Howell, J.: *Controlling Hospital Investment in Massachusetts*. Dissertation Research Proposal No. 1R03 HS 02862–01. National Center for Health Services Research. Hyattsville, Md., Aug. 1977.

Huang, L.: *An Analysis of the Effects of Demand and Supply Factors on the Utilization of Health Services in Short-Stay General Hospitals*. Final Report, Contract No. HRA 106–74–190. National Center for Health Services Research. Hyattsville, Md., Sept. 1975.

Ingbar, M.: The Consumer's Perspective, in M. Zubkoff, I. Raskin, and R. Hanft, eds. *Hospital Cost Containment, Selected Notes for Future Policy*. New York. Prodist, 1978. pp. 103–165.

Institute of Medicine: *Assessing Quality in Health Care, An Evaluation*. National Academy of Sciences. Washington, D.C., Nov. 1976a.

Institute of Medicine: *Controlling the Supply of Hospital Beds*. National Academy of Sciences. Washington, D.C., Oct., 1976b.

Keeler, E., Morrow, D., and Newhouse, J.: The demand for supplementary health insurance, or do deductibles matter? *Journal of Political Economy* 85(4): 789–801, Aug. 1977.

Klarman, H.: Health planning—progress, prospects, and issues. *Milbank Memorial Fund Quarterly* 56(1): 78–112, Winter 1978.

Lave, J., and Lave, L.: Hospital Cost Function Analysis, Implications for Cost Controls, in M. Zubkoff, I. Raskin, and R. Hanft, eds., *Hospital Cost Containment, Selected Notes for Future Policy*. New York. Prodist, 1978. pp. 538–571.

Leveson, I.: Policy Coordination and the Choice of Policy Mix, in M. Zubkoff, I. Raskin, and R. Hanft, eds., *Hospital Cost Containment, Selected Notes for Future Policy*. New York. Prodist, 1978. pp. 609–635.

Lewis, C., and Keairnes, H.: Controlling costs of medical care by expanding insurance coverage, study of a paradox. *New England Journal of Medicine* 282(25): 1405–1412, June 18, 1970.

Lipscomb, J., Raskin, I., and Eichenholz, J.: The Use of Marginal Cost Estimates in Hospital Cost-Containment Policy, in M. Zubkoff, I. Raskin, and R. Hanft, eds., *Hospital Cost Containment, Selected Notes for Future Policy*. New York. Prodist, 1978. pp. 514–537.

Lyle, C., Citron, D., Sugg, W., and Williams, O.: Cost of medical care in a practice of internal medicine, a study in a group of seven internists. *Annals of Internal Medicine* 81(1): 1–6, July 1974.

Marmor, T.: The politics of national health insurance, analysis and prescription. *Policy Analysis* 3(1): 25–48, Winter 1977.

May, J.: Utilization of Health Services and Availability of Resources, in R. Anderson, J. Kravits, and O.W. Anderson, eds., *Equity in Health Services*. Cambridge. Ballinger, 1975.

McCarthy, E., and Widmer, G.: Effects of screening by consultants on recommended surgical procedures. *New England Journal of Medicine* 291(25): 1331–1335, Dec. 19, 1974.

McCarthy, E., Finkel, M., and Kamons, A.: Second Opinion Surgical Program, A Vehicle for Cost Containment? Presentation to the AMA's National Commission on the Cost of Medical Care, Chicago, Mar. 1977.

McClure, W.: *Reducing Excess Hospital Capacity*. Pub. No. HRP–0015199, National Technical Information Service. Springfield, Va., Oct. 1976.

McNeer, J., Wagner, G., Ginsburg, P., Wallace, A., McCants, C., Conley, M., and Rosati, R.: Hospital discharge one week after acute myocardial infarction. *New England Journal of Medicine* 298(5):229–232, Feb. 2, 1978.

Mechanic, D.: *The Growth of Bureaucratic Medicine, An Inquiry into the Dynamics of Patient Behavior and the Organization of Medical Care*. New York. John Wiley & Sons, 1976.

Mitchell, B., and Phelps, C.: National health insurance, some costs and effects of mandated employee coverage. *Journal of Political Economy* 84(3): 553–571, June 1976.

Morrow, J., and Edwards, A.: U.S. health manpower policy, will the benefits justify the costs? *Journal of Medical Education* 51(10): 791–805, Oct. 1976.

National Center for Health Statistics: Volume of physician visits, United States, July 1966–June 1967, by C.S. Wilder. *Vital and Health Statistics*. Series 10—No. 49. DHEW Pub. No. (HRA) 76–1299. Health Resources Administration. Washington. U.S. Government Printing Office, Nov. 1968.

National Center for Health Statistics: Utilization of short-stay hospitals, annual summary for the United States, 1975, by L. Glickman. *Vital and Health Statistics*. Series 13—No. 31. DHEW Pub. No. (HRA) 77–1782. Health Resources Administration. Washington. U.S. Government Printing Office, Apr. 1977a.

National Center for Health Statistics: Current estimates from the Health Interview Survey, United States, 1976, by E.R. Black. *Vital and Health Statistics*. Series 10—No. 119. DHEW Pub. No. (PHS) 78–1547. Public Health Service. Washington. U.S. Government Printing Office, Nov. 1977b.

National Center for Health Statistics and National Center for Health Services Research: *Health, United States, 1976–1977*. DHEW Pub. No. (HRA) 77–1232. Health Resources Administration. Washington. U.S. Government Printing Office, 1977.

National Commission on the Cost of Medical Care: *The National Commission on the Cost of Medical Care, 1976–1977*. Chicago. American Medical Association, 1978.

Newhouse, J., and Phelps, C.: New Estimates of Price and Income Elasticities of Medical Care Services, in R. Rosett, ed., *The Role of Health Insurance in the Health Services Sector*. New York. National Bureau of Economic Research, 1976. pp. 261–313.

Noll, R.: The consequences of public utility regulation of hospitals. *Controls on Health Care*. National Academy of Sciences. Washington, D.C., 1975.

Office of Management and Budget: *Special Analyses, The Budget of the United States Government, 1979.* Executive Office of the President. Washington. U.S. Government Printing Office, 1978.

Office of Research and Statistics: National health expenditures, calendar year 1974. *Research and Statistics Note.* Note No. 5. HEW Pub. No. (SSA) 76–11701. Social Security Administration. Washington, D.C., April 14, 1976.

Public Health Service: National Guidelines for Health Planning. *Federal Register.* Vol. 43—No. 60, Part IV. DHEW. Washington, D.C., Mar. 28, 1978.

Redisch, M.: Physician Involvement in Hospital Decision Making, in M. Zubkoff, I. Raskin, and R. Hanft, eds., *Hospital Cost Containment, Selected Notes for Future Policy.* New York. Prodist, 1978. pp. 217–243.

Rice, D., and Wilson, D.: The American Medical Economy—Problems and Perspectives, in T. Hu, ed., *International Health Costs and Expenditures.* DHEW Pub. No. (NIH) 76–1067. National Institutes of Health. Washington. U.S. Government Printing Office, 1976.

Riedel, D., Walden, D., Singsen, A., Meyers, S., Krantz, G., and Henderson, M.: *Federal Employees Health Benefits Program, Utilization Study.* National Center for Health Services Research. DHEW Pub. No. (HRA) 75–3125. Health Resources Administration. Rockville, Md., 1975.

Roemer, M., and Shain, M.: *Hospital Utilization Under Insurance.* Chicago. American Hospital Association, 1959.

Rosenthal, G.: Controlling the Cost of Health Care, in M. Zubkoff, I. Raskin, and R. Hanft, eds., *Hospital Cost Containment, Selected Notes for Future Policy.* New York. Prodist, 1978. pp. 33–56.

Rothenberg, E.: *Regulation and Expansion of Health Facilities, The Certificate of Need Experience in New York State.* New York. Praeger, 1976.

Roy, W.R., editor: *Proceedings of the Conference on Effects of the Payment Mechanism on the Health Care Delivery System.* DHEW Pub. No. (PHS) 78–3227. National Center for Health Services Research. Hyattsville, Md. In press.

Russell, L.: The impact of the extended-care facility benefit on hospital use and reimbursement under Medicare. *Journal of Human Resources* 8(1): 57–72, Winter 1973.

Salkever, D., and Bice, T.: Certificate-of-Need Legislation and Hospital Costs, in M. Zubkoff, I. Raskin, and R. Hanft, eds., *Hospital Cost Containment, Selected Notes for Future Policy.* New York. Prodist, 1978, pp. 429–460.

Salkever, D., and Bice, T.: *Hospital Certificate-of-Need Controls.* Washington, D.C. American Enterprise Institute. In press.

Schlenker, R., and Ellwood, P., Jr.: Medical Inflation, Causes and Policy Options for Control. InterStudy Working Paper, Minneapolis, Minn., Mar. 1973.

Schroeder, S., Kenders, K., Cooper, J., and Piemme, T.: Use of laboratory tests and pharmaceuticals, variations among physicians and effect of cost audit on subsequent use. *Journal of the American Medical Association* 225(8): 969–73, Aug. 1973.

Schweitzer, S.: Health Care Cost-Containment Programs, An International Perspective, in M. Zubkoff, I. Raskin, and R. Hanft, eds., *Hospital Cost Containment, Selected Notes for Future Policy.* New York. Prodist, 1978. pp. 57–75.

Scitovsky, A., and McCall, N.: Changes in the costs of treatment of selected illness, 1951–1964–1971. *Research Digest Series.* National Center for Health Services Research. DHEW Pub. No. (HRA) 77–3161. Health Resources Administration. Rockville, Md., July 1976.

Scitovsky, A., and McCall, N.: Effects of coinsurance on physician services. *Social Security Bulletin* 35: 3–19, June 1972.

Sloan, F.: Physician supply behavior in the short run. *Industrial and Labor Relations Review* 28(4): 549–569, July 1975.

Sloan, F., and Steinwald, B.: Physician participation in health insurance plans, evidence on Blue Shield. *Journal of Human Resources* 13(2): 237–263, Spring 1978.

Somers, A.: Health care financing, the case for negotiated rates. *Hospitals* 52(3): 49–52, Feb. 1, 1978.

Stevens, C.: Planning and regulation, research focus. *The Program in Health Services Research.* DHEW Pub. No. (HRA) 78–3136. Health Resources Administration. Rockville, Md., Oct. 1976. pp. 22–24.

U.S. Council on Wage and Price Stability: *The Complex Puzzle of Rising Health Care Costs, Can the Private Sector Fit it Together?* Executive Office of the President. Washington. U.S. Government Printing Office, 1976.

Wagner, J., and Zubkoff, M.: Medical Technology and Hospital Costs, in M. Zubkoff, I. Raskin, and R. Hanft. eds., *Hospital Cost Containment, Selected Notes for Future Policy.* New York. Prodist, 1978. pp. 263–289.

Worthington, P.: Prospective reimbursement of hospitals to promote efficiency, New Jersey. *Inquiry* 13(3): 302–308, Sept. 1976.

27. Certificate-of-Need Legislation and Hospital Costs

DAVID S. SALKEVER and THOMAS W. BICE

Reprinted with permission from *Hospital Cost Containment: Selected Notes for Future Policy* edited by M. J. Zubkoff, I. E. Raskin, and R. S. Hanft. Published for the Milbank Memorial Fund by PRODIST, New York. © Milbank Memorial Fund 1978.

Introduction

Controls on capital investment and services are presently the cornerstone of state and federal policies for containing costs of health care. The principal rationale for these controls is that the availability of facilities and services affects utilization and costs of health care. Accordingly, limiting the availability of inpatient beds and specialized equipment and services is expected to constrain the volume of inpatient admissions and days and the use of specialized diagnostic procedures, resulting in savings in both capital and operating costs.[1] Also, it is frequently argued that uncontrolled capital and service expansion leads to duplication of facilities and services and to underutilization of capacity, which, in turn, result in higher unit costs and low quality of care. Controls on investment and services that prevent duplication are therefore deemed desirable whether or not they reduce the overall volume of services used.

Beginning in the mid-1960s, states and the federal government have adopted various forms of investment and services regulation. The general approach taken is modeled after restrictions imposed on regulated public utilities and common carriers that require firms to secure certificates of convenience and public necessity before altering their service capacities. In the health sector two main types of control are exercised—direct and indirect—each of which requires health care institutions to obtain prior approval from designated agencies of their plans for capital expenditures and/or

---

[1] Note that this conclusion is tenable even if one rejects "Roemer's Law" and accepts the argument that additional beds and equipment do not directly stimulate additional demand (Newhouse, 1974:n. 2). Although controls may not reduce demand growth, they may necessitate rationing as demand expands while capacity is limited and thereby may reduce the total volume and costs of services.

changes in service capacities. The approaches differ primarily with respect to the types of sanctions incurred by institutions that implement unapproved or disapproved capital expenditure projects. Direct controls through state certificate-of-need (CON) laws usually specify legal means to prohibit institutions from carrying out disapproved projects (for example, denial or suspension of operating licenses). Indirect controls levy only economic sanctions whereby third-party payers may refuse to reimburse institutions for costs associated with investment projects and/or service changes that fail to receive prior approval from designated agencies (Lewin and Associates, Inc., 1974).

At present, both forms of control are widespread in the United States. As of 1974, either or both direct and indirect controls were in effect in all states except Texas, Vermont, and West Virginia.[2] The first CON law was adopted in 1964 by the state of New York; by 1974, some version of CON was in force in twenty-four states, and proposals were under legislative consideration in seven others. Indirect controls are applied in thirty-seven states that participate with DHEW in so-called Section 1122 review programs. Under Section 1122 of the 1972 Amendments to the Social Security Act, reimbursements authorized by Titles V, XVIII, and XIX for depreciation, interest, and other costs associated with investments of at least $100,000 may be withheld if approval is not obtained. Similar provisions known as "conformance clauses" link Blue Cross reimbursements for capital costs to project review and approval by designated agencies in areas within nineteen states.[3]

Although direct and indirect controls are directed to the same ends and pose similar theoretical and policy issues, the present study focuses primarily on CON. Two considerations warrant this emphasis. First, it is likely that CON controls will supplant other types of investment and services regulation as the National Health Planning and Resources Development Act of 1974 (P.L. 93-641) is implemented. Section 1523 of this law requires states to enact CON statutes to be eligible for federal subsidies to support statewide and regional health planning. With this strong incentive for universal adoption of CON, it is reasonable to expect that indirect control programs will become redundant and either fall into desuetude or be merged with CON programs. Second, since CON has been in

[2] Data in this section are from a study by Lewin and Associates, Inc. (1974), which is current as of April 1974.

[3] It should also be noted that investment subsidy programs frequently require project review and approval, although sanctions are not levied on unapproved projects. All states tie eligibility for capital investment subsidies from the Hill-Burton program to prior approval from designated agencies, and forty-two states require such endorsements for assistance from their construction finance programs.

effect in sixteen states since at least 1971, we have more experience with CON than with the various forms of indirect controls. Although there is a paucity of evidence as to the functioning and efficacy of any form of investment and services regulation, the shortage is most severe with respect to the more recently appearing indirect controls.

Content of Certificate-of-Need Controls

Although CON laws are generally similar in intent, their content varies widely among states. Variations are found in (1) types of facilities covered, (2) types of changes requiring certification, (3) thresholds for review, (4) standards for review, (5) sanctions, and (6) the nature of the review process.[4]

Facilities Covered

Most CON laws cover hospitals, nursing homes, and other facilities such as outpatient clinics and laboratories. Over time, amendments to CON statutes and more recently enacted laws favor broader coverage. Only one state (Michigan) regulates only hospitals, and only one (Oklahoma) confines CON to nursing homes. In addition to Michigan and Oklahoma, two states (Colorado and Washington) and the District of Columbia exempt other facilities; according to the review by Lewin and Associates, Inc. (1974), of CON laws, Georgia's and Wisconsin's statutes are "unclear" regarding coverage of other facilities.

Changes Requiring Certification

Three broad types of changes are subject to review: changes in physical plant (facilities), equipment, or services. As with the types of facilities covered, the trend in CON statutes has been toward broader inclusion of types of changes requiring certification. Among the twenty-three states with CON in 1974 that covered hospitals (that is, excluding Oklahoma), fifteen imposed review on facilities, equipment, and services; six others attended to facilities and services. Six of the states considering CON laws in 1974 proposed to review all three types of changes, and the other intended to cover facilities and services.

All states require certification for new construction in covered facilities, although many exempt projects below a specified minimum. The clear intent of CON is thus to prevent overinvestment in new facilities, equipment, and services. However, three CON

---

[4]Information in this section is from Lewin and Associates, Inc. (1974). Other summaries are in Curran (1974) and Havighurst (1973).

programs currently in force and five of the seven proposed bills also mandate that proposed discontinuances of services be reviewed.

Thresholds

CON laws differ significantly with respect to magnitudes of changes requiring certification. For hospital facilities and equipment changes, these so-called thresholds are typically expressed in dollar amounts or as percentages of operating costs or assets. Dollar thresholds for changes in facilities range from $15,000 in Arizona to $350,000 in Kansas; thresholds for equipment changes range from $10,000 in Colorado to $100,000 in seven states. The modal threshold for facilities and equipment changes is $100,000.

Thresholds for review of bed capacity are typically more restrictive than for other types of changes. Twelve states presently require and three more propose certification for either any increase in or change of bed stock, and five others specify maximum changes allowable without certification. Changes and expansions of scope of services requiring certification are specified, albeit often vaguely, in ten CON laws.

Standards of Review

The language of CON laws as to standards is highly varied. Several statutes are silent on this point, but most mention that decisions must be derived in some manner from state or areawide health plans. As Curran (1974) notes, however, few laws are specific as to what a plan should include. Oregon's statute is uniquely detailed in this regard, listing various types of evidence that must be considered in CON reviews.

Sanctions

In all but two states, agencies' refusal to award certificates results in states' denying applicant institutions licenses to operate the proposed facilities. California prohibits implementation of the plan for one year; thereafter, institutions that implement disapproved projects are ineligible for reimbursement for associated capital costs under MediCal. Florida's law specifies no sanctions. However, as its CON provisions are virtually identical to those employed in Section 1122 review (in which Florida participates), denial of a certificate of need results in levying Section 1122 sanctions (the withholding of capital costs for Medicare, Medicaid, and Maternal and Child Health services).

Nature of the Review Process

CON involves various types of agencies in the review process. In most states, it includes the agencies that ultimately grant certificates. States differ, however, in the number of formal review steps that precede a final decision. Most employ either a two- or three-step process, beginning with an initial review by areawide Comprehensive Health Program (CHP[b]) agencies leading to final reviews and decisions by state departments of health or human services, state health commissions, or statewide CHP(a) agencies. Among the twenty-one CON states with CHP(b) agencies, seventeen vested in them responsibilities for initial reviews of applications. Four states employ no local agencies in the review, while two others allow local agencies to make final decisions.

The Political Economy of CON Regulation

As with other forms of economic regulation, the rationale for CON controls rests on assumptions about behaviors of regulatory agencies and of regulated firms. What Noll (1975) terms the "public interest theory of regulation" holds that agencies charged with administering controls are both able and willing to identify outcomes that serve the public interest and to take decisions in accordance with them. Furthermore, imposition of controls is assumed not to evoke among regulated suppliers responses that would militate against the desirable effects of regulation or, worse, exacerbate the problems it is intended to ameliorate. Were these assumptions even approximately realized in practice, one would expect CON programs successfully to contain health cost increases, to improve utilization of current service capacity, and to prevent duplication and underutilization of specialized services and facilities.

Doubting the validity of assumptions underlying the public interest theory, several critics of economic regulation in general and of CON programs in particular have recently offered alternative perspectives to explain behaviors of regulatory bodies and regulated firms. They observe that the political economy of the regulatory process creates political pressures, incentives, and constraints which cause regulatory agencies to deviate substantially from practices postulated by the public interest theory and to evoke perverse responses from providers.

Without necessarily endorsing the largely negative conclusions of critics of CON programs, we believe they offer several insights into the behavior of regulators and health providers and interactions among them that are useful when interpreting empirical data. Therefore, before presenting research findings, let us consider several of the major arguments.

The Capture Theory

The most extreme counterargument to the public interest theory of regulatory behavior is the capture theory. It asserts that regulatory bodies will generally be concerned primarily with the welfare of the regulated industry rather than with the public interest; in short, it holds that regulators are "captured" by producers. Such capture might result from overt political pressures by producers or from attempts to "buy off" regulators. As Havighurst (1973) observes, however, capture may also occur as a consequence of more subtle and pervasive forces. He suggests (p. 1119) that

> . . . even if the balance of power in an agency belongs to reasonable men, it is natural for them to develop a belief in the services rendered by the industry and sympathy for its problems, which will usually appear as obstacles to the continued improvement and wider availability of those services. In those circumstances, the compromises reached within a multimember agency will usually be in keeping with industry interests.

That regulated producers have often strongly supported and vigorously lobbied for the legislation under which they are regulated lends credence to the capture theory (Stigler, 1971). Producers' demand for regulation presumably reflects the confident expectation that their interests will be advanced by the regulatory agency. In this regard, it is noteworthy that several state hospital associations actively supported adoption of CON programs as cost control mechanisms, particularly when laws assigned major roles in the regulatory process to voluntary planning (CHP) agencies (Macro Systems, 1974:vol. 2).

Some observers note that voluntary planning agencies that implement CON programs are particularly vulnerable to provider capture. In most states CON reviews are conducted by agencies that include among their members representatives of hospitals who have access to agency personnel and influence over agency policy (Lave and Lave, 1974:168). Furthermore, hospitals often are an important source of financial contributions required for agency survival and growth, and agency staff and consumer members must rely in the review process upon providers for information and expertise (Havighurst, 1973:1183–1184).

The major implication of provider capture of the CON process is that regulatory agencies will disapprove applications for new facilities, thereby protecting existing providers from the competition of new entrants into the market. Similarly, if agencies identify with the interests of particular groups of providers (for example, nonprofit hospitals), they will discriminate against proposals from other providers (for example, proprietary hospitals or HMOs). A recent study of CON and Section 1122 controls by Lewin and Associates, Inc. (1975) lends support to these expectations. Specifically, they report that regulatory agency personnel frequently express biases against for-profit providers and are especially opposed to "outsiders" entering local health care markets. These biases are reflected in higher disapproval rates for proprietary facilities. Agency bias against HMOs, surgicenters, and other alternatives to inpatient care is less common.[5]

Although provider capture may result in discrimination against potential entrants into health care markets, it does not follow that capture precludes effective control of investments proposed by *existing* providers. Controls such as CON may actually be welcomed if they limit competition among existing providers (Posner, 1974) and enhance hospital administrators' bargaining positions vis-à-vis their medical staffs.[6] By holding that they are powerless to prevent CON agency disapproval of investment plans to which they attach low priorities, administrators gain the power necessary to forestall such plans (Schelling, 1963).

The Political-Economic Theory

Dwelling exclusively on pressures and tendencies that lead regulators to serve the interests of regulated firms, the capture theory presents a rather narrow refutation of the public interest theory. An alternative perspective on regulatory behavior, which Noll (1975) terms the "political-economic theory," holds that regulation may fail to serve the public interest even if regulatory agencies are not tools of the industries they regulate. This perspective assumes

> . . . that regulators try to serve some concept of the general public interest, rather than act as conduits for the interests of regulated firms. The problem regulators face is to identify this general public interest in a milieu in which information is uncertain, expensive, and biased, and in a society which contains

[5]Of course, the ability of CON agencies to act in accordance with these biases and blatantly to discriminate against new or other disfavored providers can be limited by procedural requirements. Well-defined standards and public disclosure of reasoning behind each decision presumably constrain agency discretion. Such procedural constraints appear to be minimal at present (Lewin and Associates, Inc., 1975).

[6]Curran's (1974) observation that medical societies, unlike hospital associations, have not been strong advocates of CON controls is of interest in this context.

numerous groups whose interests are conflicting rather than harmonious [Noll, 1975:29].[7]

Being unable clearly to identify the public interest and to defend their actions by reference to precisely articulated standards, agencies respond to political reward structures. Specifically, they seek to avoid costly conflicts[8] and highly visible failures while striving to produce clearly visible successes.

In the case of CON regulation, such behavior has important implications for the manner in which controls are applied. Without question, CON agencies typically lack well-formulated standards upon which to base decisions, a deficiency that stems from the inadequacy of routine data-reporting systems, the primitive state of the art of health planning, and a scarcity of resources for acquiring information. Although most CON laws identify state or local plans as the desired sources of standards for CON review, the reality is that few planning agencies have produced long-range, comprehensive plans in sufficient detail to serve as criteria for the conceivable variety of proposals that could emerge (Cohen, 1973). For instance, a review of planning agencies by the U.S. General Accounting Office found:

> Less than half of the 163 health planning agencies . . . indicated knowledge of 1972 needs for types of inpatient and extended and ambulatory care facilities and beds. . . . The number knowing 1975 beds was even lower. . . . Most knew the number of existing health facilities [Comptroller General of the United States, 1974:18].

A more recent study of investment controls in twenty states found agencies relying extensively on Hill-Burton plans for bed-need standards, "which are viewed as inadequate and based on obsolete data." Standards for reviewing special services, equipment, outpatient services were generally nonexistent (Lewin and Associates, Inc., 1975:ch. 3).

Lacking comprehensive plans and systematic information about needs for and use of services and having limited personnel and funds, CON agencies are unable to base each review decision on equally thorough analysis. Because agencies desire to avoid costly conflicts and to maintain credibility and legitimacy among their sponsors and constituents, political and economic considerations are

---

[7] The possibility that agencies may attempt to serve *both* the interests of regulated firms and the public interest should also be considered. This notion is consistent with Posner's (1971) thesis that agencies induce regulated providers to engage in unprofitable "public interest" activities by protecting them from competitive pressures.
[8] Hilton (1972) refers to this as the "minimal squawk" principle.

brought into their decision-making processes. Large, politically powerful institutions willing to devote considerable resources to defending their proposals through appeals, legal action, or legislative attempts to override agency decisions threaten to deplete agency resources and, if successful, tarnish the agency's public image of an effective and fair regulatory body.[9] This would suggest that CON controls will be applied selectively, with the likelihood of disapproval being inversely related to the economic and political power of the applicant institution.[10] Similar reasoning leads to the expectation of higher disapproval rates for projects that pose competitive threats to established providers, such as plans to build new hospitals or to provide lower cost alternatives to hospital care (for example, surgicenters). On this point the capture and political-economic theories agree.

Another type of selectivity deriving from the political-economic theory is the likelihood of more stringent control over the expansion of bed supplies than over new services and equipment. To some extent, this is implied by the bias against entry of new providers. However, the most compelling arguments for this hypothesis stem from the lack of review standards and information about use of and needs for services, which is especially severe with respect to new services and equipment. Although data on the supply and use of beds and estimates of bed needs are often unreliable and out of date, they are at least widely available. By contrast, information about the supply, use, and costs of special equipment and services is generally sketchy, and consistent review standards are virtually nonexistent (Lewin and Associates, Inc., 1975:ch. 3).

This informational asymmetry implies a corresponding asymmetry in the reward structures confronting CON agencies. External evaluators and legislative oversight committees concerned about the costs of acquiring information needed for developing standards and for conducting reviews tend to confine their assessment of agency

---

[9] The experience of the Massachusetts CON program demonstrates that the dangers of agency denials triggering judicial and political conflict are real. Most striking is the fact that within the four-year history of the program two agency decisions were reversed by special legislation. These are described by Reider, Mason, and Glantz (1975). Another instance of political conflict surrounding a CON decision in Maryland is detailed by West (1975).

[10] The Massachusetts experience (Reider, Mason, and Glantz, 1975) demonstrates that large institutions do not have a monopoly on political power. Community hospitals that serve well-defined population groups may effectively mobilize popular support for expansion plans (partly because these population groups bear only a fraction of the costs of expansion under existing third-party payment schemes) and translate this support into direct pressures on the CON agency or intervention by elected officials.

effectiveness to the ability to limit growth of bed supplies.[11] In consequence, agencies are rewarded more for controlling beds than for stemming the proliferation of special services and equipment. The consequences of erroneous approvals of additional beds—empty beds and low occupancy rates—are clearly visible indicators of agency failure; consequences of erroneous disapprovals (for example, longer waits for elective admissions) are less so (Pauly, 1974:158–159).

These considerations suggest that CON agencies will be predisposed to disapprove proposals for new beds and to invest considerable time and resources in reviewing them. By contrast, we expect a more lenient attitude toward proposals for new services and equipment. Moreover, since costs of acquiring information about new services or equipment proposals are high while the political rewards for building convincing cases against them are low, CON agencies have little incentive to subject such plans to careful review.

This expectation of leniency toward new services and equipment proposals is reinforced by several political and legal considerations. First, while the costs of thorough review and analysis may be prohibitive, the practice of denying such proposals after only cursory review opens the CON agency to charges of capriciously denying citizens. the fruits of medical progress. Second, disapprovals may arouse hostility toward CON agencies among groups of physicians who find their hospitals unable to offer new diagnostic or treatment technologies while colleagues with admitting privileges at other hospitals have access to them. Finally, there are significant limitations in the coverage of new services and equipment under CON laws. As we have noted, although most CON statutes require certification for new construction and for significant increases in bed capacity, other potentially important types of investment are not controlled. Several states exempt all projects below a minimum capital expenditure, and in several states expenditures for equipment or expansion of existing services or renovations that do not involve increases in beds are excluded from review.

The expectation that CON agencies will exercise strict control over bed growth while generally approving proposals for new services and equipment without detailed review is supported by several descriptive studies. Data reported by Reider and his associates (1975) and by Bicknell and Walsh (1975) show that in Massachusetts proposals for facility improvements not involving

[11]An example is the recent evaluation of Florida's CON program by the state legislature. The sole criterion upon which the evaluation is based is the extent to which the program limited bed growth to the Hill-Burton agency's need estimates (State of Florida, n.d.).

new beds were approved more often than were proposals to expand bed capacity. Furthermore, Bicknell and Walsh (1975) observed that proposals not involving new beds usually did not "attract the closer, technically more sophisticated scrutiny . . . normally reserved for bed-related applications" (p. 1057). Similar differences in approval rates under CON and Section 1122 review programs in seventeen states were found by Lewin and Associates, Inc. (1975:ch. 4). It should be noted, however, that approval rates are an imperfect index of the stringency of controls, for agencies often employ informal means to screen out projects that are likely to be disapproved prior to their formal submission. Nevertheless, these findings provide at least qualified support for our hypothesis.

Perverse Provider Responses

Several authors have noted that establishment of a CON program causes providers to alter investment plans. It is not clear, however, whether providers' responses would create more or less rapid capital expansion. Bicknell and Walsh (1975) hold that adoption of CON would reduce planned expansion, arguing (p. 1079) that

> . . . a certificate-of-need program, merely by its existence, may discourage construction and capital expenditures by causing an anticipatory reaction on the part of providers.

Others note that CON controls are similar to franchising and posit the opposite effect. According to Havighurst (1973:1171, n. 104), for instance,

> [t]here would seem to be a danger that the certificate-of-need process may actually stimulate hospital construction by causing applicants to accelerate their plans in order to pre-empt others.

This reasoning is also applied to decisions about costly innovations in services and facilities (Roth, 1974). Being the first hospital in an area to install a $400,000 brain scanner becomes especially important if the chances of approval of second and third requests are nil.

To the extent that the pre-emptive response outweighs the discouragement effect, provider responses will be perverse; that is, they will tend to increase health care costs. The possibility of a substantial perverse response appears especially probable if, as the preceding discussion of regulatory behavior implies, CON controls are applied in a selective fashion. For example, both the capture theory and the political-economic theory suggest that certain providers and groups of providers are likely to receive especially favorable treatment from CON agencies, specifically, less stringent controls over their own investments and protection from competition for patients or for donor capital. It seems reasonable to conclude that these favored providers will react by increasing their capital expenditure plans.

The expectation that investments in new equipment and services will be less stringently controlled than expansions of bed supplies also points to perverse provider responses. If the preferences of hospital trustees, administrators, and medical staff for the growth of their institution cannot be satisfied by the addition of new beds, alternative expressions of their preferences will be found among the less regulated investment options (that is, new equipment and services). An especially pessimistic view of this possibility has been expressed by Noll (1975:44):

> Controlling the number of beds will simply turn the attention of hospital administrators to other, perhaps even less desirable expenditures. Thus is the regulatory tar-baby conceived. Regulators will find their attempts to force efficiency upon a recalcitrant industry as leading only to even more detailed and expensive regulation, prohibiting a lengthening string of unnecessary expenditures, but with no apparent long-run success in dealing with the general problem of rising costs.

Implications for the Effectiveness of CON Controls

At the outset of this section we noted that the rationale for CON controls as an effective anti-inflationary device is based on the assumptions (1) that the public interest theory accurately describes behaviors of the regulatory agencies that administer CON regulations and (2) that the imposition of these controls does not evoke a substantial perverse response by providers. From our review of the capture and political-economic theories and the limited evidence pertaining to them, we believe there are reasons to doubt these assumptions. Without prejudging ultimate effects on costs of health care, experience recorded to date lends credence to the major conclusion of the capture and political-economic theories, namely, that CON controls will be applied selectively. Investment by existing providers will be less tightly controlled than will be entry of new providers. Further, we would expect more stringent controls on additional beds than on investment in services and equipment. Finally, this pattern of selective controls seems likely to stimulate perverse provider responses manifested in increased investment planning for services and equipment projects.

Whether these patterns of investment effect changes in average per diem hospital costs and total hospital expenditures depends, of course, on their cumulative effects on operating and capital costs and utilization patterns. Trade-offs between bed expansion and investment in services and equipment could increase average per diem costs as a result of higher intensity or wider scope of services while lowering the volume of inpatient days. These two factors exert opposing influences on total costs. In consequence, without detailed examination of the quantitative effects of CON on costs and use, it is impossible to predict whether CON will attain the ultimate end of controlling hospital costs.

Effects of Certificate-of-Need Controls on Hospital Investment, Costs, and Use and on Health Care Costs

Although control of health care costs is not the sole purpose of CON regulation (Reider, Mason, and Glantz, 1975), the language of most CON laws clearly indicates that it is a major objective.[12] Therefore, analysis of CON programs' impacts on hospital and other health care costs is a relevant means of assessing their effectiveness. Two strategies have been employed by researchers to study this question: a descriptive approach and an analytic approach.

The descriptive approach, illustrated by the work of Bicknell and Walsh (1975) and Lewin and Associates, Inc. (1975), focuses on the regulatory process, describing the types and numbers of applications submitted to CON agencies and the decisions taken by agencies. Although such studies provide valuable insights into health care institutions' investment priorities and CON agency behavior, they cannot directly assess CON controls' effects on investment patterns and costs. Estimates of savings based on the total costs of projects disapproved by CON agencies fail to account for projects that might have been undertaken in the absence of a CON program but for which applications were not filed because a rejection was anticipated.[13] Failure to record such projects leads to underestimates of savings effected by CON programs. Another deficiency of the descriptive approach is that it ignores program effects on types of investments that do not require agency approval. Of course, the most serious limitation of this approach is that it inevitably leads to

[12] However, Lewin and Associates, Inc. (1975), report that relatively few staff members of agencies administering CON regulation consider cost control the most important objective of these controls.

[13] Lewin and Associates, Inc. (1975), attribute the high rates of agency approval of applications partially to agencies' screening-out proposals that are highly likely to be disapproved before they reach the formal review process and to negotiations between agency staff and applicant institutions in the formulation of proposals.

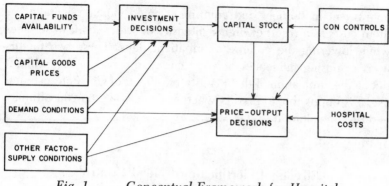

Fig. 1   Conceptual Framework for Hospital
              Cost Determination

the conclusion that CON controls reduce investment. No account is taken of the possibility of perverse provider responses.

The analytic approach estimates impacts of CON regulation by examining its effects on investment patterns and costs while statistically controlling effects of other factors that influence investment. To date, only one extensive study employing this approach has been concluded.[14] In this section we summarize its methods and findings and interpret these in light of the competing theories of CON regulation and findings from other studies of CON processes and impacts.

Evidence from our study shows that CON controls have no appreciable impact on total investment by hospitals but encourage a redirection of investment from bed expansion to growth of new services and facilities. This, in turn, leads to lower rates of utilization and somewhat higher hospital and total health care costs. In sum, CON controls do not bring about lower costs but may actually exacerbate health care cost inflation.

These conclusions derive from analyses of CON programs' effects on variables depicted in Fig. 1. We reasoned that hospital costs are affected by hospitals' capital stock and price-output decisions, both of which may be influenced by CON regulation. The former, which specify the size of a hospital's bed complement as well as the types and numbers of equipment and other capital facilities, are determined (in an environment without regulatory controls) by the availability of capital funds, prices of capital goods, demand conditions, and other factor-supply conditions (Ginsburg, 1970; Muller, Worthington, and Allen, 1975; Pauly, 1974). Price-

---

[14]As of this writing, only the analysis of investment patterns is in published form (Salkever and Bice, 1976a). The results of the overall study are in Salkever and Bice (1976b).

output decisions, which determine the prices and volumes of services rendered during a specified period, are affected by demand and factor-supply conditions and the capital stock in place during the period in question (Davis, 1973; 1974). Finally, given the nonprofit nature of the hospital industry, the aggregate price-times-volume figures will closely approximate the costs of rendering hospital services.

Following the order implied by the conceptual framework, we first examined the impact of CON controls on capital stock; next we estimated the direct effects of capital stock and CON controls on costs. By combining the results from both stages in the analysis we then computed the total (direct and indirect) effects of CON controls on costs.

Methods

Estimates of impacts of CON controls were derived from cross-section and pooled multiple regression analyses of investment, costs, and utilization of nonfederal, short-term general and other special hospitals. The data pertain to the forty-eight contiguous states and the District of Columbia and cover the period from 1968 to 1972, a period chosen because it included some exposure to CON controls in several states and was relatively free of confounding effects of Section 1122, federal price controls, and Blue Cross conformance clauses adopted subsequently.

Estimates of CON controls' impacts were obtained by two procedures. First, we specified models in which changes in dependent variables were regressed on sets of predictors specified by the conceptual framework, including a variable measuring exposure to CON controls.[15] The regression coefficient associated with the CON variable was interpreted as CON programs' direct effect on the dependent variable under investigation. A second approach estimated effects of predictors other than the CON variable, using data from non-CON states only; these estimates were then applied to data from CON states to obtain predicted values for the dependent variable. Differences between observed and predicted values were interpreted as estimates of CON programs effects. Finally, results from the regression analyses were translated into estimates of the

[15] For analyses of investment patterns, which examined a single cross-section of state data on changes in capital stock from 1968 to 1972, the CON variable was operationally defined as the fraction of that four-year period during which CON regulation was in effect. For analyses of costs and utilization, which employed pooled cross-sections of annual state data for the years 1968–1972 (or 1967–1972 in some cases), the CON variable was set equal to one if a state had a CON program in effect for two or more quarters during the year, and was zero otherwise.

magnitudes of changes in dependent variables attributable to CON controls.

Findings

Hospital Investment   Hospital investment was measured by three variables: changes in total plant assets, in total beds, and in plant assets per bed from 1968 to 1972. Changes in total plant assets represents the total dollar value of investment; changes in plant assets per bed may be viewed as an indicator of increases in the sophistication or capital-intensiveness of facilities.

In addition to the CON variable, predictors included measures of changes in demand variables (population size, income, insurance), capital funds availability factors (net revenues, Hill-Burton allocations), and factors influencing capital goods costs (construction wages). Most predictors were measured as changes for the lagged period from 1964 to 1968 as well as for the 1968–1972 period.

Results of analyses based on several specifications of the regression model showed a consistent pattern. CON coefficients for changes in total plant assets were positively signed but were generally not statistically significant, indicating that CON controls did not reduce total investment. Analyses of changes in beds and plant assets per bed revealed, however, that CON programs had a significant impact on the composition of investment. Specifically, they clearly restricted investment in new beds while encouraging investment in other services and facilities that resulted in increases in plant assets per bed. Magnitudes of these effects were relatively large. The estimated effects for the CON controls in force for the entire 1968–1972 period were a reduced growth in beds by 5.4 to 9.0 percent and a rise in the increase of plant assets per bed by 15.2 to 19.7 percent.

Findings from the second analytic approach confirmed these patterns. Eliminating the five states where CON regulation had been in effect throughout 1971 and 1972 (California, Connecticut, Maryland, New York, and Rhode Island) and deleting the CON variable, we reestimated the investment equations and used the resulting coefficients to predict changes in the dependent variables for the excluded states. Results from several specifications of the regression model showed that in almost all cases actual increases in beds in the five CON states were less than predicted increases, and actual increases in total plant assets and plant assets per bed exceeded predicted changes.

These patterns strongly suggest that investment in new equipment and facilities is substituted for expansion of bed supplies when the latter is controlled by CON regulation. The observed limitation of bed expansion is consistent with critical analyses of CON programs that point to provider domination, limitations in the coverage of CON laws, and the likely response of CON agencies to the scarcity of resources and to the asymmetry of rewards they face. Less obvious, however, is the cause of the relatively higher rate of growth in plant assets per bed in CON states. This may be due to the franchising aspect of CON controls that encourages pre-emptive investment or to the added protection from competition that regulation affords existing providers. Given the strong pressures operating within hospitals to expand services and facilities and to upgrade their quality, control of one type of investment rechannels expansionist preferences into areas not subject to stringeht control.

Hospital Costs and Utilization   Having found that CON regulation affects investment patterns (and thereby capital stock), we examined the second type of effect specified by the conceptual framework, namely, the direct influence of CON regulation and capital stock on price-output decisions. Estimates of these effects were combined with those measuring CON programs' impacts on capital stock to obtain measures of the total (direct and indirect) effects of CON regulation on hospital costs.

Although CON regulation may conceivably directly influence hospitals' price-output decisions, it is not clear what specific responses will occur. Hospitals might tend to set prices lower and run higher occupancy rates in order to be in a better position to justify proposals for expansion. Alternatively, they might set prices higher and provide a lower volume but a higher quality of services because they are protected from the competition of potential new entrants. Indeed, lower occupancy rates may facilitate blocking of entry since CON agencies will be more reluctant to permit any increases in bed supply in the market area.

To assess outcomes of CON programs' impacts on price-output decisions, several analyses were carried out in which hospital costs per capita were regressed on determinants of demand for services and factor prices, as well as on descriptors of existing capital stock (beds and assets per bed). Parallel analyses of other indicators of costs (inpatient costs per inpatient day, outpatient costs per capita) and utilization (inpatient days per capita, inpatient admissions per capita) were carried out to give a more complete picture of CON programs' impacts and to provide a check on the reasonableness of the estimates.

As in the investment analyses, estimates of CON programs' effects were derived from two different methods. First, coefficients for the CON variable and for capital stock variables were estimated for all states, and these were combined with estimates of CON programs' impacts on capital stock to calculate the average overall impact of CON regulation on the dependent variables. Second, regression equations based on data from non-CON states were combined with predictions of the 1972 levels of capital stock variables in the absence of CON in four CON states (New York, Connecticut, California, and Rhode Island) in order to obtain predicted 1972 values of the dependent variables in these states. As before, these values were compared with observed values to determine whether actual cost levels in these three CON states are different from predicted levels. If CON regulation were an effective cost control mechanism, actual costs would be less than predicted levels.

The hospital costs per capita regressions showed that increases in capital stock—beds and plant assets per bed—led to higher costs and that CON regulation also had a positive but less significant direct effect. Since increases in both capital stock variables were associated with increasing costs and CON controls affect them differently, the net indirect effect of CON regulation reflects the balancing of competing tendencies. CON controls indirectly lead to lower costs via their reducing bed expansion while contributing to cost increases by stimulating other types of investment. Adding various estimates of these indirect effects to the estimate of CON programs' direct effects resulted in a range of estimates of overall impacts on per capita costs. Using the smallest estimates of CON programs' effects on capital stock, the estimated overall influence of a CON program over the 1968–1972 period was to raise a typical state's per capita costs in 1972 by 1.54 to 2.44 percent; corresponding estimates based on the largest capital stock impacts showed reductions of per capita costs by 1.09 to 1.85 percent. Clearly, CON regulation did not substantially lower per capita costs and may have increased them slightly.

The overall effect of CON regulation on the volume of inpatient services was to reduce utilization. The direct impact of CON controls was found to be consistently negative (but not always statistically significant) for both indicators of utilization—inpatient days per capita and admissions per capita. Through its restrictions of bed expansion CON regulation led to lower utilization of inpatient services, though to a lesser extent its stimulation of other types of investment had the opposite effect. The estimated net result of these influences in combination was to lower inpatient days in a typical state having CON regulation (from 1969 to 1972) by 2.15 to 8.30 percent and to lower admissions per capita by 4.92 to 8.30 percent.[16]

[16] Inspection of deviations of predicted costs per capita based on effects of capital stock and other predictors derived from analyses of non-CON states with capital stock variables set equal to their predicted values for CON states confirmed these results. Overall, 1972 costs in the four CON states were consistently higher than

To supplement analyses of CON controls' effects on hospital costs per capita, their impacts on costs of services covered by Medicare were examined. For this purpose, we employed dependent variables measuring reimbursements for inpatient services under Part A as well as total Medicare reimbursement under both Parts A and B. Results of these analyses were similar to those found before. CON controls' direct effect was slightly positive (but not statistically significant), and influences of capital stock changes were positive but slightly smaller than those estimated for per capita hospital costs. Adding the indirect and direct effects of CON regulation results in the prediction that CON controls over the 1968–1972 period would have increased total Medicare reimbursements by 1.44 to 4.01 percent in the typical state. Because of imprecisions in the methods employed in generating these estimates, they should not be taken as conclusive proof than CON controls raise costs. However, the pattern observed across several indicators of costs clearly provides no support for the widely held presumption that these controls have reduced costs.

Results from Other Studies

Although we are not aware of other econometric studies of CON impacts on costs to which our own results could be compared, there have been several recent analyses of CON impacts on investment which should be mentioned.

Hellinger (1976) used cross-sectional state data for 1973 to estimate the impact of CON controls on total plant assets in short-term hospitals. His finding that CON did not have a significant effect is similar to our own result for total investment. In similar analyses with 1971 and 1972 data, he found that investment increased in the year in which a CON law was passed and interpreted this as the result of hospitals' efforts to undertake additional investment before the implementation date of controls. However, the results of this study must be viewed with some skepticism because of several problems with the econometric methods employed. For instance, Hellinger's regression equations incorporate the doubtful assumption that the magnitude of the CON impact is the same in all states regardless of size. It would seem more reasonable to assume that this impact varies positively with the size of the hospital industry in the state.[17] Hellinger's use of the ordinary least squares estimation

---

predicted values. To allow for the possibility that these deviations may have reflected stable characteristics rather than CON effects, we also examined residuals for the pre-CON years from three states (Connecticut, California, and Rhode Island). The fact that these residuals were always either negative or positive but smaller than the 1972 deviations confirmed our conclusion of a positive CON effect on costs.

[17] In our own total investment equations, the impact of CON on plant assets in 1972 is specified as proportional to the magnitude of plant assets in 1968.

technique is also problematic, since his regressions are based on a proportional adjustment model and therefore include the dependent variable lagged one year as a predictor. It is well known that ordinary least squares will yield biased coefficient estimates when a lagged dependent variable is used if (as is likely) autocorrelation is present.[18] Because of these and other problems in Hellinger's analysis, his findings do not provide strong corroboration of our results.

Abt Associates, Inc. (1975), used cross-sectional regression analyses of 1973 state data to estimate the impact of CON on investment in ten specialized services. Results indicated that in three cases (x-ray therapy, cobalt therapy, and radium therapy), the percentage of hospitals within a state offering a particular service was significantly reduced by CON. Although this finding seems to contradict our own evidence regarding changes in assets per bed, it may be questioned on the ground that most hospitals offering these services did so even before CON laws were in effect in their states. In other words, CON may merely be serving as a proxy for other preexisting factors omitted from the analysis. It would be interesting to test for this possibility by replicating the analysis with current data on the CON dummy variable and data for other variables from an earlier year (in the late 1960s, for example) when CON laws were nonexistent (except in New York). If this replication also revealed a significantly negative CON coefficient, its role as a proxy for preexisting factors would be confirmed.[19]

Conclusions, Limitations, and Suggestions for Further Research

Our analyses of impacts of CON regulation yield a pattern of findings that support critical arguments about the possible deleterious consequences of imposition of such controls. Contrary to expectations of the public interest theory, our findings suggest that CON controls contributed to cost increases during the 1968–1972 period. CON regulation did not deter total investment in the hospital sector; instead, it altered its composition by discouraging expansion of beds and thereby encouraging (or at least facilitating) expansionist urges of hospitals to find expression in investment in new equipment and facilities. Such findings are consistent with

[18] The high probability of bias due to positive autocorrelation in Hellinger's results is revealed by the extremely low estimates for his speed-of-adjustment parameter. Most of his estimates range between .068 and .022, implying an average lag time for investment in excess of ten years.

[19] For an example of this replication procedure in a related context, see May (1974).

observations from descriptive studies of the CON process (Bicknell and Walsh, 1975; Lewin and Associates, Inc., 1975), which reveal that CON agencies lack information and standards to guide decisions about needs for new equipment and facilities and often—because of limitations of coverage of CON controls—lack authority to review them. Under such circumstances, it is likely that equipment and facilities will diffuse among hospitals until providers themselves determine that there is no longer need for additional expansion.

Although findings from our study conform to a set of plausible predictions and are consistent with observations from other studies, several limitations of our analyses must be mentioned. First, they pertain almost exclusively to hospital services. Additional studies of other types of services such as long-term and ambulatory care and further exploration of comprehensive cost measures are required to obtain firm conclusions about CON controls' influences on health care costs. Second, our findings pertain to changes in investment and costs measured at the state level. Since CON regulation is directed initially at planning regions within states, studies of state-level impacts should be replicated for smaller geographical units to determine their possible sensitivity to the level of aggregation employed.

Furthermore, we should stress that our results pertain to a period when other approaches to cost control were not widespread. Our largely pessimistic conclusions about CON regulation may therefore apply only to situations in which CON controls were the sole or principal regulatory constraint on costs; their relevance for cases where CON regulation acts in combination with other now widely applied controls (such as PSROs and state rate-setting programs) is unknown. We would strongly suggest, however, that faith in the ameliorative possibilities of a multifaceted attack on the cost inflation problem which incorporates investment controls should not obscure the fact that this form of regulation is potentially exacerbating. Further research on the critical question of how CON regulation interacts with other controls is needed.

The reader should also note that the usefulness of our findings for predictive purposes may be further limited by selection biases resulting from systematic differences between states which adopted CON laws and those which did not. We cannot be assured that impacts of CON controls on hospital investment, costs, and use revealed in our analysis will be repeated in states that adopt CON controls in order to participate in the planning program mandated by P.L. 93-641.

Of course, there are other research questions concerning the effects of CON controls which deserve investigation. For instance, research is needed to determine whether CON programs affect the structure of the health sector by blocking entry of new competitors, retarding the growth of HMOs, and discouraging investment in less costly alternatives to hospital care. Finally, there is a need for more descriptive studies of the review process, such as those carried out by Bicknell and Walsh (1975) and Lewin and Associates, Inc. (1975), to aid in the interpretation of econometric results and to generate new hypotheses about agency behavior.

Policy Implications

In view of our finding that the failure of CON agencies to curtail hospital cost inflation is largely attributable to their inability to control investment in new equipment and facilities, one might be tempted to conclude that CON programs can be made more effective by tightening existing controls and extending them to cover most (if not all) investment projects (Abt Associates, Inc., 1975:125). The wisdom and feasibility of this approach, however, are by no means self-evident. Careful review of all certification requests, including the additional ones generated by extending the scope of CON regulation, would require large additions to agency resources. Conceivably, resources required for review might exceed costs of investment projects being reviewed. Without additional resources, simply extending the coverage of CON laws over additions to equipment and facilities makes it less likely that agencies will be able consistently to render decisions in the public interest. As we have already noted, CON agencies lack adequate information and standards for review of these additions. Burdening agencies with the responsibility of developing standards for a larger universe of conceivable projects would only exacerbate this problem.

Other seemingly straightforward options for restraining investment in new equipment and facilities may be undesirable because they are either politically infeasible or at variance with CON controls' putative objective of deterring *unnecessary* investment. For instance, CON agencies could adopt the general policy of denying certification for equipment and facilities except in cases where extreme and urgent need is demonstrable. Alternatively, substantial submission fees or even taxes on investment could be employed to discourage hospitals and other institutions from seeking certification. Although such measures have the superficial appeals of simplicity and economy, they are not particularly discriminating between needed and unneeded investments. Furthermore, they would most likely favor the large, wealthy institutions' interests even more than does the process currently in use.

Several alternative possibilities for increasing the effectiveness of CON controls are suggested by our previous discussion of the political economy of regulation. Increases in CON agencies' resources, for example, may permit more detailed reviews of proposals for new equipment or facilities and the generation of additional data relevant to these reviews. With a more substantial factual basis, agencies' decisions should be more difficult to contest and their willingness to risk conflict with providers by denying certification should therefore increase. Furthermore, the generation and promulgation of better data on the supply, costs, and use of various specialized facilities and equipment items may diminish the tendency of external evaluators to focus strictly on control of bed supplies and thereby enhance the CON agencies' incentives to control equipment and facilities investments.

Another policy option involves altering administrative procedures used in reviewing investment proposals. Presently, CON agencies render decisions in an open-ended context where, except for competing applications for the same equipment and facilities, reviews of investment plans of different institutions are treated as independent events. Placing a ceiling on allowable investment expenditures within regions and requiring agencies to select from among applications submitted during specific periods might dramatically alter the politics of the review process. Different providers, each seeking a share of the limited supply of funds, could be inclined to view others' proposals critically and to expend some effort in documenting these criticisms. In this event, agencies would have at their disposal a more complete and balanced information base for each proposed project than is typically the case at present. The use of an investment ceiling could alter the role of nonproviders as well. Decisions on the level of the ceiling, which could be made by the CON agency or another governmental body (for example, the legislature), would probably attract the participation of broad-based citizens' groups, elected officials serving large constituencies, or public agencies whose programs might be affected (for instance, Medicaid agencies). In contrast, under the current piecemeal approach, nonprovider participation frequently takes the form of one or two neighborhood or community groups lobbying for new services in their locality. Moreover, consideration of slates of competing proposals might also stimulate greater public participation in the planning process, since attention would be focused not merely on reviewing a trail of seemingly unrelated projects, each addressed to particular segments of a population, but rather on deciding which alternative means of achieving community priorities will be adopted.

While we have thus far discussed various strategies for increasing the effectiveness of CON controls, it must be acknowledged that a very different sort of policy response is also consistent with our empirical findings. Presuming that the evidence of CON's ineffectiveness reported here reflects the inevitable result of this type of regulation, one might argue for more limitations on its scope and use if only to reduce its undesirable side effects. In this spirit, Frech (1975) and Havighurst (1973) suggest exempting HMOs and other nonhospital facilities from coverage under CON laws to forestall the possibility that hospital-dominated agencies will block entry of facilities providing lower cost alternative sources of care.[20] For the same reason, critics of CON have suggested that the risk of provider capture may be reduced by alterations in the arrangements for program administration (such as placing the CON program in the control of a state agency which also has responsibility for rate regulation or for purchasing medical care under public insurance programs). Of course, the most preferred policy option for these critics is the abolition of all CON controls, although this is recognized as highly unlikely and in fact contrary to recent trends in national health policy.

Finally, we suggest that the desirability of extending CON controls should be considered within the total context of health sector regulation. Investment controls have been supplemented nationally by utilization review programs under PSROs and in several states by rate-review programs. By controlling the volume and unit costs of services (and thus total costs), these additional programs in combination may obviate the need for expanded investment controls and even make desirable their diminution or elimination.

In sum, available evidence as to the effectiveness of CON programs suggests that this form of control is not likely to bring about lower rates of cost inflation. However, research conducted to date has barely touched the range of policy questions and options advanced by proponents and critics of CON controls. Much of the reasoning employed by proponents and critics alike stems from thus far unsupported assumptions about responses of regulatory agencies and regulated firms to the political context that accompanies imposition of regulatory programs. Until the incentives created by regulatory devices such as CON programs are better understood, we will be in the position of legislating in the hope that the public interest is necessarily served by more regulation.

---

[20] Another effect of this exemption is to encourage movement of certain activities from hospitals to ambulatory facilities and thus beyond the reach of regulation. However, one suspects that this phenomenon may be limited by the fact that insurance coverage is still considerably more complete for inpatient services than for ambulatory services.

References

Abt Associates, Inc.
>
> 1975   Incentives and Decisions Underlying Hospital Adoption and Utilization of Major Capital Equipment. Cambridge, Mass.: Abt Associates, Inc.

Bicknell, W.J., and D.C. Walsh

> 1975   "Certification-of-need: The Massachusetts experience." New England Journal of Medicine 292 (May): 1054–1061.

Cohen, H.S.

> 1973   "Regulating health care facilities: The certificate-of-need process re-examined." Inquiry 10 (September): 3–9.

Comptroller General of the United States

> 1974   Comprehensive Health Planning as Carried Out by States and Areawide Agencies in Three States. Washington, D.C.: Government Printing Office.

Curran, W.J.

> 1974   "A national survey and analysis of state certificate-of-need laws for health facilities." In C.C. Havighurst, ed., Regulating Health Facilities Construction. Washington, D.C.: American Enterprise Institute for Public Policy Research.

Davis, K.

> 1969   "A Theory of Economic Behavior in Non-Profit, Private Hospitals." Ph.D. thesis, Rice University.

> 1973   "Hospital costs and the Medicare Program." Social Security Bulletin 36 (August): 18–36.

> 1974   "The role of technology, demand and labor markets in the determination of hospital cost." In Mark Perlman, ed., The Economics of Health and Medical Care. New York: John Wiley & Sons, Inc.

Feldstein, M.S.

> 1971   "Hospital cost inflation: A study of nonprofit price dynamics." American Economic Review 61 (December): 941–973.

Frech, H.E.

> 1975   "Regulatory reform: The case of the medical care industry." Paper presented at the Conference on Regulatory Reform, American Enterprise Institute, Washington, D.C., September 10–11.

Ginsburg, P.B.

> 1970   "Capital in non-profit hospitals." Ph.D. thesis, Harvard University.

Havighurst, C.C.

> 1973   "Regulation of health facilities and services by certificate-of-need." Virginia Law Review 59 (October): 1143–1232.

Hellinger, F.J.

> 1976   "The effect of certificate-of-need legislation on hospital investment." Inquiry 13 (June): 187–193.

Hilton, G.
  1972   "The basic behavior of regulatory commissions." American
          Economic Review 62 (May): 47–54.
Lave, J.R., and L.B. Lave
  1974   "The supply and allocation of medical resources: Alternative
          control mechanisms." In C.C. Havighurst, ed., Regulating
          Health Facilities Construction.
Lewin, L., and Associates, Inc.
  1974   Nationwide Survey of State Health Regulations. Washington,
          D.C., Social Security Administration.
  1975   Evaluation of the Efficiency and Effectiveness of the Section
          1122 Review Process. Washington, D.C.
Macro Systems, Inc.
  1974   The Certificate of Need Experience: An Early Assessment. Silver
          Springs, Md.
May, J.J.
  1974   "The impact of regulation on the hospital industry." Unpub-
          lished working paper, Center for Health Administration Studies,
          University of Chicago.
Muller, C., P. Worthington, and G. Allen
  1975   "Capital expenditures and the availability of funds." Interna-
          tional Journal of Health Services 5 (Winter): 143–157.
Newhouse, J.P.
  1974   Forecasting Demand for Medical Care for the Purpose of
          Planning Health Services. Santa Monica, Cal.: The RAND
          Corporation, R-1635-OEO (December).
Noll, R.G.
  1975   "The consequences of public utility regulation of hospitals." In
          Controls on Health Care. Washington, D.C. National Academy
          of Sciences, Institute of Medicine.
O'Donoghue, P., and Policy Center, Inc.
  1974   Evidence About the Effects of Health Care Regulation. Denver:
          Spectrum Research, Inc.
Pauly, M.V.
  1974   "The behavior of nonprofit hospital monopolies: Alternative
          models of the hospital." In C.C. Havighurst, ed., Regulating
          Health Facilities Construction.
Posner, R.A.
  1971   "Taxation by representation." The Bell Journal of Economics
          and Management 2 Science (Spring): 22–50.
  1974   "Certificates of need for health care facilities: A dissenting
          view." In C.C. Havighurst, ed., Regulating Health Facilities
          Construction.
Reider, A.E., J.R. Mason, and L.M. Glantz
  1975   "Certificate-of-need: The Massachusetts experience." American
          Journal of Law and Medicine 1 (March): 13–40.

Roth, E.
  1974   "Certificate of need as a part of comprehensive health planning."
          Unpublished paper, The Johns Hopkins Medical Institutions.
Salkever, D.S., and T.W. Bice
  1976a   "The impact of certificate-of-need controls on hospital invest-
          ment." Milbank. Memorial Fund Quarterly/Health and Society
          54 (Spring): 185–214.
  1976b   The Impact of Certificate-of-Need Controls on Hospital Invest-
          ment, Costs, and Utilization. Final report to the National Center
          for Health Services Research, U.S. Department of Health,
          Education, and Welfare, Contract No. HRA-106-74-57.
Schelling, T.
  1963   The Strategy of Conflict. New York: Oxford University Press.
State of Florida, House of Representatives, Committee on Health and
Rehabilitation Services
  n.d.   A Preliminary Evaluation of the Certificate of Need Program in
          Florida.
Stigler, G.J.
  1971   "The theory of economic regulation." The Bell Journal of
          Economics and Management Science 2 (Spring): 3–21.
Stuehler, G.
  1973   "Certification of need: A systems analysis of Maryland's experi-
          ence and plans." American Journal of Public Health 63 (Novem-
          ber): 966–972.
West, J.P.
  1975   "Health planning in multifunctional regional councils: Baltimore
          and Houston experience." Inquiry 12 (September): 180–192.

28. Regulating Competition in a Nonprofit Industry: The Problem of For Profit Hospitals

WILLIAM D. WHITE

Reprinted with permission of the Blue Cross Association, from *Inquiry*, Vol. XVI, No. 2 (Spring 1979), pp. 50-61. Copyright © 1979 by the Blue Cross Association. All rights reserved.

The American hospital industry is dominated by nonprofit institutions. Nonetheless, there exists a small number of forprofit hospitals.[1] These hospitals presumably maximize profits. The motives of nonprofit hospitals are not completely clear. Traditionally they have enjoyed a quasi-public utility status and, at least in theory, pursue socially desirable goals such as providing care to patients who cannot afford to pay for hospital services. The literature on the behavior of nonprofit hospitals suggests that size and status considerations and the welfare of staff physicians also may play an important role in determining the actions of these institutions.[2] However, even if nonprofit hospitals may not always try to maximize social welfare, they have played an important historical role in activities like providing subsidized care for the needy. In contrast, forprofit hospitals usually avoid providing any subsidized care unless they are forced into it by social and political constraints.[3]

To the extent that nonprofit hospitals seek objectives other than that of profit maximization, they may adopt pricing and investment policies that make them potentially vulnerable to competition from forprofit hospitals. Assuming that they do this for socially desirable reasons, this raises a basic public policy question. Should the government protect nonprofit hospitals from this kind of competition by regulating the pricing and investment behavior of forprofit hospitals?

For many years, the number of forprofit hospitals was declining in the United States and the question of regulating them did not seem like a particularly important issue. But during the last ten years, there has been a rapid growth in forprofit hospital chains, while public and private subsidies to nonprofit hospitals, which in the past have tended to give them a competitive advantage over forprofit hospitals, have been declining.[4] Meanwhile, the growth of certificate-of-need regulation, designed to limit new investments in hospital facilities, has forced policy-makers to make choices between permitting forprofit and nonprofit hospitals to expand. As a result, there has been a good deal of debate over the relative merits of the two types of hospitals and their ability to serve the needs of the communities involved.

Unfortunately, arguments in this debate have tended to be fragmented. Most empirical studies look at specific differences between forprofit and nonprofit hospitals in case mix, quality of care, and cost, rather than the impact of forprofit hospitals on the overall welfare of the consumer.[5] Critics of forprofit hospitals focus on quality and equity issues. They complain that these institutions engage in "unfair" competitive practices such as "cream skimming" (admitting patients on a selective basis that reflects their ability to pay and the ease with which they can be treated, rather than their need for medical care). They also argue that forprofit hospitals deliver less sophisticated care than nonprofit hospitals and

William D. White, Ph.D., is Assistant Professor, Department of Economics, University of Illinois at Chicago Circle, Chicago, IL 60680.

Support for this research was provided in part by a grant from the University of Illinois. The views expressed in this paper, however, are those of the author and do not necessarily reflect the position of the University. I am grateful to Carson Bays, Joseph Persky, Brian Wright and members of the Harvard University Health Economics Seminar for comments on earlier drafts of this paper. Any errors which remain, of course, are my own.

may be tempted to lower the quality of services in order to increase their earnings. Supporters of forprofit hospitals emphasize the cost side of the picture and the advantages of free markets. They argue that forprofit hospitals are more efficient than nonprofit hospitals and suggest that increased competition in the industry could keep down the rising cost of hospital care.

Because of this piecemeal approach, it is often easy to lose sight of the underlying issues in the debate and focus on details like differences in case mix. The purpose of this paper is to try to clarify the debate by presenting the main theoretical arguments for regulation of competition by forprofit hospitals on a systematic basis using simple economic models. While a full empirical analysis is beyond the scope of this paper, we will briefly consider the relevance of these arguments to current conditions in the industry and employ this discussion to suggest a number of potentially useful areas for future research.

The discussion that follows is divided into three parts. The first section briefly describes the existing structure of the hospital industry and addresses the prospects for change in the industry. The second section develops models of the behavior of nonprofit hospitals and the possible impact of competition by forprofit hospitals. These models are then used to consider the main theoretical arguments for regulating forprofit hospitals. The section also discusses the relevance of these theoretical arguments under current industry conditions. The final section summarizes our conclusions and suggests areas for future research.

In the models considered in this paper, nonprofit hospitals encounter problems with competition from forprofit hospitals because, for charitable reasons, they voluntarily deviate from profit maximizing behavior. But many of the problems of nonprofit hospitals are analogous to problems encountered with competition in regulated industries where prices are set by the government. Examples include the problems of licensed carriers with unlicensed carriers in various areas of the transportation industry as well as those of the post office with private firms which also wish to carry mail. Economists have long been interested in the problems of setting prices in regulated indus-

tries, and the discussion that follows draws extensively on the marginal cost-pricing literature.[6] At the same time, this paper may provide some insights into the problem of dealing with competition in regulated industries.

Industry Characteristics

Expenditures on hospital services account for nearly half of all expenditures on health in the United States. They have attracted widespread attention not only because of their absolute magnitude, but also because of their rapid rate of increase in price, which is now around 15% a year.

On the supply side of the market for hospital services, individual institutions tend to be small and the industry is highly decentralized. Unlike many public utilities, there is little evidence of economies of scale in hospitals above fairly low-level output, and there is no real argument for regulating them because they are natural monopolies.

On the demand side of the market, equity considerations and insurance arrangements play an important role in determining the demand for hospital services. There is a strong social preference in this country for assuring that some sort of minimum level of hospital services is available to individuals who are seriously ill, regardless of their ability to pay. In the past, most of this type of care was provided directly by public or private nonprofit hospitals in the form of free or subsidized services. More recently, the government has begun to subsidize purchases of medical care directly through programs like Medicare and Medicaid. However, there are a number of gaps in these programs and there are still significant groups in the population who have little or no access to medical care.

Over time, the demand for hospital services can fluctuate a good deal for individuals and for the industry as a whole, and these fluctuations can be difficult to predict. For example, an individual may fall ill at any time, while a natural disaster or a major accident can sharply increase the total demand for hospital services with little or no warning. Since hospital services must be consumed as they are produced and speed is often critical in determin-

Table 1. Ratio of patient revenue to direct costs of selected ancillary services, 1962–68

Year	Revenue/direct-cost ratios						
	Operating room	Delivery room	Anesthesi-ology	Radi-ology	Labora-tory	Physical therapy	Pharmacy
1962	1.43	0.97	1.62	1.37	1.70	1.27	2.12
1966	1.37	0.81	1.50	1.28	1.63	1.28	2.02
1967	1.39	0.95	1.89	1.86	1.98	1.21	2.13
1968	1.37	0.99	1.81	1.60	1.74	1.30	2.01
Average annual:							
1962–66	1.40	0.89	1.55	1.34	1.66	1.26	2.05
1967–68	1.38	0.97	1.85	1.73	1.86	1.26	2.07

Source: Davis, K., "Hospital Costs and the Medicare Program," *Social Security Bulletin* (August 1973), p. 26.

ing the value of these services to consumers, there is a strong incentive to maintain a high level of peak-load capacity in the industry to meet regular fluctuations in demand and unexpected emergencies. Difficulties in predicting demand also create an incentive for individuals to purchase insurance, and approximately 90% of Americans now have some form of hospitalization insurance.

Under existing insurance programs, patients' out-of-pocket expenditures on hospital services tend to be low and they bear only a small part of the total cost. Critics of this system, such as Martin Feldstein, argue that it is largely responsible for the rapid increase in hospital costs because it does not create any incentive for patients to try to hold down hospital expenditures.[7] At the same time, these critics emphasize that many Americans do not have adequate insurance against major medical expenditures and some have no coverage at all. They call for an overhaul of the existing insurance system not only to contain costs, but also for equity reasons. The final outcome of these reform efforts remains to be seen. But it seems likely that some form of comprehensive national health insurance will be introduced in the near future, and this possibility needs to be taken into account in any discussion of regulation in the health sector.

Arguments for Regulation

Forprofit hospitals may be able to expand their market share at the expense of nonprofit hospitals if they can offer patients the same service at a lower price or a higher quality service at the same price. Arguments for reg- ulation focus on three main types of practices that may make this possible: 1) price discrimination; 2) average cost-pricing; 3) not using least-cost techniques because of externalities. There also is a fourth point: Forprofit hospitals may be able to increase their market share if there are lags in the availability of capital to nonprofit hospitals, which do not adjust quickly to increases in the demand for hospital services.

The approach in this section is to discuss the importance of these four problems and examine arguments for regulation for each case in turn. Unfortunately, there has not been much empirical research in most of these areas and so our discussion is necessarily rather theoretical. For simplicity, we assume in this discussion that nonprofit hospitals can be treated as a group.[8] We also assume that forprofit and nonprofit hospitals are equally efficient and that there is no difference in the quality of the services they produce unless specifically stated otherwise.

Price Discrimination

Price discrimination occurs when producers charge different prices to different consumers for the same services. In the health industry this term is also used to refer to cross-subsidization where hospitals charge above cost for some types of services in order to generate profits to subsidize purchases of other types of services sold at below cost. Data in Table 1 suggest that this practice is widespread. As we can see from the table, hospitals have tended to consistently charge more than cost for services such as laboratory tests, operating room services and radiology services, while delivery room services are priced below cost.[9]

There are two main arguments for price discrimination. The first is that price discrimination may increase equity, the second that it may perform a quasi-insurance function. In the equity case, nonprofit hospitals may charge wealthy patients a premium for hospital services and use the profits from these services to subsidize purchases of services by less affluent individuals. For example, private hospital rooms, used mainly by financially better-off patients, may be priced above cost, while beds in wards used primarily by poorer patients may be priced below cost. Alternatively, as Hellenger suggests, hospitals may charge a premium for services such as diagnostic tests that generally tend to be covered by insurance, even for needy patients through programs like Medicare; these profits are then used to subsidize services that usually are not covered, such as obstetrical services.[10]

Now consider the possible impact of competition by forprofit hospitals. If patients who can pay are unwilling to bear the costs of subsidizing poor patients voluntarily, forprofit hospitals may be able to bid these patients away from nonprofit hospitals. One way they can do this is by offering lower prices. But, since most hospital care is paid through insurance, the demand for hospital services tends to be price inelastic. Even so, consumers may still be sensitive to changes in the quality of services. So may the physicians who act as patients' agents. This may encourage forprofit hospitals to compete with nonprofit hospitals by offering higher quality service at the same price, rather than lower prices. Better food, nicer rooms, and better staffing arrangements and technical services are all possible examples of quality improvements that could attract patients or physicians to forprofit hospitals.[11]

If this kind of quality competition occurs, we may not observe any direct price competition. Nevertheless, if forprofit hospitals are successful in attracting patients who have been paying for services at above cost, the only patients who will be left in nonprofit hospitals in this model are those who are either subsidized or who pay for services at cost. Unless funds are available from sources other than those based on price discrimination, non-profit institutions will face two choices: Either they can continue to treat patients who cannot pay and go bankrupt, or they can begin treating only those patients who can pay the full cost of service.

The basic equity argument for regulation in this case is that some patients lack the resources to pay for hospital care and will not receive it unless nonprofit hospitals are able to generate revenues from price discrimination. In many ways, this is similar to the argument often made for expanding regulation in industries where regulation is used as a tax along the lines described by Posner.[12] For example, this kind of argument has been used to justify regulating outside competition in order to allow the post office to do things such as subsidizing rural mail service at the expense of urban patrons. The same argument also has been used to justify protecting regulated airlines and railroads from outside competition where trunk lines are used to subsidize feeder routes.

Based on the experiences of these industries, there are two main ways to use regulation to deal with competition. One is to ban competition completely. This is the approach used by the post office for first class mail. It has the advantage of being easy to administer. But it may not be politically feasible in the hospital industry and could remove a valuable source of innovation. A second approach is to regulate the quality and price of services that are sold by forprofit hospitals. This would allow forprofit hospitals to continue to exist. But it has the disadvantage of being difficult to administer.

Under a system of price regulation, any time the price of hospital services is set above cost, there will be strong competitive pressures for forprofit hospitals to find some way to improve the quality of the services they provide so that they can either attract patients directly from nonprofit hospitals or attract them indirectly by attracting their physicians, thereby making additional profits. Conversely, any time the price of a service is set below cost, there will be strong competitive pressures for forprofit hospitals either to try to avoid offering the service or, if they are forced to offer it, to depreciate the quality of the service they provide so that patients will prefer to go to nonprofit hospitals.

The second argument for protecting price discrimination is that it enables nonprofit hospitals to perform a quasi-insurance function. Rafferty and Schweitzer suggest that nonprofit hospitals may price services so that patients with small expenditures on hospital services help subsidize patients with major illnesses.[13] This kind of price discrimination will tend to reduce the cost of major illness, while increasing the cost of minor illnesses. In effect, it amounts to a form of compulsory insurance, since everyone using these hospitals is forced to participate.

Again, pricing some services above cost and others below cost may lead to a welfare loss as a result of the underutilization or overutilization of services. The argument for price discrimination in this case is that gains from insurance effects exceed any efficiency losses that result from distorting prices. The argument for regulation is that forprofit hospitals will bid away all of the patients with less serious illnesses and nonprofit hospitals will no longer be able to perform this insurance function.

The validity of price discrimination and insurance arguments for regulating competition hinge on the availability of subsidies and insurance from other sources. A comprehensive system of national health insurance would presumably eliminate the need for regulation for equity and insurance reasons, since everyone would already have adequate insurance and be fully protected against financial hardship. In contrast, there seems to have been a strong argument for regulation during the early part of this century when direct subsidies to patients were rare and the insurance system was completely inadequate. The current situation is more difficult to evaluate. Government subsidies have increased sharply and health insurance is now widely available. But as we noted earlier, there are still gaps in the system. The key empirical question is whether nonprofit hospitals currently help fill these gaps and whether their contribution in this area is large enough to merit government intervention.

Average Cost-Pricing

Average cost-pricing occurs when producers set the price of a service equal to the average cost of producing this service. This is the standard method of pricing hospital services and it is built into most insurance reimbursement schemes. For example, the price for a hospital bed is usually set equal to the average cost of keeping a patient in a bed for a day in a hospital.

In a competitive equilibrium, average cost-pricing will have the same effect as marginal cost-pricing if consumers purchase identical services and there is no variation in costs over time. However, average cost-pricing amounts to an implicit form of price discrimination if the cost of producing a service varies either (1) within a given pricing category (i.e., consumers do not receive identical services for the same price), or (2) overtime. We can illustrate the first type of implicit price discrimination by considering the case where there is a heterogeneous patient population in a hospital.

There is no nationally accepted scheme of classifying patients by the amount of care they need. But existing studies in this area suggest that there is a good deal of variation in the amount of care hospital patients require depending upon how sick they are. For example, staffing models developed for general nursing units by Georgette, Pardee and others suggest that seriously ill patients may require twice as much nursing care as average patients, while other studies suggest that seriously ill patients make up a significant minority of the patient population in hospitals.[14]

There are several different ways in which hospitals could charge for a day in a hospital bed under these conditions. One approach is to monitor services on an individual basis and charge each individual for the cost of the services that they actually receive, including regular nursing services. In this case, seriously ill patients may end up paying considerably more than patients who are less ill. The second alternative is to use average cost-pricing and charge all patients the average cost per bed of these services. In this case, less ill, low-cost patients will end up subsidizing seriously ill, high-cost patients. This type of implicit price discrimination may result in a welfare loss if it leads low-cost patients to underutilize services and high-cost patients to overutilize them. But average cost-pricing may also increase welfare by significantly reducing monitoring costs, since hospitals need only monitor the total cost of services and the number of patients instead of the cost of providing services to each patient. The net impact on welfare will depend on the magnitude of the two types of effects.

A third type of approach, which is usually not used in hospitals, is to screen patients in advance and charge them on the basis of expected treatment costs. Screening costs are likely to vary with the level of accuracy that is desired and the type of screening. For example, it may be relatively easy for a physician to make a general qualitative judgment about whether or not a case of appendicitis will involve expensive complications. But it may be quite difficult to make a more precise evaluation. It also may be more difficult to arrive at the same kind of judgment using only quantitative data. Since third-party payers may be reluctant to pay for services on the basis of qualitative judgments, this may explain why hospitals do not use screening to set prices directly.

But they may still use it indirectly. Suppose that nonprofit hospitals use average cost-pricing. Forprofit hospitals may be able to engage in "creaming" by using screening to identify low-cost patients and bidding these patients away from nonprofit hospitals while refusing to admit expensive patients. In this case, nonprofit hospitals will be left only with the high-cost patients in each category and this will tend to push up the average cost of treatment in these hospitals. If nonprofit institutions continue to adhere to an average cost-pricing rule, they will be forced to raise prices and the process will begin again. If this process continues indefinitely, nonprofit hospitals will gradually be pushed out of the market and end up with only the most expensive patients in each category.

The most expensive patients in any category also are likely to be the patients with the most complicated illnesses. They will tend to require more sophisticated care than low-cost patients. The relative cost of caring for patients with complicated illnesses in separate facilities compared to the cost of caring for them in facilities with other patients will depend largely on the number of patients involved. In smaller communities, where the absolute number of patients is small, separating care may substantially increase costs. The argument for using regulation to protect nonprofit hospitals from creaming when they use average cost-pricing is that caring for low-cost and high-cost patients in separate facilities is inefficient.

Empirically, two main questions are involved: First, is average cost-pricing in the public interest to begin with, or have nonprofit hospitals and third-party payers simply adopted this system of pricing for their own convenience? Second, assuming that average cost-pricing is desirable for at least some categories of services, is it inefficient to treat high-cost and low-cost patients in separate facilities?

There are not many data on monitoring costs in hospitals. However, monitoring-cost arguments have sometimes been used against marginal cost-pricing in public utilities, where outputs are less complex and easier to measure than in hospitals.[15] The demand for hospital services appears price inelastic and this suggests that efficiency losses from average cost-pricing are probably relatively small. But this may be mainly the result of insurance arrangements. Feldstein suggests that demand might be a good deal more sensitive to prices if there were more coinsurance.[16] In this case, efficiency considerations might be very important. Evidence on economies of scale is not clear, although there does seem to be some positive relationship between the quality of care and the overall size of hospitals.

The cost of patient services can vary with occupancy rates in hospitals as well as with the mix of patients. As we can see from Table 2, monthly occupancy rates may vary substantially over the year. Many hospitals also report significant variations in weekly occupancy rates.[17] Maintaining excess capacity to meet peak loads can be expensive. If hospitals use average cost-pricing, this will spread the costs of maintaining peak-load capacity over the entire patient population. This amounts to a de facto form of price discrimination to the extent that patients who use hospitals in off-peak periods end up subsidizing patients who use services during peak periods. Forprofit hospitals may be able to bid patients away during off-peak periods in this case by operating institutions with no excess capacity at normal levels of demand and by offering lower prices or providing a mix of services that is more attractive to patients or physicians than is the mix offered by nonprofit hospitals.

Assuming that nonprofit hospitals continue to maintain the same amount of excess capacity as they have in the past, this will lead to an increase in the ratio of peak-load capacity to normal capacity in these hospitals during off-peak periods. As a result, average costs will rise in nonprofit hospitals, since they will now have a higher proportion of empty beds during normal periods. If nonprofit hospitals continue to follow an average cost-pricing rule, the industry will tend toward an equilibrium in which nonprofit hospitals provide peak-load services and forprofit hospitals provide normal services.

This type of situation will not necessarily be socially undesirable if the costs of providing peak-load services are independent of the normal level of operation in hospitals (i.e., there are no economies of scale). The argument for regulating forprofit hospitals is that there are in fact significant economies of scale in providing peak-load services in hospitals that also provide off-peak services.

One alternative to regulation is to use peak-load pricing. There is ample literature on peak-load pricing for public utilities which suggests that marginal cost-pricing may be socially more efficient than average cost-pricing. Feldstein and Long specifically consider this kind of problem for hospitals, while Ro suggests that multipart pricing could help shift peak loads in the industry and enable hospitals to make more efficient use of plant and equipment.[18] For example, since demand usually falls during holidays, it might be possible to increase efficiency by offering lower prices during these periods.

However, these gains may be offset by increased monitoring costs. Multipart pricing may be especially expensive to administer if fluctuations in demand cannot be predicted in advance and prices depend on stochastic variables. Furthermore, Dreze argues that some element of price discrimination will be unavoidable if demand is stochastic.[19] This means that nonprofit hospitals may still be vulnerable to competition from forprofit hospitals even if they use marginal cost-pricing. Multi-

Table 2. Monthly occupancy rates for community hospitals by bed size: 1977

Bed size	Average monthly occupancy rate for year (%)	Range in monthly occupancy rates during year (%)
Under 50	43.8	37.7–51.7
50–74	54.2	50.3–60.9
75–99	64.4	61.5–71.1
100–149	70.6	65.4–75.4
150–199	76.9	71.3–81.6
200–299	77.7	71.1–82.1
300–399	80.4	72.8–84.4
Over 400	80.9	74.0–84.5
Total	74.4	68.4–79.0

Source: National Hospital Panel Survey, American Hospital Association.

part pricing also raises equity issues. The idea of charging patients higher rates because they happen to become ill when a large number of other people are also ill is not very appealing, especially if demand is stochastic.

Unless there is a large stochastic element in demand, it is difficult to defend any pricing system that does not attempt to price services, at least in part, at marginal cost over time. However, if full peak-load pricing is not feasible for either equity or efficiency reasons, a second alternative may be for the government to use tax revenues to subsidize these services. Assuming that peak loads really are a problem this may be more efficient than using regulation to protect average cost-pricing.

Externalities and Quality Issues

Externalities occur when the actions of one individual in a market affect the welfare of others through nonmarket means. A standard example is the treatment of infectious diseases. If someone with an infectious disease goes to a hospital for treatment, that person will gain if treatment improves his or her own health status. At the same time, society as a whole may benefit if treatment limits the spread of disease to the rest of the population. These social benefits are an externality in the sense that while they are the result of a market transaction (an individual purchases medical services for his own benefit), they are not traded in the market. Precisely because they are not traded, the welfare impact of externalities may be difficult to measure because we cannot observe a price for them, although we may be able to make indirect inferences using cost-benefit analysis.

Hospital services may generate externalities in two ways: First, there may be externalities associated with the consumption of hospital services. For example, there are a number of studies in the public health literature that suggest there may be significant externalities from the treatment of infectious diseases along the lines we have just described. Second, there may be externalities from the process involved in producing hospital services in a nonprofit setting independent of any externalities from the consumption of these services per se.

In their discussions of nonprofit hospitals, Titmuss and others suggest that the act of giving for nonpecuniary motives may have a social value that is difficult to capture in market terms.[20] Underlying this view is the concept that society is ultimately a corporate venture based upon mutual cooperation and trust between individuals, rather than upon competition. Markets may increase efficiency, but they may also destroy the fabric of society by undermining socially symbolic acts that provide the means for individuals to reaffirm their participation in the social order.

Titmuss calls this kind of interaction "the gift relationship." He focuses on blood donations in his analysis of this type of relationship.[21] A direct nonmarket transfer of this sort is unusual in most other areas of the hospital. But his arguments suggest that there still may be important externalities involved in using and participating in maintaining voluntary institutions that do not occur when health care is provided in forprofit institutions. For example, there may be a much greater sense of community participation if care is produced in nonprofit hospitals than in forprofit hospitals.

We can begin our discussion of arguments for regulation by considering externalities from the consumption of hospital services. If there are externalities from subsidizing certain services, nonprofit hospitals may increase welfare by using price discrimination to finance the production of these services by charging prices above cost for services that do not involve externalities. The argument for this type of behavior is that gains from externalities outweigh any efficiency losses from

distorting prices. The argument for regulation contends that competition from forprofit hospitals makes it impossible for nonprofit hospitals to engage in this kind of activity. The main argument against regulation here is that it may be more efficient for the government to directly subsidize the production of services which result in externalities, as in fact is often done with programs like venereal disease clinics.

Turning to arguments for regulation where there are externalities from producing hospital services in a nonprofit setting, critics of nonprofit hospitals have often suggested that they are more expensive than forprofit hospitals. If this is true, nonprofit hospitals ultimately may not be able to compete with forprofits in the open market even though the social benefits of using nonprofit institutions outweigh the added costs. Therefore, it may be desirable either to regulate competition by forprofit hospitals or to subsidize nonprofits. The main empirical questions here are whether there really are important externalities from using nonprofit hospitals and the extent to which forprofit hospitals are less costly than nonprofit hospitals.

Even in the absence of externalities, critics of forprofit hospitals suggest that any apparent differences in efficiency between forprofit and nonprofit hospitals may be illusionary because of differences in the quality of services they provide. They note that forprofit hospitals have an incentive to reduce the quality of services if such action increases profits. They may be able to get away with this if quality changes are very difficult for consumers to detect because of the complexity of medical services and the high level of uncertainty about the outcomes of many of these services. In theory, consumers should be able to rely on their physicians to evaluate the quality of these services for them. However, if these physicians own stock in forprofit hospitals, this may bias their judgment. Even if they do not, hospital managers may be able to put pressure on them if physicians are employees or value their admitting privileges at forprofit hospitals. Therefore, another reason for regulating forprofit hospitals is to protect consumers against these types of abuses that can develop within the doctor-patient relationship.

Under a comprehensive system of national health insurance, it would presumably be possible to subsidize nonprofit hospitals if there really are significant externalities from the gift relationship. Nonetheless, abuses of the doctor-patient relationship do not seem very amenable to taxes or subsidies. If they are indeed a serious problem, regulation may be the only solution available. In this context, it is interesting to note that many of the issues discussed here about externalities and abuses of the agent relationship are also important in the education industry where, historically, there have been strong objections to forprofit institutions.

Adjustment Lags

Problems with adjustment lags can occur if forprofit hospitals adjust more rapidly than nonprofit hospitals to increases in the demand for hospital services. Traditionally, nonprofit hospitals have received large capital subsidies from public and private sources. These subsidies reduce capital costs and may give nonprofit hospitals a competitive advantage over forprofit hospitals. But they also may reduce flexibility, since it can be difficult to generate capital quickly from these sources. As a result, there may be significant lags before nonprofit hospitals respond to increases in demand, which Pauly estimates may be as long as four to eight years.[22]

Adjustment lags may create excess demand at existing price levels. Rafferty suggests that the usual response by nonprofit hospitals to this situation is to ration services by need, rather than by price, and to hold prices at existing levels.[23] Patients with more urgent problems are usually given preference over those with problems where treatment can be deferred. The result is that queues may form for services such as elective surgery.

This may create a large potential market for the services of forprofit hospitals. These hospitals may be able to enter the market for hospital services by providing care to patients who have been forced to wait in queues. If the response of forprofits to increases in demand is more rapid than the response of nonprofit hospitals, new capacity in the industry will take the form mainly of forprofit hospitals specializing in the treatment of paying patients

with less urgent problems. Patients with serious illnesses that require more sophisticated care, as well as those who cannot pay, will end up concentrated in nonprofit hospitals.

There is little direct evidence on the investment behavior of forprofit hospitals. But Steinwald and Neuhauser found that forprofit hospitals tend to concentrate in areas where there has been rapid growth in population and income.[24] Both variables are closely associated with increases in the total demand for hospital services and this tends to support the hypothesis that forprofit hospitals can respond more quickly to changes in demand than can nonprofits. At the same time, studies by Schweitzer and Rafferty and others have found that forprofit hospitals on average admit patients who need a less capital-intensive mix of services than patients in nonprofit hospitals.[25] This supports the hypothesis that forprofit hospitals tend to treat patients with less complicated illnesses, although it is not clear from the data whether the needs of these patients are less urgent than those of patients treated in nonprofit hospitals.

From an efficiency standpoint, investments in forprofit hospitals as a result of lags in the response time of nonprofit hospitals are undesirable if this kind of investment pattern increases the long-run cost of medical care. If forprofit hospitals are oriented toward paying patients with uncomplicated illnesses, they may invest in more comfortable, but smaller and less sophisticated facilities than nonprofit hospitals. Once this capacity is in place, it may be difficult to alter. Even if forprofit hospitals eventually convert to nonprofit status, the original investment decisions made by these institutions could shape the organization of the industry in a given area for years to come, especially if certificate-of-need legislation limits total investments in the industry.[26]

On the other hand, if forprofit hospitals can adjust more quickly to changes in demand than nonprofit hospitals, restrictions on forprofit institutions may result in longer waiting times for care for less seriously ill patients. While longer waiting times may not endanger patients' lives, longer waits may still add significantly to the pain and suffering associated with illnesses, a welfare loss that should not be overlooked.

Because of certificate-of-need legislation, the issue of whether to regulate hospital investments is largely academic. The question is whether or not regulators should limit new investments to nonprofit hospitals. The basic argument for this policy is that the short-run gains from permitting investments in forprofit facilities are less important than the long-run losses in efficiency that may result from this type of investment. An additional argument contends that a rapid increase in the number of forprofit hospitals may create a financial crisis for nonprofit hospitals if they have traditionally depended on price discrimination to finance things such as free care and peak-load capacity. This may result in a good deal of temporary disruption in the industry that may not be worth the trouble. If investment lags are really a problem for nonprofit hospitals, it may be much easier to try to improve capital markets for these institutions than to endeavor to make all the other sorts of adjustments that may be necessary if forprofit firms are allowed to enter the market. In practice, however, these types of problems seem to be largely a thing of the past. Nonprofit hospitals now have much better access to regular captial markets and enjoy far more flexibility than formerly.

Conclusions

The purpose of this paper has been to present arguments for regulation of competition by forprofit hospitals on a systematic basis and to briefly consider the implications of these arguments in light of industry conditions. The theoretical analysis suggests that it may be in the public interest to regulate competition by forprofit hospitals if nonprofit hospitals: 1) engage in price discrimination; 2) engage in average cost-pricing; 3) do not use least-cost methods of producing services for socially desirable reasons, or 4) if there are lags in the speed with which nonprofit hospitals adjust to increases in demand.

Based on this analysis, an extreme free market position (i.e., that regulation will never increase welfare) is clearly not justified a priori on theoretical grounds. However, it is also clear from our discussion that regulation of competition by forprofit hospitals will not nec-

essarily always be socially desirable. Simply because forprofit hospitals are able to increase their market share at the expense of nonprofit hospitals is not sufficient evidence that regulation is needed. For example, success of forprofit hospitals may simply reflect lax management practices by nonprofit hospitals. The impact of regulation in any given case will depend on the way in which nonprofit hospitals actually behave, on other government policies, and on market conditions.

Given this discussion, how relevant are the arguments considered in this paper for public policy in light of conditions in the industry? No attempt has been made here to carry out a full empirical analysis. But the previous section suggests several general conclusions and points up a number of areas where further research is badly needed.

Specifically, it appears on one hand that in the past there have been strong arguments for regulation because of equity considerations and problems with inadequate insurance and capital markets. On the other hand, a comprehensive system of national health insurance would probably eliminate equity problems and provide a vehicle for dealing with efficiency problems involving average cost-pricing and peak loads. In this case, the only real arguments for regulation that would remain are those involving externalities and the possible impact of competition by forprofit hospitals on the relationships between communities and hospitals and between doctors and patients.

Under current conditions, the need for regulation seems problematic. Health insurance is now widely available and government programs have reduced equity problems. But large gaps still exist in the system and nonprofit hospitals may play an important role in filling these gaps. In addition, competition by forprofit hospitals may also create problems because of externalities and the current system of average cost-pricing. As a result, it may be possible that more regulation could increase welfare.

But these issues clearly need further study. A large number of important empirical questions remain unresolved. For example, how important is price discrimination in financing care for patients who cannot pay under the current system? How large are rationing costs in the industry? Are there really serious problems with peak loads? Is there any evidence of the importance of the gift relationship in determining the behavior of nonprofit hospitals? These questions are not easy to answer. But answering them would provide a much better basis for evaluating arguments for regulation of forprofit hospitals. And even in the absence of problems with forprofit hospitals, these questions raise issues that may be important to consider if we are interested in increasing the overall efficiency of the industry and providing a more equitable system of health care delivery.

References and Notes

1 In 1974, 87% of all nonfederal general hospitals in the United States were nonprofit institutions and these hospitals accounted for 95% of all hospital assets. Only 13% of all nonfederal general hospitals were forprofit institutions and they controlled only 5% of all hospital assets.

2 See Davis, K. "Economic Theories of Behavior in Nonprofit Private Hospitals," *Economic and Business Bulletin* (Winter 1972); Harris, J. "The Internal Organization of Hospitals: Some Economic Implications," *Bell Journal of Economics*, 8:2 (Autumn 1977); Newhouse, J. "Toward a Theory of Nonprofit Institutions: An Economic Model of a Hospital," *American Economic Review* (March 1970); Pauly, M. and Redisch, M. "The Not-For-Profit Hospital as a Physicians' Cooperative," *American Economic Review* (March 1973).

3 If a forprofit hospital is the only hospital in town, social and political constraints may well force it to behave like a nonprofit hospital.

4 For example, the Hill-Burton program was recently eliminated, while third-party payers have recently begun to at least partly reimburse forprofit hospitals, as well as nonprofit hospitals, for capital costs.

5 See Bays, C. "Relative Costs and Efficiency in Private Short-Term General Hospitals," unpublished Ph.D. thesis, Department of Economics, University of Michigan, 1975; Rafferty, J. and Schweitzer, S. "Comparison of Forprofit and Nonprofit Hospitals: A Re-evaluation," *Inquiry* (December 1974); Ruchlin, H., Pointer, D. and Cannedy, L. "A Comparison of Forprofit Investor-Owned Chain and Nonprofit Hospitals, *Inquiry* (December 1973); Steinwald, B. and Neuhauser, D. "The Role of the Proprietary Hospital," *Law and Contemporary Problems* (Autumn 1970).

6 For reviews of the marginal cost-pricing literature, see Dreze, J. "Some Postwar Contributions of French Economists," *American Economic Review* (June 1964, Part 2); Farrel, M. "In Defense of Public Utility Price Theory," in Turvey, R. (ed.) *Public Enterprise* (New York: Penguin Books, 1968); Joskow, P. L. "Contributions to the Theory of Marginal Cost Pricing," *The Bell Journal of Economics* (Spring 1976).

7 Feldstein, M. "The High Cost of Hospitals and What to Do About It," *The Public Interest* (Summer 1977).

8 If the motives of nonprofit hospitals vary from hospital to hospital, it is possible that some nonprofit hospitals may engage in the same kind of practices attributed to forprofit hospitals. For example, private nonprofit hospitals in large urban areas are often accused of "dumping" a large share of their nonpaying patients on public nonprofit institutions, especially in cases where these patients are not interesting for research purposes.

9 For a general discussion of this type of behavior, see Joseph, H. "On Interdepartment Pricing of Not-For-Profit Hospitals," *Quarterly Review on Economics and Business* (Spring 1976).

10 Hellinger, F. "Hospital Charges and Medicare Reimbursement," *Inquiry* (December 1975).

11 Direct evidence of quality competition is difficult to obtain. But some studies do suggest that holding case mix fixed, forprofit hospitals tend to use more capital intensive methods of treating patients than nonprofit hospitals. See Bays, op. cit.; Schweitzer, S. and Rafferty, J. "Variations in Hospital Product: A Comparative Analysis of Proprietary and Voluntary Hospitals," *Inquiry* (June 1976).

12 Posner, R. "Taxation by Regulation," *The Bell Journal of Economics* (Spring 1971).

13 Rafferty and Schweitzer, op. cit.

14 Georgette, J. "Staffing by Patient Classification," *Nursing Clinics of North America* (June 1970); Pardee, G. "Classifying Patients to Predict Staff Requirements," *American Journal of Nursing* (March 1968). Also see Aydelotte, M. *Nurse Staffing Methodology: A Review and Critique of Selected Literature*, Division of Nursing, U.S. Public Health Service, DHEW No. (NI) 73-433 (January 1973).

15 Joskow, op. cit.

16 Feldstein, M. "The Welfare Loss of Excess Health Insurance," *Journal of Political Economy* (March/April 1973).

17 Typically, hospital occupancy rates tend to decline on weekends, at least in part because of the preferences of hospital staffs and physicians.

18 Long, M. and Feldstein, P. "Economics of Hospital Systems: Peak Loads and Regional Coordination," *American Economic Review* (May 1967); Ro, K. "Incremental Pricing Would Increase Efficiency in Hospitals," *Inquiry* (March 1969).

19 Dreze, op. cit.

20 Titmuss, R. *The Gift Relationship: From Human Blood to Social Policy* (New York: Harper and Row, 1972).

21 Titmuss, R. ibid, also suggests that markets may provide incentives for supplying low-quality blood. This conclusion is questioned by Sapolsky, J. and Finklestein, S. "Blood Policy Revisited: A New Look at the 'Gift Relationship,'" *The Public Interest* (Winter

1977). However, this is a separate issue from whether or not there are externalities from the gift relationship itself.

22 Pauly, M. "Hospital Capital Investment: The Role of Demand, Profits and Physicians," *The Journal of Human Resources* (Winter 1974).

23 Rafferty, J. "Patterns of Hospital Use: An Analysis of Short-Run Variations," *Journal of Political Economy* (January/February 1971).

24 Steinwald and Neuhauser, op. cit.

25 Schweitzer and Rafferty, op. cit.

26 Of course, nonprofit hospitals may not invest in an optimal fashion either, in which case some general kind of system of planning may be desirable. In this event, there will be no special reason for excluding forprofit hospitals as long as they are willing to produce the kinds of services that planners think are needed.

29. Evaluation of Alternative Payment Strategies for Hospitals: A Conceptual Approach

WILLIAM O. CLEVERLEY

Reprinted with permission of the Blue Cross Association, from *Inquiry*, Vol. XVI No. 1 (Summer 1979), pp. 108-118. Copyright © 1979 by the Blue Cross Association. All rights reserved.

A paragraph from Lewis Carroll's *Alice in Wonderland* aptly illustrates the focus of this paper:

"Would you tell me, please, which way I ought to go from here?" asked Alice. "That depends a good deal on where you want to go to," said the Cat. "I don't much care where," said Alice. "Then it doesn't matter which way you go," said the Cat.

It appears as though Alice and the design of payment systems in the health care industry have much in common. I'm not certain that any of the conceptual or empirical pieces on health care payment have really specified all of the criteria that should be used in evaluating which form of reimbursement or rate-setting model should be adopted. Most of the empirical studies have focused on cost, either predominantly or exclusively.[1] While cost certainly is a criterion of prime importance, it is not the only one. Nor is cost a one-dimensional standard; there are a number of constituent elements that are affected differentially by alternative reimbursement systems.[2]

In the following sections of this paper, a number of criteria useful for evaluating alternative payment systems for health care institutional providers will be posited. These criteria then will be used to analyze and evaluate alternative payment systems. It should be emphasized that the analysis of criterion attainment and the weighting of individual criteria are author-specific. Other analysts might reach different conclusions.

Criteria for Evaluating the Effectiveness of Payment Systems

In the selection of a payment system appropriate for the health care industry, the first step must be to develop desired outcomes and/or criteria. Alternative payment systems then can be evaluated on the basis of how well they attain the stated criteria. A review of the literature in the health care field suggests that a payment system should try to achieve the following objectives:[3-5]

1 Promote the efficient production of services by providers;
2 Provide a level of reimbursement to providers that will maintain their viability;
3 Require minimal administrative cost;
4 Provide for equitable reimbursement payments from multiple purchasers.

Efficient Production of Services

The rising costs of health care—especially hospital services—have been well documented in the health care literature. No additional elaboration of this point will be made here, other than to add that many individuals have concluded that a major determinant of increased hospital costs has been inefficiency in the production of hospital services.

While it may be true that health services are produced inefficiently, it seems relevant to ask: What is the relationship between payment systems and efficiency? Specifically,

William O. Cleverley, Ph.D., is Associate Professor, Graduate Program in Hospital and Health Services Administration, and Accounting, Ohio State University, Columbus, OH 43210.

does the existing system of reimbursement promote inefficiency in the health care industry? In a 1970 study, Pauly related the incentives for efficiency in the production of health services to alternative types of reimbursement.[6] In his analysis, he dealt with four dimensions of efficiency that pertain to this discussion:

1 Technical efficiency;
2 Optimal input combinations;
3 Economies of scale;
4 Optimal quantities of outputs.

In addition, we shall consider a fifth dimension mentioned by Dowling in 1974:

5 Minimum prices paid for inputs.

A discussion of the five points follows:

1 Without using economic jargon, technical efficiency simply means obtaining the maximum amount of output for a given physical level of input. Present-day retrospective cost reimbursement is believed by many to contribute to this type of inefficiency. Little incentive exists for minimizing the physical amounts of labor and capital employed in the production of services. In support of this argument, an example often cited is the wide variation in per diem costs among hospitals. This evidence is limited by the incomparability of per diem costs across institutions because of underlying differences of output. In an article published in 1974, however, Fox concluded that significant and unexplainable variation in man-hours per unit of output existed in homogeneous departments (nuclear medicine, obstetrics and emergency) across institutions.[7] A limited analysis of hospital administrative services departmental cost reports corroborates the conclusions reached in the Fox study. It is thus highly probable that technical inefficiency does exist in the health care industry and is at least partly related to the current method of payment.
2 Optimal combinations of inputs mean that inputs will be combined to produce the desired output at the lowest possible cost. For this consideration to be relevant, the production process must allow the substitution of one input for another. In most cases, economists simplify this discussion by as-

suming two inputs, capital and labor. Retrospective cost reimbursement may artificially raise the price of capital to a hospital because reimbursement is limited to historical cost depreciation.[8,9] This situation might induce hospitals to substitute labor for capital in a less than optimal manner, which is especially true for capital investments that are of a cost-saving nature.
3 In a 1970 article, Pauly classified economies of scale questions within two major dimensions.[10] The first deals with the duplication of specialized facilities, such as open heart units or nuclear medical facilities. It is widely believed that many unnecessary facilities currently exist in the hospital industry. Retrospective cost reimbursement has been blamed partly for this situation because it does not limit payment to needed facilities. Section 221 of PL 92-603 was enacted because of this perceived problem. Federal payment is now denied to new hospital programs or services that have not been approved by planning agencies. Presumably, the organizational networks created under PL 93-641 will continue and expand this activity.

The second dimension involves the appropriateness of the overall size of the institution. Berki has summarized the major findings of many econometric studies in this area.[11] Unfortunately, there is no consensus concerning the existence of economies of scale, let alone their significance. From this research, it appears that more meaningful economy of scale questions might be raised at the departmental or service level, where variation of output is not as great.
4 The optimal quantities issue also has several dimensions. First, at the total health care system level, optimal quantities of output must be produced within the various industries. Cost-minimizing substitutions must be made between inpatient acute care hospital services and inpatient skilled nursing services, between inpatient and outpatient services, and between preventive and curative care. Second, at the individual institutional level, the optimal amounts and mix of institutional services must be provided. Trade-offs between diagnostic tests and length of stay must be explored and exploited.

In most cases the consumption of health services is a decision made by the patient's physician. The importance of financial incentives, which are present in a payment system, in affecting those decisions is open to debate. Professional standards review organizations (PSROs) could have a profound effect on the importance of payment incentives in this area in the future.

5 The last area of economic efficiency deals with reasonableness of input prices. Economic theory would suggest that retrospective cost reimbursement would significantly reduce the importance of purchasing inputs at the lowest possible price. To the best of our knowledge, there is one piece of empirical research that supports this hypothesis. Emery and Halonen discovered that hospitals paid significantly higher rates of interest on borrowed funds than did comparable institutions.[12] Rumors of wide variations in prices paid for pharmaceutical items by hospitals also support the hypothesis.

Viability to Providers

A reasonable objective of any payment system should be to produce sufficient funds to allow the institution to continue to provide services. Obviously, the funds provided should be neither too little nor too much.

Failure to produce adequate funds will seriously threaten the viability of the institution. Several outcomes are possible in these circumstances. First, the institution may close its doors as a result of insufficient funds. Second, it may change its organizational structure. Specifically, the institution may change from a private to a publicly owned and operated institution. Third, it may reduce the quality and scope of services it renders. All of these outcomes may be undesirable.

At the same time, the provision of excessive funds to health care institutions is undesirable. Excessive funds are those monies paid in excess of an amount that an efficient provider of services would require to produce the same set of services. Thus, excessive transfers of funds to the health care sector will curtail both the production and consumption of goods and services in other industries.

Ideally, reimbursement should be sufficient to provide for the allowable financial requirements necessary to produce needed health care services. The American Hospital Association classified financial requirements into the following categories:[13]

A Current operating needs related to patient care:
  Direct Patient care;
  Interest;
  Educational programs;
  Research programs;
  Credit losses;
  Patients unable to pay.

B Capital needs:
  Plant capital;
    preservation and replacement;
    improvement;
    expansion;
    amortization of indebtedness;
  Operating cash needs;
  Return on investment (forprofit facilities).

Determining the financial requirements for an institution is not a difficult task, given the existing systems of accounting. In general, determining financial requirements would involve using information contained in the statement of changes in financial position, which is a readily available financial statement.

The issue of allowability, critical to the discussion of the viability criterion, is more difficult. Major reimbursement battles will be fought in this area. For example, the implementation of Section 223 of PL 92-603 serves to support this observation. For the first time, the Social Security Administration has placed ceilings on the payment of routine nursing costs. The intent is to limit costs to those required by an efficient producer of services. Thus, the level of viable payment is related to the issue of efficiency.

Administrative Costs

Another desirable objective for a payment system should be a modest level of administrative cost. This cost should encompass providers, purchasers and any other parties involved in the payment or rate-setting process.

Equity to Purchaser

Payments by purchasers should be equitable in a relative sense. This implies that one class of purchasers should not pay different amounts for identical services, assuming no underlying justification exists for those differences. The major current controversy over rates paid by cost payers (largely Medicare, Medicaid and Blue Cross Plans) and rates paid by charge payers (largely self-pay and commercial insurance) stems directly from this equity issue. Uniformity of rates will not solve this relative equity issue completely. In addition, uniformity of markups across individual services is essential. Profits earned in laboratory or radiology should not be used to subsidize other operations. This is necessary because purchasers would still be treated inequitably with differing service markups, unless all purchasers used the same relative amounts of service, e.g., a Blue Cross Plan purchases 30% of the service in each final service center.

Rate-Setting Models

This section will discuss recommendations or goals for establishing rates in the health care industry. The logic of these recommendations is based upon the relative attainment of the desired payment system outcomes specified in the foregoing section. To discuss the desirability of alternative rate-setting models, the following dimensions in the rate-setting process will be discussed:

1 Temporal:
   Retrospective;
   Prospective.
2 Rate basis:
   Cost;
   Noncost.
3 Payment unit:
   Total institution budget;
   Departmental budgets;
   Capitation;
   Case;
   Day;
   Specific services.

Temporal Basis

Efficiency. One of the major advantages cited for prospective as opposed to retrospective rate-setting is the presumed incentive provided for efficient operations. The underlying hypothesis for this expectation is that hospitals,

both proprietary and nonproprietary, are motivated by profit or surplus. To the extent, therefore, that only some hospitals are motivated by profit and no hospital is motivated to make negative profit, efficiency improvement is a reasonable expectation. Prospective rate-setting should motivate some hospitals to be more efficient producers of services; it should not motivate any hospital to be less efficient.

Research in the area of differences between forprofit and nonprofit hospitals appears to substantiate this point.[14,15] A commonly held view is that the forprofit hospital has lower costs because of its profit motivation. Earlier research studies, however, do not prove that proprietary hospitals have lower costs. The rationale for this finding could be related directly to current methods of retrospective cost reimbursement, which do not equate cost minimization with profit maximization.

The specific areas of efficiency that may be improved by prospective rate-setting are critical to this discussion. First, if the issue of economies of scale is limited to duplicated facilities, then prospective rate-setting provides no real additional motivation within the current regulatory environment. Presumably, control over capital expenditures already exists and would not be materially affected by prospective rate-setting. This observation is based on the assumed effectiveness of existing capital expenditure regulation. Such effectiveness has not, however, been established to date.[16] Second, the mere existence of prospective rate-setting does not imply an improvement in the quantities of outputs that are produced. Even if one assumes that an institutional manager has some control over the level and composition of output, the nature of the payment unit is more important than the temporal dimension of the rate-setting process. This dimension will be discussed subsequently.

Given the preceding discussion, improvements in efficiency that result from prospective rate-setting are limited in the main to improvements in technical efficiency, input combinations, or reductions in input prices. The realization of savings in these three areas largely determines the advantage that prospective rate-setting would have over retrospective rate-setting.

It should be pointed out that retrospective rate-setting may provide incentives for improving efficiency. Lampiris has noted that in situations where cost reimbursement is less than 100 percent, some potential improvement in profit is possible relative to the reductions in cost.[17] The corporate income tax rate is analogous to the proportion of cost reimbursement in this situation. In a study published in 1978, Lave et al. noted that a retrospective cost-reimbursement system, containing periodic rewards or penalties for efficient and inefficient performance, also might provide efficiency incentives.[18] In the specific case they studied, the incentive payment was based upon the retrospective actual performance of an institution relative to the retrospective actual performance of a comparable group of institutions.

All additional factors being equal, prospective rate-setting would appear more desirable than retrospective rate-setting in promoting efficiency. Because of its very nature, retrospective rate-setting is affected by measures of actual performance. Thus the amount of surplus to be earned is not as directly affected by reductions in cost as would be possible with prospective rate-setting. In addition, it is possible with prospective rate-setting to provide control over the types and amounts of expenditures made, in advance of their actual incurrence. This degree of control has been the primary motivation for capital expenditure regulation in the health care industry. Prospective rate-setting provides a mechanism for the extension of this control to all expenditures, both capital and operating.

Viability. One of the primary outcomes of prospective rate-setting is the shifting of risk from third-party payers to hospitals. This transfer of risk likely would increase the probability of failure, especially in the short run. The condition could be moderated by action, such as establishing initial high rates, allowing liberal retrospective adjustments, or reimbursing the maximum of costs or the prospectively set rates. In each case, the improvement in viability is likely to reduce the incentive for efficiency.

Analyzing this trade-off, it seems that more would be gained by prospective rate-setting in terms of improved efficiency than might be lost in terms of impaired viability. There are at least two reasons for such an assumption:

One, the present retrospective system of cost reimbursement is not conducive to long-run financial viability. Berman and Weeks and Lemer and Willman have discussed the current inadequacies of present-day retrospective cost reimbursement to meet the financial requirements of hospitals.[19,20] In sum, retrospective cost reimbursement does not provide for the expansion and replacement of capital. As a result, many hospitals have relied increasingly upon debt financing, which raises the prospect of future financial failure. Thus, while prospective rate-setting may very well present some increased risks for hospitals, it also may provide an opportunity for long-run survival not possible at present.

Two, the possible results of failure do not appear to be completely deleterious, assuming that the prospective rates established are sufficient to permit efficient production. The major risk is that an institution that provides needed services will fail. But the outcome of the failure may not be disastrous. It is possible that if the need for such services is real, the public sector will step in and provide those services either with or without some form of external subsidy. Alternatively, a private organization also may begin to deliver those services if they can be provided within the established rate limitations. In short, the risk of losing essential services that might accompany prospective rate-setting does not appear excessive.

Administrative cost. Prospective rate-setting probably would require greater administrative costs than retrospective rate-setting.[21] This difference results from the larger volume of information required for prospective rate-setting, as well as from the increased complexity in information processing that would be needed.

Prospective rate-setting probably would utilize both retrospective and prospective data in the decision-making process. At the institutional level, this certainly would be true. Sound budgeting would be essential to fiscal viability if revenues were relatively fixed and unrelated to actual cost. The increased burden at the institutional level, however, may pay dividends in terms of improved efficiency. The prospective rate-setting body also would re-quire prospective, and possibly retrospective, data. Administrative costs for the total system could be minimized if prospective information needed by the rate-setting organization could be taken directly from existing institutional budgets. This implies a need for uniform ac-counting and reporting.

Processing prospective data also is likely to be more costly than the processing of retro-spective data. The concern is more important for the rate-setting organization than for the institution where offsetting benefits are likely to occur. Intelligent utilization of prospective data requires highly competent individuals who can question forecast assumptions and methodology. The ability of rate-setting or-ganizations to attract these individuals is im-portant to the effectiveness of prospective rate-setting.

Equity to purchasers. The concept of equity to purchasers has at least two separate re-quirements, as discussed earlier. First, all pur-chasers must pay the same rate for identical services. This would eliminate differential pricing by cost-paying purchasers, such as Medicare and Medicaid. Second, all services must be priced equitably. In other words, the profit margins must be uniform for all ser-vices. This would eliminate subsidization of some services, such as obstetrics, with profit generated in other services, such as labora-tory.

Both equity requirements are related more directly to the payment unit and rate basis di-mension than to the temporal dimension of rate-setting. There is no reason why prospec-tive rates could not be as equitable as retro-spective rates.

Recommendation. Referring to Table 1, the potential improvement in efficiency possible with prospective rate-setting exceeds any im-pairment in viability or increased administra-tive costs that might be associated with it. Based on these criteria and weights, therefore, prospective payment systems are recommend-ed.

Rate Basis

Efficiency. At this juncture, it will be assumed that the alternative rate-setting models to be evaluated are prospective cost models and prospective noncost models. Prospective cost models would explicitly incorporate various measures of cost in the rate-setting process. These measures might include prior measures of actual institutional costs, budgeted mea-sures of institutional costs, normative mea-sures of cost based on peer group cost data or engineering studies, or some combination of all of the above cost categories. The major outcome would be a relationship between rates and costs that reflects either what actual costs are likely to be or what they should be in the production of services. Prospective noncost models would not explicitly incorpo-rate measures of cost in the rate-setting pro-cess. The most likely noncost base would be charges. Rates of payment might be based on projected charges adjusted by inflation screens, prior charges, or peer group charges. While using charges as the rate basis may produce a relationship between costs and rates, there is no guarantee that such a relationship could, in fact, exist.

Selecting one of these models on the basis of expected improvements in efficiency is dif-ficult. In general, incentives for efficiency in prospective rate-setting models are not affect-ed by alternative rate bases, at least not in the short run. Given the existence of a fixed-rev-enue schedule that is unrelated to actual costs, a surplus maximizing manager will try to im-prove his operating efficiency on all fronts.

If revenue is perceived by a health services manager to be related to actual cost, the in-centives for efficiency may be reduced signif-icantly. This may occur for several reasons. First, rates may be adjusted retrospectively for changes in actual cost. These retrospective adjustments remove much of the incentive for improving efficiency made possible by pro-spective rates. Second, prospective rates may be related directly to prior year actual costs. For example, the Economic Stabilization Pro-gram and the current New York State Cost Control Program both set allowed rates on the basis of prior costs. Elsewhere, Worthington has provided empirical support for this behav-ior in the New Jersey prospective reimburse-ment plan.[22] These types of programs reduce the incentive for long-run cost control because the allowed cost base would be larger for an

Table 1. Attainment of reimbursement objectives by alternative rate-setting models

	Reimbursement objectives									
	Efficiency						Admin-	Pur-	Weight-	
Rate-setting models	Tech- nical	Input combi- nations	Scale	Output combi- nations	Input prices	Via- bility	istra- tive cost	chaser equity	ed value*	Recommen- dation
Temporal Prospective	2	2	0	0	2	-2	-1	0	3	Prospective
Retrospective	-2	-2	0	0	-2	2	1	0	-3	
Basis Cost	0	0	0	0	0	2	-2	2	2	Cost
Noncost	0	0	0	0	0	-2	2	-2	-2	
Payment unit Institution budget	0	0	-1	2	0	-2	2	-2	-1	
Department budget	0	0	1	2	0	2	-2	2	5	
Capitation	0	0	-1	2	0	-2	2	-2	-1	Department budgets
Case	0	0	-1	-2	0	-2	2	-2	-5	
Day	0	0	-1	-2	0	-2	2	-2	-5	
Specific services	0	0	1	-2	0	2	-2	2	1	

Key: 2—Major relative advantage: weight = 2
  1—Slight relative advantage: weight = 1
  0—No relative advantage: weight = 0
  -1—Slight relative disadvantage: weight = -1
  -2—Major relative disadvantage: weight = -2
* Sum of individual criteria values.

inefficient producer than for an efficient producer.

Viability. Viability of any institution depends upon the relationship between revenues and costs or upon financial requirements. Basing revenues on measures unrelated to financial requirements or cost of the institution limits the ability of a rate-setting organization to establish viable rates. Rates, however, should not be based solely on actual costs; instead, they should be predicated upon measures of allowable or normative costs. Rates established on this basis will ensure viability to only a relatively efficient producer. Prospective rates that are predicated on measures of cost, both normative and actual, should promote viability relative to noncost bases.

Administrative costs. The administrative costs of supplying and analyzing data required for prospective cost-based, rate-setting models might appear to be significant. Specifically, the following data sets would be required: prospective statements of financial performance; retrospective statements of financial performance; assurances of data reliability; and normative cost measures.

Technically, only measures of normative costs would be essential if no consideration were given to the viability of the institution. Pragmatically, concern for viability would require the availability of projected and past measures of financial performance. Even during the austere Economic Stabilization Program, institutional viability was an important consideration measured by the cash hardship test.

The costs of providing the first three pieces of information noted above should be relatively low. Hospitals and most other health care organizations either currently provide or should provide all of this information. In fact, an argument might be made for reduced cost. Cohen points out that substantial savings may be realized by reducing the number of financial documents and audits currently required.[23] Rate-setting organizations could reduce administrative costs significantly at the institutional level by utilizing existing financial information systems.

Equity to purchasers. Prospective cost-based rates are more likely to be equitable to purchasers than prospective rates based on measures other than cost. Certainly, uniformity of rates to all purchasers is not conditional upon cost-based rates. The only requirement is that the rates be uniform, whatever their basis, to all purchasers. However, internal service subsidization could not be prevented with rates established on bases other than costs. Differential markups still could be allowed for those services that were produced significantly above or below normative costs so as to discourage or encourage future production.

Recommendation. Referring to Table 1, it appears that prospective rate-setting models should be cost-based. The relative attainment of viability and purchaser equity appears to more than offset any increases in administrative costs. Also, the political realities of establishing rates for health care services on bases other than cost seem to rule out noncost bases as viable alternatives. Priest and Morrissey agree that hospital rates must be related to costs or financial requirements, with adjustments for reasonableness.[24,25] In addition, the nonproprietary nature of most health care organizations implies a relationship to costs.[26]

Payment Units

Efficiency. As before, we will limit attention to prospective rate-setting models. Based upon prior analysis, it also will be assumed that prospective rates are cost-based. The following alternative payment units, discussed by Dowling, will be examined:[27]

1 Total institution budgets;
2 Departmental budgets;
3 Capitation;
4 Case;
5 Day;
6 Specific services.

The incentives for improving technical efficiency, reducing input prices, and combining inputs optimally are not differentially affected by the type of payment unit. Prospectively determined rates provide incentives for efficiency in each of these three areas.

Differing incentives may exist with respect to the economy of scale dimension of efficiency. If we assume that the primary focus should be upon the elimination of unnecessary or duplicated facilities and services, the departmental budget or specific services payment unit methods would provide explicit expenditure control. Payments for specific services could be denied or reduced far below actual costs to recognize low levels of utilization. Cohen apparently adjusted actual costs by targeted utilization levels to prompt hospitals in Maryland to discontinue underutilized services.[28] The relevance of this incentive is affected by the existing program of capital expenditure regulation. Prospective rates established for departmental budgets or specific services could expand existing capital controls from their present prospective basis to a retroactive basis. Thus, payment for prior capital expenditures could be denied. The American Hospital Association has vigorously opposed retroactive regulation of capital expenditures.[29]

The discussion of output incentives is predicated upon the existence of some control in this area by institutional managers. In other words, physician behavior must be subject to a certain amount of control by institutional managers. Dowling points to evidence that indicates this may be true.[30] In addition, the experience of New York State suggests that hospital administrators could influence length of stay decisions by physicians.[31]

Assuming that both the total budget and the departmental budget method result in fixed levels of payment, the incentive is to reduce output. Thus, a hospital would try to reduce the number of admissions, the length of stay, and the intensity of the ancillary services provided, as well as to perform more outpatient surgeries, to transfer patients to less intensive care settings, and so on. In short, the incentives appear to be in the right direction. The same observation is true, of course, for plans that use a capitation payment unit. It is interesting, however, to note that the budgetary methods produce the same incentives as the capitation method. Thus, efficient combinations of health services outputs could result from payment unit methods other than capitation. Capitation plans, nonetheless, may be more successful because of their traditionally greater involvement of physicians in the reward scheme.

The remaining three payment methods (case, day, specific services) are all based upon measures of output. Assuming that the marginal costs of producing an additional unit of that output is less than the prospective rate, there is an incentive for output expansion. All three of the payment units would provide incentives for the expansion of the delivery of inpatient curative care. Current opinion is that the health care system produces too much of this type of care.

The primary responsibility of professional standards review organizations could be materially affected by the selection of the payment unit. If the payment unit were a budgetary or capitation method, the primary responsibility would be to ensure the sufficiency of health services delivered. If the payment unit were on an output basis, the primary responsibility would be to validate the necessity of health services delivered. This would be particularly true given the existing physician incentive structure for hospitalization of patients.

Viability. Financial viability could be ensured by selecting any of the six alternative payment units. Each could generate revenue in an amount greater than the allowable financial requirements needed by the institution to survive.

The major problem in assessing viability is the measurement of normative or allowable financial requirements. It would appear that normative cost measures will be developed from both internal and external cost data. Thus, cost data between institutions must be comparable. A major problem of cost comparability, aside from some accounting measurement problems, is the nonhomogeneity of output. For example, comparing the costs of a 1,000-bed teaching hospital with the costs of a 200-bed acute care hospital is extremely difficult, if not impossible.

Macro payment units, such as the total budget, case, day or capitation method, would limit cost comparability. Assuming that comparability is essential to the development of normative cost measures, a limited, possibly nonexistent, sample of comparable institutions might be available if macro payment units were used. On this basis, it seems that the departmental budget or specific services payment unit methods would have an advantage. It should be noted, however, that recent methodology developed by Feldstein and

Shuttinga may provide a means for creating cost comparability using case-mix.[31] While cost comparisons across institutions would by no means be perfect, the relative degree of variability attributable to output variation would be significantly reduced at the departmental or service level.

Administrative costs. There is an inverse relationship between administrative costs and the fineness of the payment unit. Macro payment units would require less detailed financial data than micro payment units. Obviously, the more specific the data the greater the cost of both preparing and utilizing that data. The benefit of this finer specificity must exceed the costs.

On this basis, the advantage would be with the four macro payment units. But one point should be kept in mind: Most institutions already prepare or should prepare departmental budgets for use in their management control systems. Thus, the additional costs of preparation should be minimal, at least at the institutional level.

Equity to purchasers. Micro payment units, such as departmental budgets or specific services, appear to be more equitable to purchasers than macro payment units. Patients who pay on a per diem basis are penalized if they use few ancillary services. Short-term length of stay patients, such as those undergoing T & As, are penalized if a per case payment unit method is used. In sum, the à la carte method of pricing appears to be equitable when multipurchasers with differing relative service demands exist. If only third-party payers purchased health services and the enrollees of those plans were uniform with respect to their consumption of health services, an à la carte method of pricing would be unnecessary. Major differences between enrollees of various third-party payers do exist, however. For example, the Medicare population has distinctly different service demands than has the Blue Cross population.

Recommendation. Referring to Table 1, it appears that prospective cost-based, rate-setting models should be predicated upon approved departmental budgets. Since these budgets reflect a fixed-dollar amount, some method of apportionment among payers must be developed. For major third-party payers, such as Blue Cross Plans, Medicare and Medicaid, actual or projected percentages of departmental utilization could be used. For self-pay patients or small third-party commercial insurance companies, an actual approved unit rate could be developed by dividing the approved budget by anticipated volume. Finally, some adjustments could be made to reflect actual differences in volume or costs if they were noncontrollable, such as increases in liability insurance premiums or fuel costs.

Concluding Remarks

In this paper, alternative payment systems were evaluated according to their perceived attainment of some defined criteria. Quite possibly, different analysts would select different criteria or might perceive their relative attainment differentially. Different recommendations might thus follow.

But before payment alternatives for health care institutional providers can be selected, some delineation of criteria and their relative importance must be made. Without this framework, current recommendations have no logical base upon which to be evaluated, either conceptually or empirically. Only Dowling appears to have approached analysis of payment systems from this comprehensive decision-making, theoretic viewpoint.[33] Most other studies have focused narrowly on only one criterion, usually cost.

This paper concludes that a prospective cost-based reimbursement system predicated on departmental budgets would be the optimal form of reimbursement, given the defined alternatives and their perceived criteria attainment. It should be noted that no discussion was devoted to the administrative aspects of controlling or determining what these departmental budgets should be. This is a fatal deficiency. The only plan ever established along the recommended lines was the Connecticut Hospital Association's Social Security experiment. It was a dismal failure, largely because of inattention to this most important aspect.[34]

The Connecticut experiment was characterized by several obvious administrative flaws worth mentioning. First, the plan was peer reviewed. This meant that the budget approval boards (BABs) comprised exclusively personnel from other hospitals: three administrators; three financial officers; two nursing personnel; and one hospital director.[35] This administrative structure did not exert sufficient pressure to reduce costs. Second, the reward/penalty structure was a no-loss situation. The hospitals received the larger of approved budgets or actual costs under prior cost reimbursement formula contracts. With this type of reward/penalty structure the incentives for cost control are reduced sharply. Third, participation in the experiment was voluntary. Unquestionably, this leads to a selection bias that is conditioned by each institution's possible perception of rewards. Finally, some elements of cost that might be viewed as controllable were labeled uncontrollable and not subjected to the approval process. For example, wage rates were viewed as noncontrolled and attention was directed to number of hours worked. Unquestionably, this policy would reduce management motivation for tough negotiation with employees on compensation issues.

References and Notes

1 Gauss, C. and Hellinger, F. "Results of Prospective Reimbursement," *Topics in Health Care Financing,* Fall 1976, pp. 83–96.
2 Dowling, W. "Prospective Reimbursement of Hospitals," *Inquiry,* September 1974, pp. 163–180.
3 Ibid.
4 Lave, J., Lave, L., and Silverman, L. "A Proposal for Incentive Reimbursement for Hospitals," *Medical Care,* March–April 1973, pp. 79–90.
5 Pauly, M. "Efficiency, Incentives and Reimbursement for Health Care," *Inquiry,* March 1970, pp. 114–131.
6 Ibid.
7 Fox, R. "Service Costs and Management: The Man-Hours Variable," *Hospital Progress,* June 1974, pp. 50–53.
8 Cleverley, W. "Is Hospital Capital Being Eroded Under Cost Reimbursement," *Hospital Administration,* Summer 1974, pp. 58–73.
9 Walls, E. "Cost Reimbursement Worsens Capital Crisis," *Hospitals,* Mar. 1, 1972, pp. 81–86.
10 Pauly, op. cit.
11 Berki, S. *Hospital Economics.* Lexington, MA: Lexington Books, 1972.

12 Emery, J. and Halonen, R. "Revenue Bonds: Study Shows Hospitals Pay Higher Interest," *Hospital Financial Management*, August 1975, pp. 26–35.

13 American Hospital Association, "Statement on the Financial Requirements of Health Care Institutions and Services," Chicago, Feb. 12, 1969.

14 Health Services Foundation, *Investor Owned Hospitals: An Examination of Performance*, Chicago, 1976.

15 Hill, D. and Stewart, D. "Proprietary Hospitals Versus Nonprofit Hospitals: A Matched Sample Analysis in California," *Blue Cross Reports*, Research Series 9, March 1973.

16 O'Donoghue, P. *Evidence About the Effects of Health Care Regulation*, Spectrum Research, 1974.

17 Lampiris, L. "Hospital Industry Not So Different: Efficiency Does Equal Savings," *Hospital Financial Management*, April 1975, pp. 22–24.

18 Lave et al., op. cit.

19 Berman, H. and Weeks, L. *The Financial Management of Hospitals*, 2nd Edition, Ann Arbor, MI: Health Administration Press, 1974.

20 Lemer, R. and Willman, D. "Rate Setting," *Topics in Health Care Financing*, Winter 1974.

21 Bauer, K. G. "Information Needs for Hospital Rate Setting," *Topics in Health Care Financing*, Fall 1976.

22 Worthington, P. N. "Prospective Reimbursement of Hospitals to Promote Efficiency: New Jersey," *Inquiry*, September 1976, pp. 302–308.

23 Cohen, H. "State Rate Regulation," *Controls on Health Care*, National Academy of Sciences, 1975, pp. 123–135.

24 Priest, A. J. "Possible Adoption of Public Utility Concepts in the Health Care Field," *Law and Contemporary Problems*, Autumn 1970, pp. 839–848.

25 Morrissey, F. P. "The Dilemma of Hospitals—Is Public Utility Status the Answer," *Hospital Administration*, Fall 1971, pp. 10–19.

26 Anthony, R. N. and Herzlinger, R. *Management Control in Nonprofit Organizations* (Homewood, IL: Richard D. Irwin, Inc., 1975).

27 Dowling, op. cit.

28 Cohen, op. cit.

29 American Hospital Association, op. cit.

30 Dowling, op. cit.

31 Berry, R. E. "Prospective Rate Reimbursement and Cost Containment: Formula Reimbursement in New York," *Inquiry*, September 1976, pp. 288–301.

32 Feldstein, M. and Schuttinga, J. "Hospital Costs in Massachusetts: A Methodological Study," *Inquiry*, March 1977, pp. 22–31.

33 Dowling, op. cit.

34 Elnicki, R. "SSA-Connecticut Hospital Incentive Reimbursement Experiment Cost Evaluation," *Inquiry*, March 1975, pp. 47–58.

Index